# Essentials of Human Nutrition

# Essentials of Human Nutrition

Editor: Kristen Foley

STATES
ACADEMIC PRESS
www.statesacademicpress.com

**States Academic Press,**
109 South 5th Street,
Brooklyn, NY 11249, USA

Visit us on the World Wide Web at:
www.statesacademicpress.com



ISBN: 978-1-63989-186-3 (Hardback)



**Cataloging-in-Publication Data**

Essentials of human nutrition / edited by Kristen Foley.
p. cm.
Includes bibliographical references and index.
ISBN 978-1-63989-186-3
1. Nutrition. 2. Human physiology. I. Foley, Kristen.
QP141 .E87 2022
613.2--dc23

# Table of Contents

Preface ........ IX

Chapter 1 **Nutritional adequacy of a novel human milk fortifier from donkey milk in feeding preterm infants** ........ 1
Alessandra Coscia, Enrico Bertino, Paola Tonetto, Chiara Peila, Francesco Cresi, Sertac Arslanoglu, Guido E Moro, Elena Spada, Silvano Milani, Marzia Giribaldi, Sara Antoniazzi, Amedeo Conti and Laura Cavallarin

Chapter 2 **The effects of fatty fish intake on adolescents' nutritional status and associations with attention performance** ........ 8
Katina Handelan, Siv Skotheim, Valborg Baste, Ingvild E. Graff, Livar Frøyland, Øyvind Lie, Marian Kjellevold, Maria W. Markhus, Kjell M. Stormark, Jannike Øyen and Lisbeth Dahl

Chapter 3 **Energy, nutrient and food content of snacks in French adults** ........ 20
Wendy Si Hassen, Katia Castetbon, Christine Tichit, Sandrine Péneau, Anouar Nechba, Pauline Ducrot, Aurélie Lampuré, France Bellisle, Serge Hercberg and Caroline Méjean

Chapter 4 **Randomised controlled trial to test the effectiveness of a locally-produced ready-to-use supplementary food (RUSF) in preventing growth faltering and improving micronutrient status for children under two years** ........ 29
Bindi Borg, Seema Mihrshahi, Mark Griffin, Daream Sok, Chamnan Chhoun, Arnaud Laillou, Jacques Berger and Frank T. Wieringa

Chapter 5 **Propolis ethanolic extracts reduce adenosine diphosphate induced platelet aggregation determined on whole blood** ........ 40
Mirza Bojić, Andrea Antolić, Maja Tomičić, Željko Debeljak and Željan Maleš

Chapter 6 **Erythrocyte DHA and AA in infancy is not associated with developmental status and cognitive functioning five years later in Nepalese children** ........ 48
Sigrun Henjum, Ingrid Kvestad, Merina Shrestha, Manjeswori Ulak, Ram K. Chandyo, Andrew L. Thorne-Lyman, Prakash S. Shrestha, Marian Kjellevold, Mari Hysing and Tor A. Strand

Chapter 7 **Progress of children with severe acute malnutrition in the malnutrition treatment centre rehabilitation program** ........ 57
Anuraag Chaturvedi, Ashok K. Patwari, Deepa Soni, Shivam Pandey, Audrey Prost, Raj Kumar Gope, Jyoti Sharma and Prasanta Tripathy

Chapter 8 **Family-based intervention using face-to-face sessions and social media to improve Malay primary school children's adiposity** ........ 66
Norliza Ahmad, Zalilah Mohd Shariff, Firdaus Mukhtar and Munn-Sann Lye

Chapter 9 **Severely malnourished children with a low weight-for-height have a higher mortality than those with a low mid-upper-arm-circumference: III. Effect of case-load on malnutrition related mortality – policy implications** ........ 79
Emmanuel Grellety and Michael H. Golden

Chapter 10 **Severely malnourished children with a low weight-for-height have similar mortality to those with a low mid-upper-arm-circumference** ........ 89
Emmanuel Grellety and Michael H. Golden

Chapter 11 **Ethnic disparities of beverage consumption in infants and children 0–5 years of age: National Health and Nutrition Examination Survey 2011 to 2014** ........ 108
Elieke Demmer, Christopher J. Cifelli, Jenny A. Houchins and Victor L. Fulgoni III

Chapter 12 **A health facility based case-control study on determinants of low birth weight in Dassie town, Northeast Ethiopia: the role of nutritional factors** ........ 117
Semira Ahmed, Kalkidan Hassen and Tolassa Wakayo

Chapter 13 **Development and validation of a quantitative choline food frequency questionnaire for use with drinking and non-drinking pregnant women** ........ 127
R. Colin Carter, Sandra W. Jacobson, Sharmilah Booley, Baheya Najaar, Neil C. Dodge, Lori J. Bechard, Ernesta M. Meintjes, Christopher D. Molteno, Christopher P. Duggan, Joseph L. Jacobson and Marjanne Senekal

Chapter 14 **Dairy intake revisited – associations between dairy intake and lifestyle related cardio-metabolic risk factors in a high milk consuming population** ........ 140
Ingegerd Johansson, Lena Maria Nilsson, Anders Esberg, Jan-Håkan Jansson and Anna Winkvist

Chapter 15 **Co-morbidity, treatment outcomes and factors affecting the recovery rate of under-five children with severe acute malnutrition admitted in selected hospitals** ........ 157
Behailu Derseh, Kalayu Mruts, Takele Demie and Tesfay Gebremariam

Chapter 16 **Nutritional status of in-school children and its associated factors in Denkyembour District, eastern region, Ghana: comparing schools with feeding and non-school feeding policies** ........ 165
Mavis Pearl Kwabla, Charlotte Gyan and Francis Zotor

Chapter 17 **Effect of soy lecithin on fatigue and menopausal symptoms in middle-aged women** ........ 173
Asuka Hirose, Masakazu Terauchi, Yurika Osaka, Mihoko Akiyoshi, Kiyoko Kato and Naoyuki Miyasaka

Chapter 18 **Vitamin D status and dental caries in healthy Swedish children** ........ 181
Johanna Gyll, Karin Ridell, Inger Öhlund, Pia Karlsland Åkeson, Ingegerd Johansson and Pernilla Lif Holgerson

Chapter 19 **Association between time perspective and organic food consumption in a large sample of adults** ........ 191
Marc Bénard, Julia Baudry, Caroline Méjean, Denis Lairon, Kelly Virecoulon Giudici, Fabrice Etilé, Gérard Reach, Serge Hercberg, Emmanuelle Kesse-Guyot and Sandrine Péneau

Chapter 20 **Resistant starch lowers postprandial glucose and leptin in overweight adults consuming a moderate-to-high-fat diet** ........ 201
Mindy Patterson Maziarz, Sara Preisendanz, Shanil Juma, Victorine Imrhan, Chandan Prasad and Parakat Vijayagopal

Chapter 21 **Possible benefits of tomato juice consumption: a pilot study on irradiated human lymphocytes from healthy donors** ........ 211
Ayumi Nakamura, Chieko Itaki, Ayako Saito, Toko Yonezawa, Koichi Aizawa, Ayumi Hirai, Hiroyuki Suganuma, Tomisato Miura, Yasushi Mariya and Siamak Haghdoost

Chapter 22 **Plasma phospholipid fatty acid profile confirms compliance to a novel saturated fat-reduced, monounsaturated fat-enriched dairy product intervention in adults at moderate cardiovascular risk** ........ 222
Oonagh Markey, Dafni Vasilopoulou, Kirsty E. Kliem, Albert Koulman, Colette C. Fagan, Keith Summerhill, Laura Y. Wang, Alistair S. Grandison, David J. Humphries, Susan Todd, Kim G. Jackson, David I. Givens and Julie A. Lovegrove

**Permissions**

**List of Contributors**

**Index**

# Preface

The process by which various substances in food are transformed into tissues that provides energy for a wide range of mental and physical activities to support and sustain life and health is called human nutrition. Good nutrition is important for physical growth and biological development. A balanced diet provides the human body with optimum energy. This directly impacts the physical performance of the body. Unbalanced nutrition can result in malnutrition. This can be further divided into three categories- undernutrition, micronutrients-related malnutrition and obesity. This book provides comprehensive insights into the field of human nutrition. It strives to provide a fair idea about this discipline and to help develop a better understanding of the latest advances within this field. The extensive content of this book provides the readers with a thorough understanding of the subject.

This book is the end result of constructive efforts and intensive research done by experts in this field. The aim of this book is to enlighten the readers with recent information in this area of research. The information provided in this profound book would serve as a valuable reference to students and researchers in this field.

At the end, I would like to thank all the authors for devoting their precious time and providing their valuable contribution to this book. I would also like to express my gratitude to my fellow colleagues who encouraged me throughout the process.

**Editor**

# 1

# Nutritional adequacy of a novel human milk fortifier from donkey milk in feeding preterm infants: study protocol of a randomized controlled clinical trial

Alessandra Coscia[1], Enrico Bertino[1], Paola Tonetto[1], Chiara Peila[1*], Francesco Cresi[1], Sertac Arslanoglu[2], Guido E Moro[2], Elena Spada[1], Silvano Milani[3], Marzia Giribaldi[4,5], Sara Antoniazzi[4], Amedeo Conti[4] and Laura Cavallarin[4]

**Abstract**

**Background:** Fortification of human milk is a standard practice for feeding very low birth weight infants. However, preterm infants often still experience suboptimal growth and feeding intolerance. New fortification strategies and different commercially available fortifiers have been developed. Commercially available fortifiers are constituted by a blend of ingredients from different sources, including plant oils and bovine milk proteins, thus presenting remarkable differences in the quality of macronutrients with respect to human milk. Based on the consideration that donkey milk has been suggested as a valid alternative for children allergic to cow's milk proteins, due to its biochemical similarity to human milk, we hypothesized that donkey milk could be a suitable ingredient for developing an innovative human milk fortifier.

The aim of the study is to evaluate feeding tolerance, growth and clinical short and long-term outcomes in a population of preterm infants fed with a novel multi-component fortifier and a protein concentrate derived from donkey milk, in comparison to an analogous population fed with traditional fortifier and protein supplement containing bovine milk proteins.

**Methods:** The study has been designed as a randomized, controlled, single-blind clinical trial. Infants born <1500 g and <32 weeks of gestational age were randomized to receive for 21 days either a combination of control bovine milk-based multicomponent fortifier and protein supplement, or a combination of a novel multicomponent fortifier and protein supplement derived from donkey milk. The fortification protocol followed is the same for the two groups, and the two diets were designed to be isoproteic and isocaloric. Weight, length and head circumference are measured; feeding tolerance is assessed by a standardized protocol. The occurrence of sepsis, necrotizing enterocolitis and adverse effects are monitored.

**Discussion:** This is the first clinical study investigating the use of a human milk fortifier derived from donkey milk for the nutrition of preterm infants. If donkey milk derived products will be shown to improve the feeding tolerance or either of the clinical, metabolic, neurological or auxological outcomes of preterm infants, it would be an absolute innovation in the field of feeding practices for preterm infants.

**Keywords:** Human milk, Human milk fortifier, Donkey milk, Adjustable fortification, VLBW infants, Preterm infants, Enteral feeding, Feeding intolerance

* Correspondence: peila.chiara@gmail.com
[1]Neonatal Unit of Turin University, City of Health and Science of Turin, Via Ventimiglia 3, 10126 Turin, Italy
Full list of author information is available at the end of the article

## Background

Very preterm newborns (gestational age < 32 weeks) and Very Low Birthweight Infants (VLBWI, birthweight <1500 g) currently represent the majority of patients assisted in Neonatal Intensive Care Units (NICU) [1]. The increase of the survival rate for these newborns, due to improvements in perinatal care, has opened new perspectives regarding their outcome and has a significant impact on their health status in adulthood.

Although very preterm or VLBWI usually attain some "catch-up" growth following hospital discharge, growth deficits can persist throughout childhood and adolescence, and into adulthood. Slow postnatal growth is associated with neurodevelopmental impairment in later childhood, with poorer cognitive outcomes, and may have consequences for long-term metabolic and cardiovascular health [2–4]. Nutrition represents a fundamental factor for long-term survival and quality of life for this group of infants. The main issue is to ensure an adequate qualitative and quantitative nutrition, particularly in terms of protein intake, which is the main cause of post-natal growth deficit.

Human milk is the recommended form of enteral nutrition for all neonates including preterm infants [5]. Breast milk alone, however, does not meet the recommended nutritional needs for growth in preterm infants [6, 7]. The most common strategy in neonatal care facilities is to cope with these potential nutrient deficits by supplementing breast milk with additional nutrients (mainly proteins and minerals) to ensure a sufficient caloric intake in consideration of the special nutritional requirements [8–10]. The fortification of human milk still represents a significant challenge [11, 12]. The standard fortification strategies have been considered unsatisfactory to sustain an appropriate growth. Thus, new approaches were developed, among which Adjustable (ADJ) Fortification currently seems to be the most promising [13]. It involves the use of a protein supplement on an individualized basis, in addition to a multi-component fortifier. This method, accepted at an international level, consists of providing a variable protein intake based on the metabolic response of each single newborn by titration to the infant's blood urea nitrogen level [14, 15]. This approach requires simple, high-quality and well-tolerated protein supplements which, unfortunately, are not readily available. Most commercially available multi-nutrient fortifiers are derived from bovine milk, which has a protein composition very different from that of human milk. Moreover, cow milk protein intake in the first months of life has raised concerns because of its association with allergies [16] and some studies have observed a possible role of cow's milk proteins as a trigger of intestinal inflammation in preterm neonates. [17] Investigations on exclusive HM diets (human milk-based fortifier and donor HM, if mother's milk unavailable) have been carried out in recent years. All these studies recently underwent to a systematic review [18]; most of them were retrospective studies and not randomized clinical trials. Authors conclude that there is not strong evidence that human milk based fortifiers in otherwise exclusively human milk-fed preterm infants affect important outcomes. Consistently, milk from monogastric animals, rather than from ruminants, has been suggested during recent years to be more suitable for human nutrition based on their physiochemical properties [19]. In previous studies, our group observed on children affected by cow milk protein allergy that donkey milk (DM) was highly tolerated [20], and found that its protein and lipid fractions showed a substantial similarity to that of human milk [21, 22]. DM has an n-3 PUFA (polyunsaturated fatty acids) content equivalent to human milk, and is rich in lysozyme, a protein characterized by antibacterial properties, able to hinder pathogen growth, and milk spoilage. It has been recently demonstrated in murine models that a supplementation of the basal diet with DM decreases the accumulation of body lipids and affects glucose and lipid metabolism in a manner more similar to human milk than cow milk [23] These biological effects resulted comparable with those elicited by human milk [24] Based on the above considerations, it can be speculated that DM is more suitable than bovine milk to be an ingredient of a human milk fortifier for VLBW Infants and preterm newborns.

Our hypothesis is that feeding these newborns according to ADJ fortification principles, with human milk fortified by protein and multi-component supplements derived from DM, will improve the feeding tolerance and the clinical, metabolic, neurological and auxological outcome at short- and long-term.

We present the protocol of a study aimed to evaluate the use of DM-derived multi-component fortifier and protein concentrate for the nutrition of infants with birthweight <1500 g or gestational age < 32 weeks. This evaluation is being performed through a clinical trial (randomized, controlled, blind) by comparing it with commercial bovine milk-based multi-component fortifier and protein concentrate.

## Methods/design

The study is currently underway at the Neonatal Intensive Care Unit (NICU) of the University of Turin, and has been approved by Local Ethic Committee. Informed written consent is obtained from parents before enrollment. The trial was registered on ISRCTN Registry BioMed Central (Registration number: ISRCTN70022881).

### Study population

All patients admitted to our unit that met the following inclusion criteria were consecutively enrolled in the study.

Inclusion criteria:

- Gestational age < 32 weeks or birthweight <1500 g
- Exclusive feeding with human milk (fresh own mother's or donor milk)
- Human milk volume > 80 ml/kg/day within the first 4 weeks of life

Exclusion criteria:

- Severe gastrointestinal pathologies (diagnosed or suspected necrotizing enterocolitis, colostomy, intestinal obstruction, symptoms of peritonitis, presence of blood in the feces)
- Chromosomal abnormalities or major malformations
- Hereditary metabolic diseases
- Intravascular disseminated coagulopathy (IDC), shock
- Patent Ductus Arteriosus (PDA) requiring medical care or surgery at time of randomization
- Severe renal failure (serum creatinine >2 mg/dl)

**Study design**

Infants meeting inclusion criteria are identified and their parents approached for consent. After informed written parental consent is obtained, infants are randomized 1:1 by a software-generated list in one of the following groups:

- Control group: Adjustable Fortification with commercial multi-component fortifier (FM85 Nestlè) and protein concentrate (Protifar Nutricia), named BMC and BPC respectively, derived from bovine milk, for a minimum of 21 days (if necessary, fortification is continued after this period using the same type of product)
- Fortilat group: Adjustable Fortification with multi-component fortifier and protein concentrate derived from donkey milk, named DMC and DPC respectively, not commercially available, and prepared according to current EU legislation on Foods for special medical purposes, for a minimum of 21 days (if necessary, fortification is continued after this period using the same type of product).

The composition of BMC and DMC are provided in Table 1. Table 2 presents the composition of BPC and DPC. The experimental products were produced by ultrafiltration of pasteurized donkey milk in a pilot stainless steel plant. Retentates from the ultrafiltration processes were then pasteurized and aseptically lyophilized and packed. All the batches used for the trial were analyzed for the microbiological and chemical profile and complied with the safety criteria required by Italian legislation. The products are stored at −80 °C until used.

A nutrition protocol following the criteria of ADJ fortification is being followed to ensure that fortification advancement is consistent for all study participants. Tables 3 and 4 show the ADJ Fortification criteria for the control products (BMC and BPC) and for the test products (DMC and DPC). Since the protein concentration and energy content of the bovine milk based products differ from the donkey milk based products, the amounts of powder required to obtain the same level of fortification are different depending on the product in use (Table 4). Because the same nurses in charge of feeds preparation and administration are also in charge of evaluating signs of feeding tolerance, it is not possible to achieve a double blindness of the intervention. As caregivers are aware of the group allocation of infants, this is to be defined as a single-blind randomized controlled trial.

Advancing of enteral feeds is strictly regulated according to the feeding protocol adopted in our NICU, based on the evaluation of signs of feeding intolerance (available on demand to the authors). The criteria for hospital discharge are uniform, i.e., satisfactory weight gain while receiving full oral feeding, maintenance of adequate thermal stability and resolution of acute medical conditions.

**Table 1** Macro-composition of the multi-component fortifiers derived from bovine milk (BMC) and from donkey milk (DMC). Values per 100 g of product

| | BMC | DMC |
|---|---|---|
| Protein g (Nx6.25) | 20.0 | 22.5 |
| Carbohydrate g | 66.0 | 59.0 |
| of which: | | |
| Lactose g | 6.0 | 59.0 |
| Maltodextrine g | 60.0 | 0.0 |
| Fat g | 0.4 | 3.6 |
| Energy: | | |
| Kcal | 385 | 390 |
| kcal/g protein | 18.8 | 15.6 |
| Calcium mg | 1500 | 938 |
| Phosphate mg | 900 | 734 |
| Osmolality mOsm/Kg | 453 | 441 |

**Table 2** Composition of the protein concentrates derived from bovine milk (BPC) and from donkey milk (DPC). Values per 100 g of product

| | BPC | DPC |
|---|---|---|
| Protein g (Nx6.25) | 88.5 | 43 |
| Carbohydrate g | <1.5 | 33.5 |
| Fat g | ≤2.0 | 6.1 |
| Energy Kcal | 370 | 418 |
| Calcium mg | 1350 | 1650 |
| Phosphate mg | 700 | 1150 |

**Table 3** Adjustable Fortification criteria based on weekly blood urea nitrogen (BUN) values

| BUN (blood urea nitrogen) | |
|---|---|
| < 10 mg/dl | Increase fortification by one level |
| 10–16 mg/dl | No change |
| > 16 mg/dl | Decrease fortification by one level |

### Outcome measures

1. Primary Endpoint.
   Occurrence of at least one episode of feeding intolerance, defined as interruption of enteral feeding for at least eight consecutive hours during the observation period.
2. Secondary Endpoints.
   2.1 Gastrointestinal outcomes: Number of feeding intolerance episodes, number of feeding interruption episodes (of any duration), total hours of enteral feeding interruption, time required to reach full enteral feeding (150 ml/kg/day).
   2.2 Gastric Emptying time (ultrasonic measurements of the antral cross sectional area) [25, 26]: half-time of gastric emptying (minutes) and time of gastric emptying (minutes).
   2.3 Esophageal impedance and pH monitoring (MII/pH) [27, 28]: GER frequency (reflux events/h), bolus reflux extent (number of channels), Bolus clearance time (seconds), bolus exposure index and reflux index (percentage).
   2.4 Clinical outcomes: necrotizing enterocolitis, suspected or confirmed sepsis, mortality, hospital stay duration, intraventricular hemorrhage, retinopathy of prematurity (defined according to the Vermont Oxford Network) [29].
   2.5 Metabolic and auxological outcomes (as shown in the synoptic table) (Table 5).

**Table 4** Amount of fortifer and protein supplement at the various fortification levels, according to ADJ fortification protocol

| | Multicomponent | | | Protein concentrate | |
|---|---|---|---|---|---|
| Levels | BMC g/ml | DMC g/ml | | BPC g/ml | DPC g/ml |
| 2.5% | 0.025 | 0.02 | | – | – |
| 4% | 0.04 | 0.032 | | – | – |
| 5% | 0.05 | 0.04 | | – | – |
| 5% +1 | 0.05 | 0.04 | + | 0.004 | 0.008 |
| 5% +2 | 0.05 | 0.04 | + | 0.008 | 0.016 |
| 5% +3 | 0.05 | 0.04 | + | 0.012 | 0.024 |

#### Sample size

The sample size has been determined based on the occurrence of primary endpoint (at least one episode of interruption of enteral feeding ≥8 h). Based on the data available in our NICU from the population of VLBWI or preterm infants, about 45% of infants present at least one interruption of enteral feeding ≥8 h.

In the hypothesis that the use of a better tolerated fortifier causes a 25% reduction in the frequency of the primary endpoint, and setting the risk of type I errors and the power at the usual 5 and 80%, 62 newborns per group have been considered as required.

#### Planned recruitment rate and compliance

In the year 2014, 115 infants less than 32 weeks gestation and weighting less than 1500 g were admitted to our NICU. Breastfeeding initiation rates with mothers' own milk or donor milk were around 90% in our nursery. Therefore, around 100 infants per year were estimated to be eligible for the study, with a recruitment rate higher than 60%. We did not anticipate problems with compliance. The majority of mothers visits their baby on a regular basis, hence they are easily approached for consent as soon as the infant reaches the point to start fortification. Blood sampling required by the study protocol is consistent with the routine monitoring performed in our unit, hence there is no supplementary inconvenience for the patients and it is easily accepted by parents.

#### Data collection methods

In order to promote the data quality, it has been provided a training plan for the nurses and clinicians based on fortification protocols and evaluation of feeding tolerance. Data are being collected according to the scheme shown in the synoptic table of the study (Table 5). Weight, length and head circumference measurements are recorded at birth, and during the observation period (weight: daily; length and head circumference: weekly), at 36 ± 1 weeks of postmenstrual age, 40 ± 1 weeks of postmenstrual age, at 6, 12 and 18 months of corrected age. The collection of outcomes, baseline, and other trial data are reported in the specific form by copying them from the medical record at discharge of the newborn.

#### Estimated rate of loss to follow up

Our NICU is a tertiary level neonatal unit. Most babies in the NICU stay until discharge from hospital. Very few infants return to local hospitals prior to discharge home, and it generally is very rare that they are transferred prior to 35 weeks corrected gestational age. In addition, all infants that meet inclusion criteria for the study are planned to be followed until two years of age, as part of our follow-up program. We therefore do not expect any significant loss to follow up.

**Table 5** Synoptic table. T0: before starting the fortification; T1: day 7 after beginning the fortification (if level 3 of ADJ fortification) or as soon as level 3 is reached; T2: day 14 since beginning of fortification; T3: day 21 since beginning of fortification

| | STUDY PERIOD | | | | | | |
|---|---|---|---|---|---|---|---|
| | Enrolment | Allocation | Post-allocation | | | | Close-out |
| Timepoint | | | T0 | T1 | T2 | T3 | |
| Enrolment: | | | | | | | |
| Eligibility screen | X | | | | | | |
| Informed consent | X | | | | | | |
| Full patient history collection | X | | | | | | |
| Allocation | | X | | | | | |
| Intervention: | | | | | | | |
| BUN | | | X | X | X | X | |
| Albumin | | | X | X | X | X | |
| Creatinine | | | X | X | X | X | |
| Calcium | | | X | X | X | X | |
| Phosphate | | | X | X | X | X | |
| Alkaline Phosphatase | | | X | X | X | X | |
| Weight | | | X | X | X | X | |
| Lenght | | | X | X | X | X | |
| Head circumference | | | X | X | X | X | |
| Plasma Aminoacids | | | X | | | X | |
| Urine Aminoacids | | | X | | | X | |
| Urinary Metabolomic Profile | | | X | | | X | |
| Calprotectin | | | X | | | X | |
| pH | | | X | X | X | X | |
| BE | | | X | X | X | X | |
| $HCO_3^-$ | | | X | X | X | X | |
| MII/pH | | | | | | X | |
| Gastric emptying time | | | | | | X | |
| Assesments | | | | | | | |
| List other data variables | | | | | | | X |
| List other data variables | | | | | | | X |

## Statistical analysis

The statistical analysis will be performed by the Medical Statistics and Biometry Unit of the Clinical and Community Sciences of the University of Milan.

At the end of the recruitment, the occurrence of the primary endpoint will be evaluated on the intention-to-treat population (all randomized infants). The comparison between the two study groups will be performed with the exact Fisher test. All secondary endpoints will be modelled in the framework of generalised linear model [30] allowing, when appropriate, for relevant covariates. The number of episodes of feeding intolerance (0, 1 ... k) will be modelled as a Poisson variable. Total hours of enteral feeding interruption, time required to reach full enteral feeding, hospital stay duration, gastric emptying time and MII/pH parameters will be modelled (after proper scale transformation, if required) as normal variables. The occurrence of clinical outcomes, assesed as dychotomous variable (yes/no) will be modelled as binomial variables. Metabolic and auxological outcomes, which are repeatedly during study period, will be modelled (after proper scale transformation, if required) as normal variables, with a model allowing for repeated measures. All statistical models are fit with SAS software [31].

## Discussion

We present the protocol of a study aimed to assess the effects of a new human milk fortifier derived from donkey milk on VLBWI feeding tolerance and growth. To the best of our knowledge, this trial is unique, being the first study that investigates the use of a human milk fortifier derived from donkey milk for the nutrition of preterm and VLBWI.

In our trial all the infants received exclusively human milk (Fresh own mother's milk or Pasteurized donor milk) without any preterm formula supplementation. The trial of Sullivan, comparing a human milk based fortifier with a bovine milk based fortifier, included in the group supplemented with the bovine fortifier also subjects fed with preterm formula [32]. This represents a confounding variable masking the effects of the two different fortifiers as a sole supplement of human milk.

If the donkey milk derived fortifier will be proved to improve the feeding tolerance or some of the other outcomes (clinical, metabolic, neurological or auxological) of very preterm and VLBWI, it would be an absolute innovation in the field of feeding practices for preterm infants.

A possible limitation of our study is that it has been designed as a single-blind randomized controlled trial, being the caregivers aware of infants' allocation in the study. To try to eliminate any possible bias, a protocol about the evaluation of the signs of feeding intolerance has been introduced in our unit before the beginning of the study. A strict adhesion to the protocol was recommended to all the nursing staff.

### Abbreviations

ADJ: Adjustable Fortification; BMC: Multi-component fortifiers derived from bovine milk; BPC: Protein concentrates derived from bovine milk; BUN: Blood urea nitrogen; DMC: Multi-component fortifiers derived from donkey milk; DPC: Protein concentrates derived from donkey milk; GER: Gastroesophageal Reflux; MII/pH: Multichannel Intraluminal Impedance and pH monitoring; NICU: Neonatal Intensive Care Unit; SDS: Standard deviation score; VLBWI: Very Low Birthweight Infants

### Acknowledgements

The authors gratefully acknowledge the following partners of the Fortilat project for collaborating to the production of the donkey milk derived fortifier used in the trial: Procemsa spa (Torino, Italy), ProgeFarm srl (Novara, Italy), Eurolactis Italia srl (Corbetta, Milano, Italy), Università del Piemonte Orientale (Dipartimento di Scienze del Farmaco, Novara, Italy).

### Funding

This work was supported by Compagnia di San Paolo and by Regione Piemonte (FORTILAT project - Call "Poli di Innovazione", Por-Fesr 2007–2013 Program).

### Authors' contributions

CA and TP participated to the study design, coordinated the clinical trial and were contributors in writing the manuscript. BE and GEM are co-inventors of fortifier based on donkey milk, participated to the study design, and were contributors in writing the manuscript. PC enrolled the patients, collected the data and was a contributor in writing the manuscript. SE and MS conducted statistical analysis and were contributors in the revision of the manuscript. GM produced and analyzed the donkey milk based products and was a contributor in the revision of the manuscript. CA is a co-inventor of the fortifier based on donkey milk, participated to the study design, and was a contributor in writing the manuscript. SA produced and analyzed the donkey milk based products. CF performed pH-impedance monitoring analysis, measurements of gastric emptying by real-time ultrasound and participated to the study design. CL is a co-inventor of the fortifier based on donkey milk, participated to the study design, produced and analyzed the donkey milk based products, and was a contributor in writing the manuscript. All authors read and approved the final manuscript.

### Competing interests

EB, LC, GEM, AC have competing interest since they are the inventors of a patent on the fortifier derived from donkey milk described in the paper (Italian Patent no. n.0001421271 and international patent application no. WO2015056166 (A1)-20,150,423). No conflict of interest exists for the remaining authors.

### Author details

[1]Neonatal Unit of Turin University, City of Health and Science of Turin, Via Ventimiglia 3, 10126 Turin, Italy. [2]Italian Association of Human Milk Banks, Via Libero Temolo 4, 20126 Milan, Italy. [3]Unit of Medical Statistics and Biometry, Department of Clinical Sciences and Community Health, University of Milan, Milan, Italy. [4]Institute of Sciences of Food Production, National Research Council, Largo Braccini 2, 10095 Grugliasco (TO), Italy. [5]Research Centre for Engineering and Agro-Food Processing, Council for Agricultural Research and Economics (CREA), Strada delle cacce 73, 10135 Turin, Italy.

### References

1. Corchia C, Orzalesi M. Geographic variations in outcome of very low birth weight infants in Italy. Acta Paediatr. 2007;96(1):35–8.
2. Embleton ND. Early nutrition and later outcomes in preterm infants. World Rev Nutr Diet. 2013;106:26–32.
3. Lapillonne A, Griffin IJ. Feeding preterm infants today for later metabolic and cardiovascular outcomes. J Pediatr. 2013;162(3):S7–16.
4. Leppänen M, Lapinleimu H, Lind A, et al. Antenatal and postnatal growth and 5-year cognitive outcome in very preterm infants. Pediatrics. 2014; 133(1):63–70.
5. Johnston M, Landers S, Noble L, et al. Breastfeeding and the use of human milk. Pediatrics. 2012;129(3):e827–41.
6. Agostoni C, Buonocore G, Carnielli VP, et al. Enteral nutrient supply for preterm infants: commentary from the European Society of Paediatric Gastroenterology, Hepatology and nutrition committee on nutrition. J Pediatr Gastroenterol Nutr. 2010;50(1):85–91.
7. Embleton ND. Optimal protein and energy intakes in preterm infants. Early Hum Dev. 2007;83(12):831–7.
8. Dutta S, Singh B, Chessell L, et al. Guidelines for feeding very low birth weight infants. Nutrients. 2015;7(1):423–42.
9. Tudehope DI. Human milk and the nutritional needs of preterm infants. J Pediatr. 2013;162(3):S17–25.
10. Ziegler EE. Meeting the nutritional needs of the low-birth-weight infant. Ann Nutr Metab. 2011;58(1):8–18.
11. Arslanoglu S, Corpeleijn W, Moro G, et al. Donor human milk for preterm infants: current evidence and research directions. J Pediatr Gastroenterol Nutr. 2013;57(4):535–42.
12. Brown JV, Embleton ND, Harding JE, et al. Multi-nutrient fortification of human milk for preterm infants. In: Cochrane Database of Systematic Reviews [Internet]. John Wiley & Sons, Ltd; 2016 [cited 2016 May 17]. Available from: http://onlinelibrary.wiley.com/doi/10.1002/14651858.CD004866.pub4/full.
13. Arslanoglu S, Moro GE, Ziegler EE. Adjustable fortification of human milk fed to preterm infants: does it make a difference? J Perinatol Off J Calif Perinat Assoc. 2006;26(10):614–21.
14. Arslanoglu S, Moro GE, Ziegler EE, The Wapm Working Group On Nutrition null. Optimization of human milk fortification for preterm infants: new concepts and recommendations. J Perinat Med. 2010;38(3):233–8.
15. Arslanoglu S, Bertino E, Coscia A, et al. Update of adjustable fortification regimen for preterm infants: a new protocol. J Biol Regul Homeost Agents. 2012;26(3):65–7.
16. Sampson HA, Aceves S, Bock SA, et al. Food allergy: a practice parameter update-2014. J Allergy Clin Immunol. 2014;134(5):1016–25.

17. Abdelhamid AE, Chuang SL, Hayes P, Fell JME. In vitro Cow's milk protein-specific inflammatory and regulatory cytokine responses in preterm infants with necrotizing Enterocolitis and sepsis. Pediatr Res. 2011;69:165–9.
18. Mimouni FB, et al. The use of multinutrient human milk fortifiers in preterm infants: a systematic review of unanswered questions. Clin Perinatol. 2016; 44(1):173–8.
19. Barłowska J, Szwajkowska M, Litwińczuk Z, Król J. Nutritional value and technological suitability of milk from various animal species used for dairy production. Compr Rev Food Sci Food Saf. 2011;10(6):291–302.
20. Monti G, Bertino E, Muratore MC, et al. Efficacy of donkey's milk in treating highly problematic cow's milk allergic children: an in vivo and in vitro study. Pediatr Allergy Immunol. 2007;18(3):258–64.
21. Bertino E, Gastaldi D, Monti G, et al. Detailed proteomic analysis on DM: insight into its hypoallergenicity. Front Biosci Elite Ed. 2010;2:526–36.
22. Gastaldi D, Bertino E, Monti G, et al. Donkey's milk detailed lipid composition. Front Biosci Elite Ed. 2010;2:537–46.
23. Lionetti L, Cavaliere G, Bergamo P, et al. Diet supplementation with donkey milk upregulates liver mitochondrial uncoupling, reduces energy efficiency and improves antioxidant and antiinflammatory defences in rats. Mol Nutr Food Res. 2012;56(10):1596–600.
24. Trinchese G, Cavaliere G, Canani RB, et al. Human, donkey and cow milk differently affects energy efficiency and inflammatory state by modulating mitochondrial function and gut microbiota. J Nutr Biochem. 2015;26(11):1136–46.
25. Perrella SL, Hepworth AR, Simmer KN, Geddes DT. Validation of ultrasound methods to monitor gastric volume changes in preterm infants. J Pediatr Gastroenterol Nutr. 2013;57:741–9.
26. Newell SJ, Chapman S, Booth IW. Ultrasonic assessment of gastric emptying in the preterm infant. Arch Dis Child. 1993;69:32–6.
27. Wenzl TG. Investigating esophageal reflux with the intraluminal impedance technique. J Pediatr Gastroenterol Nutr. 2002;34:261–8.
28. Cresi F, et al. Prognostic values of multichannel Intraluminal impedance and pH monitoring in newborns with symptoms of Gastroesophageal reflux disease. J Pediatr. 2013;162:770–5.
29. Horbar JD. The Vermont Oxford network: evidence-based quality improvement for neonatology. Pediatrics. 1999;103(1):350–9.
30. Nelder JA, Wedderburn RWM. Generalized Linear Models. J R Stat Soc Ser A (General). 1972;135(3):370–84.
31. SAS Institute Inc SAS 9.4, Cary, NC, USA; 2012. http://www.sas.com
32. Sullivan S, Kim JH, Patel AL, et al. An exclusively human milk-based diet is associated with a lower rate of necrotizing Enterocolitis than a diet of human milk and bovine milk-based products. J Pediatr. 2010; 156(4):562–U83.

# 2

# The effects of fatty fish intake on adolescents' nutritional status and associations with attention performance: results from the FINS-TEENS randomized controlled trial

Katina Handeland[1,2*], Siv Skotheim[3], Valborg Baste[4], Ingvild E. Graff[1,4], Livar Frøyland[1], Øyvind Lie[1,5], Marian Kjellevold[1], Maria W. Markhus[1], Kjell M. Stormark[3,6], Jannike Øyen[1] and Lisbeth Dahl[1]

**Abstract:**

**Background:** Adolescence involves changes in dietary habits that may induce imbalances in the intake of different nutrients. Fish is an important dietary source of omega-3 (n-3) long-chain polyunsaturated fatty acids (LCPUFAs), vitamin D, several minerals and high-quality protein. By using secondary outcomes and exploratory analyses, the aims of this paper were to evaluate if nutritional biomarkers (red blood cell fatty acids, serum (s)-25(OH)D, s-ferritin and urinary iodine concentration (UIC)) were altered during a dietary intervention, and if they mediated previously reported changes in attention performance. In addition, to examine the status of the biomarkers and explore associations between dietary pattern, biomarkers and attention performance cross-sectionally at baseline.

**Methods:** The Fish Intervention Studies-TEENS (FINS-TEENS) was a three-armed intervention trial, including adolescents from eight secondary schools ($n = 415$; age: 14–15y) in Bergen, Norway. Participants were individually randomized to receive either fish meals, meat meals or n-3 LCPUFA supplements, three times a week for a total of 12 weeks. Blood and urine samples were collected pre and post intervention and attention performance was assessed with the d2 test of attention. Analyses of covariance (ANCOVA) assessed differences between groups in changes of biomarkers and linear mixed models were applied in analyses of attention performance and biomarkers. The trial is registered in ClinicalTrials.gov (NCT02350322).

**Results:** At baseline, the mean omega-3 index was 5.8 ± 1.3% and deficient status were identified for s-25(OH)D (54%), s-ferritin (10%) and UIC (40%). The intervention resulted in an increase in DHA and the omega-3 index which was larger in the supplement group compared to the fish and meat group ($P < 0.01$), and in the fish group compared to the meat group ($P < 0.01$). No differences between the groups were observed for changes in 25(OH)D, s-ferritin or UIC. None of the biomarkers mediated performance in the d2 test. The intake of fatty fish and a healthy dietary pattern was associated with scores in processing speed at baseline.

**Conclusions:** These results show that Norwegian adolescents have insufficient status of important nutrients, which may be improved with fatty fish consumption or n-3 LCPUFA supplements. However, nutritional status was not associated with scores in the d2 test of attention.

**Keywords:** N-3 LCPUFA, Vitamin D, Iron, Iodine, Fatty fish, Dietary intervention, Healthy adolescents

* Correspondence: katina.handeland@gmail.com
[1]Institute of Marine Research (IMR), P.O. Box 1870 Nordnes, 5817 Bergen, Norway
[2]Department of Clinical Medicine, Faculty of Medicine and Dentistry, University of Bergen, P.O. Box 7800, 5020 Bergen, Norway
Full list of author information is available at the end of the article

## Background

Seafood is a component of dietary patterns associated with good health, and food based dietary guidelines in almost all European countries include recommendations on fish consumption. One purpose of these recommendations is to ensure the provision of key nutrients, since fish is the main dietary source of the omega-3 (n-3) long-chain polyunsaturated fatty acids (LCPUFAs) and vitamin D, in addition to minerals and high-quality protein [1, 2]. Adolescence is a critical period involving major physiological changes, and thus, suboptimal dietary habits leading to nutritional imbalances may be of special concern in this group [3]. The cross-sectional Healthy Lifestyle in Europe by Nutrition in Adolescence (HELENA) study found that 42% had a serum 25-hydroxyvitamin D (25(OH)D) concentration < 50 nmol/L [4], which is regarded as insufficient [5]. No official cut-off for the nutritional status of n-3 LCPUFAs currently exists, but a commonly used marker for dietary intake and cardiovascular disease risk is the omega-3 index, which is the percentage of eicosapentaenoic acid (EPA) and docosahexaenoic acid (DHA) in red blood cell (RBC) fatty acids [6]. The proposed omega-3 index risk categories for cardiovascular disease in adults are: high risk, < 4%; intermediate risk, 4–8%; and low risk, > 8% [7]. Based on these cut-offs, a cross-sectional study reported that only 0.4% of 1300 Australian adolescents had an omega-3 index of > 8%, 84% had an index of 4–8%, and 15.6% had an index of < 4% [8]. The food based dietary guidelines for fish consumption generally range from 100 to 300 g per week and the European food safety authority (EFSA) recommends that the dietary advice for children aged 2–18 years should be 250 mg/d of EPA and DHA [9]. In Norway, the recommendation is 2–3 dinner portions/week, which should correspond to 300–450 g/week, of which 200 g should be fatty fish. However, data from Norway and other Western populations suggest that these recommendations are not met [1, 10].

Although the brain reaches approximately 90% of its adult size at age six, it continues to undergo changes throughout adolescence, involving e.g. myelination of axons, synaptic pruning and increased communication between the brain regions [11]. Nutrition is a key environmental factor to consider in terms of brain development and function, because it can be manipulated relatively easily [12]. To our knowledge, no previous randomized controlled trials (RCT) have provided fish to adolescents and measured nutritional status and/or cognitive performance. Two observational studies have been conducted, showing that fish consumption was positively associated with adolescents' performance at school [13] and in cognitive tests [14, 15]. Given its nutritional properties, and because increased consumption potentially could replace other foods with putative adverse health effects, it is plausible that an increased intake of fish could be more beneficial than consuming supplements. Thus, we performed a RCT to assess the effect of a 3-month dietary intervention with fatty fish meals in typically developing adolescents. Previously reported results from this study suggest that the fish meals could have led to improvements in outcomes of attention performance, although the results were difficult to interpret due to low dietary compliance [16]. By using secondary outcomes and exploratory analyses, the aims of this paper were to evaluate if nutritional biomarkers (RBC fatty acids, serum (s)-25(OH)D, s-ferritin and urinary iodine concentration (UIC)) were altered during the intervention, and if they mediated attention performance. In addition, to examine the status of nutritional biomarkers and explore associations between dietary pattern, biomarkers, and attention performance cross-sectionally at baseline.

## Methods

### Study design and ethics

Fish Intervention Studies-TEENS (FINS-TEENS) was conducted at eight lower secondary schools in Bergen, Norway, between February and May 2015. The three-armed trial used a RCT design to investigate the cognitive and nutritional effects of providing meals with fatty fish, or similar meals with meat/cheese, or fish oil supplements to adolescents.

The trial was conducted according to the declaration of Helsinki. Ethical approval was obtained from the Norwegian Data Protection Official for Research (project number: 41,030). Written informed consent was collected from all participants and one legal caregiver, and participants could withdraw from the trial without giving any reason. The trial is registered in Clinical Trials.gov (NCT02350322). The design and methods are described in detail previously [17].

### Participants and randomization

Eligible adolescents were girls and boys attending 9th grade (14–15 years-old) at the participating schools, who knew the Norwegian language orally and written. Exclusion criteria were allergy or intolerance to the study foods or supplements. The random allocation was performed individually stratified by gender, by two researchers. One researcher went through the list of participants stating only the participants' gender (boy/girl), while another (blinded from the list) drew lots marked with one of the three intervention groups from the correct box labeled either "boy" or "girl".

### Study meals and n-3 supplements

The meals were prepared by a catering service (Søtt+Salt A/S, Bergen, Norway) and were similar in content except from the meat and fish. Meals in the fish group contained salmon, mackerel and herring, whereas meals in the meat group contained chicken, turkey, beef, lamb and cheese. In addition, the meals comprised vegetables and/or salad and mainly wholegrain pasta-, focaccia-, baguette- or tortilla and sometimes dressing. Halal meat and gluten free products were provided on request. The meals had a mean weight of 230 g/portion, and the amount of fish/meat was requested to be between 80 and 100 g/portion. The number of capsules was calculated to match the weekly intake of EPA and DHA in the fish group, and was seven per serving. Capsules were Nycoplus® Omega-3, 500 mg, produced by Takeda Nycomed, Asker, Norway, bought at a public pharmacy in Bergen, Norway. Fatty acids and nutrient content in the meals and supplements were analyzed and results are summarized in Table 1.

### Procedure

The meals and supplements were delivered three times a week for a total of 12 weeks. Participants received the meals or supplements from a study worker at their school, during the lunch break (usually between 11:00 a.m. and noon). Participants in the different intervention groups ate together in their respective class-rooms. The fish and meat meals replaced the participants' usual lunch, whereas the supplement group continued to eat their habitual lunch in addition to taking the supplements. The school lunch of Norwegian adolescents is usually a packed lunch from home, containing medium dark or dark bread or crispbread with meat, cheese or liver pate as spread, and sometimes a fruit or vegetable [10, 18]. The participants were asked not to change any procedures they had besides the intervention, e.g. use of fish-oil supplements or their habitual dietary intake of fish at home. Dietary compliance was monitored throughout the trial by study staff who registered the remaining number of capsules and the amount of fish/meat eaten for each participant. The amount of fish/meat eaten was estimated by eye and registered on a scale from zero to four: '0 = nothing eaten', '1 = 1/4 eaten', '2 = 2/4 eaten', '3 = 3/4 eaten' and '4 = all eaten'.

**Table 1** Fatty acid profile and nutrient content in each portion of fish and meat meals (mean weight 230 g) and n-3 supplements

| Nutrients | Fish meals | Meat meals | Supplements[d] |
|---|---|---|---|
| Total fat[a] | 23.3 ± 9.1 | 19.3 ± 9.5 | 3.5 |
| Protein[a] | 24.8 ± 9.1 | 27.3 ± 7.7 | – |
| LA (18:2n-6)[b] | 3530.7 ± 1556.2 | 2753.1 ± 1453.4 | 35.1 ± 0.6 |
| AA (20:4n-6)[b] | 66.0 ± 36.6 | 51.3 ± 32.0 | 67.9 ± 1.1 |
| EPA (20:5n-3)[b] | 350.4 ± 456.2 | 7.3 ± 3.6 | 1079.6 ± 25.7 |
| DPA (22:5n-3)[b] | 91.7 ± 73.0 | 13.8 ± 6.5 | 119.1 ± 3.4 |
| DHA (22:6n-3)[b] | 603.2 ± 722.4 | 11.6 ± 12.0 | 743.8 ± 24.0 |
| Sum n-3[b] | 2100.6 ± 1688.1 | 434.6 ± 257.8 | 2138.5 ± 86.0 |
| Sum n-6[b] | 3738.1 ± 1557.4 | 2837.3 ± 1462.5 | 147.6 ± 1.8 |
| Vitamin $D_3^c$ | 4.9 ± 2.7 | < 0.1 ± 0.1 | – |
| Iodine[c] | 11.4 ± 20.3 | 5.9 ± 6.1 | – |
| Selenium[c] | 16.8 ± 10.7 | 12.1 ± 4.5 | – |

Abbreviations: *AA* arachidonic acid, *LA* linoleic acid, *EPA* eicosapentaenoic acid, *DPA* Docosapentaenoic acid, *DHA* docosahexaenoic acid, *n-3* omega-3, *n-6* omega-6

[a]g/portion

[b]mg/portion

[c]μg/portion

[d]1 portion = 7 capsules

Data given as mean ± SD

### Questionnaire

General information about participants (age, weight, height, and gender) and their background diet (habitual dietary intake besides the intervention) were obtained with a revised and extended version of a validated web-based food frequency questionnaire (FFQ) at pre and post intervention [19, 20]. Height and weight were not measured directly in order to prioritize the cognitive tests and blood and urine sampling. The FFQ included questions about the consumption of different fish species for dinner (never – ≥4 times/week) and in the analyses, continuous indices were made from the reported intake of salmon, herring and mackerel according to the methodology by Markhus and colleagues [19], and summarized into one continuous variable reflecting fatty fish intake (range 0.0–6.0). The questionnaire included one question about physical activity (≤30 min – 4 h or more/week) and questions regarding the frequency of using solarium (never – 2 times/week) and duration of being abroad to high-UV radiation areas (range: zero – ≥4 weeks) the past three months. The reported use of solarium was dichotomized into less than once per month or ≥once per month, and the duration of being abroad to high-UV radiation areas was dichotomized into less than one week or ≥one week. These variables were combined into solarium/high-UV exposure yes/no (categorical variable). A diet score (0–8 points) which evaluates the adherence to the current Norwegian dietary recommendations by scoring the reported intake of fruits, vegetables, wholegrain, fish, red meat, dairy products, added sugar, water and physical activity has been developed and applied to the FFQ [21]. The diet score was used in the cross-sectional analyses in the present paper.

A questionnaire sent to the caregivers by e-mail assessed parental educational level (elementary/lower secondary school – college/university ≥4 years), total household income (< 200,000 NOK – > 2000,000 NOK (100 NOK = approximately 10€/11$) and origin (participant and both parents born outside or in Norway). The mean parental educational level ((mothers' level + fathers' level)/2) (continuous variable) was used in the statistical analyses.

## Outcomes

### *Blood and urine samples, and biochemical analyses*

Authorized biomedical laboratory scientists obtained non-fasting blood samples from the elbow cavity of the participants. For preparation of RBC, venous blood was collected in BD Vacutainer® vials and centrifuged (10 min, 1000 g, 20 °C) within 30 min. RBCs were adequately separated to ensure a clean blood fraction. Venous blood for serum preparation was collected in BD Vacutainer® vials and set to coagulate for minimum 30 min before centrifuged (10 min, 1000G, 20 °C,) within 60 min. Blood samples were temporarily stored and transported on dry ice before storage in a – 80 °C freezer until analysis.

For analyzation of fatty acids, blood samples were thawed on a shaker (Nutating shaker) and prepared by the Hamilton Microlab Star Line robot. The samples were homogenized and internal standard (0.4 mg/ml Methyl Nonadecanoate in methanol) and 2% sulfuric acid in methanol were added. Samples were shaken and boiled at 105 °C for 40 min before cooled. Extraction of fatty acids was performed by adding water and heptane, and the fatty acid composition was determined on a Trace GC Ultra gas chromathograph (Thermo Corporation). The samples were analyzed on a UltraFast UFC-WAX Column (5 m × 0.1 mm × 0.1um), ThermoFischer Scientific. Helium was used as mobile phase at 0.5 ml/min constant flow. Certified reference materials were analyzed to assess the accuracy and precision of the method. A 10% difference was accepted in contents of 0.6–100% and all RBC fatty acids are expressed as weight percentage of total fatty acids. The omega-3 index was calculated as the content of EPA and DHA expressed as percent of total fatty acids [6].

S-25(OH)D concentration was determined by standardized procedures at IMR, using a liquid chromatographic-tandem mass spectrometric (LC-MS/MS) assay adding acetonitrile and internal standard ($^2$H 25(OH)$D_3$) to the samples [22]. S-ferritin was analyzed at Haraldsplass Diakonale Hospital Bergen, Norway, by an automated electrochemiluminescence immunoassay (ECLIA) on Cobas e601 (Roche). The urine samples was taken at home in the morning or at school and iodine status was determined as UIC in spot samples by Inductive Coupled Plasma Mass Spectrometry (ICP-MS) at IMR [23].

### *Cognitive tests*

The primary outcome of the study was performance on the d2 test of attention [24]. In addition, participants completed a Norwegian reading and spelling test named "Kartleggeren" and the Strengths and Difficulties Questionnaire (SDQ), which assesses mental health status, at pre and post intervention. Results from "Kartleggeren" are not reported, due to considerable ceiling effects in nearly all outcomes both pre and post intervention. Effects of the intervention on SDQ are reported in Skotheim et al. [25]. Consequently, results from the d2 test of attention only are used in the present paper, and these have also previously been presented in more detail [16].

The d2 test of attention is a pen and paper cancellation test, measuring abilities in visual scanning, processing speed and degree of accuracy, regardless of intelligence level [24, 26]. The test comprises 47 interspersed target- and distraction characters× 14 rows, and the respondents' task is to cancel out as many target characters as possible, while ignoring distraction characters. Standard outcomes of the test were included in the trial, which are: 'processing speed' (TN; total number of characters processed) and two overall measures of performance: 'total performance' (TN-E; total number of characters processed minus total errors made) and 'concentration performance' (CP; total number of correctly cancelled out target characters minus commission errors). In addition, there are two types of error-outcomes: 'omission errors' (E1; unmarked target characters) and 'commission errors' (E2; incorrectly cancelled distraction characters), and 'total errors' (E total; the sum of E1 and E2).

The same trained study staff administered the test according to standard instructions pre and post intervention. Testing was performed in classrooms between 9 and 11 a.m. Environmental factors such as noise were controlled for rigorously by the study crew and the teachers.

## Sample size

The sample size calculation was based on the design with a three armed-intervention, and pre and post intervention measurements with an assumed correlation of 0.5. The primary outcome of the trial was the d2 test of attention. To be able to reveal a meanigful effect of the intervention on the primary outcome, a small to moderate effect size (0.35) was applied. The calculated sample size was 119 participants in each group based on a power of 80% and a significance level of $\alpha = 0.05$. When taking a 20% drop out rate into account, the aim was to enroll a sample of 446 participants in the trial.

## Statistical analyses

Data are presented as either means and standard deviations (SD) or as numbers (n) and percentages (%). At baseline, differences between intervention groups were assessed with one-way ANOVA for continuous variables and Chi-square test for categorical variables.

Paired-samples *t*-tests were used for analysis of changes in nutritonal biomarkers (fatty acids, 25(OH)D, s-ferritin or UIC) within each intervention group from pre to post intervention. ANCOVA were used to test for differences between intervention groups in changes of nutritional biomarkers. The dependent variable was the value of the relevant biomarker measured at post intervention, and the model was adjusted for the same biomarker measured at pre intervention. A second model was further adjusted for dietary compliance (amount of fish, meat or n-3 supplements eaten during the trial). Pairwise comparisons with Bonferroni correction between intervention groups were performed if the overall *P*-value was significant.

To investigate if biomarkers could mediate the assosiation between intervention and TN, TN-E and E1, which as previously reported were the significant outcomes from the d2 test of attention [16], standard mediation approach was used [27] within linear mixed effects models. The association between the nutritional biomarkers at post intervention (independent variable) and the relevant d2 test outcome measured at post intervention (dependent variable) was assessed, one at a time. School class was included as random intercept and the models were adjusted for the relevant pre intervention d2 test score and pre intervention values of the relevant nutritonal biomarker.

Association with intervention groups and reported use of solarium and being abroad to high-UV radiation areas was assessed with chi-square test.

Baseline analyses assessing the associations between d2 test-scores (dependent) and nutritional biomarkers, or the reported intake of fatty fish, or the diet score from the FFQ (independent), were performed with linear mixed effects models with school class as random intercept. Unadjusted models and models adjusted for age, sex, parental educational level and physical activity were performed for the d2 test scores.

Two-tailed *P*-values < 0.05 were considered statistically significant. The analyses were performed using the Statistical Package for the Social Sciences (SPSS® Statistics version 24, IBM Corporation, US), except for the linear mixed effect models which were performed using Stata Statistical Software: Release 14. College Station, TX: (STATACorp LP®).

## Results

### Study population

Of the 785 children who were attending 9th grade at the time of recruitment and received invitation, 481 (61%) agreed to participate. Three participants withdrew from the trial at the day of baseline testing, before randomization. Thus, 478 participants were randomly allocated to intervention groups. 47 participants were lost to follow up or discontinued the intervention ($n = 22$ in the fish group, $n = 11$ in the meat group, and $n = 14$ in the supplement group) (Fig. 1). A total of 370 questionnaires (78%) were completed by the caregivers.

Participants had a mean age of 14.6 ± 0.3 years, and a mean BMI of 19.8 ± 2.9 kg/m$^2$. Most were non-immigrants, defined as the participant and both of the parents were born in Norway. The participants had a mean omega-3 index of 5.8 ± 1.3% and 95% of the sample had an index ≤8%. A total of 92%, 10% and 40% had deficient levels of s-25(OH)D, s-ferritin and UIC, respectively [5, 28, 29]. The reported baseline dietary intake of fish for dinner was on average 1.5 meals/week, of which 1 of these were fatty fish. The proportion who reported to use fish oil or other types of omega-3 supplements daily was 18%, whereas 53% reported to never use this. There were no differences between the intervention groups in baseline characteristics, nutritional status or dietary intake (Table 2).

A mean of 30 ± 6 meals were served to each participant during the intervention. As reported previously [17], the total intake (dietary compliance) was higher in the supplement group than in the meal groups, and the total intake of meat in the meat group was higher than the total intake of fish in the fish group. The proportion of participants who consumed at least half of the fish/meat/capsules during the trial was 38%, 66% and 87% in the fish, meat and supplement group, respectively [17]. There was not observed any differences between intervention groups in changes of the background diet from pre to post intervention [16].

### Change in nutritional status during the intervention

As shown in Table 3, the pairwise comparisons (with Bonferroni correction) showed that the omega-3 index and DHA increased in the supplement group compared to the fish and meat group, and that these markers also increased more in the fish group compared to the meat group. When adjusting for dietary compliance, these differences between groups were still significant for the omega-3 index, but the increase in DHA was no longer different between the supplement and fish group. The supplement group showed a decrease in AA during the intervention, compared to the two other groups. The fish group showed a mean increase in s-25(OH)D concentration of 5.3 nmol/L, whereas the increase in the meat and supplement group was 1.8 and 2.6 nmol/L respectively, and the initial analyses showed no differences between the groups. When adusting for dietary compliance, an overall difference was observed between the groups ($P = 0.032$), and the pairwise comparisons between the fish and meat group and the fish and supplement group gave $P = 0.056$ and $P = 0.060$, respectively. There were no associations between the intervention groups and the reported use of solarium and stays abroad in high-UV radiation areas during the trial. No differences between intervention groups were observed for changes in iron or iodine status from pre to post intervention.

### Associations between biomarkers of nutritional status and attention performance

None of the nutritional biomarkers were found to be associated with the post intervention value of TN, TN-E or E1, and could thereby not alone have mediated the previously reported change in these outcomes (results not shown).

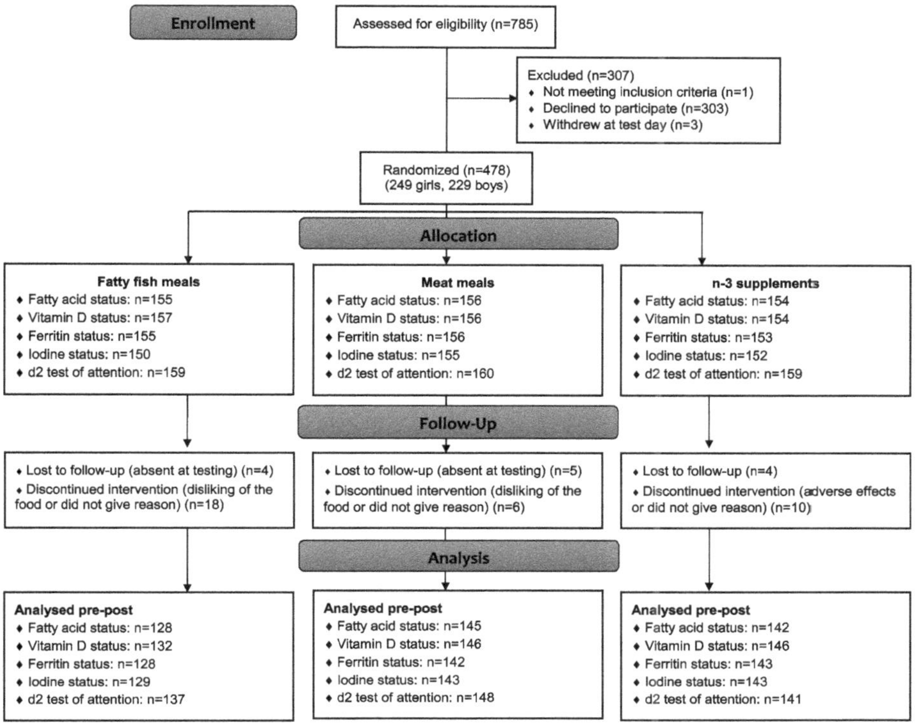


**Fig. 1** Flow chart over participants. n-3 = omega-3

Neither the unadjusted nor the adjusted cross-sectional analyses at baseline measurements showed associations between the nutritional biomarkers and performance in d2 test outcomes. An association between the participants' diet score (0–8 points reflecting low-high adherence to dietary recommendations) and CP, TN-E and TN was found in the unadjusted analyses. This association remained significant for TN after adjusting for potential confounders. An association between the reported consumption of salmon, mackerel and herring and TN was observed in the unadjusted and the adjusted analyses (Table 4).

## Discussion

This trial among school-aged adolescents showed that a 3-month dietary intervention with n-3 LCPUFA supplements or fatty fish meals increased RBC concentrations of DHA and the omega-3 index more than meat meals. No differences between groups were observed in changes of s-25(OH)D, s-ferritin or UIC concentrations from pre to post intervention. No associations between changes in nutritional biomarkers and attention performance was observed, but the cross-sectional analyses showed an association between the participants' healthy diet score and processing speed (TN) at baseline, and between the reported intake of fatty fish (salmon mackerel and herring) and TN at baseline. The proportion of participants with deficient levels were 54% for s-25(OH)D, 10% for s-ferritin and 40% for UIC.

The average omega-3 index at baseline was 5.8% in this sample of adolescents, which is slightly higher than the mean index of 4.9% found in 1300 Australian adolescents [8]. However, when compared with the categories for cardiovascular disease risk for adults [7], a larger proportion in our sample had an omega-3 index < 4% (5% in our sample compared to 0.4% in the Australian sample) and a smaller proportion had an omega-3 index > 8% (5% in our sample compared to 15.6% in the Australian sample). The mean increases in the omega-3 index of 0.6% and 1.6% in the fish and supplement group respectively, is comparable to the findings by Stonehouse et al., who reported increases between 0.8–1.8% with salmon meals (710 mg/d EPA + DHA) or salmon oil supplements (210–600 mg/d EPA+ DHA) to healthy adults for 8 weeks [30]. The proportion with vitamin D deficiency is slightly higher in this study than among European adolescents in the HELENA study [4]. This is probably because this trial started in February, which is when s-25(OH)D concentrations are almost at their lowest in high latitudes such as Bergen, Norway, (60.4°N) due to absent UV-B radiation [31]. The mean increase of 5.3 nmol/L in the fish group is nearly comparable with the results from a meta-analysis of RCTs in adults (> 18 years), showing that the average increase in fish groups relative to placebo was 4.4 nmol/L, and when only fatty fish

**Table 2** Baseline characteristics of all participants and by randomly assigned intervention groups

| Variables | Number | All | Fish | Meat | Supplement | P[a] |
|---|---|---|---|---|---|---|
| Characteristics | | | | | | |
| Gender n (%) | 415 | | | | | 0.546 |
| Male | | 195 (47.0) | 56 (43.8) | 73 (50.3) | 66 (46.5) | |
| Female | | 220 (53.0) | 72 (56.3) | 72 (49.7) | 76 (53.5) | |
| Age (years) | 415 | 14.6 ± 0.3 | 14.6 ± 0.3 | 14.6 ± 0.3 | 14.6 ± 0.3 | 0.531 |
| BMI ($kg/m^2$) | 385 | 19.8 ± 3.0 | 19.8 ± 3.4 | 19.7 ± 2.3 | 19.9 ± 3.1 | 0.940 |
| Parental education level n (%) | 341 | | | | | 0.793 |
| Elementary/vocational school | | 132 (38.7) | 41 (39.4) | 47 (40.5) | 44 (36.4) | |
| College/university | | 209 (61.3) | 63 (60.6) | 69 (59.5) | 77 (63.6) | |
| Family income in NOK[b] n (%) | 338 | | | | | 0.201 |
| < 200,000–749,999 | | 70 (20.7) | 21 (20.4) | 17 (14.8) | 32 (26.7) | |
| 750,000–1,249,999 | | 171 (50.6) | 50 (48.5) | 66 (57.4) | 55 (45.8) | |
| 1,250,000- > 2,000,000 | | 97 (28.7) | 32 (31.1) | 32 (27.8) | 33 (27.5) | |
| Immigrant[c] n (%) | 341 | 7 (2.1) | 2 (1.6) | 2 (1.7) | 3 (2.5) | 0.914 |
| Nutritional status | | | | | | |
| LA, 18:2n-6 (%) | 415 | 10.8 ± 1.3 | 10.8 ± 1.4 | 10.8 ± 1.2 | 10.9 ± 1.3 | 0.707 |
| AA, 20:4n-6 (%) | 415 | 15.6 ± 1.5 | 15.6 ± 1.4 | 15.6 ± 1.6 | 15.6 ± 1.5 | 0.958 |
| EPA, 20:5n-3 (%) | 415 | 0.9 ± 0.4 | 0.9 ± 0.3 | 0.9 ± 0.4 | 0.9 ± 0.4 | 0.960 |
| DPA, 22:5n-3 (%) | 415 | 2.4 ± 0.3 | 2.4 ± 0.3 | 2.4 ± 0.3 | 2.3 ± 0.3 | 0.110 |
| DHA, 22:6n-3 (%) | 415 | 4.9 ± 1.1 | 4.9 ± 1.0 | 5.0 ± 1.2 | 4.8 ± 1.0 | 0.171 |
| Omega-3 index[d] | 415 | 5.8 ± 1.3 | 5.8 ± 1.2 | 5.9 ± 1.4 | 5.7 ± 1.3 | 0.304 |
| ≤ 8 n (%) | | 395 (95.2) | 122 (95.3) | 135 (93.1) | 138 (97.2) | 0.271 |
| s-25(OH)D (nmol/L) | 424 | 48.8 ± 17.4 | 49.1 ± 17.1 | 49.7 ± 17.8 | 48.3 ± 17.4 | 0.671 |
| < 50 nmol/L n (%)[e] | | 229 (54.0) | 72 (54.5) | 76 (52.1) | 81 (55.5) | 0.832 |
| s-Ferritin (μg/l) | 412 | 40.7 ± 23.1 | 40.9 ± 22.4 | 41.2 ± 24.5 | 40.4 ± 22.3 | 0.953 |
| < 15 μg/l n (%)[e] | | 40 (9.7) | 12 (9.4) | 13 (9.2) | 15 (10.6) | 0.912 |
| UIC (μg/L) | 415 | 122.6 ± 63.7 | 122.6 ± 71.3 | 122.9 ± 59.3 | 125.0 ± 66.7 | 0.693 |
| < 100 μg/l[e] | | 164 (39.5) | 55 (42.6) | 49 (34.3) | 60 (42.0) | 0.282 |
| Dietary intake | 414 | | | | | |
| Fish for dinner[f] | | 1.5 (0.9) | 1.5 (1.0) | 1.4 (0.9) | 1.5 (0.9) | 0.780 |
| Herring/mackerel/salmon for dinner[f] | | 1.0 (0.9) | 1.0 (1.0) | 0.9 (0.9) | 1.0 (1.0) | 0.852 |
| Fish as bread spread[f] | | 0.6 (1.0) | 0.7 (1.0) | 0.6 (1.0) | 0.6 (0.9) | 0.620 |
| Fish oil supplements (n (%))[g] | 413 | | | | | 0.659 |
| Never | | 220 (53.3) | 60 (46.9) | 81 (56.3) | 79 (56.0) | |
| 1–3 times/month | | 53 (12.8) | 18 (14.1) | 18 (12.5) | 17 (12.1) | |
| 1–3 times/week | | 45 (10.9) | 19 (14.8) | 14 (9.7) | 12 (8.5) | |
| 4–6 times/week | | 20 (4.8) | 6 (4.7) | 5 (3.5) | 9 (6.4) | |
| Every day | | 75 (18.2) | 25 (19.5) | 26 (18.1) | 24 (17.0) | |

Abbreviations: *AA* arachidonic acid, *LA* linoleic acid, *EPA* eicosapentaenoic acid, *DPA* Docosapentaenoic acid, *DHA* docosahexaenoic acid, *25(OH)D* 25-hydroxyvitamin D, *s-Ferritin* serum ferritin, *UIC* urinary iodine concentration, *NOK* Norwegian kroner

[a]One-way ANOVA test (continuous variables) and Pearson's Chi-square test ($X^2$) (categorical variables) for comparison between treatment groups

[b]100 NOK = approximately 10€/11$

[c]Immigrant was defined as participants who's both parents and themselves were born outside Norway

[d]The content of EPA and DHA expressed as percent of total fatty acids [6]

[e]Adolescents were classified with vitamin D deficiency if s-25(OH)D < 50 nmol/L [5], with depleted iron stores if s-ferritin < 15 μg/L [29] and as iodine deficient if UIC < 100 μg/L [28]

[f]Reported meals per week (besides the intervention)

[g]N (%) of participants reporting to consume fish oil as dietary supplements

Data are given as mean ± SD if not other is indicated

**Table 3** Changes in the adolescents' fatty acids levels (% of total fatty acids), serum 25(OH)D, serum ferritin and urinary iodine concentration during the intervention

| Variables | Fish | | | Meat | | | Supplement | | | | |
|---|---|---|---|---|---|---|---|---|---|---|---|
| | Post | Change | $P^a$ | Post | Change | $P^a$ | Post | Change | $P^a$ | $P^b$ | $P^c$ |
| LA, 18:2n-6 (%) | 10.8 ± 1.4 | 0.0 ± 1.3 | 0.90 | 10.9 ± 1.2 | 0.1 ± 1.4 | 0.58 | 10.9 ± 1.3 | − 0.1 ± 1.4 | 0.64 | 0.80 | 0.77 |
| AA, 20:4n-6 (%) | 13.4 ± 1.4 | −2.2 ± 1.6 | < 0.001 | 13.7 ± 1.3 | − 1.9 ± 1.6 | < 0.001 | 12.8 ± 1.4 | − 2.8 ± 1.7 | < 0.001 | < 0.001[d,f] | < 0.001[d,f] |
| EPA, 20:5n-3 (%) | 0.8 ± 0.3 | − 0.1 ± 0.2 | 0.002 | 0.8 ± 0.4 | − 0.1 ± 0.3 | < 0.001 | 1.3 ± 0.5 | 0.5 ± 0.4 | < 0.001 | < 0.001[d,f] | < 0.001[d,e,f] |
| DPA, 22:5n-3 (%) | 2.0 ± 0.3 | − 0.3 ± 0.3 | < 0.001 | 2.0 ± 0.3 | − 0.4 ± 0.3 | < 0.001 | 2.3 ± 0.3 | 0.0 ± 0.4 | 0.59 | < 0.001[d,f] | < 0.001[d,f] |
| DHA, 22:6n-3 (%) | 5.6 ± 1.0 | 0.6 ± 0.8 | < 0.001 | 5.3 ± 1.1 | 0.3 ± 0.8 | < 0.001 | 6.0 ± 0.8 | 1.2 ± 0.9 | < 0.001 | < 0.001[d,e,f] | < 0.001[e,f] |
| Omega-3 Index[g] | 6.4 ± 1.2 | 0.6 ± 0.9 | < 0.001 | 6.1 ± 1.3 | 0.2 ± 1.0 | 0.016 | 7.3 ± 1.2 | 1.6 ± 1.1 | < 0.001 | < 0.001[d,e,f] | < 0.001[d,e,f] |
| s-25(OH)D (nmol/L) | 54.4 ± 16.7 | 5.3 ± 14.9 | < 0.001 | 51.6 ± 17.3 | 1.8 ± 12.2 | 0.07 | 50.9 ± 18.4 | 2.6 ± 11.7 | 0.009 | 0.07 | 0.032 |
| s-Ferritin (µg/l) | 39.9 ± 21.4 | − 0.7 ± 18.1 | 0.66 | 38.1 ± 22.7 | − 3.0 ± 14.8 | 0.017 | 37.0 ± 23.9 | −3.3 ± 18.7 | 0.040 | 0.40 | 0.58 |
| UIC (µg/L) | 107.7 ± 72.2 | − 11.6 ± 66.9 | 0.47 | 125.3 ± 70.3 | 2.4 ± 73.7 | 0.70 | 125.6 ± 65.8 | 0.9 ± 76.0 | 0.89 | 0.053 | 0.08 |

Abbreviations: *AA* arachidonic acid, *LA* linoleic acid, *EPA* eicosapentaenoic acid, *DPA* Docosapentaenoic acid, *DHA* docosahexaenoic acid, *s-25(OH)D* serum 25-hydroxyvitamin D, *s-Ferritin* serum ferritin, *UIC;* urinary iodine concentration
Total numbers may vary between variables due to varying numbers of missing data
[a]*P*-value for comparison within intervention groups, paired samples *t*-test
[b]*P*-value for comparison between intervention groups. ANCOVA (adjusted for the current outcome at baseline)
[c]*P*-value for comparison between intervention groups. ANCOVA (adjusted for the current outcome at baseline and dietary compliance (i.e. the total intake of fish, meat or supplements)) during the trial
[d]$p < 0.01$ fish - supplement, [e] $p < 0.01$ fish - meat, [f] $p < 0.01$ supplement - meat (Bonferroni correction for post-hoc comparison between intervention groups)
[e]The content of EPA and DHA expressed as percent of total fatty acids [6]
Data given as mean ± SD

interventions was considered, the difference increased to 6.8 nmol/L [32]. Mostly white meat was served to the meat group, which may explain the decreased level of s-ferritin in this group, although no differences between groups were evident. We did not measure puberty stage, but it is unlikely that the onset of menarche should have affected s-ferritin levels during the relatively short duration of 12 weeks. The median UIC in this sample of adolescents was 111.8 µg/L, which is just above the epidemiologic criteria for sufficient iodine status in populations given by WHO [28]. However, it is considerably lower than the median of 200 µg/L found in Icelandic adolescent girls ($n = 112$, 16–20 y) [33]. This could be because Iceland in the past has been known for its high iodine status due to a high intake of fish and milk. The large percentage with UIC below 100 µg/L in the present trial give cause for concern, and some of the explanation might be that iodized salt is not commonly used in households, and not used at all in the Norwegian food industry. The reason why no change in UIC was observed in the fish group from pre to post intervention is possibly because we used fatty fish, whereas lean fish is usually higher in iodine contents [34].

As mentioned, this is to our knowledge the first study that has provided fish to adolescents to measure the effect on attention performance. Associations between the d2 test of attention and RBC fatty acid status (the omega-3 index) have been investigated in two other studies, one RCT in healthy school children [35] and one cross-sectional study in healthy adolescents [36]. They reported contradictory (a positive [35] and a negative [36]) associations between the omega-3 index and errors of omission (E1 errors). The RCT also found associations between the omega-3 index and scores in concentration performance (CP) and total performance (TN-E) at baseline, but not in the correlation analyses between the intervention-induced changes. Thus, the results from previous studies using the d2 test of attention are inconclusive, which brings into question whether the test assesses performance in brain areas affected by n-3 LCPUFA status. The cross-sectional analyses in the present study suggesting that there is an association between TN and fatty fish intake, and a healthier dietary pattern is interesting. Other studies in healthy young participants have reported associations between cognitive outcomes and fish intake [13, 15] and between a healthy diet or intake of healthy foods [37–40]. However, because the present results are based on cross-sectional analyses, we cannot make statements on causality; although it is tempting to make the interpretation that TN was driven by the diet measures, the opposite may be true, such that higher scores in TN may implicate better dietary choices. In future studies, a more sensitive measure of processing speed e.g. response times in milliseconds may be useful to assess the potential association between fish or dietary intake and processing speed.

Given a 100% dietary compliance rate, the consumption of three portions/week of the fatty fish meals would have provided the participants in this trial with a weekly mean dose of approximately 1050 mg EPA and 1800 mg DHA. Divided by seven this corresponds to a daily mean dose of

**Table 4** Associations between adolescents' cognitive test-performances and nutritional variables or FFQ data at baseline

| | Unadjusted[a] | | | Adjusted[b] | | |
|---|---|---|---|---|---|---|
| | Number | ß (95% CI) | P | Number | ß (95% CI) | P |
| Omega-3 Index[c] | 460 | | | 367 | | |
| Concentration performance (CP) | | 0.62 (−1.75, 2.99) | 0.61 | | −1.43 (−4.07, 1.20) | 0.29 |
| Total performance (TN-E) | | −0.09 (−5.28, 5.11) | 0.97 | | −3.56 (−9.42, 2.31) | 0.23 |
| Processing speed (TN) | | −0.67 (− 6.36, 5.02) | 0.82 | | −2.93 (−9.36, 3.51) | 0.37 |
| s-25(OH)D | 462 | | | 368 | | |
| Concentration performance (CP) | | −0.04 (−0.21, 0.14) | 0.69 | | −0.08 (− 0.28, 0.11) | 0.41 |
| Total performance (TN-E) | | −0.11 (− 0.50, 0.27) | 0.56 | | −0.18 (0.62, 0.26) | 0.43 |
| Processing speed (TN) | | −0.17 (− 0.58, 0.25) | 0.44 | | −0.18 (0.66, 0.31) | 0.47 |
| s-Ferritin | 459 | | | 365 | | |
| Concentration performance (CP) | | 0.07 (−0.06, 0.20) | 0.30 | | 0.08 (−0.08, 0.22) | 0.32 |
| Total performance (TN-E) | | 0.13 (−0.17, 0.42) | 0.40 | | 0.15 (−0.19, 0.49) | 0.38 |
| Processing speed (TN) | | 0.06 (−0.23, 0.40) | 0.60 | | 0.13 (−0.24, 0.50) | 0.50 |
| UIC | 452 | | | 359 | | |
| Concentration performance (CP) | | 0.04 (−0.01, 0.08) | 0.13 | | 0.01 (−0.04, 0.06) | 0.68 |
| Total performance (TN-E) | | 0.03 (−0.08, 0.13) | 0.63 | | −0.02 (− 0.14, 0.09) | 0.70 |
| Processing speed (TN) | | −0.02 (− 0.13, 0.09) | 0.75 | | −0.05 (− 0.18, 0.07) | 0.39 |
| Diet score[d] | 465 | | | 368 | | |
| Concentration performance (CP) | | 2.61 (0.54, 4.69) | 0.014 | | 1.09 (−1.31, 3.48) | 0.38[e] |
| Total performance (TN-E) | | 5.76 (1.35, 10.27) | 0.012 | | 4.32 (−1.00, 9.64) | 0.11[e] |
| Processing speed (TN) | | 5.54 (0.61, 10.48) | 0.028 | | 6.05 (0.24, 11.85) | 0.04[e] |
| Fatty fish consumption[f] | 463 | | | 368 | | |
| Concentration performance (CP) | | 1.51 (−1.78, 4.81) | 0.37 | | 1.92 (−1.67, 5.52) | 0.29 |
| Total performance (TN-E) | | 5.86 (−1.23, 12.95) | 0.11 | | 6.98 (−0.98, 14.93) | 0.09 |
| Processing speed (TN) | | 8.51 (0.80, 16.23) | 0.031 | | 10.08 (1.42, 18.74) | 0.023 |

Abbreviations: *FFQ* food frequency questionnaire, *25(OH)D* 25-hydroxyvitamin D, *s-Ferritin* serum ferritin, *UIC* urinary iodine concentration
[a]Linear mixed effects model with school class as random intercept
[b]Linear mixed effects model with school class as random intercept, adjusted for age, sex, parental educational level and physical activity level
[c]The content of EPA and DHA expressed as percent of total fatty acids [6]
[d]A score including the reported intake of fruits, vegetables, wholegrain, fish, red meat, dairy products, added sugar, water and physical activity according to the Norwegian dietary recommendations. Range: 0–8 points [21]
[e]Not adjusted for physical activity
[f]Reported frequency of eating salmon, herring and mackerel from the FFQ

150 mg EPA and 257 mg DHA. This dose is lower compared to other RCTs that used supplements [41–43], but slightly higher than the daily recommendation of 250 mg/d EPA and DHA advised by EFSA [9]. However, the relatively low dietary compliance in the fish group means that these participants were exposed to a lower dose, which is probably why we observed a greater mean increase of DHA and the omega-3 index in the supplement group than in the fish group. It is possible that the dose of n-3 LCPUFAs used in the present trial was too low and the duration too short for the intervention to result in brain modifications measurable with a cognitive test. However, a RCT in healthy boys found that supplementing with both 400 mg/d DHA (which is comparable to the dose used in our study) and 1200 mg/d DHA for only eight weeks increased the amount of DHA in RBC, and that this correlated with prefrontal cortex activation as measured with fMRI [44]. The low proportion of participants found to be iron deficient may explain why we did not see any association between iron and performance in the d2 test of attention.

### Strengths and limitations

Strengths of this trial include the use of RBC fatty acids as biomarker, since this has shown to be a valid and objective indicator of fatty acid intake the prior weeks, and it is not altered in the fed state [45, 46]. Furthermore, the use of LC-MS/MS method for determination of s-25(OH)D and ICP-MS for determination of UIC is a strength because these are considered methods of high trueness and precision [47, 48]. The fact that the whole meal was homogenized and analyzed for its nutrients content after cooking gives a more accurate assessment of actual nutrient intakes by the participants compared to analyses of the plain or raw filet. In addition, the close follow-up of the participants throughout the dietary intervention provided us with useful data on dietary compliance. An important limitation of this trial was the low study dietary compliance particularly observed in the fish group. One of the main reasons for this is perhaps that we had to serve the meals cold due to practical reasons. Thus, future studies should emphasize that meals have high quality and tastiness in order to achieve acceptable compliance. Another limitation is the ceiling effect in the reading and writing test that left us with only one test on cognitive performance. A test-battery measuring other cognitive functions than just attention could have potentially revealed associations that were undetected in this trial. Furthermore, the EPA and DHA content was not equal between the fish and supplement group, although that was the aim. Paradoxically, the fish meals also had a slightly higher total content of n-6 PUFAs compared to meat, which was mainly due to a high content of LA in the farmed salmon. It could be argued that a 12 weeks duration was not sufficient, since RBC n-3 fatty acids do not plateau until around 6 months [49]. However, it has been noticed in supplementation studies that the greatest increase is achieved within the first 4–8 weeks [49, 50]. Still, it is questionable whether the duration was sufficient to achieve a clinically meaningful change in the brain that could be fully translated into performance in a cognitive test.

## Conclusions

In conclusion, the intake of n-3 supplements and fatty fish meals increased RBC levels of DHA and the omega-3 index more than meat meals, but n-3 supplements also increased more in these parameters than the fish meals, possibly due to differences in dietary compliance. None of the nutritional biomarkers were found to be associated with performance in the d2 test of attention. Baseline measurements showed deficient levels of s-25(OH)D and UIC in addition to suboptimal levels of EPA + DHA in RBC (based on adult cut-offs) in a considerable number of participants. The longer-term implications for the suboptimal nutritional status found in these adolescents is unknown, however, they give cause for concern and should be given increased attention in future studies.

### Abbreviations

25(OH)D: Serum 25-hydroxyvitamin D; AA: Arachidonic acid; CP: Concentration performance; DHA: Docosahexaenoic acid; DPA: Docosapentaenoic acid; E total: Total errors; E1: Errors of omission; E2: Errors of commission; EPA: Eicosapentaenoic acid; FFQ: Food frequency questionnaire; FINS: Fish intervention studies; LA: Linoleic acid; LCPUFA: Long-chain polyunsaturated fatty acids; n-3: Omega-3; RBC: Red blood cells; RCT: Randomized controlled trial; s-Ferritin: Serum ferritin; TN: Processing speed; TN-E: Total performance; UIC: Urinary iodine concentration

### Acknowledgements

We thank the participants and their parents for their participation in the trial. We are also grateful for the support and assistance from fieldworkers, teachers and principals of the schools. A special thanks to Runa Borgund Barnung, Nina Wollertsen, Annie Fürstenberg and Elisabeth Rasmussen Ødegård for technical contribution during data collection.

### Funding

This trial was financially supported by The Norwegian Seafood Research Fund (FHF) (grant number: 900842) after consideration by the Research Council of Norway (grant number 222648). This study is a part of the FINS project supported by FHF. Marine Harvest A/S (MH) and Pelagia A/S supported FINS with fish used in the diets. FHF, MH and Pelagia A/S had no role in the design of the study, in the collection, analyses, or interpretation of data, in the manuscript writing, or in the decision to publish the results.

### Authors' contributions

IEG, ØL, LF, LD, KMS, MWM, MK, KH, SS and JØ designed the research; LD, KH and SS conducted the research; VB, JØ and KH performed the statistical analyses; KH wrote the paper; all authors read and critically revised the manuscript and approved the final manuscript, and had primary responsibility for final content.

### Competing interests

The authors declare that they have no competing interests.

### Author details

[1]Institute of Marine Research (IMR), P.O. Box 1870 Nordnes, 5817 Bergen, Norway. [2]Department of Clinical Medicine, Faculty of Medicine and Dentistry, University of Bergen, P.O. Box 7800, 5020 Bergen, Norway. [3]Regional Centre for Child and Youth Mental Health, Uni Research Health, P.O. Box 7810, 5020 Bergen, Norway. [4]Present Address: Uni Research Health, P.O. Box 7810, 5020 Bergen, Norway. [5]Present Address: Directorate of Fisheries, P.O. Box 185 Sentrum, 5804 Bergen, Norway. [6]Department of Health Promotion and Development, University of Bergen, P.O. Box 7807, N-5020 Bergen, Norway.

### References

1. EFSA: Scientific Opinion on health benefits of seafood (fish and shellfish) consumption in relation to health risks associated with exposure to methylmercury. 2014. [https://www.efsa.europa.eu/en/efsajournal/pub/3761]. Accessed 24 Jan 2018.
2. Dahl L, Bjorkkjaer T, Graff IE, Malde MK, Klementsen B. Fish-more than just omega 3. Tidsskr Nor Laegeforen. 2006;126:309–11.
3. Moreno LA, Gottrand F, Huybrechts I, Ruiz JR, González-Gross M, DeHenauw S. Nutrition and lifestyle in european adolescents: the HELENA (healthy lifestyle in Europe by nutrition in adolescence) study. Adv Nutr. 2014;5:615S–23S.
4. González-Gross M, Valtueña J, Breidenassel C, Moreno LA, Ferrari M, Kersting M, De Henauw S, Gottrand F, Azzini E, Widhalm K, et al. Vitamin D status among adolescents in Europe: the healthy lifestyle in Europe by nutrition in adolescence study. Br J Nutr. 2012;107:755–64.

5. Braegger C, Campoy C, Colomb V, Decsi T, Domellof M, Fewtrell M, Hojsak I, Mihatsch W, Molgaard C, Shamir R, et al. Vitamin D in the healthy European paediatric population. J Pediatr Gastroenterol Nutr. 2013;56:692–701.
6. Harris WS, Von Schacky C. The Omega-3 index: a new risk factor for death from coronary heart disease? Prev Med. 2004;39:212–20.
7. Harris WS. The omega-3 index as a risk factor for coronary heart disease. Am J Clin Nutr. 2008;87:1997S–2002S.
8. O'Sullivan TA, Ambrosini GL, Mori TA, Beilin LJ, Oddy WH. Omega-3 index correlates with healthier food consumption in adolescents and with reduced cardiovascular disease risk factors in adolescent boys. Lipids. 2011;46:59–67.
9. EFSA: Scientific Opinion on Dietary Reference Values for fats, including saturated fatty acids, polyunsaturated fatty acids, monounsaturated fatty acids, trans fatty acids, and cholesterol. 2010. [https://www.efsa.europa.eu/en/efsajournal/pub/1461]. Accessed 11 Apr 2017.
10. Hansen LB, Myhre JB, Johansen AMW, Paulsen MM, Andersen LF: UNGKOST 3 Landsomfattende kostholdsundersøkelse blant elever i 4. -og 8. klasse i Norge, 2015 [UNGKOST 3 Nationwide dietary survey among pupils in 4th -and 8th grade in Norway, 2015]. 2016. [https://www.fhi.no/globalassets/dokumenterfiler/rapporter/ungkost-rapport-24.06.16.pdf]. Accessed 16 Dec 2016.
11. Casey B, Jones RM, Hare TA. The adolescent brain. Ann N Y Acad Sci. 2008;1124:111–26.
12. Isaacs E, Oates J. Nutrition and cognition: assessing cognitive abilities in children and young people. Eur J Nutr. 2008;47:4–24.
13. JI K, Winkvist A, Åberg MA, Åberg N, Sundberg R, Torén K, Brisman J. Fish consumption and school grades in Swedish adolescents: a study of the large general population. Acta Paediatr. 2010;99:72–7.
14. Åberg MA, Åberg N, Brisman J, Sundberg R, Winkvist A, Torén K. Fish intake of Swedish male adolescents is a predictor of cognitive performance. Acta Paediatr. 2009;98:555–60.
15. de Groot RHM, Ouwehand C, Jolles J. Eating the right amount of fish: inverted U-shape association between fish consumption and cognitive performance and academic achievement in Dutch adolescents. Prostaglandins Leukot Essent Fatty Acids. 2012;86:113–7.
16. Handeland K, Oyen J, Skotheim S, Graff IE, Baste V, Kjellevold M, Froyland L, Lie O, Dahl L, Stormark KM. Fatty fish intake and attention performance in 14-15 year old adolescents: FINS-TEENS - a randomized controlled trial. Nutr J. 2017;16:64.
17. Skotheim S, Dahl L, Handeland K, Frøyland L, Lie Ø, Øyen J, Kjellevold M, Stormark KM, Graff IE. Design of the FINS-TEENS study: a randomized controlled trial assessing the impact of fatty fish on cognitive performance in adolescents. Scand J Public Health. 2017;45:621–9.
18. Norges forskningsråd [Norwegian Research Council]: Hva spiser elevene på skolen? [What do students eat at school?]. 2011. [http://arrangor.forskningsdagene.no/binfil/download.php?tid=884034]. Accessed 23 Mar 2017.
19. Markhus MW, Graff IE, Dahl L, Seldal CF, Skotheim S, Braarud HC, Stormark KM, Malde MK. Establishment of a seafood index to assess the seafood consumption in pregnant women. Food Nutr Res. 2013;57
20. Dahl L, Maeland CA, Bjorkkjaer T. A short food frequency questionnaire to assess intake of seafood and n-3 supplements: validation with biomarkers. Nutr J. 2011;10:127.
21. Handeland K, Kjellevold M, Wik Markhus M, Eide Graff I, Frøyland L, Lie Ø, Skotheim S, Stormark KM, Dahl L, Øyen J. A diet score assessing Norwegian Adolescents' adherence to dietary recommendations-development and test-retest reproducibility of the score. Nutrients. 2016;8
22. Kissmeyer A-M, Sonne K, Binderup E. Determination of the vitamin D analog EB 1089 (seocalcitol) in human and pig serum using liquid chromatography–tandem mass spectrometry. J Chromatogr B Biomed Sci Appl. 2000;740:117–28.
23. Dahl L, Meltzer HM, Opsahl JA, Julshamn K. Iodine intake and status in two groups of Norwegians. Food Nutr Res. 2003;47
24. Brickenkamp R, Zillmer E. d2 test of attention manual. Göttingen: Hogrefe & Huber Publishers; 2003.
25. Skotheim S, Handeland K, Kjellevold M, Oyen J, Froyland L, Lie O, Eide Graff I, Baste V, Stormark KM, Dahl L. The effect of school meals with fatty fish on adolescents' self-reported symptoms for mental health: FINS-TEENS - a randomized controlled intervention trial. Food Nutr Res. 2017;61:1383818.
26. Bates ME, Lemay EP. The d2 test of attention: construct validity and extensions in scoring techniques. J Inter Neuropsych Soc. 2004;10:392–400.
27. Baron RM, Kenny DA. The moderator-mediator distinction in social psychological research: conceptual, strategic, and statistical considerations. J Pers Soc Psychol. 1986;51:1173–82.
28. WHO: Urinary iodine concentrations for determining iodine status deficiency in populations. 2013. [http://apps.who.int/iris/bitstream/10665/85972/1/WHO_NMH_NHD_EPG_13.1_eng.pdf]. Accessed 14 Mar 2017.
29. WHO: Serum ferritin concentrations for the assessment of iron status and iron deficiency in populations. 2011. [http://www.who.int/vmnis/indicators/serum_ferritin.pdf]. Accessed 31 Mar 2017.
30. Stonehouse W, Pauga MR, Kruger R, Thomson CD, Wong M, Kruger MC. Consumption of salmon v. Salmon oil capsules: effects on n −3 PUFA and selenium status. Br J Nutr. 2011;106:1231–9.
31. Christensen MH, Lien EA, Hustad S, Almas B. Seasonal and age-related differences in serum 25-hydroxyvitamin D, 1,25-dihydroxyvitamin D and parathyroid hormone in patients from western Norway. Scand J Clin Lab Invest. 2010;70:281–6.
32. Lehmann U, Gjessing HR, Hirche F, Mueller-Belecke A, Gudbrandsen OA, Ueland PM, Mellgren G, Lauritzen L, Lindqvist H, Hansen AL, et al. Efficacy of fish intake on vitamin D status: a meta-analysis of randomized controlled trials. Am J Clin Nutr. 2015;102:837.
33. Gunnarsdottir I, Gunnarsdottir BE, Steingrimsdottir L, Maage A, Johannesson AJ, Thorsdottir I. Iodine status of adolescent girls in a population changing from high to lower fish consumption. Eur J Clin Nutr. 2010;64:958–64.
34. NIFES: Seafood data. [https://sjomatdata.nifes.no/#search/]. Accessed 29 June 2017.
35. Sørensen LB, Damsgaard CT, Dalskov SM, Petersen RA, Egelund N, Dyssegaard CB, Stark KD, Andersen R, Tetens I, Astrup A. Diet-induced changes in iron and n-3 fatty acid status and associations with cognitive performance in 8–11-year-old Danish children: secondary analyses of the optimal well-being, development and health for Danish children through a healthy new Nordic diet school meal study. Br J Nutr. 2015;114:1623–37.
36. van der Wurff IS, von Schacky C, Berge K, Zeegers MP, Kirschner PA, de Groot RH. Association between blood Omega-3 index and cognition in typically developing Dutch adolescents. Nutrients. 2016;8. https://doi.org/10.3390/nu8010013
37. Cohen JFW, Gorski MT, Gruber SA, Kurdziel LBF, Rimm EB. The effect of healthy dietary consumption on executive cognitive functioning in children and adolescents: a systematic review. Br J Nutr. 2016;116:989–1000.
38. Haapala EA, Eloranta AM, Venäläinen T, Schwab U, Lindi V, Lakka TA. Associations of diet quality with cognition in children–the physical activity and nutrition in children study. Br J Nutr. 2015;114:1080–7.
39. Khan NA, Raine LB, Drollette ES, Scudder MR, Kramer AF, Hillman CH. Dietary fiber is positively associated with cognitive control among prepubertal children. J Nutr. 2015;145:143–9.
40. Nyaradi A, Foster JK, Hickling S, Li J, Ambrosini GL, Jacques A, Oddy WH. Prospective associations between dietary patterns and cognitive performance during adolescence. J Child Psychol Psychiatry. 2014;55:1017–24.
41. Kirby A, Woodward A, Jackson S, Wang Y, Crawford MA. A double-blind, placebo-controlled study investigating the effects of omega-3 supplementation in children aged 8-10 years from a mainstream school population. Res Dev Disabil. 2010;31:718–30.
42. Stonehouse W, Conlon CA, Podd J, Hill SR, Minihane AM, Haskell C, Kennedy D. DHA supplementation improved both memory and reaction time in healthy young adults: a randomized controlled trial. Am J Clin Nutr. 2013;97:1134–43.
43. Kennedy DO, Jackson PA, Elliott JM, Scholey AB, Robertson BC, Greer J, Tiplady B, Buchanan T, Haskell CF. Cognitive and mood effects of 8 weeks' supplementation with 400 mg or 1000 mg of the omega-3 essential fatty acid docosahexaenoic acid (DHA) in healthy children aged 10-12 years. Nutr Neurosci. 2009;12:48–56.
44. McNamara RK, Able J, Jandacek R, Rider T, Tso P, Eliassen JC, Alfieri D, Weber W, Jarvis K, DelBello MP. Docosahexaenoic acid supplementation increases prefrontal cortex activation during sustained attention in healthy boys: a placebo-controlled, dose-ranging, functional magnetic resonance imaging study. Am J Clin Nutr. 2010;91:1060–7.
45. Harris WS, Thomas RM. Biological variability of blood omega-3 biomarkers. Clin Biochem. 2010;43:338–40.
46. Harris WS, Varvel SA, Pottala JV, Warnick GR, McConnell JP. Comparative effects of an acute dose of fish oil on omega-3 fatty acid levels in red blood cells versus plasma: implications for clinical utility. J Clin Lipidol. 2013;7:433–40.
47. Stepman HCM, Vanderroost A, Van Uytfanghe K, Thienpont LM. Candidate reference measurement procedures for serum 25-Hydroxyvitamin D3 and 25-Hydroxyvitamin D2 by using isotope-dilution liquid chromatography–tandem mass spectrometry. Clin Chem. 2011;57:441–8.

48. Julshamn K, Dahl L, Eckhoff K. Determination of iodine in seafood by inductively coupled plasma/mass spectrometry. J AOAC Int. 2001;84: 1976–83.
49. Katan MB, Deslypere JP, van Birgelen AP, Penders M, Zegwaard M. Kinetics of the incorporation of dietary fatty acids into serum cholesteryl esters, erythrocyte membranes, and adipose tissue: an 18-month controlled study. J Lipid Res. 1997;38:2012–22.
50. Cao J, Schwichtenberg KA, Hanson NQ, Tsai MY. Incorporation and clearance of omega-3 fatty acids in erythrocyte membranes and plasma phospholipids.(Lipis, Lipoproteins and Cardiovascular Risk Factors). Clin Chem. 2006;52:2265.

3

# Energy, nutrient and food content of snacks in French adults

Wendy Si Hassen[1*], Katia Castetbon[2], Christine Tichit[3], Sandrine Péneau[1], Anouar Nechba[1], Pauline Ducrot[1], Aurélie Lampuré[1], France Bellisle[1], Serge Hercberg[1,4] and Caroline Méjean[1,5]

**Abstract**

**Background:** Snacking raises concern since it may lead to an additional energy intake and poor nutrient quality. A snacking occasion can be defined as any eating occasion apart from main meals, regardless of the amount or type of foods consumed. We described the frequency of snacking occasions according to daily timing in French adults, and compared them between each other, and with the main meals, in terms of energy intake, energy and nutrient density, and food content.

**Methods:** This cross-sectional analysis included 104,265 adults from the NutriNet-Santé cohort. Food intake was estimated using 24-h records of weekdays. For each eating occasion, nutrient density and energy content and density were computed.

**Results:** After weighting, 47.6% of our sample were men and mean age was 45.6 (15.3). Overall, 68% of participants ate at least one snack during the reported record, mainly in the morning or afternoon. Overall snack had a lower nutrient density [22.8 (SD = 278.3)] than main meals [25.8 (36.9) to 30.0 (30.4)]; but higher energy density [222.2 (163.3) kcal/100 g] than meals [133.9 (57.3) to 175.9 (99.6) kcal/100 g]. Morning snack was the snacking occasion with the lowest energy density [211 kcal/100 g], the lowest energy intake [104.1 kcal] and the highest nutrient density [60.1]. Afternoon and evening snacks had the highest energy loads [192.4 kcal and 207.6 kcal], but low nutrient scores [16 and 13, respectively]. The main food groups contributing to energy intake from snacks were fatty-sweet and sugary foods, fruit, hot beverages, and bread.

**Conclusions:** Our findings highlight the frequency of snacking and the varying nutritional quality of snacks over the day. The morning snack was shown to be healthier than afternoon and evening snacks.

**Trial registration:** This study was conducted according to guidelines laid down in the Declaration of Helsinki, and all procedures were approved by the Institutional Review Board of the French Institute for Health and Medical Research (IRB Inserm No. 0000388FWA00005831) and the French Data Protection Authority (Commission Nationale Informatique et Libertés No. 908450 and No. 909216). Electronic informed consent was obtained from all participants (Clinical Trial no. NCT03335644).

**Keywords:** Snack, Meal, Eating patterns, Eating occasions, Nutritional content

* Correspondence: w.sihassen@eren.smbh.univ-paris13.fr
[1]Université Paris 13, Sorbonne Paris Cité, Centre de Recherche en Epidémiologie et Statistique, Equipe de Recherche en Epidémiologie Nutritionnelle, Inserm (U1153), Inra (U1125), Cnam, 74 rue Marcel Cachin, F-93017 Bobigny, France
Full list of author information is available at the end of the article

## Background

Snacking behavior, defined as any eating occasion apart from main meals, regardless of the amount or type of food consumed [1], is a common practice in Western countries [2–6]. Although the pattern of eating three main meals, characterized by structure and conviviality, continues to prevail in France [7–10], previous studies had shown that snacking is frequent among French adults and children [5, 11]. The effects of snacking and eating frequency on dietary quality, nutrient intake and health are ambiguous [1, 12]. In some studies, snacking or eating frequency were associated with better dietary quality and higher intake of vitamins, potassium or magnesium, but also carbohydrates [13–17]; others found inconsistent associations with intake of protein and fat [13, 16]. One Finnish study showed that when daily energy intake came mainly from snacking, daily dietary intake had lower nutrient quality, associated with higher intake of fructose and lower intake of micronutrients such as potassium and vitamin C [18]. Most studies have focused on the nutrient content of snacking. Previous works reported that the main foods consumed during snacking varied, i.e. desserts, sweet and fat products, juice and fruits, sweetened beverages, salty snacks, coffee, milk, nuts, etc. [3, 19, 20]. However, little is known about the contribution of foods to snacking in terms of energy and dietary quality [21, 22]. In a study conducted in the United States among working adults in 2010–2013 [21], energy intake from snacks came mainly from desserts and sweets, chips, crackers and fruits, while the major contributors to energy intake in Finnish adults in 2002 were sweet bakery goods, bread and milk products [18]. Such differences highlight the importance of social and cultural contexts in snacking practices. Differences in nutritional content may also vary according to the daily timing of snacking in the two countries. However, up until now, no study has explored together the nutrient content, energy density and food group intake associated with snacking according to time of day.

Snacking may represent a large percentage of the daily energy intake and may contribute to a positive energy balance [2, 19, 23] that could consequently lead to weight gain [24, 25]. The contribution of snacking to energy and food intake thus needs to be further elucidated. Our objectives were to describe the frequency of snacking occasions according to daily timing in French adults, and to compare them between each other, and with the main meals, in terms of energy intake, energy and nutrient density, and food content.

## Methods

### Sample and study design

Subjects were participants in the NutriNet-Santé study, a large web-based prospective observational cohort launched in France in May 2009. The study was implemented in the French general population targeting internet-using volunteers aged ≥18 years. The design, methods and rationale have been described previously [26]. Briefly, participants were included in the cohort once they had completed a baseline set of questionnaires assessing dietary intake, physical activity, socioeconomic and health status. As part of their follow-up, the participants completed the same set of questionnaires every year. This study was conducted according to guidelines laid down in the Declaration of Helsinki, and all procedures were approved by the Institutional Review Board of the French Institute for Health and Medical Research (IRB Inserm No. 0000388FWA00005831) and the French Data Protection Authority (Commission Nationale Informatique et Libertés No. 908450 and No. 909216). Electronic informed consent was obtained from all participants.

This cross-sectional study focused on 104,265 participants included in the NutriNet-Santé cohort study between May 2009 and January 2015, living in the French metropolitan area, who had completed at least two 24-h dietary records at baseline and with no missing data for the weighting procedure.

Socioeconomic (education, occupation, household income) and demographic (age, area of residence, marital status and presence of children in the household) data were collected at baseline using a web-based self-completed questionnaire, using categories consistent with the French National Institute of Statistics definitions and demographic variables [27–29]. The highest attained diploma defined the educational level [27]. The reported monthly household income was then divided by the number of household units (HU) [30].

### Assessment of dietary behaviors

At baseline, participants were invited to fill in 3 non-consecutive web-based 24-h dietary records, randomly assigned over a 2-week period (2 weekdays and 1 weekend day) [26, 31, 32]. The dietary record was completed via a validated interactive interface and designed for self-administration on the Internet [33]. The web-based dietary assessment method relies on an event-based approach, recording all foods and beverages (type and quantity) consumed at all eating occasions. On the web-based interface, only 4 initial categories of eating occasions are suggested and named as follows: breakfast, lunch, dinner, and "other eating occasion". Participants were also asked to indicate time of each eating occasion. The participants estimated portion sizes for each reported food and beverage according to standard measurements (e.g., home containers, grams indicated on the package) or using validated photographs [34]. Values for energy, macronutrients and micronutrients were estimated using published nutrient databases and completed for recent market foods and recipes [35].

#### Definition of meals and eating occasions

We categorized the eating occasions according to their nutritional content and self-reported time. Our first step was to associate all eating occasions with time periods. After noticing that almost all self-reported main meals (breakfast, lunch, and dinner) were occurring during specific time slots, we chose to define the following time periods: early morning slot (2 AM to 5 AM), breakfast slot (5 AM to 10 AM), late morning slot (10 AM to 11 AM), midday or lunch slot (11 AM to 2 PM), afternoon slot (2 PM to 6 PM), dinner slot (6 PM to 10 PM) and late night slot (10 PM to 2 AM).

Then, we analyzed the content of the self-reported main meals (breakfast, lunch and dinner): reported main meals which contain only a beverage or seasoning or only contain one food item which quantity consumed was lower than 20 g for breakfast or 50 g for lunch or dinner, were recoded as "other eating occasion". When one or several other eating occasions and a main meal were reported in the same time slot, we compared the energy content of the other occasions to that of the main meal. The eating occasion with the highest energy value was considered as the main meal and the remaining ones were recoded as "other eating occasions".

Finally, 8 categories of eating occasions were used: 3 main meals (breakfast, lunch, dinner) and 5 snacks (morning, midday, afternoon, evening and night snacks). Morning snacks include all other eating occasions than main meals occurring during the breakfast and late morning time slots. Midday snacks include all other eating occasions than main meal occurring during the midday slot. Afternoon snacks include all other eating occasions than main meals occurring during the afternoon time slot. Evening snacks include all eating occasions other than main meals occurring during the dinner time slot. Night snacks include all eating occasions other than main meals occurring during the late night and early morning time slots.

Daily overall snacking was defined by the occurrence of at least one snacking occasion during the 24 h record. All snacking occasions occurring at different times during a 24 h record were then pooled to define the content and quality of overall daily snacking.

#### *Computation of nutritional indicators of eating occasions*

**Energy intake and energy density** The total energy intake of each eating occasion was calculated by summing the energy intake of all food items ingested on that occasion. Energy density was defined as the ratio of energy intake by the weight of the eating occasion*100 [36]. Low-calorie beverages (first decile of energy per 100 g) were excluded from computation.

**Nutrient density** To assess the nutrient density of eating occasions, the NRF9.3 index proposed by Fulgoni et al. [37] was used. The NRF9.3 is a score based on nine beneficial nutrients (protein, fibre, vitamins A, C and E) and minerals (magnesium, potassium, iron and calcium), and three nutrients that should be limited (saturated fat, added sugars and sodium). For each eating occasion, the total amount of each considered nutrient per 100 kcal was calculated using a published nutrient database [35] (without inclusion of dietary supplement intake); daily values defined by the Food and Drug Administration [38] were used to score each eating occasion using the NRF9.3 algorithm. A high positive score reflects dietary intake that provides large amounts of beneficial nutrients.

$$\text{Algorithm}: NRF9.3_{100\ \text{kcal}} = \sum\nolimits_{i=1-9}(\text{Nutrient}_i/\text{RDV}_i) * 100 - \sum\nolimits_{i=1-3}(\text{Nutrient}_i/\text{MDV}_i) * 100$$

RDV = recommended daily values; MDV : maximum daily values

#### Contribution of food groups to total energy intake

We also computed the contribution of the food groups to energy intake by summing up the energy intake of each food item. Contribution in percent of food groups to energy intake on an eating occasion was assessed by calculating the amount of energy from each food group and dividing by the total energy intake of the eating occasion.

#### Statistical analysis

Comparisons of demographic and socioeconomic characteristics between excluded and included participants were performed using chi-square or Fischer tests as appropriate. Data were weighted according to the French population socio-demographic distribution. Weighting was calculated separately for each sex using an iterative proportional fitting procedure and national census data on age, educational level, employment status, marital status, area of residence and presence of any children in the household [39]. Because of variable and unusual eating behaviors on the weekend, we focused our analysis on weekdays.

We used weighted percentages of individuals to describe occurrence of eating occasions and weighted means or medians for nutritional indicators to describe their nutritional quality.

Comparisons of energy intake, energy and nutrient densities between main meals, between snacks and between overall snack and main meals were performed using analysis of variance. Data pre-treatment and statistical analyses were performed using SAS (version 9.3; SAS Institute, Inc., Cary, NC, USA).

## Results

Among 144,746 individuals with available dietary data at baseline, we excluded individuals who were pregnant and those who did not provide at least two 24-h dietary records ($n$ = 19,987; 13.8%), underreporting subjects ($n$ = 15,785; 10.9%) and individuals with missing data for the weighting procedure ($n$ = 4709; 3.3%), leaving 104,265 individuals for analysis. Among 104,265 individuals, after weighting, 47.6% were men and 52.4% were women; 20.6% of participants were ≤30 years and 26.4% were > 60 years; 27.7% had a primary school education level, while 13.0% had a postgraduate level (Table 1). Proportions of young subjects (18–30 years), individuals with primary school level, manual workers, employees and never employed persons, those belonging to the lowest income class were higher in excluded participants than those included in the sample while proportions of older subjects, those with postgraduate education, managerial staff individuals, and those belonging to the highest income class were lower (date not shown).

### Snacking occasions of weekdays

On weekdays, around 28% of participants snacked in the morning, 8% at midday, 45% during the afternoon, 18% in the evening and 10% at night. The highest values for energy intake from snacks and the lowest scores for nutrient density were found for afternoon, evening and late-night snacks while the morning snack showed the lowest mean energy load, the lowest mean energy density and the highest nutrient density score (Table 2). Hot beverages contributed most to the energy load of the morning snack (33%), followed by fatty-sweet and sugary products (13.6% and 15%) and fruits (8%) (Table 3). Fatty-sweet products contributed most to the energy intake of afternoon snacks (33%), followed by fruits (16%), hot beverages (11.4%) and sweet foods (9%) (Table 3). The main contributors to the energy content of the evening snack were fatty-sweet products (26%), fruits (11%), alcoholic beverages (9%) and sweet foods (8%) (Table 3). The highest contribution of sweetened drinks to energy intake from beverages was observed in the afternoon snack (34%) and the highest contribution of alcoholic beverages to energy intake from beverages was observed for the evening snack (27%) (Table 4).

### Overall snack and main meals of weekdays

Overall, 68% of subjects snacked on at least one occasion while 86% of participants ate breakfast and around 96% ate lunch and 96% dinner during weekdays (Table 2).

Total energy intake from overall daily snacks (around 260 kcal) was lower than these from main meals (Table 2). Overall snack had a lower nutrient density score (22.8) than main meals (breakfast: 25.8 to lunch: 30.0); the mean energy density of overall daily snacks

**Table 1** Demographic and socioeconomic characteristics of the sample (weighted data) ($n$ = 104,265)

| | Weighted data (%) |
|---|---|
| Sex | |
| Men | 47.6 |
| Women | 52.4 |
| Age class | |
| 18–30 y | 20.6 |
| 31–45 y | 27.9 |
| 46–60 y | 25.1 |
| < 60 y | 26.4 |
| Educational level | |
| Primary | 27.7 |
| Secondary | 47.4 |
| Undergraduate | 11.9 |
| Postgraduate | 13.0 |
| Occupational categories [b] | |
| Never employed | 3.2 |
| Self-employed (craftsman, shopkeeper company manager, farmer) | 7.5 |
| Managerial staff | 19.6 |
| Employees | 32.4 |
| Manual workers | 15.2 |
| Intermediate professions | 22.1 |
| Household income per consumption unit | |
| Unwilling to declare | 11.8 |
| < 1200 euros | 24.0 |
| 1200–1800 euros | 292 |
| 1800–2700 euros | 20.2 |
| > 2700 euros | 14.8 |
| Living area | |
| Rural | 24.7 |
| 20,000 inhabitants. | 16.6 |
| 20,000–200,000 inhabitants. | 18.6 |
| > 200,000 inhabitants | 40.1 |
| Household composition | |
| Living alone | 16.2 |
| Living with other adult(s) but no child | 47.2 |
| Living with at least one child | 36.6 |

[a]Weighting accounted for socio-demographic characteristics compared with the national population census (age, occupational category, household including at least one child or not and living area)
[b]Unemployed and retired individuals were asked to indicate their last occupation status. In this particular case, the previous status was used to assess the occupation in the analyses

**Table 2** Nutritional characterization of meals and snacks of weekdays ($N = 104{,}265$)

| Eating occasion | Subjects reporting the eating occasion (%) | Mean energy (SD) kcal | Median NRF9.3 score (SD) | Mean energy density without low-calorie beverages[a] (kcal/100 g) (SD) |
|---|---|---|---|---|
| Meals | | | | |
| Breakfast | 86.0 | 414.0[b, d] (233.8) | 25.8[b, d] (36.9) | 175.9[b, d] (99.6) |
| Lunch | 95.6 | 734.6[b, d] (350.6) | 30.0[b, d] (30.4) | 137.9[b, d] (52.5) |
| Dinner | 96.3 | 734.0[b, d] (390.3) | 25.9[b, d] (29.4) | 133.9[b, d] (57.3) |
| Snacks | | | | |
| Overall | 68.0 | 260.8[d] (284.6) | 22.8 (278.3) [d] | 222.2 (163.3) [d] |
| Morning | 27.8 | 104.1[c] (155.0) | 60.1 [c] (385.1) | 211.3 [c] (170.2) |
| Midday | 8.3 | 117.9 [c] (173.1) | 53.1[c] (328.8) | 227.7 [c] (159.7) |
| Afternoon | 44.5 | 192.4 [c] (203.5) | 16.36[c] (269.3) | 223.9 [c] (156.3) |
| Evening | 17.8 | 207.6[c] (231.3) | 12.8[c] (595.2) | 220.1 [c] (164.0) |
| Night | 9.8 | 161.8[c] (226.3) | 11.1[c] (1218.5) | 223.9 [c] (179.1) |

[a]10% lowest caloric beverages
[b]$P$-value < 0.001 (comparisons between main meals using analysis of variance)
[c]$P$-value < 0.001 (comparisons between snacks using analysis of variance)
[d]$P$-value < 0.001 (comparisons between overall snack and main meals using analysis of variance)

(222.2 kcal/100 g) was higher than main meals (dinner: 133.9 (57.3) to breakfast: 175.9 (99.6) kcal/100 g).

Mean energy intake at breakfast was around 414 kcal, and 734 kcal for both lunch and dinner. Median nutrient density score was higher for lunch compared to breakfast and dinner, while energy density was higher for breakfast than for lunch and dinner (Table 2).

Overall, fatty-sweet products (30%), fruits (13.1%), hot beverages (11.3%), sweet foods (9%) and bread (6%) contributed most to the energy intake from daily weekday snacks (Table 3). Hot or sweetened beverages and milk were the main contributors to the total energy intake of beverages for overall snack (Table 4).

Regarding breakfast on weekdays, food groups that contributed most to energy intake were bread, fatty-sweet products, sweet foods, butter, milk and breakfast cereals (Additional file 1: Table S1). The major contributors to total energy intake from beverages were hot beverages, milk and juices (Additional file 2: Table S2). For lunch and dinner on weekdays, fish, meat, poultry and eggs contributed most to the energy intake of for these meals (24 and 18%) (Additional file 1: Table S1). The other main food groups were starches and bread, followed by vegetables, fruits, cheese, sauces, fats and fatty-sweet products (Additional file 1: Table S1). During lunch and dinner, hot beverages, sweetened and "diet" drinks and alcoholic beverages were the main sources of energy intake from beverages. (Additional file 2: Table S2).

## Discussion

Our study showed that almost all adults ate the traditional three main meals (breakfast, lunch and dinner) on weekdays, while more than two-thirds of them also snacked at least once during the day, especially in the afternoon and, to a lesser extent, in the morning. Overall

**Table 3** Contribution (%) of food groups to energy intake of weekday snacking occasions

| | Morning % (SD) | Midday % (SD) | Afternoon % (SD) | Evening % (SD) | Night time % (SD) | Overall % (SD) |
|---|---|---|---|---|---|---|
| Fruit | 8.5 (26.5) | 11.7 (27.7) | 15.9 (32.0) | 11.1 (26.9) | 11.0 (29.5) | 13.1 (28.0) |
| Bread | 4.7 (16.6) | 3.8 (14.1) | 5.6 (16.8) | 5.4 (16.0) | 2.9 (12.6) | 6.0 (16.4) |
| Milk and milk substitutes | 7.2 (22.0) | 2.1 (11.3) | 2.7 (12.2) | 2.1 (11.6) | 4.8 (19.2) | 3.9 (14.7) |
| Fatty-sweet products (pastry, cookies, chocolate, etc.) | 13.6 (31.8) | 15.2 (30.9) | 33.3 (41.1) | 25.9 (38.8) | 27.3 (41.9) | 29.6 (38.2) |
| Sweet foods (honey, candy, jam, etc.) | 15.0 (32.0) | 13.5 (29.1) | 8.9 (23.8) | 8.1 (23.7) | 12.6 (30.5) | 9.0 (22.5) |
| Hot beverages (coffee, tea, cappuccino, etc.) | 32.9 (44.7) | 24.7 (38.0) | 11.4 (29.3) | 5.9 (21.7) | 7.1 (24.3) | 11.3 (28.5) |
| Juices (fruit or vegetable) | 5.3 (19.9) | 4.3 (17.5) | 2.3 (12.4) | 3.1 (15.3) | 4.0 (18.8) | 3.5 (14.8) |
| Sweetened and light beverages (non- alcoholic) | 3.4 (16.7) | 5.1 (19.1) | 4.6 (18.0) | 5.0 (19.0) | 7.1 (24.6) | 4.4 (16.6) |
| Alcoholic beverages | 0.1 (2.8) | 2.6 (13.5) | 1.9 (12.1) | 9.2 (24.5) | 6.0 (22.3) | 3.2 (14.2) |
| Oleaginous seeds, appetizer | 0.9 (8.7) | 3.0 (13.9) | 1.8 (11.1) | 5.4 (18.4) | 1.8 (12.1) | 2.6 (12.6) |

**Table 4** Contribution of beverages to total energy intake of beverages (%) of weekday snacking occasions

| | Morning snack % (SD) | Midday snack % (SD) | Afternoon snack % (SD) | Evening snack % (SD) | Night time snack % (SD) | Overall snack % (SD) |
|---|---|---|---|---|---|---|
| Milk and milk substitutes | 22.9 (44.1) | 7.3 (24.2) | 13.3 (32.0) | 8.2 (26.8) | 18.8 (46.8) | 13.0 (31.1) |
| Sweetened and light beverages (non-alcoholic) | 6.0 (25.8) | 26.9 (41.7) | 34.2 (45.0) | 29.8 (45.0) | 26.4 (53.0) | 13.1 (31.7) |
| Hot beverages (coffee, tea, cappuccino, etc.) | 58.0 (52.9) | 53.6 (46.7) | 35.6 (45.4) | 27.3 (43.8) | 15.3 (41.2) | 55.3 (47.3) |
| Juice (fruit or vegetable) | 13.1 (35.5) | 11.5 (30.1) | 12.9 (31.6) | 8.0 (26.7) | 17.7 (44.7) | 9.8 (27.7) |
| Alcoholic beverages | 0.1 (3.3) | 0.7 (7.7) | 4.0 (18.8) | 26.7 (43.5) | 21.7 (50.3) | 8.8 (26.8) |

snack had lower nutrient density but higher energy density than main meals on weekdays. Energy density, nutrient density and food groups eaten strongly varied according to snack time. The morning snack represented the snacking occasion with the lowest energy density and the highest nutrient density, with high intake of hot beverages, fatty-sweet products and sugary foods while afternoon and evening snacks had the highest energy load, with high intake of fatty-sweet products and fruits. In addition, sweetened beverages strongly contributed to energy intake from beverages in afternoon and evening snacks. Alcoholic beverages were also an important contributor to energy intake from beverages in the evening snack.

Our findings confirm that snacking is a very frequent behavior among French adults during the week; indeed, 68% snacked at least once a day. This high percentage of individuals who snacked attained levels observed in previous work in the US [3]. Contrary to other countries, the French daily eating pattern is fairly synchronized [40], with three main meals per day [8], generally at set times and based on social eating habits [41]. Compared to a French representative survey, percentages of individuals eating a morning or an afternoon snack were higher in our study (28% and 45% vs. 10% and 35%) [42]. Such differences could be explained by important variations in data collection methods. The earlier study was based on a telephone interview and pre-defined questions. Moreover, some inherent biases in studies based on interviews, such as social desirability may be different in a web-based study. In particular, judgement bias due to higher perceived anonymity is probably lower in web-based studies and may encourage individuals to report more food items [33].

Contributions of fruits, sweetened beverages and fatty-sweet products to energy intake for overall snacking were higher in our study than in previous American and Finnish studies in adults, whereas the contribution of dairy products and bread was lower [18, 21]. In agreement with previous studies in adults in Finland and the United States [22, 43], our findings highlighted that energy intake and nutrient density are lower for most snacking occasions than for main meals, while energy density is higher. These results suggest that snacking is associated with less healthy choices. In addition, the fact that overall snack represented around 13% of total daily energy intake shows the importance of a better characterization of snacking occasions. The main food groups contributing to energy intake varied greatly between main meals and snacks. The major contribution of fatty-sweet products and sweet foods to the energy intake of snacking leads to intake of added sugars, lipids, saturated fatty acids and sodium, explaining the higher energy density and lower nutrient density of snacking compared to main meals. This important contribution of foods rich in nutrients that should be limited, along with high energy density during snacking, raise concern about the effect of snacking on weight and health status [44–48]. Mixed results, however, have been observed for associations between snacking and body mass index [12, 17, 19, 43, 49]. Further prospective analyses could help to define whether snacking involving high energy density is a risk factor of weight gain.

Snacking occasions had lower nutrient density (< 17) than main meals, except for morning and midday snacks. Evening and afternoon snacks only weakly contributed to the intake of recommended nutrients (fibre, vitamins, proteins and minerals), but provided nutrients the consumption of which should be limited based on dietary recommendations, such as saturated fatty acids, added sugars and sodium. This finding is related to the foods consumed on these eating occasions: fatty-sweet products, but also sweet foods and alcoholic beverages. Since percentages of individuals snacking in the evening and afternoon were relatively high in our sample, the associations between such behaviors and health events should be investigated to assess potential adverse effects. In contrast, fruits strongly contribute to the energy intake of snacks and may be beneficial [50]. Targeting both snacking and meal behaviors in public health messages is thus important.

The finding that most participants reported eating the main meals in a French population is concordant with previous studies conducted in French adults, which showed that the three-meal pattern continues to prevail among adults [9, 42, 51]. In our study, lunch was the main meal with the highest nutrient density. The higher contribution of cheese, alcoholic beverages and fast foods explains the lower nutrient density of dinner compared with lunch. As expected, food groups that contributed most to energy intake during lunch and dinner are animal foods (fish, meat, poultry and eggs) and cereals (starches and bread), followed by vegetables, fruits, cheese, sauces/added fats and fatty-sweet products. Our findings are concordant with previous studies regarding fish, meat and starches [5, 18], but differ in the contributions of fruits, vegetables and bread, which were higher in our population, while the contribution of milk was lower [18]. In France, main meals are generally structured into two or three courses, which could explain the wider variety of foods during a meal [42].

Since intakes of sugar-sweetened products, sugary drinks during snack eating occasions but also those of beneficial products such as fruits, appropriate actions are needed to promote consumption of healthy foods and limit other non-recommended items [1, 52]. Since snacking occasions are common, promoting intakes consumption of certain foods such as fruit when snacking, rather than banning snacks might be worth exploring. Since snacking could help to reduce hunger and improve satiety, favoring healthy snacks could potentially help to avoid overconsumption or to reduce energy intake during the subsequent meal, balancing daily intakes [12, 53–57]. In addition, a separate analysis showed that snacking behavior varies across demographic and socioeconomic subgroups. Although snacking was less prevalent in low socioeconomic categories and young adults, their snacks had higher energy content and were of poorer nutrient density. When focusing on public strategies regarding snacking behavior, policy makers should take into account these demographic and socio-economic disparities to implement specific actions – either through professional networks or education programs for instance.

### Strengths and limitations

A major strength of our study lies in its assessment of eating habits of French adults, taking into account both meals and snacks. Characterizing eating occasions on their daily timing allowed us to describe snacks more precisely. Further analyses are however needed to assess potential correlations between multiple snacking occasions within subjects that may have affected the variability of our results. The different parameters used to assess the nutritional content of such eating occasions (contribution of different food groups to snacking energy, nutrient and energy densities) constitute an original contribution; indeed, previous works had mainly focused on content of specific nutrients and energy. Since the $NRF9.3_{100kcal}$ has been validated and can be applied to individual food, meals, menus and even the daily diet, this nutrient index enabled us to assess the nutrient density of the different eating occasions [37, 58]. The strength of this score lies in the fact that it includes both positive and negative components. Since the NutriNet-Santé cohort includes volunteers, subjects had a healthier lifestyle and were probably more interested in nutrition than the general population. Thus, caution is needed when interpreting and generalizing results. Analyses, however, were weighted according to French population socio-demographic distribution, which allows bias to be limited. A web-based design may affect internal validity by inducing misreporting. However, studies investigating the validity of our web-based, self-reported dietary record tool against biomarkers showed that our tool performs well at estimating several nutrients and food intakes [31, 32]. Because of the lack of a consensual definition of snacking, our definition based on time of day, along with our analytical choices, is subject to caution. Because of variable and unusual eating behaviors on weekends, we chose to relate findings of weekdays only. Further analyses describing and comparing all eating occasions on weekends could usefully complement our current results. Contrary to previous work, the definition of snacking was not based on consumed food items or the participant's definition of snacking. In addition, the fact that the volunteers did not declare snacking occasions as such (but only eating occasions in general) may have reduced the desirability bias, since snacking is often viewed as unhealthy behavior.

## Conclusions

This study highlights the common practice of snacking among French adults, but indicates that most individuals still eats the three main meals. Snack content varies greatly according to timing. The morning snack appears to be heathier than afternoon and evening snacks. The high prevalence of energy-dense, low-nutrient snacks raises concern, as it may be a risk factor in weight gain [47]. Snacking was associated with intake of foods and nutrients whose consumption should be limited, but also foods recommended for a healthy diet, such as fruits. Better knowledge of the effect of snacking behavior on weight and health status is crucial for defining public action in promoting healthy eating habits.

#### Abbreviations

MDV: Maximum daily values; NRF9.3 $_{100kcal}$: Nutrient-rich food index 9.3 per 100 kcal; RDV: Recommended daily values

#### Acknowledgements

The authors thank the scientists, dietitians, technicians, and assistants who helped carry out the NutriNet-Santé Study. We especially thank Younes Esseddik, Thi Duong Van, Frédéric Coffinieres, Mac Rakotondrazafy, Régis Gatibelza, Paul Flanzy, Paul Flanzy, Mohand Ait Oufella, and Yasmina Chelghoum (computer scientists), Nathalie Arnault, Véronique Gourlet, Fabien

Szabo, Charlie Menard, Laurent Bourhis (data-manager/biostatisticians), and the dieteticians Cédric Agaesse and Claudia Chahine, for their technical contribution to the NutriNet-Santé study. We thank all the volunteers of the NutriNet-Santé cohort. We are grateful to Jerri Bram for English editing of the manuscript.

### Funding

Wendy Si Hassen was funded by a PhD grant from the Université Paris 13. The NutriNet-Santé study is supported by the following public institutions: Ministère de la Santé, Institut de Veille Sanitaire (InVS), Institut National de la Prévention et de l'Education pour la Santé (INPES), Fondation pour la Recherche Médicale (FRM), Institut National de la Santé et de la Recherche Médicale (INSERM), Institut National de la Recherche Agronomique (INRA), Conservatoire National des Arts et Métiers (CNAM) and Université Paris 13. This research benefits from the joint assistance of the French National Health Insurance Fund for Employees (CNAMTS), the French Directorate General of Health (DGS), the Arc Foundation for Cancer Research, the French National Cancer Institute (INCA), the French National Institute for Prevention and Education in Health (INPES), the French National Institute of Health and Medical Research (INSERM), the French Inter-Departmental Agency for the Fight against Drugs and Addictive Behaviors (Mildeca) and the French Social Security Scheme for Liberal Professionals (RSI) as part of the "Primary Prevention" call for proposals issued by IReSP and INCA in 2013. The funders had no role in study design, data collection and analysis, decision to publish or preparation of the manuscript.

### Authors' contributions

WSH designed the study, performed statistical analysis, interpreted data and wrote the manuscript. KC was involved in the design of the study, interpretation of data, and helped to draft the manuscript. AN was involved in the statistical analysis. CT, FB SP, PD and AL were involved in interpretation of data, and helped to draft the manuscript. SH designed and coordinated the cohort study and supervised the study. CM was involved in the conception and design of the study, supervision of statistical analysis and interpretation of data, and helped to draft the manuscript. All authors read and approved the final manuscript.

### Competing interests

The authors declare that they have no competing interests.

### Author details

[1]Université Paris 13, Sorbonne Paris Cité, Centre de Recherche en Epidémiologie et Statistique, Equipe de Recherche en Epidémiologie Nutritionnelle, Inserm (U1153), Inra (U1125), Cnam, 74 rue Marcel Cachin, F-93017 Bobigny, France. [2]Université Libre de Bruxelles, Ecole de Santé publique, Centre de Recherche en Epidémiologie, Biostatistique et Recherche Clinique, Route de Lennik 808 – CP 598, 1070 Brussels, Belgium. [3]Institut National de la Recherche Agronomique (INRA) – UR 1303 Alimentation et Sciences Sociales ALISS, 65 boulevard de Brandebourg, F-94025 Ivry sur Seine, France. [4]Département de santé publique, Hôpital Avicenne, 125 rue de Stalingrad, F-93000 Bobigny, France. [5]MOISA, Université de Montpellier, INRA, CIRAD, CIHEAM-IAMM, Montpellier SupAgro, Montpellier, France.

### References


1. Hess JM, Jonnalagadda SS, Slavin JL. What is a snack, why do we snack, and how can we choose better snacks? A review of the definitions of snacking, motivations to snack, contributions to dietary intake, and recommendations for improvement. Adv Nutr. 2016;7:466–75.
2. Bellisle F. Meals and snacking, diet quality and energy balance. Physiol Behav. 2014;134:38–43.
3. Piernas C, Popkin BM. Snacking Increased among U.S. adults between 1977 and 2006. J Nutr. 2010;140:325–32.
4. Poulain JP. The contemporary diet in France: "de-structuration" or from commensalism to "vagabond feeding". Appetite. 2002;39:43–55.
5. Bellisle F, Dalix AM, Mennen L, Galan P, Hercberg S, de Castro JM, Gausseres N. Contribution of snacks and meals in the diet of French adults: a diet-diary study. Physiol Behav. 2003;79:183–9.
6. Zizza C, Siega-Riz AM, Popkin BM. Significant increase in young adults' snacking between 1977-1978 and 1994-1996 represents a cause for concern! Prev Med. 2001;32:303–10.
7. Volatier J.L. Le repas traditionnel se porte encore bien. Crédoc Consommation et modes de vie. 1999.
8. Riou J, Lefevre T, Parizot I, Lhuissier A, Chauvin P. Is there still a French eating model? A taxonomy of eating behaviors in adults living in the Paris metropolitan area in 2010. PLoS One. 2015;10:e0119161.
9. Mathé T, Tavoularis G, Pilorin T. La gastronomie s'inscrit dans la continuité du modèle alimentaire français. Cahiers de recherche du Credoc. 2009;3. https://scholar.google.fr/scholar?hl=fr&as_sdt=0%2C5&q=Math%C3%A9+T.%3B+Tavoularis+G.%3B+Pilorin+T.+La+gastronomie+s%E2%80%99inscrit+dans+la+continuit%C3%A9+du+mod%C3%A8le+alimentaire+fran%C3%A7ais.+Cahiers+de+recherche+du+Credoc.+2009+3.&btnG=.
10. Holdsworth M. The French paradox: fact or fiction? - how important are differences in national eating. Dialog Cardivasc Med. 2008;13:200–8.
11. AFSSA - French Agency for Food, E.a.O.H.&.S. Étude Individuelle Nationale des Consommations Alimentaires 2 (INCA 2) 2006–2007. 2009.
12. Miller R, Benelam B, Stanner SA, Buttriss JL. Is snacking good or bad for health: an overview. Nutr Bull. 2013;38:302–22.
13. Kerver JM, Yang EJ, Obayashi S, Bianchi L, Song WO. Meal and snack patterns are associated with dietary intake of energy and nutrients in US adults. J Am Diet Assoc. 2006;106:46–53.
14. Murakami K.; Livingstone M.B. Associations between meal and snack frequency and diet quality in US adults: National Health and nutrition examination survey 2003–2012. J Acad Nutr Diet. 2016;267.
15. Zizza CA, Arsiwalla DD, Ellison KJ. Contribution of snacking to older adults' vitamin, carotenoid, and mineral intakes. J Am Diet Assoc. 2010;110:768–72.
16. Zizza CA, Tayie FA, Lino M. Benefits of snacking in older Americans. J Am Diet Assoc. 2007;107:800–6.
17. Drummond SE, Crombie NE, Cursiter MC, Kirk TR. Evidence that eating frequency is inversely related to body weight status in male, but not female, non-obese adults reporting valid dietary intakes. Int J Obes Relat Metab Disord. 1998;22:105–12.
18. Ovaskainen ML, Reinivuo H, Tapanainen H, Hannila ML, Korhonen T, Pakkala H. Snacks as an element of energy intake and food consumption. Eur J Clin Nutr. 2006;60:494–501.
19. Hampl JS, Heaton CL, Taylor CA. Snacking patterns influence energy and nutrient intakes but not body mass index. J Hum Nutr Diet. 2003; 16:3–11.
20. Duffey KJ, Pereira RA, Popkin BM. Prevalence and energy intake from snacking in Brazil: analysis of the first nationwide individual survey. Eur J Clin Nutr. 2013;67:868–74.
21. Barnes TL, French SA, Harnack LJ, Mitchell NR, Wolfson J. Snacking behaviors, diet quality, and body mass index in a community sample of working adults. J Acad Nutr Diet. 2015;115:1117–23.
22. Ovaskainen ML, Tapanainen H, Pakkala H. Changes in the contribution of snacks to the daily energy intake of Finnish adults. Appetite. 2010;54:623–6.
23. de GC. Effects of snacks on energy intake: an evolutionary perspective. Appetite. 2006;47:18–23.
24. Plachta-Danielzik S, Landsberg B, Bosy-Westphal A, Johannsen M, Lange D, Muller J. Energy gain and energy gap in normal-weight children: longitudinal data of the KOPS. Obesity (Silver Spring). 2008;16:777–83.
25. Prentice A, Jebb S. Energy intake/physical activity interactions in the homeostasis of body weight regulation. Nutr Rev. 2004;62:S98–104.
26. Hercberg S, Castetbon K, Czernichow S, Malon A, Mejean C, Kesse E, Touvier M, Galan P. The Nutrinet-Sante study: a web-based prospective study on the relationship between nutrition and health and determinants of dietary patterns and nutritional status. BMC Public Health. 2010;10:242.
27. INSEE (French National Institute of Statistics) definition of qualification level. Available online: https://www.insee.fr/fr/metadonnees/definition/c1785. Accessed 13 May 2016.
28. Vergnaud AC, Touvier M, Mejean C, Kesse-Guyot E, Pollet C, Malon A, Castetbon K, Hercberg S. Agreement between web-based and paper versions of a socio-demographic questionnaire in the NutriNet-Sante study. Int J Public Health. 2011;56:407–17.

29. INSEE (French National Institute of Statistics) Definition of occupational categories. Available online: https://www.insee.fr/fr/information/2406153. Accessed 28 May 2016.
30. INSEE (French National Institute of Statistics) Definition of consumption unit. Available online: http://www.insee.fr/en/methodes/default.asp?page=definitions/unite-consommation.htm. (Accessed on 12 Feb 2015).
31. Lassale C, Castetbon K, Laporte F, Camilleri GM, Deschamps V, Vernay M, Faure P, Hercberg S, Galan P, Kesse-Guyot E. Validation of a web-based, self-administered, non-consecutive-day dietary record tool against urinary biomarkers. Br J Nutr. 2015;113:953–62.
32. Lassale C.; Castetbon K.; Laporte F.; Deschamps V.; Vernay M.; Camilleri G.M.; Faure P.; Hercberg S.; Galan P.; Kesse-Guyot E. Correlations between fruit, vegetables, fish, vitamins, and fatty acids estimated by web-based nonconsecutive dietary records and respective biomarkers of nutritional status. J Acad Nutr Diet. 2016.
33. Touvier M, Kesse-Guyot E, Mejean C, Pollet C, Malon A, Castetbon K, Hercberg S. Comparison between an interactive web-based self-administered 24 h dietary record and an interview by a dietitian for large-scale epidemiological studies. Br J Nutr. 2011;105:1055–64.
34. Le Moullec N, Deheeger M, Preziosi P, Montero P, Valeix P, Rolland-Cachera MF, Potier de Courcy G, Christides JP, Galan P, Hercberg S. Validation du manuel photos utilisé pour l'enquête alimentaire de l'étude SU.VI.MAX. Cah Nutr Diet. 1996;31:158–64.
35. Arnault N, Caillot L, Castetbon K, Coronel S, Deschamps V, Fezeu L, Figuette M, Galan P, Guénard-Charpentier F, Hercberg S, Houet D, Julia C, Kesse-Guyot E, Lanotte M, Lisi A, Lucas F, Méjean C, Mohtadji A, Péneau S, Poulhès L, Salanave B, Tisseron E, Touvier M, Vernay M, Voegtlin C. Table de composition des aliments NutriNet-santé. Paris: Editions Économica; 2013.
36. Ello-Martin JA, Ledikwe JH, Rolls BJ. The influence of food portion size and energy density on energy intake: implications for weight management. Am J Clin Nutr. 2005;82:236S–41S.
37. Fulgoni VL III, Keast DR, Drewnowski A. Development and validation of the nutrient-rich foods index: a tool to measure nutritional quality of foods. J Nutr. 2009;139:1549–54.
38. U.S.Food & Drug Administration Guidance for Industry: A Food Labeling Guide Available online: https://www.fda.gov/downloads/Food/GuidanceRegulation/GuidanceDocumentsRegulatoryInformation/UCM265446.pdf. Accessed 2 Dec 2016.
39. INSEE La MACRO SAS CALMAR. Available online: https://www.insee.fr/fr/information/2021902. (Accessed on 1 Oct 2016).
40. Eurostat. How Europeans spend their time-everyday life of women and men-data 1998–2002. Luxembourg: Office for Official Publications of the European Communities; 2004.
41. Rozin P. The meaning of food in our lives: a cross-cultural perspective on eating and well-being. J Nutr Educ Behav. 2005;37(Suppl 2):S107–12.
42. Escalon H., Bossard C., Beck F., and dir. Baromètre santé nutrition. Baromètre santé. 2009 : 424 p. 2009. Saint-Denis, coll.
43. Murakami K, Livingstone MB. Energy density of meals and snacks in the British diet in relation to overall diet quality, BMI and waist circumference: findings from the National Diet and Nutrition Survey. Br J Nutr. 2016;116:1479–89.
44. Hammad S, Pu S, Jones PJ. Current evidence supporting the link between dietary fatty acids and cardiovascular disease. Lipids. 2016;51:507–17.
45. Mozaffarian D, Appel LJ, Van HL. Components of a cardioprotective diet: new insights. Circulation. 2011;123:2870–91.
46. Kant AK, Graubard BI. Energy density of diets reported by American adults: association with food group intake, nutrient intake, and body weight. Int J Obes. 2005;29:950–6.
47. Bes-Rastrollo M, van Dam RM, Martinez-Gonzalez MA, Li TY, Sampson LL, Hu FB. Prospective study of dietary energy density and weight gain in women. Am J Clin Nutr. 2008;88:769–77.
48. Mendoza JA, Drewnowski A, Christakis DA. Dietary energy density is associated with obesity and the metabolic syndrome in U.S. adults. Diabetes Care. 2007;30:974–9.
49. Hartmann C, Siegrist M, van der Horst K. Snack frequency: associations with healthy and unhealthy food choices. Public Health Nutr. 2013;16:1487–96.
50. Hung HC, Joshipura KJ, Jiang R, Hu FB, Hunter D, Smith-Warner SA, Colditz GA, Rosner B, Spiegelman D, Willett WC. Fruit and vegetable intake and risk of major chronic disease. J Natl Cancer Inst. 2004;96:1577–84.
51. Lhuissier A, Tichit C, Caillavet F, Cardon P, Masullo A, Martin-Fernandez J, Parizot I, Chauvin P. Who still eats three meals a day? Findings from a quantitative survey in the Paris area. Appetite. 2013;63:59–69.
52. Zizza CA. Healthy snacking recommendations: one size does not fit all. Physiol Behav. 2014;134:32–7.
53. Speechly DP, Buffenstein R. Greater appetite control associated with an increased frequency of eating in lean males. Appetite. 1999;33:285–97.
54. de GC, Hulshof T. Effects of weight and energy content of preloads on subsequent appetite and food intake. Appetite. 1996;26:139–51.
55. Njike VY, Smith TM, Shuval O, Shuval K, Edshteyn I, Kalantari V, Yaroch AL. Snack food, satiety, and weight. Adv Nutr. 2016;7:866–78.
56. Rolls BJ, Kim S, McNelis AL, Fischman MW, Foltin RW, Moran TH. Time course of effects of preloads high in fat or carbohydrate on food intake and hunger ratings in humans. Am J Phys. 1991;260:R756–63.
57. Allirot X, Saulais L, Seyssel K, Graeppi-Dulac J, Roth H, Charrie A, Drai J, Goudable J, Blond E, Disse E, Laville M. An isocaloric increase of eating episodes in the morning contributes to decrease energy intake at lunch in lean men. Physiol Behav. 2013;110-111:169–78.
58. Drewnowski A. Defining nutrient density: development and validation of the nutrient rich foods index. J Am Coll Nutr. 2009;28:421S–6S.

# 4

# Randomised controlled trial to test the effectiveness of a locally-produced ready-to-use supplementary food (RUSF) in preventing growth faltering and improving micronutrient status for children under two years in Cambodia

Bindi Borg[1,7*], Seema Mihrshahi[1], Mark Griffin[2], Daream Sok[3,4], Chamnan Chhoun[4], Arnaud Laillou[5], Jacques Berger[6] and Frank T. Wieringa[6]

**Abstract**

**Background:** Existing ready-to-use supplementary and therapeutic foods (RUSFs and RUTFs) have had limited acceptance and effectiveness in Cambodia. This has hampered the treatment and prevention of child malnutrition. An innovative, locally produced, multiple micronutrient fortified lipid-based nutrient supplement (LNS) has been developed for use as an RUSF. Unlike most RUSFs, which contain milk, this product contains fish as the animal protein. Few RUSFs have been formulated using non-milk animal-source foods and they have not been widely tested. An acceptability trial that was conducted on this novel RUSF in June 2015 demonstrated that children will eat the RUSF and that caregivers will feed it to their children. The current trial aims to evaluate the effectiveness of the RUSF in preventing growth faltering and improving micronutrient status in Cambodian children.

**Methods and analysis:** This trial is a six-month, prospective, cluster randomised, non-blinded controlled trial among infants in peri-urban Phnom Penh. The trial aims to establish the superiority of the novel RUSF, compared to three alternatives (Corn-Soy Blend Plus Plus (CSB++) and Sprinkles micronutrient powders as active comparators, and the unimproved diet as a control). The allocation ratio is 1:1. Healthy children (N = 540) aged six to eleven months will be recruited. Data will be collected at baseline, and monthly thereafter for a period of six months. Participants will be provided with a monthly supply of the food to which their village has been allocated.

(Continued on next page)

* Correspondence: bindi_borg@yahoo.com.au
[1]School of Public Health, Faculty of Medicine, University of Sydney, Sydney, Australia
[7]c/o Pascal Marino, European Union Delegation in Cameroon, BP 847 Yaoundé, Cameroon
Full list of author information is available at the end of the article

(Continued from previous page)

**Discussion:** There is an urgent need to develop locally produced and culturally acceptable RUSFs, and to compare these with existing options in terms of their potential for preventing malnutrition, in Cambodia and elsewhere. This trial will contribute much-needed data on the effectiveness of supplementary foods with an animal-source food other than milk, by comparing a novel RUSF based on fish to one that uses milk (CSB++). Moreover, it will deepen the understanding of the impact of multiple micronutrients provided with or without macronutrients, by comparing the novel RUSF and CSB++, which combine macronutrients with multiple micronutrients, to Sprinkles, which contains no macronutrients. In addition, it will augment the body of evidence.from Asia.

**Keywords:** Ready-to-use supplementary food (RUSF), Lipid-based nutrient supplement (LNS), Childhood malnutrition, Growth faltering, Corn-Soy Blend Plus Plus (CSB++), Supercereal Plus, Sprinkles micronutrient powders, Cambodia

## Background and rationale

Undernutrition is an underlying cause in almost half of all deaths in children under five years [1]. In Cambodia, rates of malnutrition remain stubbornly high [2] with 32% of all children under five years (and 40% of three to four year-olds) stunted, 10% wasted, and 24% underweight [2]. Suboptimal infant feeding practices, in particular, poor complementary feeding, result in inadequate energy and nutrient intakes to achieve optimal growth and micronutrient status, and consequently, childhood malnutrition.

Adequate complementary feeding can prevent malnutrition [3]. In Cambodia, the traditional weaning food is a white rice porridge called *borbor*, which has very low nutrient density. Special supplementary foods, containing a source of protein and lipids such as powered milk, soy or peanuts, and multiple micronutrients, can be used to improve complementary feeding. Supplementary foods can be either foods requiring preparation e.g. fortified blended products, such as Corn-Soy Blend++ (CSB++, now called Supercereal Plus), that is mixed with water to make a porridge; or ready-to-use e.g. biscuits, such as BP5. Until fairly recently, prevention of malnutrition relied on fortified blended products. However, increasingly, ready-to-use foods are lipid-based nutrient supplements (LNSs) which are often pastes, such as the peanut-based Plumpy'Doz™. These energy-dense ready-to-use supplementary foods (RUSFs) contain both macro and micronutrients [4, 5]. These new RUSFs are proving effective, as they have a higher energy content, and have a longer shelf life, and, since they require no preparation, are more convenient [5, 6]. Another common nutrition intervention is multiple micronutrient supplements such as Sprinkles, used solely to combat micronutrient deficiencies. These are individually-packed powders that can be added to food. Micronutrients are more likely to achieve growth outcomes when they are combined with energy, for example, in lipid-based nutrient supplements; there is no evidence that micronutrient powders alone contribute to sustained improvements in linear growth [7–12].

In Cambodia, various supplements and supplementary or therapeutic foods, including micronutrient powders, CSB++, BP100, and Plumpy'Nut™ have been used or trialled. The United Nations World Food Program (WFP) in Cambodia distributed CSB++ to children under two years to prevent malnutrition. Micronutrient powders (Sprinkles) have also been distributed through the public health system, though coverage is limited. These products are relatively expensive to procure and ship to Cambodia and in the case of Sprinkles, are not as effective as foods that contain macronutrients [9, 10]. Plumpy'Nut™, which is produced in France by Nutriset, was trialled in Cambodia in 2009 and was not well accepted [13]. Nor was CSB++ very well accepted in practice [14]. Due to lack of acceptability, and also due to budget constraints, WFP phased out distribution of CSB++ in Cambodia in June 2014. In addition, BP100, which is currently used in Cambodia to treat severe acute malnutrition, has not been well accepted [15].

For these reasons, the Cambodian Ministry of Health sought a ready-to-use food (in both therapeutic and supplementary versions) containing macro and micronutrients that was locally-produced and therefore more likely to be acceptable and cheaper than imported products.

In 2009 in Vietnam, UNICEF, IRD (Institute of Research for Development) and the National Institute of Nutrition developed a supplementary food from mainly local ingredients including rice, soy, mung beans, sugar, milk powder, oil and multiple micronutrients (called HEBI). This product proved more acceptable and as effective as Plumpy'-Nut™ and is now widely used in Vietnam [16]. In mid-2013, IRD, partnering with UNICEF and the Cambodian Department of Fisheries Post-harvest Technologies and Quality (DFPTQ), began developing a novel RUSF based on the same concept as the Vietnamese product.

WHO recommends daily consumption of animal-source foods for their high protein, energy, and micronutrient availability, which plant-based complementary food alone cannot provide [17]. Animal-source foods have been associated with greater micronutrient status, linear growth and non-fat mass gain compared to non-animal-source food [18, 19]. Usually, milk or whey powder is the animal-source food most commonly used in supplementary foods including CSB++ and various RUSFs [20, 21]. However, milk powder is an expensive (and often imported) ingredient. Therefore, it could perhaps be replaced with a cheaper, local source of animal protein that is widely accepted by the target population. There are precedents for replacing milk in supplementary foods for cost effectiveness [22], but until now, only a handful of supplementary foods have used meat, fish or eggs and they have generally not been tested for effectiveness on a wide scale [23–27]. The only known effectiveness study involving a supplementary food with fish compared a peanut and soy-based fortified spread to a corn porridge fortified with fish powder with six to eighteen month old children, and found that children consuming the porridge with fish powder gained less weight from six to eleven months, but otherwise the two supplementary foods performed similarly in terms of weight gain from twelve to eighteen months and linear growth [28]. In a number of studies, supplementing with meat or milk (as opposed to a supplementary food product containing no meat or milk), the nutritional improvement was less than expected, and sometimes was only the slowing of growth faltering [29, 30]. A study in Kenya is the only one to have compared milk and meat, and found meat had a greater impact, perhaps because milk inhibited iron and zinc uptake [29]. In all of these studies, the limited impact of meat or milk may have been because the additional food did not contain a sufficient range or quantity of micronutrients to overcome deficiencies.

In Cambodia, fish is inexpensive, readily available and highly acceptable to local tastes, and could therefore replace milk in a supplementary food. Combined with rice, soy, mung beans, oil and sugar, the resulting product should be less expensive and more acceptable to Cambodians. IRD developed the first version of this product in paste form in early 2014. It was compared to BP100, and found to be equally acceptable in younger children, although older children preferred BP100's milky taste to the fishy flavour of the RUSF.

The product was revised to reduce the fish smell and make it into a snack. It was then tested for acceptability in comparison to CSB++ and Sprinkles with *borbor* in June 2015. That trial demonstrated that children will eat the RUSF and that caregivers will feed it to their children. The next step is to assess the effectiveness of the food in preventing malnutrition, and promoting optimal growth and development. Therefore, a six-month effectiveness trial will be conducted. The impact of the product on children aged six to seventeen months will be compared to the impact of CSB++, Sprinkles, and to a control group consuming an unsupplemented diet, typically *borbor* at an early age (e.g. six to nine months) and thereafter, family foods.

## RUSF formulation

The RUSF has been formulated and produced locally, using local inputs. Small freshwater fish were cleaned, dried, roasted and ground. Soy and mung beans were roasted and ground, then mixed with the fish and coconut. This mix was extruded, then combined with multiple micronutrient premix (DMS), icing sugar, maltodextrin and canola oil to create the RUSF paste. Wafers were hand-made from rice flour, eggs, water, sugar, salt and coconut with small amounts of vanilla or sesame seeds for added flavour. The wafer is a hollow cylinder between 8.5-9 cm long with an internal diameter of 0.4–0.5 cm. Such wafers, unfilled, are a popular Cambodian snack. The ingredients of the RUSF are detailed in Table 1.

Although there are no definitive guidelines for supplementary foods, the RUSF was developed with the recommended guidelines for the nutritional composition of RUTFs in mind [31]. RUTFs should provide 520-550 kcal/100 g with 10–12% and 45–60% of the total energy coming from proteins and lipids respectively. Our RUSF contains 484 kcal/100 g, with 11% and 45% of the total energy coming from proteins and lipids respectively. The energy content of the paste is 499 kcal/100 g. The wafer, filled with the RUSF paste, yields a final snack weighing approximately 10-11 g, including 7 g of paste and 3-4 g of wafer, with an energy content of approximately 48 kcal/piece.

**Table 1** Ingredients of RUSF snack (paste and wafer)

| Ingredients | g/100 g |
|---|---|
| Small indigenous fish | 5.9 |
| Mung beans | 9.6 |
| Rice | 4.2 |
| Soy beans | 12.2 |
| Icing sugar | 10.3 |
| Maltrodextrin | 9.3 |
| Canola oil (g) | 3.7 |
| Palm vegetable shortening | 14.0 |
| Desiccated coconut | 1.5 |
| Rice bran | 2.2 |
| Vitamin and mineral mix | 0.9 |
| Rice flour | 9.0 |
| Duck eggs | 2.5 |
| Refined sugar | 7.2 |
| Coconut | 7.2 |
| Salt | 0.0 |
| Flavour (vanilla or sesame seeds | 0.1 |
| Oil for cooking | 0.4 |

All processing has been conducted in quality-certified facilities. The novel RUSF will be tested for microbiological safety (first five batches and every fifth batch thereafter) at the Pasteur Institute in Phnom Penh.

## Design and methods

### Objective and Hypothesis

This trial aims to evaluate the effectiveness of the locally produced RUSF on children aged six to seventeen months in preventing growth faltering and improving micronutrient status. The impact of the product will be compared to CSB++, Sprinkles, and to a control group consuming an unsupplemented diet.

Based on trials with other RUSFs, and the Cambodian experience with CSB++ [14], it is expected that this novel RUSF will be as effective as CSB++, and more effective than Sprinkles or the standard diet in promoting growth and preventing stunting [32, 33].

### Trial Design

The trial is a prospective, cluster randomised, non-blinded controlled trial among infants six to seventeen months of age. The trial aims to establish the superiority of the novel RUSF, using CSB++, and Sprinkles as active comparators and the unimproved diet as a control. The allocation ratio is 1:1. The study will take place over six months.

### Comparators

The RUSF will be compared with:

1. CSB++: CSB++ has been chosen as a comparator because it is currently the standard supplementary food. WFP usually provides CSB++ for children aged six months to two years to prevent malnutrition.
2. Sprinkles: Sprinkles micronutrient powders have been chosen since they are a commonly provided supplement in developing countries, such as Cambodia, with low dietary diversity, and complementary foods with low nutrient density [34].
3. Control: An unsupplemented diet, typically *borbor* and family foods, has been chosen as a control because this is the standard diet in Cambodia. *Borbor* is the traditional food for weanlings (children transitioning from exclusively milk diets to diets that include complementary foods) and is often the only food given until about nine months.

The active comparators comply with WFP and UNICEF standards for supplementary foods, and have been used and tested in Cambodia and elsewhere [18, 33, 35]. They have been found to be safe and to have no unintended side-effects. The table below contrasts the characteristics of the RUSF and comparators (Table 2).

The potential comparators that will not be used are BP100 (because it is designed to treat severe acute malnutrition) and peanut-based RUSFs. The latter will not be included because they are thought to be less acceptable, and are too expensive from current producers. Moreover, including peanuts in a locally produced Cambodian RUSF is not advisable as local production standards may not be adequate to safeguard against aflatoxin contamination, given that the rate of aflatoxin contamination of peanuts in South-East Asia is probably quite high [36–38].

### Outcomes and their measurement

The main outcome of interest is anthropometric status, i.e. length/height-for-age (L/HAZ), weight-for-height (WHZ) and weight-for-age (WAZ), calculated through monthly weight and height measurements. A HAZ $< -2$ indicates stunting, a WAZ $< -2$ indicates underweight, and a WHZ $< -2$ indicates wasting. A secondary outcome is children's body composition. Body composition, like linear growth, gives an indication of the quality of nutritional recovery, inasmuch as non-fat or lean tissue growth requires balanced nutrition while fat gain requires only calories [39]. Body composition will be calculated using triceps and subscapular skinfolds [40, 41]. Another secondary outcome is biochemical status, including iron status and anaemia, infection measured by C-reactive protein (CRP) and alpha-2 acid glycoprotein (AGP), and parasite infestation. An additional outcome is cognitive development and achievement of developmental milestones.

### Blinding

This will be an open trial with no blinding, since the three foods will be visibly different to data collectors, caregivers and children. The principal investigator (who will do supervision in the field) and the staff administering the intervention will know which food has been allocated to a given village.

### Study setting

The study will be conducted in northern peri-urban Phnom Penh (Khan Russey Keo, Mekong Health District). This area has a large population of urban poor whose children experience higher than average rates of underweight and stunting [42, 43].

### Allocation sequence generation and concealment

Randomisation of the interventions will occur at site level. Using UNICEF data on health centre coverage, potential villages and their populations (including the expected population of children aged 6–11 months) will be listed. Villages receiving Sprinkles or CSB++ will be excluded based on information provided by UNICEF, WFP and the

**Table 2** Characteristics of the RUSF and comparators

| CHARACTERISTIC | RUSF | CSB++ | Sprinkles |
|---|---|---|---|
| Daily serving size | 40-110g* | 100 g dry CSB++ | 1 sachet (1 g) |
| Animal-source food | Fish | Milk | – |
| Energy (kcal/100 g) | 484 | 410 | – |
| Protein (g/100 g) | 13 | 16 | – |
| Carbohydrates (g/100 g) | 52 | 67 | – |
| Lipids (g/100 g) | 24 | 9 | – |
| Fibre (g/100 g) | 1.6 | 3 | – |
| Vitamin A | 1080 µg | 540 µg | 400 µg |
| Vitamin D | 60 µg | 4.6 µg | 5 µg |
| Vitamin B1 (thiamine) | 0.59 mg | 0.47 mg | 0.5 mg |
| Vitamin B2 (riboflavin) | 0.89 mg | 0.84 mg | 0.5 mg |
| Vitamin B6 | 0.84 mg | 2.1 mg | 0.5 mg |
| Phosphorus | 474 mg | 530 mg | – |
| Calcium | 366 mg | 260 mg | – |
| Pantothenic acid | 1.75 mg | 7.3 mg | – |
| Copper | 1.6 mg | – | 0.56 mg |
| Vitamin E | 10.9 mg | 9.8 mg | 5 mg |
| Folic acid | 230 µg | 115 µg | 150 µg |
| Iron | 8 mg | 8.9 mg | 10 mg |
| Magnesium | 137 mg | | – |
| Vitamin B3 (niacin) | 9.63 mg | 7.2 mg | 6 mg |
| Vitamin C | 53.4 mg | 100 mg | 30 mg |
| Zinc | 8.4 mg | 7.5 mg | 4.1 mg |
| Potassium | 806 mg | 990 mg | – |
| Vitamin B12 | 10 µg | 2.3 µg | 0.9 µg |
| Biotin | 0.37 mg | – | – |
| Selenium | 90 µg | – | 17 µg |
| Iodine | – | 60 mg | 90 µg |
| Vitamin K | 3 µg | 115 µg | – |
| Taste | Fishy | Creamy, sweet, smooth [52] | Should not have a taste [53] |
| Preparation | No | 10 mins cooking | No |
| Acceptability in Cambodia | Yes | Acceptable in trial [52], but not in practice [14] | Yes [35] |
| Effectiveness in reducing malnutrition | To be tested | Not inferior to peanut-based RUSFs, which are the most effective in promoting linear growth and weight gain [18, 33] | Improves micronutrient status but not linear growth or weight gain [5, 12, 35] |
| Intra-household sharing | To be tested | Yes [33] | None noted [35] |
| Packaging | To be determined | Packaging may encourage sharing [5, 39] | Looks like "medicine" thus may discourage sharing [5, 39] |
| Local production capacity | Unknown | None [5] | None |
| Cost | To be determined. Goal is <US$0.10/day | Less expensive than peanut-based RUSFs if produced locally [18], but also have to consider logistics, time to treat, relapse [39] | Very cheap to produce at US$0.025/daily dose [11], but also have to consider logistics |

*RUSF daily serving size depends on the child's age, i.e. 6-8 m – 4 pieces, 40 g; 9-11 m – 6 pieces, 60 g; 12-17 m – 11 pieces, 110 g

Ministry of Health. Small villages that are close to each other may merged into one site, or large villages split into multiple sites, in order to create sites of similar sizes. Sites will then be randomised to one of the arms.

Thus, participants will not be individually randomised. All subjects in a given site will be in the same intervention group to avoid potentially confounding social interaction, such as inter-household sharing of different foods, and to ensure better compliance [44]. Sites will be randomly allocated to one of the foods, using an Excel random number table and a randomised incomplete block design. The principal researcher will generate the allocation sequence. At least three sites will be allocated to each food.

### Sample size

The main outcome of interest is anthropometric status (WHZ, WAZ and L/HAZ), calculated through changes in weight and length/height for the novel RUSF in comparison to the CSB++, Sprinkles, and the control after six months of the interventions. An overall required sample size of 424 subjects, or 106 subjects per group, was calculated, based on the assumptions of a difference in mean z-scores of 0.1 between the groups (95%CI), an SD = 0.8, and an assumption that subjects provide five measurements (out of a possible total of seven), with a precision of 0.05, power of 0.8. This is in keeping with similar effectiveness studies which have aimed to detect a difference in mean z-scores of 0.16 between groups, assuming SD = 0.8 [45], or a difference in mean z-scores of 0.1 and SD = 0.8 [20]. Therefore, detection of difference in mean z-scores of 0.1 between groups is reasonable.

In similar studies, retention has been high at [22, 28, 35]. Therefore, we can assume a maximum attrition of 25% with confidence. The total number of subjects enrolled will therefore be 530, or approximately 133 children in each group. This will be rounded up to 135 children/group for a total of 540 subjects, which should be adequate. See Fig. 1 for the planned site selection, recruitment and enrolment of children.

### Eligibility criteria

Children must be between six to eleven months of age at enrolment. It is expected that there will be approximately equal numbers of female and male children. Subjects must be normally nourished or only moderately malnourished (mid-upper arm circumference, MUAC> 115 mm, WHZ score > − 3), and healthy. Their iron status should be normal or only moderately anaemic; children with severe anaemia (haemoglobin, Hb < 70 g/l) will be referred for treatment. Any children who have been using Sprinkles or CSB++, are regularly consuming or receiving other food or micronutrient supplementation, are enrolled in any other research or supplementary feeding program, or have received therapy for acute malnutrition within one month prior to recruitment, will be excluded. Children with

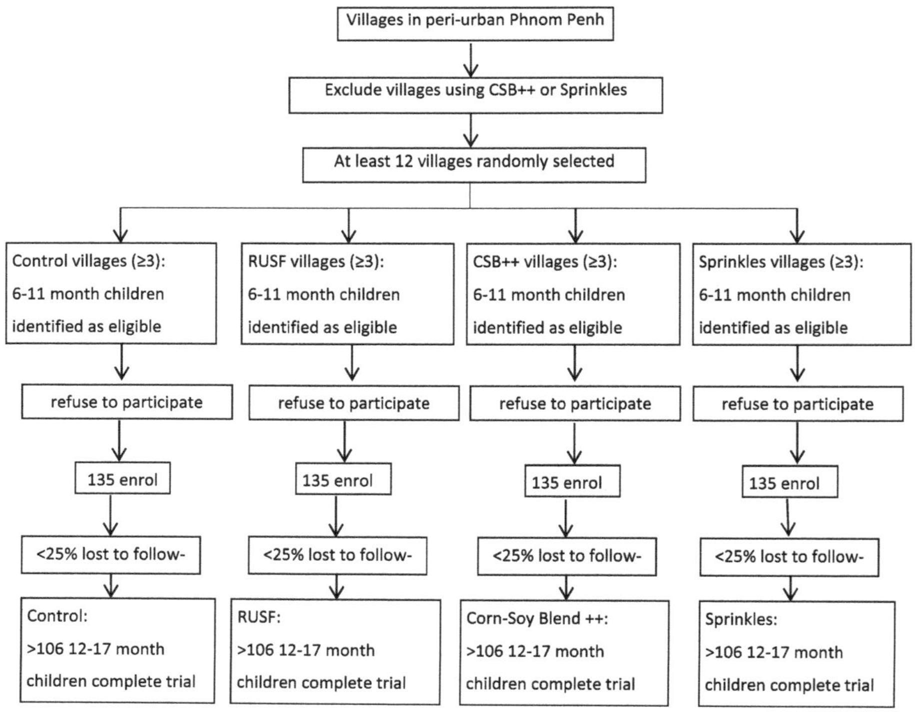


**Fig. 1** Site selection, recruitment and enrolment of children

known food intolerances will also be excluded. Caregivers must be healthy, and must give informed signed consent for their children to be included.

**Recruitment, Enrolment and Consent**

Village Health Support Group members (local health volunteers) will assist with recruitment, initially by inviting potential caregivers and children to participate in the trial. The data collection team will use a screening form to assess initial eligibility of participants. Some participants may be excluded at this point (e.g. on the basis of age or unwillingness to participate). Those who are excluded for severe acute malnutrition, anaemia or illness will be referred for treatment.

Those who are eligible will be provided with written and verbal information about the trial in Khmer language. If the participant is willing to continue, they will be asked to provide their verbal and signed (or fingerprinted) consent for them and their children to participate. It will be made clear that potential participants have the option of not joining the study. If they consent to participate, it will be made clear that they can ask questions, make complaints, or withdraw at any time.

**Data collection**

After informed consent and enrolment, baseline data will be collected. This will include demographics, morbidity, anthropometry (weight, height, MUAC, skinfolds), biochemical samples (blood, stool), dietary data (breastfeeding, food frequency and dietary diversity), and developmental milestone achievement. Participants may still be excluded if they are malnourished (MUAC< 115 mm, WHZ score < – 3) or severely anaemic.

Participants in the intervention groups will then be provided with a one-month supply of the food to which their site has been allocated. Thereafter, participants will be provided with food on a monthly basis, and they will continue to consume the food over a six-month period. Data will be collected monthly (anthropometry, morbidity, developmental milestones), and/or at endline (biochemical).

Staff will inform the Village Health Support Group members in advance of monthly data collection sessions, and the latter will arrange for participants to be present. If caregivers are not present, they will be followed up by mobile phone and/or by the Village Health Support Group members and home visits will be conducted.

***Anthropometric data***

Anthropometric measurements will include weight to the nearest 0.1 kg, recumbent length to the nearest 0.1 cm, skinfolds to the nearest 1 mm, and MUAC to the nearest 1 mm. Weight will be measured with a SECA scale, length will be measured on wooden UNICEF height boards, MUAC will be measured with a flexible UNICEF insertion tape and skinfolds will be measured with a standard caliper (Holtain, United Kingdom). Anthropometry will be measured monthly. Children with MUAC < 115 mm and WHZ < – 3 at enrolment or at any time during the study will be excluded from the study and referred to the health centre for treatment.

***Morbidity data***

Data on diarrhoea and respiratory infections will be collected at the beginning of the study and monthly thereafter. Children with serious illnesses or severe malnutrition will be excluded from the study and referred to the health clinic for treatment.

***Biochemical samples***

Blood samples (4mls) will be drawn at baseline and endline by trained nurses who are skilled and experienced in taking paediatric blood samples. One to two drops will be used immediately to measure haemoglobin (using a HemoCue HB301 photometer). Of the remaining blood, 2mls will be placed in a trace element sodium heparin vacuette for further micronutrient analysis. The remaining blood will be placed in Ethylenediamine tetraacetic acid (EDTA) tubes for fatty acid analysis, then 40 μl will be pipetted onto pre-treated chromatography paper to be analysed as a dried blood spot. Blood samples will be stored, transported and analysed appropriately to avoid contamination and deterioration. Analysis will be conducted for micronutrient status including haemoglobin (g/l), ferritin (μg/l), transferrin receptor (mg/l), retinol-binding protein (vitamin A status) (μmol/l), zinc (μmol/l), C reactive protein (mg/l), using internationally accepted indicators [46].

Stool samples will be taken and tested for parasites. Stool containers will be distributed to caregivers and collected the following day. Analysis will be conducted using FLOTAX method.

***Cognitive data and developmental milestones***

The mental and motor development and behaviour of the participants will be tested monthly using the Bayley Scales of Infant Development (BSID), an internationally recognised standard of determining children's developmental progress. In addition, a more detailed assessment will be conducted at endline.

***Compliance data***

Data on consumption, sharing, and adherence will be gathered monthly. Subjects will be provided with a month's supply of food at this time.

***Dietary data***

Dietary data including breastfeeding status, food frequency and dietary diversity for caregivers and children will be collected monthly, using the Cambodian Demographic and Health Survey (CDHS) questionnaires as a model.

***Endline data***

Endline data will be collected on infants aged twelve to seventeen months at the end of the study.

### Timeline

The study will take place in 2016–2017 (see Table 3).

### Statistical analysis

All data will be double-entered in Excel. Data will be analysed in the statistical software required by the PhD candidates' respective universities. Thus, anthropometric data will be analysed by one PhD candidate in the statistical software STATA version 13.1, and biochemical and cognitive/developmental data will be analysed by another PhD candidate in SPSS and R.

Since most of the measures being taken are repeated on a monthly basis, the assumption of independence is not satisfied. Therefore, a mixed effect model, which is appropriate for repeated measurements, will be used. Predictor variables will be checked for normality and linearity, and manipulated and recoded as necessary. Outcome variables will be manipulated and recoded if necessary to deal with non-normality and/or for easier interpretation. Initial univariate screening will be conducted at $p \leq 0.2$ level using simple logistic regression to screen for variables that could have an effect, and collinearity assumptions will be checked, in order to determine which covariates to include in the model. A complete mixed effects logistic regression will then be fit to the data. Significance levels will be considered $p < 0.05$. Any missing data will be treated as "missing at random" and accounted with the mixed effect model.

***Anthropometric status***

The main outcome of interest is change in anthropometric status. The independent variables are the food, sex and age, and the dependent variables are the mean weight-for-height (WHZ), height/length-for-age (H/LAZ) and weight-for-age (WAZ). Anthropometric indices for children will be calculated using World Health Organisation (WHO) 2006 standards (ANTHRO version 3.2.2 January 2011) and expressed as z-scores for weight-for-height (WHZ), height/length-for-age (H/LAZ) and weight-for-age (WAZ). Thus, multiple means will be compared, and changes will be analysed using a mixed effects model to determine whether there are statistically significant changes in WHZ, H/LAZ and WAZ of participants consuming the different foods.

***Body composition***

A second outcome is body composition measured by skinfold thickness. The independent variable is the food and the dependent variable will be the mean of skinfold thickness. The data will be analysed using a mixed effects model to determine whether there is a statistically significant difference in the body composition of participants eating the different foods.

***Enrolment data***

Enrolment data describing the characteristics of the recruited participants (e.g. sex, age, anthropometric and biochemical status, morbidity, breastfeeding status) will be reported as means ± SD for continuous measures.

## Ethics and consent

Ethics approval was received from the University of Queensland Medical Research Ethics Committee and the National Ethics Committee for Health Research (NECHR)

**Table 3** Schedule of enrolment, interventions and assessments

| | STUDY PERIOD | | | | | |
|---|---|---|---|---|---|---|
| | Enrolment | Allocation | Post-allocation | | | Close-out |
| TIMEPOINT | *Feb 2016* | *Feb 2016* | *Feb 2016* | *Mar-Sept 2016* | *Oct 2016* | *Early 2017* |
| ENROLMENT: | X | | | | | |
| Eligibility screen | X | | | | | |
| Informed consent | X | | | | | |
| Allocation | | X | | | | |
| INTERVENTIONS: | | | | | | |
| *Baseline* | | | X | | | |
| *Monthly data collection* | | | | X | | |
| *Endline* | | | | | X | |
| DOCUMENTATION: | | | | | | |
| *Anthropometry* | | | | | | X |
| *Micronutrients* | | | | | | X |

in Cambodia. Written informed consent will be obtained from all the caregivers or parents of the participating children before recruitment into the study. Based on the experience of similar trials [20, 22, 28, 45], and given the inclusion and exclusion criteria, no harm is expected from trial participation. However, morbidity data will be collected every month, and this will record any harm (nausea, etc.) that could come from participation in the trial.

## Discussion

The development and comparison of new supplementary foods with current fortified blends and existing RUSFs in terms of their potential for preventing growth faltering and malnutrition responds to a need noted by various researchers [5, 22, 47–49] as well as to a programmatic need. Such products need to be affordable, effective, and acceptable in terms of preparation as well as taste [23]. The novel RUSF has proved acceptable and this trial will test its effectiveness, in terms of the main outcomes, namely, anthropometric measures, body composition and biochemical status.

Six months is sufficient time to see changes in the main outcome, that is, in anthropometric measures. Similar effectiveness studies (considering weight and length outcomes) have ranged from as little as four weeks [20], with many studies taking twelve weeks to compare three to eight food supplementation regimes [18, 22, 29, 32, 33, 50], and others taking six months [39]. The INCAP study in Guatemala provided supplementary food to children for up to seven years, but nevertheless noted a detectable difference after three and six months of supplementation [10]. With respect to linear growth, healthy infants grow approximately 1.25 cm each month from six to eleven months [51]. Golden notes that although the maximum rate of height gain is as yet unknown, catch-up growth can easily be three times the rate of normal growth. Thus, a malnourished child less than one year of age can gain one z-score in two to four weeks if receiving adequate nutrition [4]. The mean HAZ-score for a Cambodian child of six months is − 0.5, for twelve to seventeen month-olds is − 1.3 and for eighteen to twenty-three month-olds is − 1.8 [2]. Therefore, s/he loses around 0.8 z-score in six to eleven months, or approximately 0.07 z-score per month. In our trial, if the intervention stops or slows growth faltering, we could see a difference in HAZ-scores of up to 0.42 over six months between intervention and control groups.

Since it is not uncommon nowadays to find stunted but overweight individuals [4], a recent Cochrane review recommended that future research report results on body composition [49]. Among stunted, non-wasted children, prevention is preferable to treatment [5]. In either treatment or prevention of malnutrition, the aim is to increase non-fat mass (bones, muscles) in preference to fat mass, and one should therefore see linear growth as well as increased weight, since linear growth is a better indicator of nutritional recovery than weight gain [4]. Therefore, body composition will also be an important outcome of our trial.

The effectiveness trial of our novel RUSF will determine how a ready-to-use, fish-based, supplementary food compares with CSB++, Sprinkles, and an unsupplemented diet in terms of preventing of growth faltering and improving micronutrient status. This trial will contribute much-needed data on the effectiveness of supplementary foods with an animal-source food other than milk, by comparing a supplementary food with fish (the RUSF) and one with milk (CSB++). Moreover, it will deepen the understanding of the impact of multiple micronutrients provided with or without macronutrients, by comparing the RUSF and CSB ++, which combine macronutrients with multiple micronutrients, and Sprinkles, which contains no macronutrients. Moreover, most studies on supplementary foods are from Africa, so this research will be an important contribution to the body of evidence from Asia [49].

There are two limitations of this trial. First, the data on consumption and compliance is based on self-reporting, and therefore risks response bias. It could be expected that any response bias would favour over-reporting of consumption, which may suggest lower effectiveness of the interventions. Similarly, sharing of foods with family members would likely be under-reported, again leading to underestimation of effectiveness. The second limitation is related to the generalisability of the findings to non-urban Cambodian populations, and to other South East Asian populations. Rural areas of Cambodia experience higher levels of malnutrition and poorer infant and young child feeding practices than urban [2]. Therefore, in rural settings, it would be difficult to predict if the interventions would appear more efficacious, or less.

From a programmatic point of view, if the novel RUSF proves successful, not only would it provide an acceptable, effective product for preventing childhood malnutrition. It might also simplify interventions in maternal and child nutrition in Cambodia and in countries where similar products could be produced, since, because of its composition, it could be used with pregnant and lactating women as well as children aged six months to two years.

### Abbreviations

AGP: Alpha-2 acid glycoprotein; BSID: Bayley Scales of Infant Development; CDHS: Cambodian Demographic and Health Survey; CRP: C-reactive protein; CSB++: Corn-Soy Blend Plus Plus, now called Supercereal Plus; DFPTQ: (Cambodian) Department of Fisheries Post-harvest Technologies and Quality; EDTA: Ethylenediamine tetraacetic acid; Hb: Haemoglobin; L/HAZ: Length/

height-for-age z-score; LNS: Lipid-based nutrient supplement; MUAC: Mid-upper arm circumference; NECHR: National Ethics Committee for Health Research; RUSF: Ready- to-use supplementary food; RUTF: Ready- to-use therapeutic food; SD: Standard deviation; WAZ: Weight-for-age z-score; WFP: United Nations World Food Program; WHO: World Health Organisation; WHZ: Weight-for-height z-score

**Acknowledgements**
The authors thank Remco Peters, Sanne Sigh, Marjoleine Dijkhuizen and Lyndon Paul (Vissot) for their work on product development. BB thanks Dr Eliana Jimenez Soto for her support and comments on early versions of the protocol and data collection tools.

**Funding**
This work is supported by UNICEF Cambodia; Department of Fisheries Post-Harvest Technologies and Quality Control (DFPTQ), Fisheries Administration, Ministry of Agriculture, Forestry and Fisheries, Cambodia; and IRD France.

**Authors' contributions**
BB developed the original research design, and refined it with FTW, SM, MG, DS, CC, JB and AL. BB wrote the initial draft protocol and all authors subsequently contributed to, commented on, and approved the final version.

**Competing interests**
The authors declare that they have no competing interests.

**Author details**
[1]School of Public Health, Faculty of Medicine, University of Sydney, Sydney, Australia. [2]School of Public Health, University of Queensland, Brisbane, Australia. [3]Department of Nutrition, Exercise and Sports, Faculty of Science, University of Copenhagen, Copenhagen, Denmark. [4]Department of Fisheries Post-Harvest Technologies and Quality Control, Fisheries Administration, Ministry of Agriculture, Forestry and Fisheries, Phnom Penh, Cambodia. [5]Child Survival and Development Section, UNICEF, Phnom Penh, Cambodia. [6]UMR Nutripass, Institut de Recherche pour le Développement, IRD/UM/SupAgro, Montpellier, France. [7]c/o Pascal Marino, European Union Delegation in Cameroon, BP 847 Yaoundé, Cameroon.

**References**

1. Black RE, Martorell R, Uauy R, Victora CG, Walker SP, Bhutta ZA, et al. Maternal and child undernutrition and overweight in low-income and middle-income countries. Lancet. 2013;382(9890):427–51.
2. National Institute of Statistics Directorate General for Health, and ICF International. Cambodia Demographic and Health Survey 2014. Phnom Penh, Cambodia, and Rockville, Maryland, USA: National Institute of Statistics, Directorate General for Health, and ICF International; 2015.
3. Bhutta ZA, Das JK, Rizvi A, Gaffey MF, Walker N, Horton S, et al. Evidence-based interventions for improvement of maternal and child nutrition: what can be done and at what cost? Lancet. 2013;382(9890):452–77.
4. Golden MH. Proposed recommended nutrient densities for moderately malnourished children. Food Nutr Bull. 2009;30(3 Suppl):S267.
5. de Pee S, Bloem MW. Current and potential role of specially formulated foods and food supplements for preventing malnutrition among 6-to 23-month-old children and for treating moderate malnutrition among 6-to 59-month-old children. Food Nutr Bull. 2009;30(3):S434–S63.
6. de Pee S, Manary M, Ashorn P. The devil is in the details. Nutr Rev. 2011;69(2):116–7.
7. Imdad A, Sadiq K, Bhutta ZA. Evidence-based prevention of childhood malnutrition. Current Opinion in Clinical Nutrition and Metabolic Care. 2011;14(3):276–85.
8. Dewey KG, Yang Z, Boy E. Systematic review and meta-analysis of home fortification of complementary foods. Maternal and Child Nutrition. 2009;5(4):283.
9. Adu-Afarwuah S, Lartey A, Brown KH, Zlotkin S, Briend A, Dewey KG. Randomized comparison of 3 types of micronutrient supplements for home fortification of complementary foods in Ghana: effects on growth and motor development. Am J Clin Nutr. 2007;86(2):412.
10. Rivera JA, Habicht J-P. Effect of supplementary feeding on the prevention of mild-to-moderate wasting in conditions of endemic malnutrition in Guatemala. Bull World Health Organ. 2002;80(12):926.
11. Zlotkin S. Overview of Efficacy, Effectiveness and Safety of MNPs: UNICEF; 2009 [Available from: http://nutritioncluster.net/wp-content/uploads/sites/4/2013/12/Revised_UNICEF_CombinedOverview_of_Efficacy_Effectiveness_and_Safety_of_MNPs.pdf.
12. Dewey KG, Adu-Afarwuah S. Systematic review of the efficacy and effectiveness of complementary feeding interventions in developing countries. Matern child nutr. 2008; 4 Suppl 1(s1): 24–85.
13. Boudier F. Socio-anthropological Investigation Related to the Acceptability of Plumpy'nut® in Cambodia. Paris: IRD; 2009.
14. WFP. Personal communication. Cambodia: Phnom Penh; 2014.
15. Wieringa F. Personal communication. Cambodia: IRD; 2014.
16. Peters R. Acceptability and impact on nutritional status of locally produced Ready-To-Use-Food (RUF) in preschool children in Cambodia (unpublished). 2014.
17. PAHO/WHO. Guiding Principles for Complementary Feeding of the Breastfeed Child. Washington DC: Pan American Health Organization/World Health Organization; 2002.
18. Manary MC, Cindy Y. Comparing Milk Fortified Corn-Soy Blend (CSB++), Soy Ready-to-Use Supplementary Food (RUSF), and Soy/Whey RUSF (Supplementary Plumpy®) in the Treatment of Moderate Acute Malnutrition. Washington, DC: FANTA-2 Bridge/FHI 360; 2012.
19. Neumann CG, Jiang L, Weiss RE, Grillenberger M, Gewa CA, Siekmann JH, et al. Meat supplementation increases arm muscle area in Kenyan schoolchildren. Br J Nutr. 2013;109(7):1230–11.
20. Nga T,T, Nguyen M, Mathisen R, Hoa DTB, Minh NH, Berger J, et al. Acceptability and impact on anthropometry of a locally developed ready-to-use therapeutic food in pre-school children in Vietnam. Nutr J. 2013;12(1):120.
21. Adu-Afarwuah S, Lartey A, Zeilani M, Dewey KG. Acceptability of lipid-based nutrient supplements (LNS) among Ghanaian infants and pregnant or lactating women. Maternal and Child Nutrition. 2011;7(4):344–56.
22. Kuusipalo H, Maleta K, Briend A, Manary M, Ashorn P. Growth and Change in Blood Haemoglobin Concentration Among Underweight Malawian Infants Receiving Fortified Spreads for 12 Weeks: A Preliminary Trial. J Pediatr Gastroenterol Nutr. 2006;43(4):525–32.
23. Anderson AK, Bediako-Amoa B, Steiner-Asiedu M. Acceptability of chicken powder in home prepared complementary foods for children in Ghana. Afr J Food Agric Nutr Dev. 2014;14(2):1–12.
24. Pachón H, Domínguez MRL, Creed-Kanashiro H, Stoltzfus RJ. Acceptability and Safety of Novel Infant Porridges Containing Lyophilized Meat Powder and Iron-Fortified Wheat Flour. Food Nutr Bull. 2007;28(1):35–46.
25. Bogard JaHT, S.. Using nutrient-rich local ingredients in the development of a complementary food. Bangladesh: WorldFish.
26. Nurhasan MT, Bun; Skau, Jutta; Roos, Nanna; Wieringa, Frank; Friis, Henrik; Michaelsen, Kim Fleischer; Chhoun, Chamnan, Münke, Christopher; Thea, Lach WinFood Cambodia: Improving Child Nutrition through Utilization of Local Food.
27. Skau J, Bunthang T, Chamnan C, Wieringa FT, Dijkhuizen MA, Roos N, et al. The use of linear programming to determine whether a formulated complementary food product can ensure adequate nutrients for 6- to 11-month-old Cambodian infants. Am J Clin Nutr. 2014;99(1):130–8.
28. Lin CA, Manary MJ, Maleta K, Briend A, Ashorn P. An energy-dense complementary food is associated with a modest increase in weight gain when compared with a fortified porridge in Malawian children aged 6-18 months. J Nutr. 2008;138(3):593.
29. Grillenberger M, Neumann CG, Murphy SP, Bwibo NO, van't Veer P, Hautvast JGAJ, et al. Food supplements have a positive impact on weight gain and the addition of animal source foods increases lean body mass of Kenyan schoolchildren. J Nutr. 2003;133(11 Suppl2):3957S.
30. Krebs NF, Mazariegos M, Chomba E, Sami N, Pasha O, Tshefu A, et al. Randomized controlled trial of meat compared with multimicronutrient-

fortified cereal in infants and toddlers with high stunting rates in diverse settings. The American journal of clinical nutrition [Internet]. 2012;96(4):840–7.
31. FAO/WHO. Proposed Draft Guideline for Ready-to-Use Therapeutic Foods. Hamburg Germany: Joint FAO/WHO Food Standards Programme CODEX Committee on Nutrition and Foods for Special Dietary Uses; 2016.
32. Ackatia-Armah RS. Community-based management of acute malnutrition in Malian children: A cluster randomized trial. Ann Arbor: ProQuest Dissertations Publishing; 2013.
33. LaGrone LN, Trehan I, Meuli GJ, Wang RJ, Thakwalakwa C, Maleta K, et al. A novel fortified blended flour, corn-soy blend "plus-plus," is not inferior to lipid-based ready-to-use supplementary foods for the treatment of moderate acute malnutrition in Malawian children. American journal of clinical nutrition [Internet]. 2012;95(1):212–9.
34. HF-TAG. Programmatic Guidance Brief on Use of Micronutrient Powders (MNP) for Home Fortification. In: Home Fortification Technical Advisory Group; 2011. https://www.unicef.org/nutrition/files/HFTAG_Micronutrient_Powder_Program_Guidance_Brief.pdf.
35. Jack SJ, Ou K, Chea M, Chhin L, Devenish R, Dunbar M, et al. Effect of Micronutrient Sprinkles on Reducing Anemia. Archives of Pediatrics & Adolescent Medicine. 2012;166(9):842–50.
36. Tran-Dinh N, Kennedy I, Bui T, Carter D. Survey of Vietnamese peanuts, corn and soil for the presence of Aspergillus flavus and Aspergillus parasiticus. Mycopathologia. 2009;168(5):257–68.
37. Shank RC, Wogan GN, Gibson JB. Dietary aflatoxins and human liver cancer. I. Toxigenic moulds in foods and foodstuffs of tropical south-east asia. Food and Cosmetics Toxicology. 1972;10(1):51–60.
38. Binder EM, Tan LM, Chin LJ, Handl J, Richard J. Worldwide occurrence of mycotoxins in commodities, feeds and feed ingredients. Anim Feed Sci Technol. 2007;137(3):265–82.
39. Nackers F, Broillet F, Oumarou D, Djibo A, Gaboulaud V, Guerin PJ, et al. Effectiveness of ready-to-use therapeutic food compared to a corn/soy-blend-based pre-mix for the treatment of childhood moderate acute malnutrition in Niger. J Trop Pediatr. 2010;56(6):407–13.
40. Yeung DC-s, SS-c H. Validity and reliability of skinfold measurement in assessing body fatness of Chinese children. Asia Pac J Clin Nutr. 2010;19(3):350–7.
41. Garza C, de Onis M. Rationale for developing a new international growth reference. Food Nutr Bull. 2004;25(1 Suppl):S5.
42. Municipality PP. The Phnom Penh Urban Poor Assessment: A baseline survey on the social and economic situations and capacity of existing services in urban poor communities. Phnom Penh: Phnom Penh Municipality; UNICEF. In: NCDD; 2012.
43. UNICEF. People In Need. Phnom Penh Multiple Indicator Assessment of the Urban Poor. Phnom Penh: UNICEF; 2014.
44. Van Hoan N, Van Phu P, Salvignol B, Berger J, Trèche S. Effect of the consumption of high energy dense and fortified gruels on energy and nutrient intakes of 6–10-month-old Vietnamese infants. Appetite. 2009;53(2):233–40.
45. Pham VP, Berger J, Nguyen VH, Salvignol B, Treche S, Wieringa FT, et al. A six-month intervention with two different types of micronutrient-fortified complementary foods had distinct short- and long-term effects on linear and ponderal growth of Vietnamese infants. J Nutr. 2012;142(9):1735.
46. Gorstein JSK, Parvanta I, Begin F. Indicators and Methods for Cross-Sectional Surveys of Vitamin and Mineral Status of Populations. Atlanta: The Micronutrient Initiative (Ottawa) and the Centers for Disease Control and Prevention; 2007.
47. Manary MJ. Local production and provision of ready-to-use therapeutic food (RUTF) spread for the treatment of severe childhood malnutrition. Food Nutr Bull. 2006;27(3 Suppl):S83.
48. Ali E, Draguez B, Delchevalerie P, Harries AD, Zachariah R, Dahmane A, et al. Peanut-based ready-to-use therapeutic food: acceptability among malnourished children and community workers in Bangladesh. Public Health Action. 2013;3(2):128–35.
49. Lazzerini M, Rubert L, Pani P. Specially formulated foods for treating children with moderate acute malnutrition in low- and middle-income countries. The Cochrane database of systematic reviews. 2013;6:CD009584.
50. Wang RJ, Trehan I, LaGrone LN, Weisz AJ, Thakwalakwa CM, Maleta KM, et al. Investigation of food acceptability and feeding practices for lipid nutrient supplements and blended flours used to treat moderate malnutrition. J Nutr Educ Behav. 2013;45(3):258–63.
51. Foote JM, Mohr PJ, Schultheis DS, Walker BS, Phillips KT, Brady LH, et al. Development of an evidence-based clinical practice guideline on linear growth measurement of children. J Pediatr Nurs. 2011;26(4):312–24.
52. Skau JN. Marie; Sok, Daream; Wieringa, Frank Acceptability Study Of Fortified Blended Food Products Among Children 12–36 Months Old Children And Caregivers In Cambodia (unpublished). Phnom Penh: WFP; 2012.
53. Salam RA, Macphail C, Das JK, Bhutta ZA. Effectiveness of Micronutrient Powders (MNP) in women and children. BMC public health 2013; 13 Suppl 3(Suppl 3):S22.

5

# Propolis ethanolic extracts reduce adenosine diphosphate induced platelet aggregation determined on whole blood

Mirza Bojić[1*], Andrea Antolić[2], Maja Tomičić[3], Željko Debeljak[4,5] and Željan Maleš[6]

## Abstract

**Background:** Propolis is a well-known bee product containing more than 2000 identified compounds. It has many beneficial effects on human health that include antibacterial, antiviral, anticancer and hepatoprotective justifying its use as a dietary supplement. Platelet aggregation plays crucial role in thrombus formation that can cause stroke or heart attacks. As cardiovascular diseases, including those caused by thrombus formation, are related to 50% of deaths of Western population, the objective of this study was to determine antiaggregatory activity of propolis on platelet aggregation on the whole blood samples.

**Methods:** Twenty one propolis samples from Southeast Europe were characterized by spectrophotometric methods to determine content of the total flavonoids and phenolic acids. High performance liquid chromatography coupled with diode array detection was used to identify and quantify individual polyphenols. Platelet aggregation was tested by impedance aggregometry on the whole blood samples of ten healthy volunteers.

**Results:** The mean content of total polyphenols was 136.14 mg/g and ranged from 59.23 to 277.39 mg/g. Content of total flavonoids ranged between 6.83 and 55.44 mg/g with the mean value of 19.28 mg/g. Percentage of total phenolic acids was in the range 8.79 to 45.67% (mean 26.63%). Minimal antiaggregatory concentration, representing the lowest concentration of propolis extract sample that can cause statistically significant reduction of aggregation, ranged from 5 μM to 10.4 mM. Samples of propolis with lower content of luteolin and higher content of pinocembrin-7-methyleter showed better antiplatelet activity i.e. lower values of minimal antiaggregatory concentration.

**Conclusions:** This is the first study that shows antiaggregatory potential of propolis ethanolic extracts on the whole blood samples in the low micromolar concentrations suggesting that propolis supplementation may influence platelet aggregation and consequently thrombus formation. Further in vivo studies are needed to confirm the beneficial effects in prevention of cardiovascular diseases.

**Keywords:** Propolis, Flavonoids, Phenolic acids, Platelet aggregation, Thrombus formation, Cardiovascular diseases

* Correspondence: mbojic@pharma.hr
[1]Faculty of Pharmacy and Biochemistry, Department of Medicinal Chemistry, University of Zagreb, A. Kovačića 1, 10000 Zagreb, Croatia
Full list of author information is available at the end of the article

## Background

Propolis is a well-known bee produced wax mixture containing more than 2000 identified compounds [1]. It is collected from by honeybees (*Apis mellifera* L.) from plants, primarily from flowers and leaf buds [2]. Chemical composition of this resinous mixture varies depending of the origin and plant species but in principle contains up to 45–55% polyphenols (flavonoids, phenolic acids and it esters), 25–35% beeswaxes (waxes and fatty acids), 10% volatile substances (essential oils), 5% pollen containing amino acids and 5% of other substances like minerals, vitamins and sugars [2].

Propolis has many beneficial effects on human health that justify its use as a dietary supplement. It is mainly used due to its antioxidant properties and along with wine represents the most significant source of polyphenols in Western world [3]. Many in vitro and in vivo animal studies have shown antibacterial [4], antiviral [1], hepatoprotective [5], immunomodulatory [6], anticancer [7] and other biological effects of propolis. These positive effects are primarily related to the content of flavonoids and phenolic acids [5]. Our group has extensively studied Croatian and other European propolis and found that propolis ethanolic extracts possess antibacterial activity against *Staphylococcus aureus* and antifungal activity against yeast *Candida albicans* [4]. Antioxidant activity assessed using diphenylpicrylhydrazyl, a colored free stable radical, was related to the content of *p*-coumaric acid, tectochrysin, and kaempferol [4]. The content of tectochrysin, galangin, pinocembrin chrysin, apigenin, and kaempferol was significantly correlated with antimicrobial activity while p-coumaric acid, apigenin, and kaempferol were significantly correlated with the activity of propolis against *C. albicans* [5]. Antitumoral activity against HeLa cell lines was related to the high concentrations of ferulic and *p*-coumaric acid, galangin and pinocembrin [8].

Cardiovascular diseases are related to 50% of deaths of Western population [9]. Direct and indirect costs of cardiovascular diseases are estimated to total more than $316 billion [9]. As people get more conscientious of their wellbeing and health protection, many opt for dietary supplements containing functional foods and nutraceuticals. One of the approaches is to prevent platelet aggregation i.e. primary step in blood clot (thrombus) formation that can cause heart attack [10], brain stroke [11], pulmonary embolism [12] and deep-vein thrombosis [13]. For this purpose, aspirin (acetylsalicylic acid) is often used, but as medicines are accompanied with significant side effects new regulators of platelet aggregation are of interest [14]. It has been shown that flavonoids [15] and phenolic acids [16] can prevent platelet aggregation.

By now, there have been two reports of antiaggregatory effect of propolis. Zhang et al. [17] tested platelet aggregation on platelet rich plasma and our group conducted preliminary research on whole blood [18]. However, in both studies concentration (dry mass expressed as molar equivalents of quercetin per volume of extract) that caused statistically significant reduction of aggregation induced by adenosine diphosphate were above 30 μM. As maximal concentration of flavonoids that can be found in blood goes up to 7.6 μM [19], further studies are needed to determine minimal concentrations at which propolis extracts prevent platelet aggregation.

Thus, the objective of this work was to characterize propolis extracts by spectrophotometric and high-performance liquid chromatography (HPLC) methods, and explore influence of propolis on platelet aggregation based on adenosine diphosphate (ADP) induced aggregation testing on the whole blood samples of healthy volunteers.

## Methods

### Materials and propolis extracts

All standards of flavonoids and phenolic acids were obtained from Extrasynthese (Genay, France) and Sigma Aldrich (St. Louis, MO, USA), respectively, and were used as methanolic solutions. Organic solvents were obtained from Fisher Scientific (Hampton, NH, USA) and Kemika (Zagreb, Croatia). Propolis samples were obtained commercially; 19 samples were from Croatia to reflect different composition of propolis between continental and costal part, as well as one from Macedonia and one from Bosnia and Herzegovina for a comparison. Ethanolic extracts of propolis were prepared at room temperature using 80% ethanol (*V/V*) [20]. 1 g of raw propolis was extracted with solvent for one hour, filtered and as such used for chemical characterization. For the purpose of platelet aggregation functional testing extracts were dried using rotary vapor and reconstituted in dimethyl sulfoxide.

### Total polyphenols, flavonoids and phenolic acids

Total content of polyphenols was determined by Folin-Ciocalteu method according to the method described by Slinkard and Singleton [21]. The method is based on the reduction of $MoO^{4+}$ to $MoO^{3+}$ and absorbance is recorded at 765 nm. The results are expressed as equivalents of gallic acid from the calibration curve.

Total flavonoids were determined by Christ-Müller's method [22]. After acid hydrolysis flavonoids were determined as liberated aglycones spectrophotometrically at 425 nm as a complex with aluminum in a methanol-ethyl acetate-acetic acid medium. Results were expressed as equivalents of quercetin based on calibration curve of quercetin standard.

Total phenolic acids were determined based on European Pharmacopoeia [23] procedure. Phenolic acids form a complex with sodium molybdate-sodium nitrite that has absorbance maximum at 505 nm. Result is expressed as percentage, an equivalent of rosmarinic acid based on formula: Phenolic acids (%) = 0.5 x $A$ / $m$, where $A$ is measured absorbance and $m$ mass of sample used in the analysis.

#### HPLC-DAD analysis

HPLC analysis was performed on Agilent 1100 chromatograph equipped with a diode array detector using Agilent Zorbax SBC18 column (250 mm × 4.6 mm, particle size 5 μm) with Zorbax SB-C18 guard column (12.5 mm × 4. 6 mm, particle size 5 μm). Mobile phase A consisted of water/methanol/formic acid in volume ratio 93:5:2 and mobile phase B of water/methanol/formic acid in ratio 3: 95:2. Flow rate was set to 1 mL/min (volume injected was 10 μL and temperature was set to 40 °C. Following gradient was used: 0 min, 20% mobile phase B, with linear increases to10 min, 40%, 35 min, 50%, 47 min, 50%, 70 min, 80%, followed by re-equilibration to 20% for 10 min. Chromatograms were recorded at 270, 290, 320 and 350 nm. Content of polyphenols was determined using calibration curves of individual flavonoid and phenolic acid [24].

#### Platelet aggregation functional test

This study was approved by Ethical committee of the Croatian Institute of Transfusion Medicine (CITM). A total number of 10 volunteers participated in this research, 5 males median age 34 (minimal age 28, maximal age 42) years and 5 females median age 35 (minimal age 28, maximal age 51) years, taking no antiaggregatory medications at least 10 days before giving a blood sample. The main inclusion criteria were: healthy status, age of 18–55 years, no history of thrombosis, known thrombophilia, bleeding diathesis of coagulopathy. These were volunteers that met the legal requirements related to the blood donors' selection in CITM and were willing to give additional 4.5 mL of blood (calcium citrate used as anticoagulant). Volunteers gave informed written consent.

All blood samples were tested within two hours after collection by treating them with propolis extracts or solvent as a control. Blood samples showed normal aggregation with ADP potentiator (38 to 85 units) measured by Multiplate® (Roche, Switzerland) functional analyzer under the standardized and firmly controlled in vitro conditions in Hemostasis laboratory of CITM. All consumables used in platelet assays were disposed as biological waste under the principles of good laboratory practice and current national regulations (Official Gazette of the Republic of Croatia no. 50/2005).

Platelet aggregation was analyzed by impedance analyzer. General analysis procedure was used: 300 μL of citrate blood was incubated for 3 min with 20 μL of extract solution and 300 μL of calcium chloride saline physiological solution. Analysis was conducted at a temperature of 37 °C. Untreated sample – negative control contained 20 μL of dimethyl sulfoxide. Final concentration of solvent in all experiments was below 3%. Aggregation was initiated by addition of 20 μL of adenosine diphosphate reagent (ADPtest) and was measured for 6 min. Results, expressed as area under curve in arbitrary units (AU), were used for determination of minimal antiaggregatory concentration (*MINaAC*). *MINaAC* represents the lowest concentration of sample that can cause statistically significant reduction of aggregation and was determined as previously reported by our group [15]. Briefly, aggregation of untreated sample (solvent control) and the sample of propolis are measured. If the difference of the recorded aggregation values is greater than 5% the measurement of additional two citrate bloods is performed. Otherwise, double concentration of propolis is taken and the first step is repeated. If the propolis sample in the analyzed concentration shows statistically lower aggregation compared to the untreated sample (assessed by $t$-test) the analyzed concentration is equal to minimal antiaggregatory concentration (*MINaAC*). If not, analysis is performed from the beginning with double the concentration of propolis extract. This presumes that the analyzed concentration is not the first analyzed, else, the analysis is performed from beginning using the half of the concentration of flavonoid.

Difference between means of the control and propolis sample was determined by Student's $t$-test (at statistical significance $\alpha = 0.05$) [25]. To be able to use $t$-test, normal distribution of aggregation was assessed using Shapiro-Wilk test ($p = 0.501$) justifying the use of $t$-test [15].

To determine the relationship between *MINaAC* and the content of total flavonoids, phenolic acids, polyphenols, and individual polyphenols, Pearson's correlation coefficient was calculated as well as its statistical significance (at $\alpha = 0.05$) assessed using SocSciStatistics online software [25].

## Results

#### Chemical characterization of propolis ethanolic extracts

All propolis samples were characterized using spectrophotometric methods on total content of polyphenols, flavonoids and phenolic acids. Individual polyphenols have been determined by liquid chromatography. Results of this spectrophotometry and chromatography analysis are presented in Tables 1 and 2, respectively.

**Table 1** Content of total polyphenols, flavonoids and phenolic acids determined in propolis extracts by spectrophotometric methods

| No | Propolis sample | Polyphenols (mg/g) [a] | Phenolic Acids (%) [b] | Flavonoids (mg/g) [c] |
|---|---|---|---|---|
| 1 | Beli Manastir | 126.65 | 16.33 | 18.17 |
| 2 | Bjelovar | 159.14 | 25.3 | 27.5 |
| 3 | Daruvar | 112.11 | 20.99 | 20.35 |
| 4 | Garešnica | 142.73 | 21.24 | 17.55 |
| 5 | Gospić | 248.01 | 31.78 | 6.84 |
| 6 | Hercegovina | 102.65 | 31.88 | 14.56 |
| 7 | Karlovac 1 | 163.66 | 17.22 | 20.69 |
| 8 | Karlovac 2 | 277.39 | 38.67 | 25.61 |
| 9 | Kumanovo (FYRM) | 62.42 | 19.86 | 13.03 |
| 10 | Lika | 155.47 | 40.71 | 33.95 |
| 11 | Lisice (BiH) | 128.63 | 30.3 | 17 |
| 12 | Metković | 59.23 | 15.45 | 9.98 |
| 13 | Okučani | 143.51 | 37.45 | 6.83 |
| 14 | Osijek | 153.09 | 42.77 | 31.68 |
| 15 | Pregrada | 141.61 | 8.79 | 7.35 |
| 16 | Costal Croatia | 72.05 | 19.56 | 7.91 |
| 17 | Sisak | 62.09 | 12.2 | 9.27 |
| 18 | Slavonija | 176.61 | 45.67 | 30.2 |
| 19 | Varaždin | 112.15 | 30.69 | 14.55 |
| 20 | Virovitica 1 | 142.65 | 20.45 | 16.52 |
| 21 | Virovitica 2 | 117.16 | 31.88 | 55.44 |

[a]Total polyphenols are expressed as gallic acid equivalents
[b]Total phenolic acids are expressed as percentage of rosmarinic acid equivalents
[c]Total flavonoids are expressed as quercetin equivalents

### Antiaggregatory effect of propolis

The effect of propolis extracts on platelet aggregation is shown in Table 3. To include biological variability, minimal antiaggregatory concentration (*MINaAC*) of propolis ethanolic extracts was determined. It includes statistical *t*-test between control and sample and represents concentration of sample that can cause statistically significant decrease of platelet aggregation. As it has previously been reported in μM values, propolis ethanolic extracts concentrations were expressed in molar concentrations taking into account molecular weight of quercetin ($M_w = 302.236$). *MINaAC* ranged between 5 μM and 10.4 mM.

## Discussion

### Chemical characterization of propolis ethanolic extracts

Propolis is extremely rich in polyphenols with content of 59.23 to 277.39 mg of GAE per g of raw propolis (Table 1). This is in accordance with extensive study of ethanolic extracts of propolis collected worldwide by Kumazawa et al. in which quantity of total polyphenols varied between 31 and 299 mg/g also determined by Folin-Ciocalteu method [26].

Content of phenolic acids varies between 8.79 and 45.67% (Table 1). These values are much higher when compared with the results of Kalogeropoulos et al. [27] who attributed phenolic acids to 1 to 9% of total polyphenols. This can be attributed to different methodology of determination GC-MS vs. spectrophotometry as well as fact that spectrophotometric method for determination of phenolic acids in European Pharmacopeia expresses phenolic acids as equivalent of rosmarinic acid ($M_w = 360.32$) while most of the phenolic acids found in propolis are much lower molecular weight e.g. caffeic acid ($M_w = 164.05$).

Flavonoids ranged between 6.83 and 55.44 mg per gram of propolis (Table 1). As it has been previously shown [26], propolis extracts of different geographical origin have different profile of polyphenols. Generally European propolis has lower quantities of total flavonoids and based on Christ-Müller's method goes up to 5.5% (propolis sample 21). Ratio of flavonoids in Greek and Cyprus propolis ranged from 4 to 31% of total polyphenols among determined and quantified classes of polyphenolic compounds based on gas chromatography coupled with mass spectrometry analysis [27].

**Table 2** Content of individual flavonoids and phenolic acids determined in propolis extracts by liquid chromatography. Results are expressed in mg per gram of propolis sample

| | | Phenolic Acids | | | | Flavonoids | | | | | | | | | |
|---|---|---|---|---|---|---|---|---|---|---|---|---|---|---|---|
| No. | Propolis sample | Caffeic Acid | *p*-Coumaric Acid | Ferulic Acid | Isoferulic Acid | Apigenin | Chrysin | Galangin | Kaempferol | Luteolin | Morin | Naringenin | Pinocembrin | Pinocembrin-7-methylether | Quercetin |
| 1 | Beli Manastir | 2.753 | 2.347 | 3.743 | 2.959 | 0.751 | n.d | 12.038 | 1.281 | 9.845 | n.d. | 1.339 | 1.509 | n.d. | n.d. |
| 2 | Bjelovar | 11.248 | 11.410 | 13.616 | 9.648 | 1.418 | n.d. | 27.950 | 4.604 | 8.174 | n.d. | 3.756 | 4.577 | n.d. | 1.033 |
| 3 | Daruvar | 2.362 | 0.931 | 0.926 | n.q. | 0.895 | 11.713 | n.d. | n.d. | 0.930 | n.d. | 0.004 | n.d. | n.d. | 0.460 |
| 4 | Garešnica | 3.524 | 2.477 | 1.345 | n.q. | 0.610 | 11.628 | n.d. | n.d. | 0.213 | n.d. | 0.343 | n.d. | n.d. | n.d. |
| 5 | Gospić | 1.307 | 11.016 | 14.704 | 2.017 | 0.280 | 8.224 | n.d. | 3.501 | 0.642 | 0.839 | n.q. | 1.590 | 6.128 | 3.549 |
| 6 | Hercegovina | 0.772 | 2.838 | 3.837 | 1.163 | 0.371 | 0.959 | n.d. | 1.332 | 0.882 | n.d. | 0.766 | n.d. | n.d. | n.d. |
| 7 | Karlovac 1 | 3.797 | 9.115 | 9.581 | 4.929 | 0.927 | 12.891 | n.d. | n.d. | 2.262 | 3.126 | 2.070 | 1.684 | n.d. | 2.096 |
| 8 | Karlovac 2 | n.d. | 2.037 | 2.064 | 0.591 | 2.679 | n.d. | 8.151 | n.d. | 1.195 | n.d. | n.d. | n.d. | n.d. | 0.577 |
| 9 | Kumanovo (FYRM) | 1.812 | 0.590 | 0.177 | 1.886 | 0.490 | 9.090 | 0.644 | 0.706 | 1.616 | n.d. | 0.896 | 0.489 | 4.817 | n.d. |
| 10 | Lika | 8.639 | 2.076 | 1.885 | 5.314 | 1.571 | n.d. | 26.600 | 3.521 | 6.950 | n.d. | 3.741 | 4.033 | n.d. | 1.225 |
| 11 | Lisice (BiH) | 2.198 | 3.028 | 1.065 | 0.056 | 1.399 | 7.844 | n.d. | n.d. | 0.642 | 0.004 | 0.032 | 0.429 | n.d. | n.d. |
| 12 | Metković | 0.130 | 0.578 | 0.522 | 0.113 | 0.229 | 15.468 | n.d. | 0.245 | 0.063 | n.d. | 0.545 | n.d. | n.d. | n.d. |
| 13 | Okučani | 0.780 | 7.089 | 8.693 | 0.793 | 1.043 | n.d. | n.d. | n.d. | 1.370 | n.d. | 0.149 | n.d. | n.d. | 0.224 |
| 14 | Osijek | 8.332 | 3.161 | 1.682 | 0.306 | 2.405 | n.d. | 0.538 | n.d. | 1.757 | n.d. | 0.719 | n.d. | n.d. | 0.724 |
| 15 | Pregrada | n.q. | 1.215 | 1.544 | 0.249 | 0.134 | 3.905 | n.d. | n.d. | 1.428 | 0.730 | 0.220 | n.d. | n.d. | n.d. |
| 16 | Costal Croatia | n.q. | 2.091 | 2.649 | 0.674 | 0.237 | n.d. | 4.894 | 0.827 | 0.236 | n.d. | 0.249 | n.d. | n.d. | 1.430 |
| 17 | Sisak | 0.110 | 1.201 | 1.332 | 0.720 | 0.310 | 20.690 | 1.445 | 0.438 | 0.941 | n.d. | n.d. | n.d. | n.d. | n.d. |
| 18 | Slavonija | 6.084 | 4.241 | 4.908 | 4.461 | 0.868 | 51.839 | 1.135 | 2.049 | 9.734 | n.d. | 3.580 | n.d. | n.d. | 0.548 |
| 19 | Varaždin | 3.304 | 3.372 | 3.672 | 2.347 | 1.165 | 47.355 | n.d. | 3.416 | 7.837 | n.d. | 1.410 | n.d. | 1.697 | n.d. |
| 20 | Virovitica 1 | 1.249 | 5.134 | 6.310 | 1.769 | 0.348 | n.d. | 7.043 | 0.912 | 1.644 | 0.338 | 0.794 | 1.232 | 2.471 | 1.217 |
| 21 | Virovitica 2 | 5.286 | 1.499 | 2.255 | n.q. | 3.038 | 6.311 | n.d. | 7.772 | 1.606 | n.d. | 0.076 | n.d. | n.d. | 0.599 |

*n.d.* not detected, *n.q.* not quantified

**Table 3** Minimal antiaggregatory concentrations of propolis extracts (*MINaAC*) determined by impedance aggregometry induced by ADP

| No | Propolis sample | *MINaAC* (μM) | *p* |
|---|---|---|---|
| 1 | Beli Manastir | 10,432 | 0.028 |
| 2 | Bjelovar | 326 | 0.001 |
| 3 | Daruvar | 41 | 0.002 |
| 4 | Garešnica | 41 | 0.011 |
| 5 | Gospić | 20 | 0.029 |
| 6 | Hercegovina | 5 | 0.034 |
| 7 | Karlovac 1 | 163 | 0.013 |
| 8 | Karlovac 2 | 41 | 0.006 |
| 9 | Kumanovo (FYRM) | 41 | 0.018 |
| 10 | Lika | 41 | 0.009 |
| 11 | Lisice (BiH) | 652 | 0.001 |
| 12 | Metković | 163 | 0.004 |
| 13 | Okučani | 41 | 0.001 |
| 14 | Osijek | 326 | 0.002 |
| 15 | Pregrada | 41 | 0.001 |
| 16 | Costal Croatia | 20 | 0.002 |
| 17 | Sisak | 163 | 0.021 |
| 18 | Slavonija | 41 | 0.003 |
| 19 | Varaždin | 163 | 0.002 |
| 20 | Virovitica 1 | 81 | 0.003 |
| 21 | Virovitica 2 | 41 | 0.001 |

*p*-value determined by Student's *t*-test

Out of four detected phenolic acids (Table 2) the most abundant was ferulic that was accounted to from 0.2 to 14.7 mg/g (propolis sample 5). This is above values found in Greek and Cyprus propolis (0.1–1.8 mg/g) and lower than those of Polish propolis samples (19.3–44.5 mg/g) [27, 28]. *p*-Coumaric, as well as ferulic, was detected in all samples and content was lower than the one reported for Polish propolis (0.6–11.4 mg/g vs. 37.5–117.0 mg/g) and higher than reported by Barbarić et al. [8] (0.01–0.16 mg/g). Content of caffeic acid was in the range of 0.1 to 11.2 mg/g which is similar to the values observed by Kumazawa et al. [26] (0.2–3.3 mg/g) and Socha et al. [28] (7.7–20.1 mg/g). Isoferulic acid was detected in propolis samples from Serbia [29]. In our study isoferulic acid ranged from 0.1 to 9.6 mg/g.

A total of ten flavonoids have been detected and quantified in propolis ethanolic extracts. Main flavonoids found in all propolis samples were luteolin and apigenin, ranging from 0.1 to 9.8 and 0.1 to 3.0 mg/g, respectively. Both were previously reported as constituents of propolis, and quantities of apigenin are in the range reported for Greek propolis samples (0.25–15.85 mg/g) [27]. Other flavonoids determined in more than a half of analyzed propolis samples were naringenin, kaempferol, chrysin and quercetin with quantities of up to 3.8, 7.8, 51.8 and 3.5 mg/g, respectively. These results are similar to the ones obtained by Socha et al. [28] that determined naringenin, kaempferol, chrysin and quercetin in Polish propolis samples ranging 1.4–21.3 mg/g, 2.4–8.0 mg/g, 13.4–45.5 mg/g and 4.1–7.9 mg/g. Pinocembrin and its 7-methyleter (pinostrobin) were found in eight (0.4–4.6 mg/g) and four (1.7–6.1 mg/g) samples. These concentrations are similar to previously reported values in Croatian propolis; pinocembrin 0.1–7.7 mg/g, and slightly higher for pinostrobin that was reported 0.02–0.25 mg/g [8]. Morin was found in four propolis samples within range of 0.004–3.126 mg/g that is similar in value reported for samples of Chinese propolis of 0.076–0.172 mg/g [30]. Chemical characterization of propolis samples used in this study showed comparable results of Croatian propolis to those reported for propolis samples derived from Eurasia.

When compared to values reported for individual flavonoids of 0.2 to 122 μM in the platelet functional test induced by ADP, propolis shows significant potential to influence platelet aggregation.

As flavonoids are major propolis constituents responsible for pharmacological activity, the mechanism of antiplatelet activity of propolis as well as targeted signaling pathways are the same. Flavonoids inhibit platelet aggregation induced by thromboxane A2, ADP, thrombin and collagen [31]. Underlying mechanisms that prevent platelet aggregation that were reported for individual flavonoids include inhibitions of intracellular signaling pathways through inhibition of the enzymatic activities of phospholipase C [32, 33], phospholipase A2 [34] and cyclooxygenase 1 [35], reducing the oxidative burst and decreasing nitric oxide production [36].

Propolis samples with lowest *MINaAC* values were 5, 6 and 16. Sample 5 had *MINaAC* of 20 μM and it contained pinocembrin-7-methylether as most dominant flavonoid for which *MINaAC* of 0.95 μM was reported [15]. Sample 6 was the most potent in preventing platelet aggregation (*MINaAC* = 5 μM) and it contained luteolin, apigenin and chrysin with *MINaAC* values of 7.6, 3.8 and 3.8 μM [15]. While in samples 5 and 6 comparable values of *MINaAC* between propolis and pure substances was observed, sample 16 contained mainly galangin for which *MINaAC* of 122.17 μM is reported [15]. This could indicate that individual flavonoids can have synergistic effect in propolis enhancing its antiplatelet activity and could be rationalized by different mechanism of action on how individual polyphenol exhibits its biological activity.

When all 21 propolis samples have been taken account and *MINaAC* (Table 3) was related to quantities of individual polyphenol constituents (Table 2), only content of luteolin showed week connection to *MINaAC* that was statistically significant (Pearson's correlation coefficient 0.4831, $p = 0.0266$). If statistical significance was set to α = 0.1, pinocembrin-7-methyleter would show strong negative correlation to *MINaAC* ($r = -0.9146$, $p = 0.0855$) [37]. However, this should be considered with caution as pinocembrin-7-methyleter was found only in 4 while luteolin was quantified in all propolis samples. More potent propolis samples have lower *MINaAC* values, consequently samples of propolis with lower content of luteolin and higher content of pinocembrin-7-methyleter showed better antiplatelet activity.

In our preliminary studies we have observed antiplatelet activity of propolis in concentrations of 200 mg/L [18] while Zhang et al. reported 100 mg/L [17] when using ADP as inductor of platelet aggregation. Disadvantage of both studies was testing only arbitrary concentrations of propolis, not a range on which either $IC_{50}$ values or *MINaAC* determination can be based of. Moreover, study by Zhang et al. was performed on one propolis sample by optical densitometry assay on platelet rich plasma which can be regarded inadequate as composition of propolis is highly variable [3]. Advantage of this study is that we have analyzed 21 propolis sample of different origin and conducted platelet aggregation assays on whole blood which better reflects in vivo conditions.

Propolis is rich source of polyphenols commonly used as dietary supplement i.e. functional food. Most commonly active components, flavonoids and phenolic acids are extracted with mixtures of ethanol and water in different ratios (optimal 70–80%). This is the first study that shows antiaggregatory potential of propolis ethanolic extracts in low micromolar concentrations on the whole blood that can be attributed to some extent to polyphenolic constituents of propolis in vitro. Results of this study suggest that propolis supplementation can influence function tests of platelet aggregation in vitro. Further studies are needed to confirm beneficial effect in prevention of cardiovascular diseases in vivo.

## Conclusions

Propolis is rich source of polyphenols commonly used as dietary supplement i.e. functional food. Most commonly active components, flavonoids and phenolic acids are extracted with mixtures of ethanol and water in different ratios (optimal 70–80%). This is the first study that shows antiaggregatory potential of propolis ethanolic extracts on the whole blood in the low micromolar concentrations that can be attributed to some extent to polyphenolic constituents of propolis. Results of this study suggest that propolis supplementation can influence function tests of platelet aggregation as well as may have potential beneficial effect in prevention of cardiovascular diseases if proven in human studies.

### Abbreviations

ADP: Adenosine diphosphate; CITM: Croatian Institute of Transfusion Medicine; HPLC: high performance liquid analysis; *MINaAC*: Minimal antiaggregatory concentration

### Funding

This work was supported by University of Zagreb (Z1111 – M.B.)

### Authors' contributions

MB and ŽD designed the study; AA and MB did HPLC analysis; AA, MT and ŽD performed the platelet aggregation experiments; ŽM and MB analyzed the data and wrote the paper. All authors read and approved the final manuscript.

### Competing interests

The authors declare that they have no competing interests.

### Author details

[1]Faculty of Pharmacy and Biochemistry, Department of Medicinal Chemistry, University of Zagreb, A. Kovačića 1, 10000 Zagreb, Croatia. [2]Faculty of Science, PDS Biology, University of Zagreb, Rooseveltov trg 6, 10000 Zagreb, Croatia. [3]Department of Platelet and Leukocyte Immunology, Croatian Institute of Transfusion Medicine, Petrova 6, 10000 Zagreb, Croatia. [4]Institute of Clinical Laboratory Diagnostics, Osijek University Hospital Center, Josipa Huttlera 4, 31000 Osijek, Croatia. [5]Faculty of Medicine, University J. J. Strossmayer of Osijek, Josipa Huttlera 4, 31000 Osijek, Croatia. [6]Faculty of Pharmacy and Biochemistry, Department of Pharmaceutical Botany, University of Zagreb, Schrottova 39, 10000 Zagreb, Croatia.

### References

1. Kujumgiev A, Tsvetkova I, Serkedjieva Y, Bankova V, Christov R, Popov S. Antibacterial, antifungal and antiviral activity of propolis of different geographic origin. J Ethnopharmacol. 1999;64:235–40.
2. Krell R. Value-added products from beekeeping. Rome: Food and Agriculture Organization; 1996.
3. Medić-Šarić M, Bojić M, Rastija V, Cvek J. Polyphenolic profiling of Croatian Propolis and wine. Food Technol Biotechnol. 2013;51:159–70.
4. Tlak Gajger I, Pavlović I, Bojić M, Kosalec I, Srečec S, Vlainić T, Vlainić J. The components responsible for the antimicrobial activity of Propolis from continental and Mediterranean regions in Croatia. Czech J Food Sci. 2017;35:376–85.
5. Banskota AH, Tezuka Y, Kadota S. Recent progress in pharmacological research of propolis. Phytother Res. 2001;15:561–71.
6. Sforcin JM. Propolis and the immune system: a review. J Ethnopharmacol. 2007;113:1–14.
7. Banskota AH, Tezuka Y, Adnyana IK, Midorikawa K, Matsushige K, Message D, Huertas AA, Kadota S. Cytotoxic, hepatoprotective and free radical scavenging effects of propolis from Brazil, Peru, the Netherlands and China. J Ethnopharmacol. 2000;72:239–46.
8. Barbarić M, Mišković K, Bojić M, Lončar MB, Smolčić-Bubalo A, Debeljak Ž, Medić-Šarić M. Chemical composition of the ethanolic propolis extracts and its effect on HeLa cells. J Ethnopharmacol. 2011;135:772–8.
9. Benjamin EJ, Virani SS, Callaway CW, Chang AR, Cheng S, Chiuve SE, Cushman M, Delling FN, Deo R, de Ferranti SD, Ferguson JF, Fornage M, Gillespie C, Isasi CR, Jiménez MC, Jordan LC, Judd SE, Lackland D, Lichtman JH, Lisabeth L, Liu S, Longenecker CT, Lutsey PL, Matchar DB, Matsushita K,

Mussolino ME, Nasir K, O'Flaherty M, Palaniappan LP, Pandey DK, Reeves MJ, Ritchey MD, Rodriguez CJ, Roth GA, Rosamond WD, UKA S, Satou GM, Shah SH, Spartano NL, Tirschwell DL, Tsao CW, Voeks JH, Willey JZ, Wilkins JT, Wu JH, Alger HM, Wong SS, Muntner P. Heart disease and stroke Statistics-2018 update: a report from the American Heart Association. Circulation. 2018;137: e67–e492.

10. Singer DE, Albers GW, Dalen JE, Fang MC, Go AS, Halperin JL, Lip GYH, Manning WJ. Antithrombotic therapy in atrial fibrillation. Chest. 2008;133:546S–92S.
11. Amarenco P, Cohen A, Tzourio C, Bertrand B, Hommel M, Besson G, Chauvel C, Touboul PJ, Bousser MG. Atherosclerotic disease of the aortic arch and the risk of ischemic stroke. N Engl J Med. 1994;331:1474–9.
12. Torbicki A, Perrier A, Konstantinides S, Agnelli G, Galiè N, Pruszczyk P, Bengel F, Brady AJ, Ferreira D, Janssens U, Klepetko W, Mayer E, Remy-Jardin M, Bassand JP. Guidelines on the diagnosis and management of acute pulmonary embolism: the task force for the diagnosis and management of acute pulmonary embolism of the European Society of Cardiology (ESC). Eur Heart J. 2008;29:2276–315.
13. Kearon C, Kahn SR, Agnelli G, Goldhaber S, Raskob GE, Comerota AJ. Antithrombotic therapy for venous thromboembolic disease. Chest. 2008; 133:454S–545S.
14. Bojić M, Sedgeman CA, Nagy LD, Guengerich FP. Aromatic hydroxylation of salicylic acid and aspirin by human cytochromes P450. Eur J Pharm Sci. 2015;73:49–56.
15. Bojić M, Debeljak Z, Tomičić M, Medić-Šarić M, Tomić S. Evaluation of antiaggregatory activity of flavonoid aglycone series. Nutr J. 2011;10:73.
16. Maleš Ž, Antolić A, Babić I, Jurić S, Bojić M. Quantitative analysis of phenolic acids and antiplatelet activity of *Melissa officinalis* leaf extracts. Nat Prod Commun. 2017;12:93–4.
17. Zhang YX, Yang TT, Xia L, Zhang WF, Wang JF, Wu YP. Inhibitory effect of Propolis on platelet aggregation in vitro. J Healthc Eng. 2017;2017:3050895.
18. Bojić M, Antolić A, Tomičić M. The effect of ethanolic extracts of propolis on platelet aggregation. Pharmacia. 2015;18:163.
19. Manach C, Williamson G, Morand C, Scalbert A, Rémésy C. Bioavailability and bioefficacy of polyphenols in humans. I. Review of 97 bioavailability studies. Am J Clin Nutr. 2005;81:230S–42S.
20. Cvek J, Medić-Sarić M, Jasprica I, Zubcić S, Vitali D, Mornar A, Vedrina-Dragojević I, Tomić S. Optimisation of an extraction procedure and chemical characterisation of Croatian propolis tinctures. Phytochem Anal. 2007;18:451–9.
21. Slinkard K, Singleton VL. Total phenol analysis: automation and comparison with manual methods. Am J Enol Vitic. 1977;28:49–55.
22. Maleš Ž, Plazibat M, Bilušić Vundać V, Žuntar I. Qualitative and quantitative analysis of flavonoids of the strawberry tree - *Arbutus unedo* L. (Ericaceae). Acta Pharma. 2006;56:245–50.
23. Council of Europe. European Pharmacopoeia. 6th ed. Strasbourg: Council of Europe; 2007.
24. Medić-Šarić M, Rastija V, Bojić M. Recent advances in the application of high performance liquid chromatography in the analysis of polyphenols in wine and propolis. J AOAC Int. 2011;94:32–42.
25. Social Science Statistics. 2017. http://www.socscistatistics.com. Accessed 30 Sep 2017.
26. Kumazawa S, Hamasaka T, Nakayama T. Antioxidant activity of propolis of various geographic origins. Food Chem. 2004;84:329–39.
27. Kalogeropoulos N, Konteles SJ, Troullidou E, Mourtzinos I, Karathanos VT. Chemical composition, antioxidant activity and antimicrobial properties of propolis extracts from Greece and Cyprus. Food Chem. 2009;116:452–61.
28. Socha R, Gałkowska D, Bugaj M, Juszczak L. Phenolic composition and antioxidant activity of propolis from various regions of Poland. Nat Prod Res. 2015;29:416–22.
29. Ristivojević P, Trifković J, Gašić U, Andrić F, Nedić N, Tešić Ž, Milojković-Opsenica D. Ultrahigh-performance liquid chromatography and mass spectrometry (UHPLC-LTQ/Orbitrap/MS/MS) study of phenolic profile of Serbian poplar type propolis. Phytochem Anal. 2015;26:127–36.
30. Huang S, Zhang CP, Wang K, Li GQ, Hu FL. Recent advances in the chemical composition of propolis. Molecules. 2014;19:19610–32.
31. Bojić M, Debeljak Ž, Medić-Šarić M, Tomičić M. Interference of selected flavonoid aglycons in platelet aggregation assays. Clin Chem Lab Med. 2012;50:1403–8.
32. Hubbard GP, Wolffram S, Lovegrove JA, Gibbins JM. Ingestion of quercetin inhibits platelet aggregation and essential components of the collagen-stimulated platelet activation pathway in humans. J Thromb Haemost. 2004; 2:2138–45.
33. Wright B, Moraes LA, Kemp CF, Mullen W, Crozier A, Lovegrove JA, Gibbins JM. A structural basis for the inhibition of collagen-stimulated platelet function by quercetin and structurally related flavonoids. Br J Pharmacol. 2010;159:1312–25.
34. Gómez-Betancur I, Pereañez JA, Patiño AC, Benjumea D. Inhibitory effect of pinostrobin from Renealmia alpinia, on the enzymatic and biological activities of a PLA2. Int J Biol Macromol. 2016;89:35–42.
35. Jin YR, Han XH, Zhang YH, Lee JJ, Lim Y Chung JH, Yun YP. Antiplatelet activity of hesperetin, a bioflavonoid, is mainly mediated by inhibition of PLC-gamma2 phosphorylation and cyclooxygenase-1 activity. Atherosclerosis. 2007;194:144–52.
36. Faggio C, Sureda A, Morabito S, Sanches-Silva A, Mocan A, Nabavi SF, Nabavi SM. Flavonoids and platelet aggregation: a brief review. Eur J Pharmacol. 2017;807:91–101.
37. Udovičić M, Baždarić K, Bilić-Zulle L, Petrovečki M. What we need to know when calculating the coefficient of correlation? Biochem Med. 2007;17:10–5.

# 6

# Erythrocyte DHA and AA in infancy is not associated with developmental status and cognitive functioning five years later in Nepalese children

Sigrun Henjum[1*], Ingrid Kvestad[2], Merina Shrestha[3], Manjeswori Ulak[3], Ram K. Chandyo[4], Andrew L. Thorne-Lyman[5,6], Prakash S. Shrestha[3], Marian Kjellevold[7], Mari Hysing[2] and Tor A. Strand[8,9]

**Abstract**

**Background:** Long chain polyunsaturated fatty acids (LCPUFA) especially docosahexaenoic acid (DHA) and arachidonic acid (AA) are crucial for normal brain development in utero and in early infancy. Data on fatty acid status and cognitive development in infants and children from low-income countries are scarce.

**Methods:** We examined the association between the DHA and AA status in infancy ($n = 320$) and developmental status and cognitive functioning five years later. At five years of age, we measured development by the Ages and Stages Questionnaire 3rd. ed. (ASQ-3) and cognitive functioning by subtests from the neuropsychological test battery NEPSY II. In addition, infant fatty acid composition in red blood cells (RBC) was analyzed. In multiple linear and logistic regression models, we estimated the associations between DHA and AA status in infancy and scores on the ASQ-3 and the NEPSY II subtests.

**Results:** There were no notable associations between infant AA and DHA status, and the scores on the ASQ-3 and the NEPSY II subtests five years later. It should be noted that we found better than expected concentrations of erythrocyte DHA and AA among the infants, and the ASQ scores were left-skewed, which limited the ability to identify associations.

**Conclusion:** DHA and AA status in infancy is seemingly not related to neurodevelopment measured 5 years later in this peri-urban population from Nepal.

**Keywords:** Polyunsaturated fatty acids, Plasma phospholipids, DHA, AA, Developmental status, Cognitive functioning, Follow up study, Nepalese children

## Background

Adequate nutrition, especially during pregnancy and infancy, is necessary for normal brain development [1, 2]. Long chain polyunsaturated fatty acids (LCPUFA) such as docosahexaenoic acid (DHA) and arachidonic acid (AA) are crucial in this process [2–5]. DHA and AA represent over 30% of all fatty acids in the gray matter of the human brain and the highest concentrations are found in the synapses of the neurons, where they have an important role in signal transduction [6]. DHA regulates numerous neuronal and glial cell processes including neurogenesis, neuroplasticity, neurite outgrowth, synaptogenesis and membrane fluidity, which in turn supports membrane protein functions affecting the speed of signal transduction and neurotransmission [7–10]. DHA and AA influence neurotransmission as precursors in the eicosanoid metabolism, and are important for normal function of the brain [11]. AA and DHA can either be supplied by dietary intake or synthesized from their essential precursors linoleic acid (LA) or a-linolenic acid (ALA), respectively. The conversion of ALA to eicosapentaenoic acid (precursor of DHA) is assumed to be low, and this may explain why

* Correspondence: sigrun.henjum@hioa.no; shenjum@oslomet.no
[1]OsloMet – Oslo Metropolitan University, Postboks 4, St. Olavs plass, Oslo, Norway
Full list of author information is available at the end of the article

formula-fed infants not consuming DHA have lower levels of DHA in brain compared to breast-fed infants [12]. Postpartum levels of DHA in the mother have been shown to be determined by DHA levels in pregnancy [13]. Thus, both insufficient maternal fatty acid status in pregnancy and the infants dietary sources of DHA after birth can put the infant at risk for deficiency in a critical period for the development of the central nervous system (CNS) [2, 12].

In the scientific literature, the role of LCPUFA on cognitive development is not conclusive. There is some evidence that LCPUFA supplementation has an effect on cognition among preterm [1, 3, 14–16] and low birth weight (LBW) infants [3, 4], in those who are LCPUFA deficient, [17, 18] or at risk for deficiency [6]. In full-term infants, however, beneficial effects of LCPUFA on cognition have been found in some [16, 18–20], but not in all studies [3, 6, 14, 21, 22]. The lack of an association of LCPUFA on cognition may have several explanations including differences in DHA and AA concentration of supplements/formula, duration of intervention, the type of development assessments, age at assessment, and the possibility of effect modification by unmeasured genetic polymorphisms (FADS) [23]. Emerging data demonstrate that the presence of FADS polymorphisms among study populations introduces substantial variation not recognized in initial studies in this field [23]. Few studies conducted in low-income countries have examined associations between fatty-acid status in infants and their longer-term development [1, 3, 24, 25].

In Bhaktapur, Nepal, despite low dietary intake of LA, ALA and LCPUFA, many infants and women had better DHA and AA status than expected [26, 27]. We observed a wide range of DHA and AA status, potentially making this a useful population to study associations with outcomes, such as child development and cognitive functioning. The aim of the present study is therefore to examine the association between the AA and DHA status in infancy and developmental status and cognitive functioning 5 years later in a representative sample of children from Nepal. In a recently published paper from the same study, we demonstrated that vitamin B12 status was significantly associated with these cognitive outcomes [28].

## Methods

### Design, recruitment, and participants

We used a two-stage cluster sampling procedure whereby 66 neighborhoods ("toles") were randomly selected as the primary sampling unit from 160. We listed all women living in these toles, and randomly selected women and infant pairs. The inclusion criteria for the study were that both mothers and children had no on-going clinically assessed infections that the infants were between 2 and 11 months, resided in the selected clusters, were willing to provide their household information, and consented to participate. Details of the selection criteria and a flow chart of the recruitment of the study subjects have been published elsewhere [29]. The study obtained ethical clearance from the institutional review board at the Institute of Medicine in Kathmandu, Nepal and the Regional Committee for Medical and Health Research Ethics in Norway. In 2012 and 2013, approximately five years after the first inclusions, we approached 330 of the children from the initial cohort of 500 women-child pairs for inclusion to developmental and neuropsychological assessment (Study 2) (Fig. 1). Of these 330, 10 children did not perform the Ages and Stages Questionnaire 3rd edition (ASQ-3) and 11 did not performed the NEPSY II. One child was excluded from the analysis due to the suspicion of a medical condition that undermined the validity of the assessment of that specific child, and the final number of valid assessments was 320 for ASQ-3 and 319 for the NEPSY II. In 36 children, we were not able to obtain sufficient blood at baseline, and thus the number of children in the regression analysis is 282 and 283. There were no major differences between the current subsample and the original sample in the demographic features such as child characteristics, child nutritional status and family situation at baseline, results are presented elsewhere [28]. Written consent was obtained from mothers at baseline and for the follow-up visits.

### Laboratory procedures

A trained phlebotomist drew approximately 3 mL of whole blood from the cubital vein at enrolment when the infant were between 2 and 11 months, into olypropylene tubes with lithium heparin (Sarstedt, Germany). The samples were then centrifuged (760×g, for 10 min, room temperature) and plasma was allocated into polypropylene vials (Eppendorf, Hinz, Germany). Samples were stored at − 20 °C at the field site laboratory until they were transported with an ice pack to the central laboratory in Kathmandu at the end of each day. There, samples were stored at − 80 °C until transport on dry ice to Norway. The fatty acid composition of total RBC was determined by ultrafast gas chromatography (UFGC) (Thermo Electron Corporation, Massachusetts, USA), using a method developed by Araujo P, Nguyen TT, Froyland L, Wang J and Kang JX [30]. Briefly, 50 μl homogenized samples were mixed with boron trifluoride (BF3) and internal standard (19:0 methyl ester), followed by extraction with hexane. The fatty acid composition was calculated using a labdataprogram (Chromeleon 6.80, Dionex Corporation, California, USA), connected to the UFGC and identification ascertained by standard mixtures of methyl esters (Nu-Chek, Minnesota, USA). Limit of quantification was 10 μg fatty acid/g samples (wet weight. *w*/w). The certified reference materials (CRM) CRM 162 (soy oil) and CRM 163 (pig fat) controlled the analytical quality of the method and systematic errors. The fatty acid composition

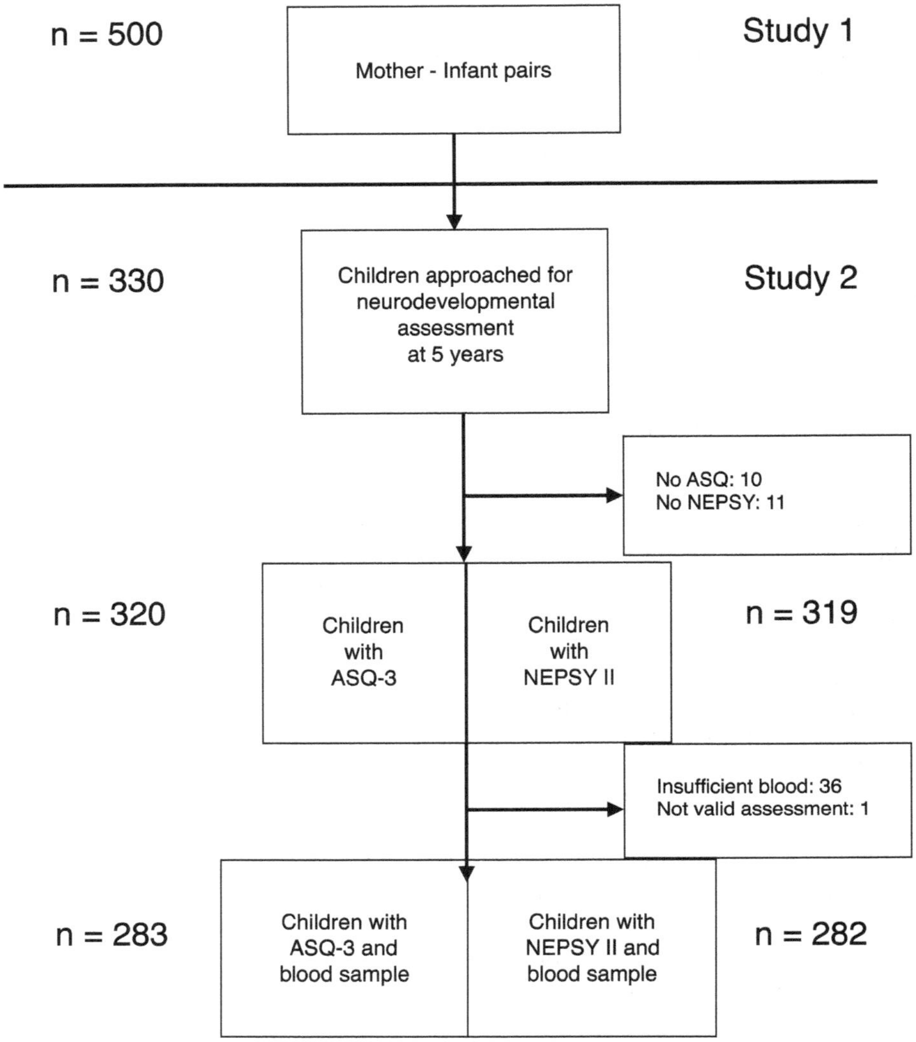


**Fig. 1** Flowchart of the study participants

of cooking oils was analyzed by gas liquid chromatography (GLC, Trace GC 2000, Termo) according to previously described method [31]. Total lipid content was extracted, filtered, evaporated, saponified and fatty acids were esterified. The methyl esters were separated using Auto-GC (Instrument-Teknikk AS, Norway), equipped with a 50 m CP sil 88 (Chrompack) fused silica capillary column (id:0.32 mm), using "cold on column" injection, temperature program (60 °C (25 °C/min) to 160 (25 °C/min) to 190 (25 °C/min) to 220) and flame ionization detector. The fatty acid composition was calculated using a labdataprogram (Turbochrom Navigator, Version 6.1), connected to the GLC and identification as ascertained by standard mixtures of methyl esters (Nu-Chek, Elyian, USA). Nonadecanoic acid (19:0) methyl ester was used as internal standard. Limit of quantification (LOQ) was 10 μg fatty acid/g sample (wet weight, *w*/w).

### Cognitive assessments

We used the Ages and Stages Questionnaire 3rd. edition and subtests from the NEPSY II, to assess neurodevelopment and cognitive functioning in the present study. A local pediatrician and a psychologist, both experienced in child development assessment, were trained to perform the assessments by two Norwegian clinical psychologists. The local psychologist performed most of the assessments under close supervision. Assessments were conducted at the study clinic in a well-lit room free from distractions. The children were followed to the clinic by their caregivers, and the caregivers had the opportunity to sit in the back of the room during the assessments. The sessions lasted for approximately one hour. A detailed description of the translation, training and assessment procedures are presented elsewhere [28].

The ASQ-3 is a comprehensive developmental screening, standardized for children 1–66 months with age-appropriate questionnaires [32]. The questionnaires contain 30 items that sums up to five subscales: communication, gross motor, fine motor, problem solving and personal-social (possible scores range from 0 to 60), and a total score (possible score range from 0 to 300). The ASQ-3 is designed to be answered by caregivers, but can also be used for direct assessment of the child by a trained professional [33] as we did in the current study. The examiner (the trained psychologist) aimed to answer the items in the questionnaire during the sessions and used a collection of standardized material (e.g. large and small balls, pen, paper and scissors) in the assessments. If the examiner could not answer the items through direct observation during the sessions, the response relied on answers from the caregiver. The 60 months questionnaire (age range 57–66 months) was used for the present study. In total, 160 of the 320 participants were above 66 months at the time of the assessment; however, we decided to perform the ASQ-3 for all children in the sample. The mean (SD) age in months at testing was 66.7 (3.4). The questionnaire was translated and back translated and culturally adapted particularly for this Nepalese setting according to standard procedures. A detailed description of the translation, training and assessment procedures are presented elsewhere [28].

The NEPSY-II is a comprehensive neuropsychological test battery that consists of 32 subtests in six functional domains for children aged 3 to 16 years [34]. The battery is flexible and allows for individual administration. The following six age–appropriate subtests were administrated in the present study: Inhibition, Statue, Visuo-motor Precision, Affect Recognition, Geometric Puzzles and Block construction. Since norms are not available for the Nepalese population, we calculated the scaled scores based on the American norms [34]. The NEPSY II scaled scores have a total possible range from 1 to 19, with 10 (3) as the mean (SD).

### Anthropometric measurements

Children were weighed on a UNICEF electronic pediatric scale (SECA, Germany) and length was measured using a locally made wooden board with an accuracy of ±0.1 cm. The Z-scores for height-for-age (HAZ) and weight-for-age (WAZ) were calculated using WHO growth reference standard from 2006 [35]. Children were classified as stunted or underweight if their HAZ or WAZ was <– 2 SD, respectively.

### Data management and statistics

Data were analysed using STATA version 14 (StataCorp., College Station,TX, USA). Data were expressed both as means (±SD) and median (IQR). We used multiple linear and logistic regression models to estimate the association between fatty acid status in infancy and the scores on ASQ-3 and the NEPSY II subtests approximately 5 years later. DHA and AA concentrations were used as the exposure variables in the different regression models both as linear variables and categorized in tertiles. The ASQ-3 subscales were highly skewed, and we dichotomized the scores at the 25th percentile and used logistic regression when analysing the subscales. An OR more than one indicates an increased risk of being in the lowest 25th percentile for each increment of a biomarker unit. We also undertook the multiple regression analyses adjusting for variables listed in Table 1, only variables that changed the exposure-outcome relationships by more than 15% were included in the final models. The variables included in the multiple regression models are sex, age at baseline, weight-for-age-z-score and age at testing. We present only the analyses of the linear exposure variables, and present both crude and adjusted estimates. The effect estimates are expressed as linear regression coefficient and odds

**Table 1** Variables assessed in the multiple regression models to measure the association between fatty acids (AA and DHA) and the ASQ-3 and NEPSY II scores

| | Continuous | Categorical |
|---|---|---|
| Sex | | male or female |
| Age at enrollment | months | |
| Exclusive breastfeeding at enrollment | – | yes or no |
| Iron status at enrollment | μmol/L | – |
| Height-for-age z-scores at enrollment | z scores | |
| Weight-for-height z-scores at enrollment | z scores | |
| Weight-for-age z-scores at enrollment | z scores | |
| Parity | | 1–2 or 2 and more |
| Energy intake mother at enrollment | Kcal /day | |
| Folate supplementation in pregnancy | | yes or no |
| Living in joint family | | yes or no |
| Family owns land | | yes or no |
| Number of rooms in the home | number | – |
| Mothers age | years | – |
| Level of education, mother | | less than 10th grade or 10th grade and more |
| Level of education, father | | less than 10th grade or 10th grade and more |
| Occupation, mother | | no work/agricultural or other work |
| Occupation, father | | no work/agricultural or other work |

ratios (OR), and a *p*-value-threshold of 0.05 was used to denote statistical significance. Post hoc, we stratified the analyses on children with birthweight less than 2500 g and children 2500 g and above.

## Results

Child, household and maternal characteristics and family situation at baseline are presented in Table 2. The mean (SD) age of the children at baseline was 7.0 (2.9) months and birthweight was 2872 (476) grams. Fourteen percent of the children had a birthweight below 2500 g. In total, 5% of the children were classified as underweight and 9% as stunted. Around half of the mothers and 70% of the fathers had more than 10th grade.

Median (IQR) and mean (range) for the total ASQ-3 score and the five subscales are presented in Table 3. The median (IQR) for the total score was 270 (255–285). Mean (SD) for the total raw and corresponding scaled NEPSY II scores in the 319 children are shown in Table 4. The mean scaled scores range from 5.9 (2.8) to 12.5 (1.7), with the lowest scores in the Visuo-motor precision total completion time subtest, and the highest in the Statue total score subtest.

Fatty acid composition of red blood cells in infants is presented in Table 5. The mean concentrations of DHA and AA for all infants were 116 and 311 μg/g, respectively. DHA was the main n-3 fatty acid, as AA was the major n-6 fatty acid.

Associations between DHA and AA and the total and subscale scores of the ASQ-3 in the Nepalese preschoolers are presented in Table 6. In both the multiple adjusted linear and logistic regression analysis we found no associations between ASQ-3 total and subscale scores with either AA or DHA. None of our analytical approaches (i.e. exposures categorized on tertiles) revealed any significant associations between developmental scores and fatty acid status. Low birth weight did not modify any of the associations (data not shown).

Associations between DHA and AA and the NEPSY II subtests in the Nepalese preschoolers are presented in Table 7. We found no notable associations between the

**Table 2** Child, parent, and household characteristics at baseline (n = 320)

| Characteristics | % (n) |
|---|---|
| Boys | 55.9 (179) |
| Age infant, months[a] | 7.0 (2.9) |
| Birth weight[a] | 2872 (476) |
| Birth weight < 2500 g | 14 (45) |
| Exclusively breast at enrolment | 13.6 (43) |
| Underweight (<−2 z score weight for age) | 5 (16) |
| Stunted (<−2 z score length for age) | 9 (27) |
| Mother: | |
| Age mother[a] | 26.1 (4.2) |
| Less than grade 10 of schooling | 48.2 (147) |
| 10th grade and more | 51.8 (158) |
| Working outside home | 26.2 (80) |
| Father: | |
| Less than grade 10 | 30.3 (94) |
| 10th grade and more | 69.7 (216) |
| Working outside home | 93.1 (281) |
| Household: | |
| Joint family | 53.8 (170) |
| Own land | 57.6 (182) |

[a]Mean (SD)
Characteristics of the total sample is presented elsewhere (24)

**Table 3** ASQ-3 total and subscale scores in 320 Nepali children

| Characteristics | Median (IQR) | Mean (Range) |
|---|---|---|
| Total ASQ-3 | 270 (255–285) | 265.8 (45–300) |
| Subscales: | | |
| Communication | 50 (40–55) | 47.9 (0–60) |
| Gross motor | 60 (60–60) | 57.6 (20–60) |
| Fine motor | 50 (45–55) | 49.1 (0–60) |
| Problem solving | 60 (55–60) | 55.9 (0–60) |
| Personal Social | 60 (50–60) | 55.1 (15–60) |

Total possible range is 0–300 for total score and 0–60 for the subscale score

**Table 4** NEPSY-II raw and scaled scores in 319 Nepali Children

| | | Raw scores (SD) | Mean scaled scores (SD)[a] | Range scaled scores |
|---|---|---|---|---|
| Attention and Executive Functioning | | | | |
| 1 | Inhibition-Naming Completion Time Total | 95.0 (23.9) | 10.2 (2.9) | 1–19 |
| | Inhibition-Inhibition Completion Time Total | 138.8 (38.6) | 9.8 (2.8) | 1–19 |
| | Inhibition Total Errors | 20.8 (16.3) | 8.7 (4.3) | 1–19 |
| 2 | Statue Total Score | 27.9 (2.8) | 12.5 (1.7) | 5–14 |
| Sensorimotor | | | | |
| 3 | Visuo-motor Precision Total Completion Time | 184.3 (56.3) | 5.9 (2.8) | 1–19 |
| | Visuo-motor Precision Combined Scaled Score | | 10.3 (2.2) | 4–19 |
| Social Perception | | | | |
| 4 | Affect Recognition Total Score | 14.5 (3.3) | 7.6 (3.3) | 1–15 |
| Visuospatial Processing | | | | |
| 5 | Block Construction Total Score | 7.4 (1.7) | 7.9 (2.5) | 1–15 |
| 6 | Geometric Puzzles Total Score[b] | 13.3 (3.0) | | |

[a]The NEPSY II scaled scores are calculated based on US norm. The scaled scores have a total possible range from 1 to 19, with 10(3) as mean (SD)
[b]Scaled scores are not available for this age range

**Table 5** Fatty acid composition of red blood in infants ($n$ = 303)[a]

| | Infants (n = 303) (µg/ml) | % |
|---|---|---|
| Total SAFA | 948 (99) | 41 |
| Total MUFA | 449 (76) | 19 |
| Total PUFA | 906 (158) | 38 |
| Total *n*-6 PUFA | 685 (128) | 29 |
| Total *n*-3 PUFA | 222 (44) | 9.4 |
| 18:2 *n*-6 (LA) | 269 (76) | 11.3 |
| 18:3 *n*-3 (ALA) | 5.4 (5) | 0.2 |
| 20:4 *n*-6 (AA) | 311 (59) | 13.2 |
| 20:5 *n*-3 (EPA) | 8.3 (4) | 0.3 |
| 22:6 *n*-3 (DHA) | 116 (22) | 4.9 |
| 22:5 *n*-3 (DPA) | 37 (11) | 1.6 |
| n-6/n-3 PUFA *Ratio* | 3.2 (0.6) | |
| Sum fatty acids | 2345 (293) | |
| Omega 3 index %[b] | | 5.2 |

Mean ± SD
[a]Has been presented elsewhere (21)
[b]Sum %EPA + %DHA (% of sum of total fatty acids)

NEPSY II subtests with either AA or DHA in the linear regression models.

## Discussion

Overall, we did not find any associations between early DHA and AA status and developmental status by ASQ-3 and cognitive functioning by NEPSY II five years later in a sample of 303 children from Nepal.

The lack of associations between early DHA and AA status and neurodevelopmental scores in our study is in accordance with literature that report no beneficial effect of n-3 LCPUFA supplementation on cognitive function in full-term infants [14, 21, 22, 36–39]. However, four recent reviews reported that n-3 LCPUFA supplementation in term infants might have a potential effect on later child development [2, 16, 18, 23]. Few studies have in general investigated the long-term associations between early fatty acid status and cognitive function. A longitudinal examination of the relationship over time may be needed given that the subtle effects of fatty acids on the brain may not show up until later in childhood [3]. Two studies have reported beneficial effects on some specific aspects of cognition (attention, speed of processing, and problem solving), suggesting that the effects of LCPUFA supplementation in early life may be better detectable at a later age for specific cognitive functions [40, 41]. Some other studies assessed cognitive development of children between 6 or 9 years of age and found no overall positive effect of fatty acids on general cognitive functioning [42–44].

According to Carlson, the effect of DHA and AA status and supplementation in infancy has been largely evaluated through global developmental assessments focused on attainment of normative milestones, although more granular measures of specific cognitive function may be more sensitive markers of the effects of

**Table 6** Associations between DHA and AA and the total and subscale scores of the ASQ-3 in Nepali preschoolers

| VARIABLES | | N | AA | | | DHA | | |
|---|---|---|---|---|---|---|---|---|
| Linear regression | | | Coeff. | CI | *P* | Coeff. | CI | *P* |
| Total ASQ-3 | crude | 283 | 3.61 | (− 0.28, 7.50) | 0.07 | 8.48 | (−2.30, 19.27) | 0.12 |
| | adjusted[a] | 282 | −0.56 | (− 4.40, 3.29) | 0.77 | − 1.60 | (− 11.39, 8.209 | 0.75 |
| Logistic regression | | | OR | | | | | |
| Total ASQ-3 | crude | 283 | 0.56 | (0.36, 0.87) | 0.01 | 0.26 | (0.08, 0.81) | 0.02 |
| | adjusted[a] | 282 | 0.85 | (0.52, 1.40) | 0.52 | 0.65 | (0.20, 2.13) | 0.48 |
| Subscales | | | OR | | | | | |
| Communication | crude | 283 | 0.44 | (0.23, 0.82) | 0.01 | 0.10 | (0.02, 0.51) | 0.01 |
| | adjusted[a] | 282 | 0.72 | (0.35, 1.46) | 0.36 | 0.28 | (0.04, 1.90) | 0.19 |
| Gross motor | crude | 283 | 0.83 | (0.46, 1.50) | 0.54 | 0.39 | (0.09, 1.73) | 0.22 |
| | adjusted[a] | 282 | 1.11 | (0.58, 2.12) | 0.75 | 0.73 | (0.13, 4.19) | 0.72 |
| Fine motor | crude | 283 | 1.01 | (0.68, 1.79) | 0.70 | 1.33 | (0.40, 4.45) | 0.64 |
| | adjusted[a] | 282 | 1.40 | (0.87, 2.26) | 0.16 | 2.38 | (0.71, 8.01) | 0.16 |
| Problem Solving | crude | 283 | 0.71 | (0.42, 1.21) | 0.21 | 0.49 | (0.10, 2.32) | 0.37 |
| | adjusted[a] | 282 | 1.01 | (0.60, 1.72) | 0.96 | 1.03 | (0.24, 4.37) | 0.97 |
| Personal Social | crude | 283 | 1.07 | 0.52, 2.23) | 0.85 | 1.62 | (0.28, 9.40) | 0.59 |
| | adjusted[a] | 282 | 1.34 | (0.64, 2.78) | 0.44 | 2.78 | (0.45, 17.14) | 0.27 |

Linear and logistic regression models adjusted for clustering
[a]Adjusted for sex, age at baseline and weight-for-age z-scores at baseline and age at testing
OR > 1 indicates an increased risk of being in the lowest 25th percentile for each increment of one biomarker units

**Table 7** Crude and adjusted[b] associations between AA and DHA and the NEPSY-II subtests in Nepali preschoolers[a]

| VARIABLES | | | AA | | | DHA | | |
|---|---|---|---|---|---|---|---|---|
| | | N | Coefficient | CI | *P* | Coefficient | CI | *P* |
| Attention and Executive Functioning | | | | | | | | |
| Inhibition-Naming Completion Time Total - raw | crude | 282 | −3.34 | (−7.91, 1.23) | 0.15 | −2.90 | (−14.18, 8.38) | 0.61 |
| | adjusted | 281 | −3.26 | (−7.44, 0.93) | 0.12 | −1.95 | (− 12.85, 8.96) | 0.72 |
| Inhibition-Inhibition Completion Time Total- raw | crude | 282 | −6.00 | (−12.01, 0.02) | 0.03 | −10.60 | (−27.63, 6.44) | 0.22 |
| | adjusted | 281 | −6.84 | (−13.59, − 0.09) | 0.05 | − 11.99 | (− 30.27, 6.29) | 0.19 |
| Inhibition Total Errors - raw | crude | 282 | −0.41 | (−3.33, 2.52) | 0.78 | 1.96 | (−4.55, 8.48) | 0.55 |
| | adjusted | 281 | 0.19 | (−2.49, 2.86) | 0.89 | 3.43 | (−2.88, 9.74) | 0.28 |
| Statue Total Score - raw | crude | 282 | −0.11 | (−0.56, 0.34) | 0.64 | 0.00 | (−1.31, 1.31) | 1.00 |
| | adjusted | 281 | −0.13 | (− 0.61, 0.35) | 0.60 | − 0.03 | (−1.40, 1.33) | 0.96 |
| Sensorimotor | | | | | | | | |
| Visuo-motor Precision Total Completion Time - raw | crude | 282 | 4.69 | (−6.23, 15.62) | 0.39 | 4.69 | (−22.81, 32.18) | 0.73 |
| | adjusted | 281 | 3.69 | (−6.73, 14.11) | 0.48 | 3.38 | (−22.71, 29.47) | 0.80 |
| Social Perception | | | | | | | | |
| Affect Recognition Total Score - raw | crude | 282 | 0.33 | (−0.46, 1.14) | 0.40 | 0.93 | (−1.22, 3.07) | 0.39 |
| | adjusted | 281 | 0.20 | (−0.56, 0.95) | 0.61 | 0.69 | (−1.34, 2.72) | 0.50 |
| Visuospatial Processing | | | | | | | | |
| Geometric Puzzles - raw | crude | 282 | 0.63 | (0.06, 1.21) | 0.03 | 1.80 | (0.22, 3.40) | 0.03 |
| | adjusted | 281 | 0.60 | (0.03, 1.16) | 0.04 | 1.70 | (0.07, 3.32) | 0.04 |
| Block Construction - raw | crude | 282 | 0.24 | (−0.05, 0.53) | 0.10 | 0.31 | (−0.50, 1.13) | 0.44 |
| | adjusted | 281 | 0.21 | (−0.06, 0.49) | 0.12 | 0.22 | (−0.60, 1.03) | 0.60 |

[a]All models are adjusted for clustering
[b]Adjusted for sex, age at baseline and weight-for-age z score at baseline and age at testing

LCPUFA supplementation [19]. Researchers now have access to techniques to measure brain electrical interconnectivity and brain structure and function; these techniques were not used in the early studies of DHA and AA supplementation and could explain the lack of an effect [23].

Trials have found a positive effect of n-3 LCPUFA supplementation on cognitive function in low birth weight (LBW) infants at risk of deficiency in certain fatty acids, including DHA [3, 4]. Regional estimates of LBW include 28% in South Asia [45]. In our study sample, 14% of the infants had LBW, however, we did not find any difference in either essential fatty acid concentration or the ASQ-3 and NEPSY II scores when the analyses was stratified on children less than 2500 g and children 2500 g and above.

From the literature, there are some evidence for a favorable effect of n-3 LCPUFA in children deficient in fatty acids [17, 18]. In many low to middle-income countries, including Nepal, diets are lacking EFA and low fatty acids status would be expected. Despite substantial variability in fatty status, we found better than expected concentrations of erythrocyte DHA and AA among breastfeeding women and their infants in Nepal [26], and this may explain the lack of associations between early DHA and AA status and developmental scores five years later in the current study. The main dietary source of fat among the Nepali women was sunflower, soybean, sesame, and mustard oils. The relatively high concentration of LA in the cooking oils ensured a substantial intake of this essential fatty acid in their diet. For ALA, the concentration in cooking oil was considerably lower, giving a much lower total intake of ALA. Cooking oils and ghee had very low concentrations of AA; no item provided more than 1 mg/g, and DHA was not detected in any of the analyzed food items. Some of the vegetable oils commonly used in food preparation contained EPA and may be a significant dietary source [27]. Analysis of differences in genetic polymorphisms (FADS) should be taken into consideration in future studies [23]. Further, child development may be influenced by several other nutritional inadequacies, such as undernutrition, iron- zinc and B-vitamin deficiency, in addition to inadequate childcare and home environment [1]. Our multivariable models were adjusted for potential confounders including age, nutritional status, exclusive breastfeeding, maternal education and family situation (Table 1), however, given the observational nature of our dataset we cannot rule out the possibility for unmeasured negative confounding that may have led to bias in our study.

Even though we did not find any association between DHA and AA status and the neurodevelopmental scores five years later in this follow-up study, it is well established that fatty acids are crucial for optimal brain development [1]. DHA and AA are major components of the brain, and play an important role in the structure and function of all cell membranes [6] through neuron proliferation, synapse formation, pruning, and myelination [1]. Why then is the crucial role of fatty acids in brain development not reflected in the numerous RCT and epidemiological studies aiming to link fatty acids and cognitive performance, and why do systematic reviews and meta-analyses often show conflicting results? Firstly, comparison of results from different studies is often compromised by differences in age of supplementation, different dosages and different lengths of supplementation, lack of consideration of FADS polymorphisms, the inclusion of populations only of a specific age, or exclusion of healthy individuals only. Secondly, the large heterogeneity in cognitive tests may complicate the comparison of the potential effect of fatty acid status on brain development [3, 16, 19, 23].

To the best of our knowledge, this is one of the first studies on fatty acid status and child development in South Asia and the first from Nepal. In addition to a representative sample of children, one of the strengths of our study is that fatty acid status of the infants was measured in the infants' red blood cells, as recommended [18], not maternal fat intake or maternal fatty acid status during pregnancy and lactation. A trained local psychologist performed the neurodevelopmental assessment by the ASQ-3 and NEPSY II; however, it should be noted, that these tools have not been validated for a Nepalese setting. The assessment has been used previously in similar settings and the psychometric properties are comparable to those of other studies [33]. The fact that 160 of the children were above the recommended age range for the ASQ-3 assessment may have compromised our results and could explain the null findings in the models with the ASQ-3 scores. In spite of the limitation that approximately half of the children where above the recommended age range for the ASQ-3, the data has previously yielded findings in a study on vitamin B-12 status and child development, which give support to the validity of the developmental variables [28].

In conclusion, no notable associations between early DHA and AA status and overall developmental status and cognitive functioning five years later, were found in this study among children from a peri-urban area of Nepal. It should be noted that better than expected concentrations of erythrocyte DHA and AA were found, and the ASQ scores were left-skewed, which limited the ability to identify associations.

#### Abbreviations

AA: arachidonic acid; ALA: a-linolenic acid ASQ-3: Ages and Stages Questionnaire 3rd. ed.; CNS: central nervous system; DHA: docosahexaenoic acid; HAZ: height-for-age; LA: linoleic acid LBW: low birth weight; LCPUFA: long chain polyunsaturated fatty acids; RBC: red blood cells; WAZ: weight-for-age

#### Acknowledgments

We want to thank the children and their families for participating in this study. We are also grateful to the staff at Siddhi Memorial Hospital and the fieldworkers.

#### Funding

Supported by Research Council of Norway (project No. 172226), and a grant from the GCRieber Funds, South-Eastern Norway Regional Health Authority (grant No. 2012090) and by the USAID Feed the Future Innovation Laboratory for Nutrition (USAID grant number AID-OAA-L-1-00005).

#### Authors' contributions

The contributions of the authors were as follows: TAS, IK, MH, PS, RKC and MS designed and conducted the research; IK, TAS and SH analysed the data; SH wrote the paper; IK, MK, MH, ALT-L and MU contributed to writing the paper. SH had primary responsibility for the final content. All authors read and approved the final manuscript.

#### Competing interests

The authors declare that they have no competing interests.

#### Author details

[1]OsloMet – Oslo Metropolitan University, Postboks 4, St. Olavs plass, Oslo, Norway. [2]Regional Center for Child and Youth Mental Health and Child Welfare, West, Uni Research Health, Bergen, Norway. [3]Department of Child Health, Tribhuvan University Teaching Hospital, Kathmandu, Nepal. [4]Department of Community Medicine, Kathmandu Medical College, P.O. Box 21266, Kathmandu, Nepal. [5]Center for Human Nutrition, Department of International Health, Johns Hopkins Bloomberg School of Public Health, Baltimore, MD, USA. [6]Harvard T.H. Chan School of Public Health, Boston, MA, USA. [7]Institute of Marine Research, 5817 Bergen, Norway. [8]Division for Medical Services, Innlandet Hospital Trust, Lillehammer, Norway. [9]The Center for International Health, University of Bergen, Bergen, Norway.

#### References

1. Prado EL, Dewey KG. Nutrition and brain development in early life. Nutr Rev. 2014;72:267–84.
2. Lauritzen L, Brambilla P, Mazzocchi A, Harslof LB, Ciappolino V, Agostoni C. DHA effects in brain development and function. Nutrients. 2016;8:6.
3. Koletzko B, Boey CC, Campoy C, Carlson SE, Chang N, Guillermo-Tuazon MA, Joshi S, Prell C, Quak SH, Sjarif DR, et al. Current information and Asian perspectives on long-chain polyunsaturated fatty acids in pregnancy,

lactation, and infancy: systematic review and practice recommendations from an early nutrition academy workshop. Ann Nutr Metab. 2014;65:49–80.
4. Harris WS, Baack ML. Beyond building better brains: bridging the docosahexaenoic acid (DHA) gap of prematurity. J Perinatol. 2015;35:1–7.
5. Karr JE, Alexander JE, Winningham RG. Omega-3 polyunsaturated fatty acids and cognition throughout the lifespan: a review. Nutr Neurosci. 2011;14: 216–25.
6. van de Rest O, van Hooijdonk LW, Doets E, Schiepers OJ, Eilander A, de Groot LC. B vitamins and n-3 fatty acids for brain development and function: review of human studies. Ann Nutr Metab. 2012;60:272–92.
7. Horrocks LA, Farooqui AA. Docosahexaenoic acid in the diet: its importance in maintenance and restoration of neural membrane function. Prostaglandins Leukot Essent Fatty Acids. 2004;70:361–72.
8. Innis SM. Dietary (n-3) fatty acids and brain development. J Nutr. 2007;137: 855–9.
9. Luchtman DW, Song C. Cognitive enhancement by omega-3 fatty acids from child-hood to old age: findings from animal and clinical studies. Neuropharmacology. 2013;64:550–65.
10. Tassoni D, Kaur G, Weisinger RS, Sinclair AJ. The role of eicosanoids in the brain. Asia Pac J Clin Nutr. 2008;17(Suppl 1):220–8.
11. Wauben IP, Wainwright PE. The influence of neonatal nutrition on behavioral development: a critical appraisal. Nutr Rev. 1999;57:35–44.
12. Cunnane SC, Francescutti V, Brenna JT, Crawford MA. Breast-fed infants achieve a higher rate of brain and whole body docosahexaenoate accumulation than formula-fed infants not consuming dietary docosahexaenoate. Lipids. 2000;35:105–11.
13. Markhus MW, Rasinger JD, Malde MK, Froyland L, Skotheim S, Braarud HC, Stormark KM, Graff IE. Docosahexaenoic acid status in pregnancy determines the maternal docosahexaenoic acid status 3-, 6- and 12 months postpartum. Results from a longitudinal observational study. PLoS One. 2015;10:e0136409.
14. Makrides M, Collins CT, Gibson RA. Impact of fatty acid status on growth and neurobehavioural development in humans. Matern Child Nutr. 2011;7:80–8.
15. Qawasmi A, Landeros-Weisenberger A, Bloch MH. Meta-analysis of LCPUFA supplementation of infant formula and visual acuity. Pediatrics. 2013;131: e262–72.
16. Jiao J, Li Q, Chu J, Zeng W, Yang M, Zhu S. Effect of n-3 PUFA supplementation on cognitive function throughout the life span from infancy to old age: a systematic review and meta-analysis of randomized controlled trials. Am J Clin Nutr. 2014;100:1422–36.
17. Cooper RE, Tye C, Kuntsi J, Vassos E, Asherson P. Omega-3 polyunsaturated fatty acid supplementation and cognition: a systematic review and meta-analysis. J Psychopharmacol. 2015;29:753–63.
18. Stonehouse W. Does consumption of LC omega-3 PUFA enhance cognitive performance in healthy school-aged children and throughout adulthood? Evidence from clinical trials. Nutrients. 2014;6:2730–58.
19. Carlson SE, Colombo J. Docosahexaenoic acid and arachidonic acid nutrition in early development. Adv Pediatr. 2016;63:453–71.
20. Birch EE, Garfield S, Hoffman DR, Uauy R, Birch DG. A randomized controlled trial of early dietary supply of long-chain polyunsaturated fatty acids and mental development in term infants. Dev Med Child Neurol. 2000;42:174–81.
21. Simmer K, Patole SK, Rao SC. Long-chain polyunsaturated fatty acid supplementation in infants born at term. Cochrane Database Syst Rev. 2011: CD000376.
22. Qawasmi A, Landeros-Weisenberger A, Leckman JF, Bloch MH. Meta-analysis of long-chain polyunsaturated fatty acid supplementation of formula and infant cognition. Pediatrics. 2012;129:1141–9.
23. Lien EL, Richard C, Hoffmann DR. DHA and ARA addition to infant formula: current status and future research directions. Prostaglandins Leukotrienes and Essential Fatty Acids. 2018;128:26–40.
24. Walker SP, Wachs TD, Grantham-McGregor S, Black MM, Nelson CA, Huffman SL, Baker-Henningham H, Chang SM, Hamadani JD, Lozoff B, et al. Inequality in early childhood: risk and protective factors for early child development. Lancet. 2011;378:1325–38.
25. Huffman SL, Harika RK, Eilander A, Osendarp SJ. Essential fats: how do they affect growth and development of infants and young children in developing countries? A literature review Matern Child Nutr. 2011;7(Suppl 3):44–65.
26. Henjum S, Lie O, Ulak M, Thorne-Lyman AL, Chandyo RK, Shrestha PS, W WF, Strand TA, Kjellevold M. Erythrocyte fatty acid composition of Nepal breast-fed infants. Eur J Nutr. 2017;
27. Henjum S, Torheim LE, Thorne-Lyman AL, Chandyo R, Fawzi WW, Shrestha PS, Strand TA. Low dietary diversity and micronutrient adequacy among lactating women in a peri-urban area of Nepal. Public Health Nutr. 2015;18:3201–10.
28. Kvestad I, Hysing M, Shrestha M, Ulak M, Thorne-Lyman AL, Henjum S, Ueland PM, Midttun O, Fawzi W, Chandyo RK, et al. Vitamin B-12 status in infancy is positively associated with development and cognitive functioning 5 y later in Nepalese children. Am J Clin Nutr. 2017;105:1122–31.
29. Henjum S, Manger M, Skeie E, Ulak M, Thorne-Lyman AL, Chandyo R, Shrestha PS, Locks L, Ulvik RJ, Fawzi WW, Strand TA. Iron deficiency is uncommon among lactating women in urban Nepal, despite a high risk of inadequate dietary iron intake. Br J Nutr. 2014;112:132–41.
30. Araujo P, Nguyen TT, Froyland L, Wang J, Kang JX. Evaluation of a rapid method for the quantitative analysis of fatty acids in various matrices. J Chromatogr A. 2008;1212:106–13.
31. Lie O, Lambertsen G. Fatty acid composition of glycerophospholipids in seven tissues of cod (Gadus morhua), determined by combined high-performance liquid chromatography and gas chromatography. J Chromatogr. 1991;565:119–29.
32. Squires J, Bricker D. Ages & stages questionnaires [R], (ASQ-3 [TM]): a parent-completed child-monitoring system. Brookes Publishing Company. 2009;
33. Kvestad I, Taneja S, Kumar T, Bhandari N, Strand TA, Hysing M, Study G. The assessment of developmental status using the ages and stages questionnaire-3 in nutritional research in north Indian young children. Nutr J. 2013;12:50.
34. Brooks BL, Sherman EMS, Strauss E. NEPSY-II: a developmental neuropsychological assessment, second edition. Child Neuropsychology. 2009;16:80–101.
35. de Onis M, Onyango AW, Borghi E, Siyam A, Nishida C, Siekmann J. Development of a WHO growth reference for school-aged children and adolescents. Bull World Health Organ. 2007;85:660–7.
36. Drover JR, Hoffman DR, Castaneda YS, Morale SE, Garfield S, Wheaton DH, Birch EE. Cognitive function in 18-month-old term infants of the DIAMOND study: a randomized, controlled clinical trial with multiple dietary levels of docosahexaenoic acid. Early Hum Dev. 2011;87:223–30.
37. Scott DT, Janowsky JS, Carroll RE, Taylor JA, Auestad N, Montalto MB. Formula supplementation with long-chain polyunsaturated fatty acids: are there developmental benefits? Pediatrics. 1998;102:E59.
38. Hoffman DR, Boettcher JA, Diersen-Schade DA. Toward optimizing vision and cognition in term infants by dietary docosahexaenoic and arachidonic acid supplementation: a review of randomized controlled trials. Prostaglandins Leukotrienes & Essential Fatty Acids. 2009;81:151–8.
39. Eilander A, Hundscheid DC, Osendarp SJ, Transler C, Zock PL. Effects of n-3 long chain polyunsaturated fatty acid supplementation on visual and cognitive development throughout childhood: a review of human studies. Prostaglandins Leukotrienes & Essential Fatty Acids. 2007;76:189–203.
40. Colombo J, Carlson SE, Cheatham CL, Shaddy DJ, Kerling EH, Thodosoff JM, Gustafson KM, Brez C. Long-term effects of LCPUFA supplementation on childhood cognitive outcomes. Am J Clin Nutr. 2013;98:403–12.
41. Willatts P, Forsyth S, Agostoni C, Casaer P, Riva E, Boehm G. Effects of long-chain PUFA supplementation in infant formula on cognitive function in later childhood. Am J Clin Nutr. 2013;98:536S–42S.
42. Bakker EC, Hornstra G, Blanco CE, Vles JS. Relationship between long-chain polyunsaturated fatty acids at birth and motor function at 7 years of age. Eur J Clin Nutr. 2009;63:499–504.
43. Drover JR, Felius J, Hoffman DR, Castaneda YS, Garfield S, Wheaton DH, Birch EE. A randomized trial of DHA intake during infancy: school readiness and receptive vocabulary at 2-3.5 years of age. Early Hum Dev. 2012;88:885–91.
44. de Jong C, Kikkert HK, Fidler V, Hadders-Algra M. Effects of long-chain polyunsaturated fatty acid supplementation of infant formula on cognition and behaviour at 9 years of age. Dev Med Child Neurol. 2012;54:1102–8.
45. World Health Assembly. Global nutrition targets 2025. Low birth weight policy brief vol. In: Accessed 31th of; January 2018. http://www.who.int/nutrition/topics/globaltargets_lowbirthweight_policybrief.pdf.

# 7

# Progress of children with severe acute malnutrition in the malnutrition treatment centre rehabilitation program: evidence from a prospective study in Jharkhand, India

Anuraag Chaturvedi[1*], Ashok K. Patwari[2], Deepa Soni[1], Shivam Pandey[3], Audrey Prost[4], Raj Kumar Gope[5], Jyoti Sharma[3] and Prasanta Tripathy[5]

## Abstract

**Background:** In Jharkhand, Malnutrition Treatment Centres (MTCs) have been established to provide care to children with severe acute malnutrition (SAM). The study examined the effects of facility- and community based care provided as part the MTC program on children with severe acute malnutrition.

**Method:** A cohort of 150 children were enrolled and interviewed by trained investigators at admission, discharge, and after two months on the completion of the community-based phase of the MTC program. Trained investigators collected data on diet, morbidity, anthropometry, and utilization of health and nutrition services.

**Results:** We found no deaths among children attending the MTC program. Recovery was poor, and the majority of children demonstrated poor weight gain, with severe wasting and underweight reported in 52 and 83% of the children respectively at the completion of the community-based phase of the MTC program. The average weight gain in the MTC facility ($3.8 \pm 5.9$ g/kg body weight/d) and after discharge ($0.6 \pm 2.1$ g/kg body weight/d) was below recommended standards. 67% of the children consumed food that met less than 50% of the recommended energy and protein requirement. Children experienced high number of illness episodes after discharge: 68% children had coughs and cold, 40% had fever and 35% had diarrhoea. Multiple morbidities were common: 50% of children had two or more episodes of illness. Caregiver's exposure to MTC's health and nutrition education sessions and meetings with frontline workers did not improve feeding practices at home. The take-home ration amount distributed to children through the supplementary food program was inadequate to achieve growth benefits.

**Conclusions:** Recovery of children during and after the MTC program was suboptimal. This highlights the need for additional support to strengthen MTC program so that effective care to children can be provided.

**Keywords:** Wasting, Assessment of nutritional status, Severe acute malnutrition, Malnutrition treatment centers, Food and nutrient intake, India

* Correspondence: anuraag7@gmail.com
[1]Public Health Foundation of India, Gurugram, India
Full list of author information is available at the end of the article

## Background

Wasting in children is the result of recent rapid weight loss or failure to gain weight due to hunger and/or disease. Children suffering from wasting have low immunity, are susceptible to developmental delays and face an increased risk of death [1]. The prevalence of severe wasting (WHZ less than − 3 of the median WHZ in WHO Child Growth Standards) in the state of Jharkhand (located in Eastern India) is high and greater than the national average: in 2016, 11.4% of children aged 0–35 months were severely wasted in Jharkhand, compared to a national average of 7.5%. Therefore, at any point of time, around 0.6 million children in the state are severely wasted [2].

To address this challenge, Jharkhand's State government has established 88 malnutrition treatment centres (MTCs) through the National Health Mission (NHM), where children with severe acute malnutrition (SAM)—severe wasting and/or mid-upper arm circumference (MUAC) < 115 mm and/or bilateral pitting oedema— receive medical and therapeutic care based on the WHO and Indian Academy of Pediatrics protocols [3–5]. Detection of children with SAM in the community is done by the Anganwadi workers (AWWs) of the Integrated Child Development Services (ICDS) program. Once at the MTC, children are again screened for SAM and admitted to MTC if they meet the admission criterion. After admission, children are treated for their medical complications and fed locally prepared therapeutic formula F-75 every 2 h for 2 days, and subsequently, F-100 six time daily for 48 h.[1] After completing 4 days at the MTC, children are alternately fed F-100 and locally prepared semi-solid therapeutic food until the child is discharged from the centre. During stabilization phase, nurses conduct health and nutrition education sessions for caregivers on child feeding, illness management, immunization and hygiene. Children are discharged from MTC when they have (a) no signs of bilateral pitting oedema, fever and/or infection, and (b) gained at least 5 g/kg body weight/d. After discharge, children are transitioned to the community phase of the program, where they are followed up in the community by frontline workers; enrolled into the ICDS supplementary nutrition program; and returned for three follow-up visits to the MTC every 15 days during the 2 months following discharge.

Between July 2009–June 2011, 3595 children were treated in the 48 MTCs of Jharkhand [6]. MTC results highlight the following challenges: high defaulting rates; poor weight gain once children are back in the community; and low attendance rate in the follow-up visits. However, there is limited about the reasons for this persistent challenges [6]. Current literature on MTC, or Nutrition rehabilitation centers (NRCs) as they are called in other parts of India, have mainly reported treatment outcomes for the facility-based phase of the program. During the community-based phase however, children often return to an environment where optimal care for children remains a challenge. The objective of our study is to describe children's outcomes for both phases of the program, determine access and utilization of post-discharge services, and measure compliance of health and nutrition practices advised by MTC in order to inform future implementation of the MTC and broader nutrition programs in India.

## Methods

### Study sites and participants

We randomly selected 14 out of the 48 MTCs operating before March 2011 for the study. A total of 150 children admitted to these MTCs between December 20, 2011 and January 31, 2012 were enrolled and followed at three points: at admission (first contact), discharge (second contact), and after completion of 2 months of community phase of the program (third contact). We interviewed 116 children and their caregivers at discharge (34 defaulted and left the MTC against the advice of the MTC staff), and 100 children after completion of community phase of the program (18 had migrated and 2 could not be located).

### Data collection

We obtained data on the health and nutritional status of children at admission and discharge from MTC records. Caregivers (mothers) were interviewed by local trained investigators after obtaining their written informed consent. In case respondents could not read or write, alternate witnessed consent process was followed. We pretested the study instruments in the community and collected data on: (a) mothers' socio-economic and demographic characteristics; (b) children's morbidity during first and third contact (c) dietary intake in the past 24 h during third contact; (d) utilisation of Integrated child development services(ICDS) and health services during first and third contact; (e) knowledge, attitude and practice of caregivers on child feeding during all three conatcts; (f) anthropometric measurements at all three contacts.

All anthropometric assessments were conducted as per WHO (2006) protocol. Anthropometric measurements were conducted by trained field investigators. Children were weighed without clothes on portable electronic scales accurate to the nearest 0.1 kg that were calibrated daily. Portable infantometers and stadiometers accurate to 0.1 cm were used to record length and height respectively. Mid upper-arm circumference was measured using MUAC tapes supplied by UNICEF.

Anthropometric measurements were taken twice and the mean value was recorded.

Dietary information was obtained using 24-h dietary recall by probing caregivers in detail. Using standardized kitchen utensils, cut outs and kitchen weighing scales, investigators recorded the food amount, ingredients and feeding time. For any reported outside snacks, samples of packaged local snacks were collected for measurement reference. Knowledge of caregivers on MTC recommended child feeding practices was assessed through structured open ended questions and categorized as right or wrong. The feeding practices were evaluated from children's 24-h dietary recall survey.

## Data analysis

Statistical analysis was performed using SPSS, version 19 (SPSS Inc., Chicago). We used Anthro software, WHO version 3.0.1, to generate anthropometric indices. Diet analysis was conducted by trained nutritionists. We converted dietary data into individual raw food weights and analyzed these using Diet Soft version 1.1.9. The diet's energy and protein nutrient adequacy was compared against recommendations for catch up growth (at least 150 kcal/kg/day and 4 g protein/kg/day). [7] Analysis of variance (ANOVA) and chi-square tests were used to test for statistical significance and changes in anthropometric indices were tested with repeated measure ANOVA tests.

Poisson regression was used to identify factors associated with follow-up visits to MTC, and McNemar's test was applied to analyze change in child feeding knowledge of caregivers after admission in the MTC program.

## Results

Children admitted in MTC were very young (Table 1); 85% of children were in the 6–23 months' age group.

**Table 1** Characteristics of children and their mothers in the MTC program

| | First Contact (Admission) | Second contact (Discharge) | Third Contact (Community- based phase) | Defaulted & Loss to follow-up |
|---|---|---|---|---|
| Children's Sex (%) | | | | |
| Male | 46 | 46.2 | 47 | 44 |
| Female | 54 | 53.8 | 53 | 56 |
| Children's Age, months (%) | | | | |
| 6–11 | 38.7 | 33.9 | 25 | 32 |
| 12–23 | 45.3 | 49.2 | 55 | 46 |
| 24–35 | 12 | 14.4 | 14 | 16 |
| 36+ | 4 | 2.5 | 6 | 6 |
| Mother's religion(%) | | | | |
| Hindu | 29.3 | 30.5 | 30 | 28 |
| Muslim | 6 | 5.1 | 6 | 4 |
| Sarna | 54 | 56.8 | 55 | 60 |
| Others | 10.7 | 7.6 | 9 | 8 |
| Mother's caste(%) | | | | |
| SC | 9.3 | 11 | 10 | 10 |
| ST | 68 | 70.3 | 71 | 72 |
| OBC | 15.3 | 14.4 | 14 | 12 |
| General | 7.4 | 4.2 | 5 | 6 |
| Mother's age (%) | | | | |
| 18–25 | 46.7 | 47.5 | 47 | 42 |
| 26–30 | 24 | 22.9 | 24 | 26 |
| 31+ | 29.3 | 29.7 | 29 | 32 |
| Mother's education (%) | | | | |
| No schooling | 67.3 | 66.1 | 66 | 70 |
| 1–8 | 26.1 | 29 | 29 | 28 |
| 9+ | 6.6 | 5.2 | 5 | 2 |
| Total children and mothers | 150 | 116 | 100 | 50 |

Over half (54%) of children were girls, and 68% belonged to scheduled tribe(ethnic/tribal) families. The majority of caregivers were 18–25 years' old and had received no formal schooling. Enrollment characteristics—socio-demographic and wasting status—of children who defaulted were similar to those who completed the 2 months' follow-up.

### Child growth

Tables 2 describes the anthropometric indices of children and their growth status at discharge and follow up. Out of 150 children admitted, 116 (77.3%) children completed their treatment at the MTC, their average length of stay at MTC was 16.2(SD: ±4.9) days. About 22% of children achieved the recommended weight gain of 8 g/kg/day in MTC, with the average weight gain being 3.8 g/kg/day (SD: ±5.9). WHZ and WAZ scores improved significantly between admission and discharge, though all children remained in the severe underweight category (WAZ < – 3) at discharge. After transition of the children to community-based phase of the program, their average weight gain per day reduced to 0.6 g/kg/day (SD: ±2.1) and many became undernourished again. At follow-up, more children were severely undernourished than at discharge; 52% of children were severely wasted (mean WHZ: – 3.1 ± 1.5) and 83% were underweight (mean WAZ: – 4.0 ± 1.1) at follow-up.

### Dietary intake by children

Table 3 describes the mean macronutrient and micronutrient intake of children as well as the nutrition adequacy of their diet during community phase of the program. The recommendations for adequate energy and protein intake for children are at least 150 Kcal/kg bodyweight/day, and 4 g/Kg bodyweight/day, respectively. 67 and 63% children consumed food that met less than 50% energy and protein requirement on the day preceding the survey. We found no significant association between the children's age or sex and energy and protein adequacy levels. The energy and protein intake of severely wasted children was significantly lower compared to that of moderately wasted children and normal children. The mean iron and zinc intake in the previous day's diet was inferior to recommended daily allowances for all age groups. Mean meal frequency was similar among severely wasted (2.4 ± 2.0), moderately wasted (2.8 ± 2.1) and normal children (3.5 ± 2.7).

### Morbidity

We assessed morbidity among children in last 2 months preceding the survey (results not shown). Caregivers reported episodes of cold or cough in 68% of children (median episode:1; average duration 6.6 ± 3.8 days), followed by fever in 40% children (median episodes:1.5; average duration 4.5 ± 2.1 days) and diarrhoea in 35% children (median episode:1; average duration 4.8 ± 3.2 days). Multiple morbidities were common in children after discharge from MTCs: About 15% children reported all three morbidities; while 26% reported two morbidities during last 2o months preceding the survey. Few children remained free from illness: 21% children reported no illness. Highest reported morbidities were found in the 12–23 months' age group: 74% cough and cold incidences, 38% diarrhoea, and 34% fever were reported from this age group. No significant association was observed between illness and gender.

### Follow up visits to MTCs

Sixteen children were lost to follow-up due to migration in the community-based phase of the study. Out of the 100 children, 19% attended all three follow-up visits to MTC. 19% of children attended two and 21% children attended one follow-up visits. 41% of children did not attend any follow-up visit. The Poisson regression analysis

**Table 2** Anthropometric indices of children and weight gain during facility-based and community-based phase of the MTC program

| | Facility based Phase | | | Community–based phase | *p*-value |
|---|---|---|---|---|---|
| | Admission *N* = 150 | Discharge *N* = 116 | *p*-value | *N* = 100 | |
| WHZ (mean ± SD) | −3.2 ± 1.9 | −2.8 ± 1.1 | 0.001 | −3.1 ± 1.5 | 0.018[‡] |
| Severe (%) | 54 | 40 | | 52 | |
| Moderate (%) | 46 | 38 | | 27 | |
| Normal (%) | – | 22 | | 21 | |
| WAZ (mean ± SD) | −4.2 ± 1.2 | −3.8 ± 1.1 | < 0.001 | −4.0 ± 1.1 | 0.001[‡] |
| Severe (%) | 84 | 71 | | 83 | |
| Moderate (%) | 16 | 26 | | 14 | |
| Normal (%) | – | 3 | | 3 | |
| Average weight gain/body weight/day (grams) | | 3.8 ± 5.9 | | 0.6 ± 2.1 | < 0.001[‡] |

[‡]Significant difference between community-based phase and discharge

**Table 3** Mean macro and micronutrient intake of children after discharge by age group and growth status, and nutrient adequacy from home diet on the day preceding the survey

| | Energy intake (mean Kcal ± SD) | *P*-value | Protein intake (mean g ± SD) | *P*-value | Iron intake (mean mg ± SD) | *P*-value | Zinc intake (mean mg ± SD) | *P*-value |
|---|---|---|---|---|---|---|---|---|
| Age group | | | | | | | | |
| 6–11 months | 266.8 ± 135.3 | | 7.7 ± 4.7 | | 1.4 ± 0.9 | | 0.9 ± 0.5 | |
| 12–23 months | 459.7 ± 211.8 | < 0.001[1] | 12.0 ± 6.5 | 0.05 | 2.5 ± 1.9 | 0.01[1] | 1.4 ± 0.8 | 0.01[1] |
| ≥ 24 months | 484.0 ± 163.1 | | 12.4 ± 7.4 | | 3.6 ± 4.2 | | 1.6 ± 0.6 | |
| WHZ status | | | | | | | | |
| Severe | 365.1 ± 198.9 | | 9.1 ± 6.1 | | 2.6 ± 3.0 | | 1.3 ± 0.7 | |
| Moderate | 465.3 ± 168.1 | 0.01[1] | 11.7 ± 5.7 | 0.05 | 2.2 ± 2.1 | 0.8 | 1.3 ± 0.7 | 0.4 |
| Normal | 504.0 ± 221.9 | | 13.9 ± 6.8 | | 2.6 ± 1.7 | | 1.6 ± 0.8 | |
| Nutrient adequacy (%)[2] | | | | | | | | |
| < 50% | 67% | | 63% | | | | | |
| 50–66% | 22% | | 18% | | | | | |
| 66–100% | 11% | | 19% | | | | | |

[1]Significant difference between groups; ANOVA, [2]Energy adequacy: subject's calorie intake/(150 Kcal/kg bodyweight); Protein: subject's protein intake/(4 g/kg bodyweight)

after adjusting socio-demographic factors, mother's education, growth status at discharge, child morbidities and length of stay at MTC, indicated that increased number of follow-up visits to MTC was significantly ($p < 0.05$) associated with awareness about the need for three follow-up visits (adjusted PR: 4.3; 95%CI: 2.0–9.1); caregivers being accompanied by someone to MTC (adjusted PR: 2.1; 95% CI: 1.4–3.1); and children having MUAC< 115 mm at discharge (adjusted PR: 1.9; 95% CI: 1.1–3.6).

### Knowledge and practice about child feeding and hygiene practices

We measured and analyzed caregivers' knowledge on child feeding and hygiene at three time intervals: at admission; at discharge; and again during community phase to assess retention of MTC delivered messages (Table 4). McNemar's test determined that compared to pre-admission knowledge, more caregivers had correct knowledge on diet modification at discharge (21% vs 52%; $p < 0.001$) and food quantity (1% vs 35% $P < 0.001$), while no difference was observed for knowledge on feeding frequency and food consistency. Caregivers retained this knowledge during the community phase; the proportion of caregivers with correct knowledge on child feeding practices was similar at discharge and in the community-based phase. We examined children's diet in the previous day before the survey in the community-based phase; this showed a gap between caregiver's knowledge and practice; 37% caregivers knew that children should be fed five or more times per day, but only 14% of the caregivers practiced this.

### Linkages with local nutrition and health services after discharge

Jharkhand's Integrated Child Development Services (ICDS) programme mandates free distribution of double amount of take-home ration (THR) of rice, daal (lentils), soyabean, oil and sugar to all children after their discharge from MTC. The majority of caregivers received less than one-third of the entitled THR (Table 5). The majority of caregivers reported contact by frontline workers after discharge from MTC—60% Anganwadi

**Table 4** Caregivers correct knowledge and practice on child feeding and hygiene at three time intervals

| | At Admission | At discharge | *P*-value[1] | At follow-up | *P*-value[2] |
|---|---|---|---|---|---|
| Knowledge about feeding frequency (%) | 30 | 34 | 0.60 | 37 | 0.75 |
| Gave at least five meals to the child in last 24 h (%) | – | – | – | 14 | – |
| Knowledge about dietary modification (%) | 21 | 52 | < 0.001 | 56 | 0.6 |
| Modified child's food in last 24 h (%) | – | – | | 0 | – |
| Knowledge about food consistency (%) | 53 | 57 | 0.5 | 60 | 0.7 |
| Knowledge about food quantity (%) | 2 | 35 | < 0.001 | 33 | 0.8 |
| Awareness of six MTC promoted hygiene practices | – | 2.8 ± 1.8 | | 4.4 ± 2.1 | < 0.001 |

[1]Difference between admission and discharge, [2]Difference between follow-up and discharge

**Table 5** Linkages between caregivers and frontline workers and services received in the community-based phase of the program

| Distribution of Take Home Ration (THR) in the previous month (%) | ≤ 1/3 amount | 1/3–2/3 amount | Full amount | Mean amount (grams ± SD) |
|---|---|---|---|---|
| Rice (3000 g) | 81 | 19 | – | 1129 ± 362.5 |
| Lentils (750 g) | 78 | 22 | – | 269.4 ± 92.5 |
| Soyabean (500 g) | 63 | 37 | – | 171.1 ± 94.6 |
| Cooking oil (250 g) | 16 | 60 | 24 | 123.5 ± 66.1 |
| Sugar (1900 g) | 100 | – | – | 249.1 ± 104.5 |
| Contact with Frontline workers in last 2 months (%) | None | One contact | Two contacts | Three or more contacts |
| AWW | 12 | 28 | 38 | 22 |
| ASHA (Sahiya) | 21 | 25 | 33 | 21 |
| ANM | 36 | 29 | 28 | 7 |
| Weight measurement by frontline workers in last two months (%) | Not weighed | Weighed once | Weighed twice | Weighed thrice |
| | 31 | 33 | 26 | 10 |

workers (AWW) and 54% ASHA (Sahiya) contacted caregivers two or more times in last 2 months preceding the survey. About 36% caregivers reported monthly weight measurement of children, while 31% said that child had not been weighed (Table 5). Consumption of Iron supplementation by children was reported by 26% caregivers and deworming by 15% caregivers after discharge from MTC.

## Discussion

This study examines children's progress in the MTC program—in facility, and after discharge in the community-based phase of the program. Our result show, children gained weight below the national standards of care, suffered multiple morbidities, defaulted on follow-up visits, and received food supplements that were inadequate to meet their needs. These are important findings and strengthens the need for finding appropriate solutions to provide effective care for SAM children in the program.

MTC or NRC program in India has shown high survival outcomes (< 5% child deaths) [6, 8] and a similar performance was observed in our study. In spite of many children being severely wasted at discharge, we found no deaths among children in the program. A study in rural India that followed 409 severely wasted children reported low case-fatality (1.2–2.7%) among children without community management of acute malnutrition [9].

Recovery among children remained poor as majority of the children demonstrated poor weight gain during both phases of the program. The children's average weight gain in the MTC facility and after discharge was below the recommended national and international standards [10, 11], and lower than that achieved by other programs in India [12] and Community Based Management of Acute Malnutrition (CMAM) programs elsewhere [13]. The poor weight gain suggests of sub-optimal quality of the therapeutic food in MTC, and low energy and protein dense foods at home. In our study, two out every three children received less than 50% of the energy required (at least 150 Kcal/kg body weight/day) and protein required (4 g/Kg body weight/day) from their previous day's home diet. Consumption of high energy density meals is known to result in higher weight gains, and when small meals are consumed, their energy density becomes even more important [14, 15]. Dietary analysis of children highlighted inadequacy of energy-and-nutrient dense foods in their meals. Caregivers fed foods of thin consistency, minimal diversity, and fed small portion in main meals. In our study, caregivers typically fed children 2–3 meals (rice with lentils or vegetable gravy) in a day, and provided occasional snacks (biscuits, local savories and *murhi*-rice puffs) between meals. While we did not assess household food security(HHFS), this has been shown to affect diet, nutrition and infant feeding practices. Better HHFS status has been reported to be associated with the type of complementary foods given to the infants [16], and was also observed as a significant predictor of receiving a minimally acceptable diet for infants [17].

Morbidity was common post-discharge, about 50% of all children reported more than two illnesses in the 2 months of the community phase of the program. Micronutrient deficiencies could have led to morbidity by impairing immune function. We found that children's diet was essentially vegetarian and micronutrient intake (iron, zin and calcium) remained inferior to recommended daily allowances for all age groups. In the 2 months after discharge from MTC facility, no micronutrient supplements were provided except vitamin A under routine immunization program. Diarrhoea remains a common health problem after treatment of SAM [18, 19] which is unsurprising given that children return to the same environment characterised by inadequate food, poor access to sanitation and safe water. Khanum and Ashworth observed that 92% children after treatment of SAM in Bangladesh experienced diarrhoea (mean:7episodes; range 0–30) during 1 year and weight gain tended to be lower in children who experienced more episodes of diarrhoea. [20]

Our results showed no difference in the weight gain of children who did not attend any follow-up visit compared to those who visited MTC after discharge. Caregivers defaulted on their follow-up visit to MTC due to low awareness about the need for re-visits and non-availability of family members or acquaintance to accompany caregivers to MTC. The low attendance rate for follow-up visits was similar to a previous study in Jharkhand where 62.4% of the 2770 discharge children did not return for any follow-up visits, and only 14.9% children completed the three follow-up visits. Caregiver's awareness about the services and their opportunity cost are important factors as they may influence the health seeking behavior. Puett and Guerrero [21] in a study in Pakistan and Ethiopia observed that caregiver's low awareness about the services, distance to the facility and the accompanying transportation cost negatively impacted the access to CMAM services. Role of frontline workers has shown to be central in reducing default rates. In the neighboring state of Bihar, involvement of ASHA contributed to the sharp decline in default rate to < 20%. [22] In our study, frontline workers played a major role in the identification and admission of SAM children to MTCs but became inactive during the follow-up visits: ASHA and AWWs identified 51 and 40% SAM cases; accompanied caregivers to MTC for admission in 44 and 31% cases; but in follow-up visits accompanied caregivers only in 13 and 5% cases respectively. Effective actions are required to improve compliance to the follow-up visits. Improved community messaging regarding follow-up visits and integration of follow-up visit with existing incentive based health delivery services of health workers could improve follow-up visits of caregivers to MTC.

Health and nutrition education sessions conducted by nurses at MTC showed mixed results. Caregiver's awareness about the child feeding practices improved for few topics, but many still remained unaware about the correct feeding practices at the time of discharge. The result underscores the need for support to strengthen the content and delivery of MTC education sessions. Our results also showed that majority caregivers did not adopt optimal feeding practices known to them. In-depth interviews (data not reported) with caregivers showed feeding frequent meals remained a challenge due to competing demands of siblings; workload in the house and field; and limited cooking resources at home. Discrepancies between maternal knowledge and practice had been found to be related with psychological and social factors that included cultural experiences, existing norms and expectations, available support, time constraints and work load. [23] We also observed that the regular contact between caregivers and frontline workers did not improve the child feeding practices at home. A capacity assessment study of AWWs in Gujarat observed that AWWs had adequate knowledge on infant young child feeding practices but could not engage effectively with caregivers, lacked the skills to assess child's breastfeeding and complementary feeding practices and provided general advice to caregivers irrespective of child's condition [24]. As observed elsewhere, frontline workers consider weight measurement in the growth monitoring sessions as an end in itself, and fail to discuss with caregivers the reasons for growth faltering and solutions to address it [25, 26]. A literature search of successful community-based rehabilitation programs for the period from 1980 to 2005 found involvement of motivated and trained staff who taught caregivers about child feeding and health promotion through structured program; had sessions that required caregivers to practice what they had learned; and provided continuous reinforcement to caregivers through home visits. [7] Sub-optimal child feeding practices of caregivers despite their regular contact with frontline workers calls for strengthening the counseling capacity of frontline ICDS and NHM workers so that caregivers could be guided for compliance to the MTC promoted feeding and hygiene practices.

All severely underweight children and those discharged from MTCs are entitled for double THR amount. That distribution of THR amount was inadequate for the children to realize growth benefits. Previous studies on ICDS have attributed poor coverage of take-home ration to low demand for the product due to poor ration quality; distribution to non-eligible households; and insufficient stocks at AWCs [27, 28]. Intra-household sharing of ration targeted at the children remains a challenge for food based programs. Results from our previous study showed that out of the reduced THR received by severely underweight children, 70% was further shared with other family members [29]. For better targeting of children in the community-based phase, the existing ICDS provision of hot cooked meals to 3–6 years' age children can be modified and extended to children with SAM so to provide them with cooked meals comprising of essential macro and micronutrients.

Our study had several limitations: (a) Fifty children had defaulted after admission to MTC and could not be traced. Mortality among defaulted children remains unknown. Although no differences existed between children who defaulted and those who continued in the program, the study instruments might not have captured all the differences; (b) Morbidity information is subject to uncertainty as it was not validated, and caregivers might have failed to accurately recall illness episodes due to 2 month's recall period. (c) Breastmilk volume consumed by children was not assessed, the inclusion of which would have improved the reported nutrient intake among the children (d) About three-fourth of the study children belonged to the tribal families, caution must be taken to generalize the findings to SAM children treated at rehabilitation centres in general. (e) Data on complicated and non-complicated SAM at MTC was not available, analysis of which could have provided more insights about the children's recovery in the program.

## Conclusions

To date facility- based management remains the accepted strategy to treat children with SAM in India. The following suggestions could be summarized from this study to improve the performance of MTC program.

1. Provide appropriate therapeutic foods in MTC to ensure minimum average weight gain. At home, aim to provide high-energy, high-protein diet to children for rapid weight gain
2. Set up a responsive system at community level to provide health services during morbidity episodes. Provide micronutrient supplementation after discharge to improve immune function
3. Invest in improving the technical and counseling skills of MTC nurses and frontline workers so that active support can be extended to caregivers on child feeding and health care practices.
4. Modify and extend hot cooked meals served to 3–6 years' age children under ICDS supplementation program to children with SAM so to provide them with meals comprising of essential macro and micronutrients

## Endnotes

[1]Composition of locally prepared F-75(per 1000 ml): cow's milk or toned milk (300 ml), sugar (60 g), vegetable oil (25 g) puffed rice (25 g), water (to complete 1000 ml). Composition of F-100 (per 1000 ml): cow's milk or toned milk (750 ml), sugar (25 g), vegetable oil (20 g), puffed rice (70 g), water (to complete 1000 ml). Composition of locally prepared semi-solid therapeutic food (per 100 g): roasted groundnuts (25.5 g), milk powder (30.6 g), coconut oil (15.3 g) and sugar (28.6 g)

#### Abbreviations

ANM: Auxiliary Nurse Midwife; ASHA: Accredited Social Health Activist; AWW: Anganwadi Workers; CMAM: community based management of acute malnutrition; HAZ: Height for age z score; ICDS: Integrated Child Development Services; MTC: Malnutrition Treatment Centre; NHM: National Health Mission; SAM: Severe Acute Malnutrition; THR: Take Home Ration; WAZ: Weight for age Z score; WHZ: weight for height z score

#### Acknowledgements

We would like to acknowledge John M. Pile, Chief of Party MCH-STAR initiative for his support during study implementation. The support of NHM Jharkhand and MTC staff members is acknowledged sincerely.

#### Funding

The study was supported by MCH-STAR (CARDNO EMG), initiative of United States Agency for International Development (USAID); grant number 4390-000-PHFI-00-ROG-06. Funding agency had no involvement in study design, data collection, analysis, or in this manuscript writing.

#### Authors' contributions

AC as principal investigator conceived, designed and implemented the study and prepared the draft manuscript. PKT and RKG implemented the study in Jharkhand and critically reviewed the draft. DS wrote the draft manuscript with AC and SP helped in statistical analysis. AKP provided oversight to the study, reviewed study instruments and manuscript. AP and JS reviewed interim analysis and interpretation and helped in manuscript writing. All authors read and approved the final manuscript.

#### Competing interests

The authors declare that they have no competing interests.

#### Author details

[1]Public Health Foundation of India, Gurugram, India. [2]Hamdard Institute of Medical Sciences and Research and H.A.H.Centenary Hospital, Hamdard University, New Delhi, India. [3]Indian Institute of Public Health, Gurugram, India. [4]University College London, London, UK. [5]Ekjut, Chakradharpur, Jharkhand, India.

#### References

1. Schaible UE, Kaufmann SHE. Malnutrition and infection: complex mechanisms and global impacts. PLoS Med. 2007;4:e115.
2. National Family Health Survey 4 - State Fact Sheet: Jharkhand. http://rchiips.org/NFHS/pdf/NFHS4/JH_FactSheet.pdf. Accessed 20 June 2017.
3. List of Malnutrition Treatment Centre. http://mtc.dreamworksinfotech.com/Downloads.aspx. Accessed 7 Jan 2017.
4. Bhatnagar S, Lodha R, Choudhury P, Sachdev HP, Shah N, Narayan S, Wadhwa N, Makhija P, Kunnekel K, Ugra D. IAP guidelines 2006 on hospital based management of severely malnourished children (adapted from the WHO guidelines). Indian Pediatr. 2007;44:443–61.
5. WHO. Guideline: update on technical aspects of the management of severe acute malnutrition in infants and children. Geneva: World Health Organization; 2013.
6. Aguayo VM, Jacob S, Badgaiyan N, Chandra P, Kumar A, Singh K. Providing care for children with severe acute malnutrition in India: new evidence from Jharkhand. Public Health Nutr. 2014;17:206–11.
7. Ashworth A. Efficacy and effectiveness of community-based treatment of severe malnutrition. Food Nutr Bull. 2006;27:S24–48.
8. Singh K, Badgaiyan N, Ranjan A, Dixit H, Kaushik A, Kushwaha K, Aguayo V. Management of children with severe acute malnutrition: experience of nutrition rehabilitation centers in Uttar Pradesh, India. Indian Pediatr. 2014; 51:21–5.
9. Sachdev HS, Sinha S, Sareen N, Pandey RM, Kapil U. Survival and recovery in severely wasted under-five children without Community Management of Acute Malnutrition Programme. Indian Pediatr. 2017;54(10):817-24.

10. MoHFW. Operational guidelines on facility-based management of children with severe acute malnutrition. New Delhi: India Government of India; 2011.
11. The Sphere Project. Humanitarian charter and minimum standards in humanitarian response: 2011 edition.. Bangalore, India The Sphere; 2011.
12. Aguayo VM, Agarwal V, Agnani M, Das Agrawal D, Bhambhal S, Rawat AK, Gaur A, Garg A, Badgaiyan N, Singh K. Integrated program achieves good survival but moderate recovery rates among children with severe acute malnutrition in India. Am J Clin Nutr. 2013;98:1335–42.
13. Collins S, Sadler K, Dent N, Khara T, Guerrero S, Myatt M, Saboya M, Walsh A. Key issues in the success of community-based Management of Severe Malnutrition. Food Nutr Bull. 2006;27:S49–82.
14. Brown KH, Sanchez-Grinan M, Perez F, Peerson JM, Ganoza L, Stern JS. Effects of dietary energy density and feeding frequency on total daily energy intakes of recovering malnourished children. Am J Clin Nutr. 1995; 62:13–8.
15. Brooke OG, Wheeler EF. High energy feeding in protein-energy malnutrition. Arch Dis Child. 1976;51:968–71.
16. Owais A, Kleinbaum DG, Suchdev PS, Faruque A, Das SK, Schwartz B, Stein AD. Household food security and infant feeding practices in rural Bangladesh. Public Health Nutr. 2016;19:1875–81.
17. Saha KK, Frongillo EA, Alam DS, Arifeen SE, Persson LA, Rasmussen KM. Household food security is associated with infant feeding practices in rural Bangladesh. J Nutr. 2008;138:1383–90.
18. Munthali T, Jacobs C, Sitali L, Dambe R, Michelo C. Mortality and morbidity patterns in under-five children with severe acute malnutrition (SAM) in Zambia: a five-year retrospective review of hospital-based records (2009–2013). Arch Public Health. 2015;73(1)
19. Kumar R, Singh J, Joshi K, Singh HP, Bijesh S. Co-morbidities in hospitalized children with severe acute malnutrition. Indian Pediatr. 2014;51:125–7.
20. Khanum S, Ashworth A, Huttly SR. Growth, morbidity, and mortality of children in Dhaka after treatment for severe malnutrition: a prospective study. Am J Clin Nutr. 1998;67:940–5.
21. Puett C, Guerrero S. Barriers to access for severe acute malnutrition treatment services in Pakistan and Ethiopia: a comparative qualitative analysis. Public Health Nutr. 2015;18:1873–82.
22. Burza S, Mahajan R, Marino E, Sunyoto T, Shandilya C, Tabrez M, Kumari K, Mathew P, Jha A, Salse N, Mishra KN. Community-based management of severe acute malnutrition in India: new evidence from Bihar. Am J Clin Nutr. 2015;101:847–59.
23. Brodribb W. Barriers to translating evidence-based breastfeeding information into practice. Acta Paediatr. 2011;100:486–90.
24. Chaturvedi A, Nakkeeran N, Doshi M, Patel R, Bhagwat S. Capacity of frontline ICDS functionaries to support caregivers on infant and young child feeding (IYCF) practices in Gujarat, India. Asia Pac J Clin Nutr. 2014;23(Suppl 1):S29–37.
25. Gerein NM, Ross DA. Is growth monitoring worthwhile? An evaluation of its use in three child health programmes in Zaire. Soc Sci Med. 1991;32:667–75.
26. George SM, Latham MC, Frongillo EA, Abel R, Ethirajan N. Evaluation of effectiveness of good growth monitoring in south Indian villages. Lancet. 342:348–52.
27. Ramakrishnan U, Lowe A, Vir S, Kumar S, Mohanraj R, Chaturvedi A, Noznesky EA, Martorell R, Mason JB. Public health interventions, barriers, and opportunities for improving maternal nutrition in India. Food Nutr Bull. 2012;33:S71–92.
28. Leyvraz M, Wirth JP, Woodruff BA, Sankar R, Sodani PR, Sharma ND, Aaron GJ. High coverage and utilization of fortified take-home rations among children 6-35 months of age provided through the integrated child development services program: findings from a cross-sectional survey in Telangana, India. PLoS One. 2016;11:e0160814.
29. Chaturvedi A, Sharma J, Patwari AK, Prost A, Pandey S, Gope RK, Tripathy P: How do children with severe acute malnutrition progress after discharge from malnutrition treatment Centres? Evidence from Jharkhand, India. Manuscript submitted for publication. 2017.

# 8

# Family-based intervention using face-to-face sessions and social media to improve Malay primary school children's adiposity: a randomized controlled field trial of the Malaysian REDUCE programme

Norliza Ahmad[1], Zalilah Mohd Shariff[2], Firdaus Mukhtar[3] and Munn-Sann Lye[1*]

**Abstract**

**Background:** Social media may be an effective medium by which parents could be trained to promote healthy eating behaviour and physical activity for their children. This trial evaluates the effectiveness of a family-based intervention using social media in combination with face-to-face sessions - the REDUCE (REorganise Diet, Unnecessary sCreen time and Exercise) programme - on adiposity of Malay children.

**Methods:** Five primary schools in an urban area in Selangor, Malaysia participated in this two-arm randomized controlled field trial. Participants were parents ($n = 134$) and their primary school-going children 8–11 years of age who were either overweight or obese. These parent-child dyads were randomly allocated to intervention and wait-list control groups and were blinded to group assignment. The intervention was a four-week training programme using two face-to-face sessions and two Facebook sessions followed by weekly booster sessions over a three-month period using WhatsApp. The primary outcome was body mass index (BMI) z-score. Height, body weight, waist circumference and percentage of body fat were measured by blinded assessors. Data were collected at baseline (T1), immediately post-training (T2) and at three- (T3) and six-month post training (T4) and were analysed using generalized linear mixed modelling adjusted for covariates to estimate the intervention effects. Subgroup analysis was conducted for overweight and obese children.

**Results:** Ninety-one percent of parents completed the study, 64 in intervention group and 58 in wait-list group. At the sixth month post-training, BMI z-scores were significantly reduced in the intervention group compared to the wait-list group, for the all children (overweight and obese children) and within the obese subgroup (($F(6, 517) = 2.817$, $p = 0.010$) and ($F(6, 297) = 6.072$, $p < 0.001$) respectively. For waist circumference percentile and body fat percentage, the intervention group experienced a significant reduction compared to the wait-list group, within the obese subgroup (($F(6, 297) = 3.998$, $p = 0.001$) and within the overweight subgroup ($F(6, 201) = 2.526$, $p = 0.022$).

**Conclusions:** The four-month REDUCE intervention programme was effective in reducing childhood adiposity. Further research using this approach needs to be conducted including cost-effectiveness studies before implementing it in a child obesity prevention programme.

(Continued on next page)

* Correspondence: lyems9@yahoo.com; lyemunn@upm.edu.my
[1]Department of Community Health, Faculty of Medicine and Health Sciences, Universiti Putra Malaysia, Level 1, Block B (Academic), 43400 UPM, Serdang, Selangor, Malaysia
Full list of author information is available at the end of the article

(Continued from previous page)

**Keywords:** Paediatric obesity, Social media, Body mass index, Waist circumference, Body fat percentage, Parents intervention, Primary school children

## Background

The prevalence of overweight and obesity among children 5 to 19 years of age was reported to have experienced a tenfold increase worldwide from 11 million in 1975 to 124 million in 2016 [1]. Developing countries are now experiencing such a trend where the relative percentage increase was 59% between the year 1980 and 2013 compared to 41% increase in developed countries [2]. In Malaysia - a developing country - the childhood obesity prevalence increased from 3.9% in 2011 to 11.9% in 2015 [3, 4]. Because childhood obesity is associated with negative health effects, it warrants serious public health attention to prevent further increase in its prevalence [5].

Some ethnic groups are more affected by obesity and in Malaysia, the Chinese have the highest prevalence of obesity (13.0%), followed by Indians (12.6%) and Malays (11.8%). However, in terms of absolute numbers, Malays form the largest group as they are the ethnic majority in Malaysia and thus are more greatly affected in terms of disease burden. The ethnic composition in Malaysia consists of Malay (52.9%), Chinese (27.8%), Indian (13.3%) and other ethnic groups (6%) [6]. Healthy lifestyle programmes that are socio-culturally customized may be more effective [7] and thus this intervention programme was tailored to the Malay ethnicity.

Parents can influence the eating behaviour and physical activities of their children; thus intervention programmes that targeted parents as the agent of change had their roots decades ago [8–19]. However, parents often had other commitments that hindered their adherence to face-face intervention programmes [20]. New approaches to educate parents in nutrition and physical activity have emerged - there is an increasing trend in using social media as a mode of communication among young people and adults. As of April 2018, the most common social networking site worldwide was Facebook (2.2 billion), followed by WhatsApp (1.5 billion), You Tube (1.5 billion) and Facebook Messenger (1.3 billion) [21]. About 76.9% of Malaysians use the Internet, and 97.3% of them are Facebook users [22]. Systematic reviews of experimental studies on health behaviour intervention concluded that this platform could be effectively used to promote behaviour change [23, 24]. Thus, the use of social networking as a platform to provide health education and impart relevant skills could be feasible and appropriate. Studies have incorporated social media in body weight management [25–28] but using this modality among parents to influence their children is a fairly new concept [23, 29]. Currently overweight and obese children in Malaysia are referred for treatment only if they developed complications. Thus developing a child obesity prevention programme which is parent-friendly and provider-friendly is justified and timely to help curb the increasing prevalence of childhood obesity in Malaysia.

The aim of this study is to evaluate the effectiveness of using social media and face-to-face sessions in a family-based intervention on the primary outcome of body mass index (BMI) z-score and secondary outcomes of waist circumference percentile and percentage total body fat. We also assessed parental factors which include parental knowledge, healthy lifestyles, parental feeding style and parental self-efficacy as well as child factors which include children's eating behaviours, food and beverages consumption (fruit and vegetable, snacks and sugar-sweetened beverages), physical activity and screen time. However, parental factors and child factors are not reported here. We hypothesize that in comparison with the wait-list group, children in the intervention group will have reduced BMI z-score, waist circumference percentile and percentage of total body fat.

## Methods

A detailed elaboration of the methodology of this field trial, has been published elsewhere [30]. However, a summary of the methodology is described here.

### Participants and design

This is a two-armed, parallel, randomized controlled field trial conducted in an urban area in one of the states in Malaysia. An urban area was chosen as the Malaysia National Health and Morbidity Survey (2015) [4] showed that prevalence of childhood obesity was slightly higher in the urban areas than in the rural areas.

All five primary government schools in this area were selected for this study. Before the study was conducted, BMI z-scores of school children in those schools were not available as there was no standardized reporting and referral upon detecting childhood overweight and obesity unless there were complications. Thus the number of children with overweight and obesity were unknown prior to the study. Brochures were sent to all the five schools informing parents about the intervention and the study and requesting them for consent to measure weight and height of their school-going children aged 7 to 10 years from August to September 2014. Those children whose parents gave written consent were screened for BMI z-score eligibility in October 2014. Parents who agreed to participate also provided consent on behalf of their children. Parents whose children with BMI z-score of more than 1 standard deviation (SD) were then invited to participate in the study. Parent-child dyads of Malay ethnicity who were computer literate, had access to the internet, were willing to use social media for interaction and children 7 to 10 years of age were recruited. Parents who reported children having co-morbidities, chronic diseases, physical disabilities, learning disabilities, on medication for chronic illness or participated in other research were excluded.

Individual randomisation was used over cluster design as contamination was expected to be low, because parents in the study setting hardly intermingle. In addition, the distribution of schools across intervention and control groups would be unequal because there are five schools and differences in distribution of sociodemographic characteristics and children with weight problems were unknown prior to the study. Each parent-child dyad from all five schools was number coded by the first author (NA) and sent to a research assistant who performed a computer generated randomization list which allocated parents into intervention or wait-list control groups using a simple randomization procedure of an online software (Research Randomiser) [31] with 1:1 allocation. This ensured the concealment of allocation from the rest of the researchers and participants. The list was then provided to the first author to invite the intervention group for the REDUCE intervention program.

Participating parents were informed that the intervention would be done in stages. So, parents would have the understanding that some of them would be participating earlier than others. Eventually all in the wait-listed control group would undergo the same intervention as parents in the intervention group after the final data collection. Parents in the wait-list control group were not informed of the starting of the intervention for the intervention group. The intervention group was informed not to share their social media experience with other parents; in addition they did not know who were in the wait-listed group, hence minimizing contamination. The face-to-face sessions for the intervention group were conducted in the Faculty of Medicine and Health Sciences, UPM without the knowledge of the wait-listed control group.

The researcher (NA) as the implementer of the intervention was not involved in the measurement of the children's weight, height, waist circumference and body fat percentage and data entry.

The sample size was based on a power of 80% and a level of significance (α) of 0.05 to detect a BMI z-score difference between intervention and wait-list control groups of 0.24 with standard deviation of 0.48 based on a previous study [32]. The dropout rate after randomization was assumed to be 15% requiring a minimum sample size of 56 parents per arm. The parent-child dyad was based on a 1:1 ratio – one parent to one child. All except two parents had one eligible child who was overweight or obese. For those two parents, the parents were requested to volunteer one other child for the study.

#### Intervention

The REDUCE (REorganise Diet, Unnecessary sCreen time and Exercise) intervention programme to impart information and skills was a newly developed programme by the researchers (NA, ZMS and FM) using social cognitive theory (SCT) [33]. The programme trained the parents on children's nutrition, physical activity, behaviour modification techniques and parenting skills to improve their children's health behaviours. The SCT posits behaviour as a reciprocal interaction between the person and environmental factors. The person is the child and the environment is the home environment and the parental factors that are conducive to the children's behaviour change. The child's ultimate daily targeted behaviours included no consumption of sugar-sweetened beverages (SSB) and unhealthy snacks, intake at least five servings of fruit and vegetables (two servings of fruit and three servings of vegetables), a minimum of 30 min of moderate to vigorous physical activity and a maximum of 120 min of screen time (watching television and playing video games). However, parents and children were empowered to choose which of the five targets to start working towards, first starting with the more manageable to achieve targets and to make small changes, one at a time. The elements of behaviour modification skills in the SCT include self-monitoring, goal setting, self-efficacy, problem solving, relapse prevention, and stimulus control. Parents were encouraged to acquire authoritative parenting skills, practise healthy behaviours and improve self-efficacy of child's healthy behaviours. The four-month REDUCE intervention programme consisted of 4 weeks of weekly training and 3 months of weekly booster.

The four-week training phase of the REDUCE intervention module was comprised of 8 units; 2 units were delivered through half-day face-to-face sessions (session one) followed by 2 units delivered weekly via Facebook for 2 weeks, and finally the last 2 units delivered via half-day face-to-face sessions (session two). The face-to-face sessions were conducted at the Faculty of Medicine and Health Sciences, University Putra Malaysia. All 4 units delivered in the face-to-face sessions were subsequently uploaded on the Facebook after each session. The training contents are summarized in Table 1. All the training sessions were delivered by the first author (NA) who is a public health physician except for the exercise tips in unit 8 which was conducted by a sports medicine specialist. All units were delivered to parents only, except for units 7 and 8 which were delivered to parents and children.

The booster phase of the REDUCE intervention programme were weekly one-hour sessions using parents' dedicated WhatsApp group that lasted for 12 weeks. The aims of the booster phase were to strengthen parents' knowledge and skills in promoting the targeted behaviours of the REDUCE programme. In this phase the first author (NA) posted on WhatsApp key information and skills provided in the training phase but in the form of a poster, responded to any queries by parents and provided feedback on the adiposity progress of the children based on the measurements taken. Parents were encouraged to enquire and discuss with the researcher (NA) and to interact with other parents in the intervention group in order to promote programme adherence and maintain motivation using this platform. The total contact time between researcher and participants was 22 h. Programme adherence was assessed by percentage of parents who attended the face-to-face sessions, and accessed the information in the Facebook as well as messages in the WhatsApp. Parents' responses were also compared between Facebook and What sApp.

The wait-list control group received the intervention after the completion of the final 6-month follow-up. To minimize attrition among intervention and wait-list control groups, small incentives (mainly stationeries) were given to the children each time they participated in the physical measurements and returned the parent-administered questionnaires.

#### Parents' involvement

In the pilot testing of the REDUCE intervention module, Malay parents of obese and overweight primary school children were involved in providing feedback on the module's duration, mode of delivery and the performance feedback of the children's progress over an eight-week training programme delivered only via Facebook.

In the randomized controlled trial, parents in the intervention group were informed of their children's progress via WhatsApp after each data collection immediately post-training, at 3 months and 6 months post-training while parents in the wait-listed group received feedback at similar times after the study ended. Feedback was obtained from parents in the intervention group regarding the burden or otherwise of the intervention.

#### Measures

The primary outcome was BMI z-score while waist circumference percentile and percentage of total body fat were secondary outcomes. BMI z-score which was determined using the WHO Anthroplus software [34] with weight in kg, height in cm, gender and age. Height was measured using a portable Seca stadiometer to the nearest 0.1 cm with bare feet. Weight was measured using the Omron Karada Scan (model HBF 212) to the nearest 0.1 kg with light clothing on and empty pockets.

Waist circumference was measured using Seca non-extensible tape meter at the approximate midpoint between the lower margin of the last palpable rib and the top of the iliac crest at the end of normal expiration [35]. The waist circumference was then converted to waist circumference percentile for Malaysian children by reading off the table on percentile values of WC (cm) by age and gender [36]. Percentage of body fat was measured after weight measurement using the same scale to

**Table 1** Contents of REDUCE intervention module

| Week | Unit | Approach | Themes | Behaviour modification techniques |
|---|---|---|---|---|
| 1 | 1 | Face-to-face session one | Introduction, obesity overview, parenting skills and role modelling | Goal setting, self-monitoring, self-efficacy, problem solving and stimulus control |
| | 2 | | Sugar-sweetened beverages | |
| 2 | 3 | Facebook | Fruits and vegetables | Goal setting, self-monitoring, self-efficacy, problem solving and stimulus control |
| | 4 | | Unhealthy snacks | |
| 3 | 5 | | Physical activity | |
| | 6 | | Screen time | |
| 4 | 7 | Face-to-face session two | Risky situations and review of performance | Relapse prevention |
| | 8 | | Further roles and actions, exercise tips and success stories | |

the nearest 0.1%. All physical measurements were performed by trained research assistants who were blinded regarding the allocation status of these children. The implementer of the intervention (NA) was not involved in any of these measurements. Each type of measurement was assigned to a designated trained research assistant to minimize inter-rater measurement bias. For example, a research assistant who did waist circumference only measured waist circumference. Assessments were completed at baseline, immediate post-training, 3 months and 6 months post-training.

Sociodemographic information was collected at baseline comprising of child's data on birth date, gender, number of siblings, order in the family and parents' data on marital status, education level and income. Parents' self-report on weight and height were also collected at baseline to determine parents' BMI.

### Statistical analysis

Data were analysed using SPSS version 22.0. Tests for normality were done using skewness, kurtosis, and graphs (histogram with normal distribution curve, whisker boxplot, and Q-Q and P-P plots) before further analyses were conducted. Non-normally distributed data were log transformed first before further analysis. Differences between intervention and wait-list control at baseline were tested using independent t-test (continuous variables) or chi-square test or Fischer's exact test (categorical variables) to examine the homogeneity between groups. All follow-up outcomes were analysed with intention-to-treat analysis.

Changes in BMI z-score, waist circumference percentile and percentage of total body fat were compared between intervention and wait-list control groups using independent t-test for continuous variables. The effectiveness of the intervention was evaluated using generalized linear mixed modelling adjusted for baseline covariates. Covariates included were variables that could affect body weight - child's age, child's gender, parents' BMI, parents' education, family income, and child's adiposity baseline measurements (BMI z-score, waist circumference percentile and percentage body fat). Subgroup analysis was conducted for overweight and obese children. The level of significance was set at $\alpha = 0.05$, and the null hypothesis rejected when $p \leq 0.05$. The CONSORT checklist of this study is in the Additional file 1.

## Results

One hundred and twenty-two parents completed this study giving an overall response rate of 91% among parents (64 parents in the intervention group and 58 parents in the wait-list control group were available for analysis). Parents who did not return the questionnaire after defaulting three follow-up sessions were considered dropouts. There was no significant difference between parents who remained in the study and parents who dropped out in terms of sociodemographic characteristics, parental BMI and the anthropometric measurements of their children. There was complete data for anthropometry and body fat percentage of all the children at all the four time points. The CONSORT flow diagram of parent-child participation is shown in Fig. 1.

Table 2 shows the baseline measurements of the respondents. There was no significant difference between the intervention and control groups at baseline. There was no unintended effect reported by the participants in the intervention and wait-list groups.

### Programme adherence

96.9% of parents participated in WhatsApp and 81.3% in Facebook respectively, compared to 68.8% for session one and 42.2% for session two of the face-to-face sessions. Since all the material used in the face-to-face sessions was uploaded on the Facebook after each session, the contents of the face-to-face sessions thus were available for all parents in the intervention group. Parents' adherence in WhatsApp was by counting the number of times they accessed the messages. Table 3 shows parents' participation and characteristics in WhatsApp and Facebook. One quarter of the parents' responses (82/356) expressed support for the programme. Examples of texted support included: expressing thanks for having the programme, welcoming other group members, texting phrases such as 'to make healthy and happy family' and congratulating group members who managed to reduce their children's BMI. One fifth of the responses (77/356) shared the parents' or their child's progress. For example, they reported on their children's improvement in reducing sugar-sweetened beverages, their ways of doing so and their children's activities. Another one fifth of the responses (75/356) gave simple replies. Examples included thank you, thumbs up and a smiley emoji.

### Impact on children's adiposity

Changes in children's adiposity for the intervention and wait-list control groups over the course of the study are shown in Table 4. There were increases in mean differences between intervention and wait-list control groups observed in BMI z-score and waist circumference percentile over the study period and these differences were significant at the end of 6 months ($p = 0.045$ and $p = 0.021$ respectively).

Table 5 shows the changes in adiposity between baseline and six-month follow-up for the whole sample, overweight and obese subgroups. The mean decrease in BMI z-score was $0.10 \pm 0.26$ for whole sample and $0.11 \pm 0.14$ for obese subgroup in the intervention group. The wait-list control group had higher increment in

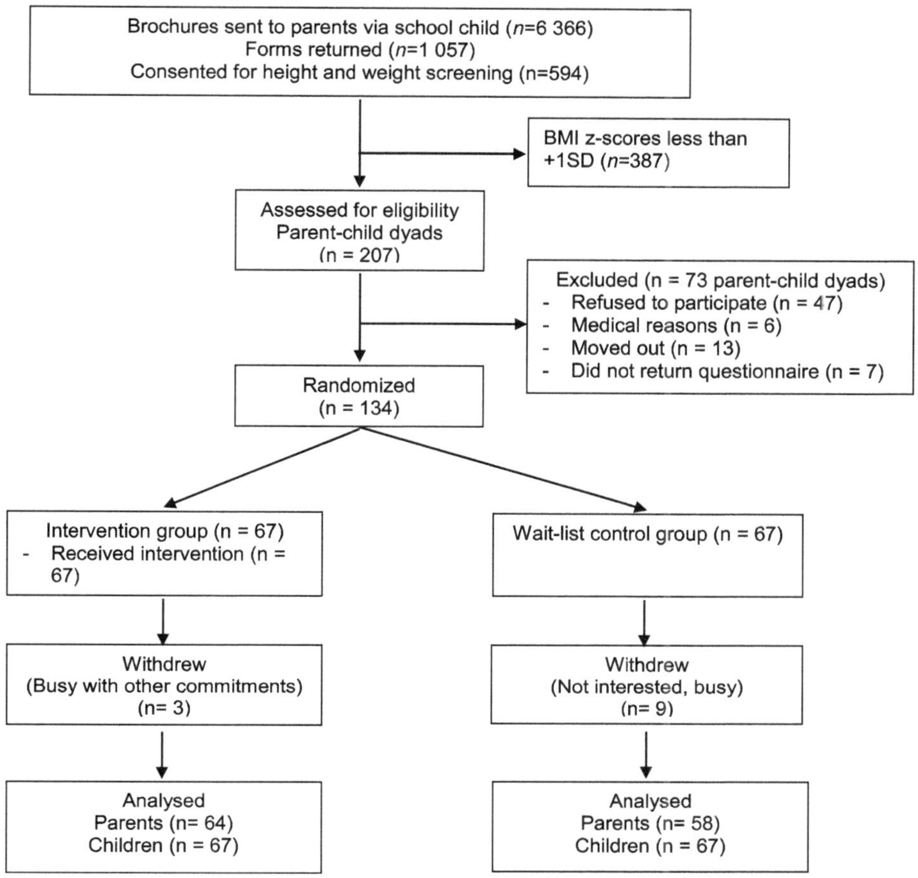


**Fig. 1** CONSORT flow diagram of parent-child's participation throughout study period

**Table 2** Baseline characteristics of the sample

| Characteristics | Intervention (n = 67) | | Wait-list control (n = 67) | | P value |
|---|---|---|---|---|---|
| | n (%) | Mean ± SD | n (%) | Mean ± SD | |
| Parent | | | | | |
| Age (years) | | 39.8 (3.6) | | 41.3 (5.7) | 0.079 |
| Gender - female | 39 (58.2) | | 37 (55.2) | | 0.862 |
| BMI (kg/m$^2$) | | 27.4 (4.41) | | 27.8 (4.27) | 0.622 |
| Child | | | | | |
| Age (years) | | 9.6 (1.2) | | 9.6 (1.2) | 0.826 |
| Gender - female | 40 (59.7) | | 38 (56.7) | | 0.861 |
| Height (cm) | | 136.1 (8.6) | | 135.6 (9.2) | 0.753 |
| Weight (kg) | | 47.0 (10.5) | | 48.2 (12.0) | 0.537 |
| BMI | | 25.2 (3.5) | | 25.7 (3.9) | 0.272 |
| BMI z-score | | 2.0 (0.4) | | 2.1 (0.4) | 0.381 |
| BMI z-score category | | | | | 0.861 |
| Overweight | 28 (41.8) | | 27 (40.3) | | |
| Obese | 39 (58.2) | | 40 (59.7) | | |
| Waist circumference (cm) | | 77.7 (8.8) | | 78.8 (9.1) | 0.465 |
| Waist circumference percentile | | 90.2 (8.0) | | 91.3 (7.0) | 0.410 |
| Total body fat | | 37.9 (4.2) | | 37.6 (4.1) | 0.740 |

**Table 3** Parents' participation and characteristics in WhatsApp and Facebook

| Characteristics | WhatsApp n (%) | Facebook n (%) |
|---|---|---|
| Initial number of parents at start of study, n (%) | 64 (96) | 64 (96) |
| Number of parents who left group, n (%) | 3 (4) | 3 (4) |
| Total responses by parents | 356 | 135 |
| Total posts and responses by researcher | 179 | 34 |
| Responses by parents: | | |
| Request clarification on the post | 9 | – |
| Support programme | 82 | 45 |
| Sharing of their problems or progress or child's progress | 77 | 8 |
| Request regarding child's progress | 20 | 3 |
| Sharing information about food and physical activity | 24 | 2 |
| Simple replies (e.g. thank you, thumbs up, smiley emoji) | 75 | 73 |
| Suggestions to improve children's obesity issue at school level and national level | 6 | – |
| Enquiry about other health issues | 4 | – |
| Others | 59 | 4 |
| Responses per parent: | | |
| 1–5 | 35 | 36 |
| 6–10 | 18 | 14 |
| ≥11 | 11 | 14 |

**Table 4** Changes in child's adiposity between intervention and wait-list groups from baseline to 6-month post-training

| Variables | Data ($N = 134$) Means ± SD | | | |
|---|---|---|---|---|
| | Baseline | Immediately post-training | 3-month post-training | 6-month post-training |
| BMI z-scores | | | | |
| Intervention group ($n = 67$) | 2.05 ± 0.40 | 2.03 ± 0.38 | 1.99 ± 0.41 | 1.95 ± 0.45 |
| Wait-list group ($n = 67$) | 2.11 ± 0.39 | 2.10 ± 0.36 | 2.11 ± 0.35 | 2.09 ± 0.35 |
| t-test ($p$-value) | - 0.879 ($p = 0.381$) | −1.158 ($p = 0.249$) | −1.730 ($p = 0.086$) | −2.025 ($p = 0.045$)[a] |
| Mean difference | − 0.06 | − 0.07 | −0.11 | − 0.14 |
| 95% CI for mean difference | −0.194 to 0.075 | − 0.200 to 0.052 | −0.244 to 0.016 | - 0.278 to - 0.003 |
| Waist circumference percentile | | | | |
| Intervention group ($n = 67$) | 90.21 ± 7.98 | 91.09 ± 7.71 | 90.06 ± 9.56 | 89.37 ± 9.26 |
| Wait-list group ($n = 67$) | 91.28 ± 7.04 | 93.82 ± 4.31 | 92.25 ± 6.11 | 92.55 ± 6.20 |
| t-test ($p$-value) | − 0.826 ($p = 0.410$) | − 2.532 ($p = 0.013$)[a] | − 1.583 ($p = 0.116$) | −2.335 ($p = 0.021$)[a] |
| Mean difference | − 1.07 | −2.73 | − 2.19 | −3.18 |
| 95% CI for mean difference | −3.647 to 1.498 | −4.871 to −0.592 | −4.940 to 0.552 | −5.876 to − 0.482 |
| Percentage of body fat | | | | |
| Intervention group ($n = 67$) | 37.87 ± 4.20 | 37.68 ± 4.14 | 36.66 ± 4.75 | 36.75 ± 4.75 |
| Wait-list group ($n = 67$) | 37.63 ± 4.09 | 37.23 ± 4.50 | 37.65 ± 4.25 | 37.25 ± 4.46 |
| t-test (p-value) | 0.333 ($p = 0.740$) | 0.603 ($p = 0.548$) | −1.263 ($p = 0.209$) | − 0.630 ($p = 0.530$) |
| Mean difference | 0.24 | 0.45 | −0.98 | −0.50 |
| 95% CI for mean difference | −1.178 to 1.654 | − 1.027 to 1.927 | −2.524 to 0.557 | − 2.077 to − 1.074 |

[a]Significant at $p \le 0.05$, *SD* standard deviation, *CI* confidence interval

**Table 5** Comparison of changes in adiposity within groups between baseline and six-month follow-up

| | Mean difference ± SD baseline vs 6-month[c] | t | *p*-value [a] |
|---|---|---|---|
| BMI z-score | | | |
| Whole sample | | | |
| Intervention group ($n = 67$) | 0.100 ± 0.257 | 3.190 | 0.002[b] |
| Wait-list group ($n = 67$) | 0.019 ± 0.172 | 0.907 | 0.368 |
| Overweight children | | | |
| Intervention group ($n = 28$) | 0.087 ± 0.367 | 1.257 | 0.220 |
| Wait-list group ($n = 27$) | − 0.067 ± 0.185 | −1.887 | 0.070 |
| Obese children | | | |
| Intervention group ($n = 39$) | 0.109 ± 0.136 | 5.022 | < 0.001[b] |
| Wait-list group ($n = 40$) | 0.077 ± 0.138 | 3.545 | 0.001[b] |
| Waist circumference percentile | | | |
| Whole sample | | | |
| Intervention group ($n = 67$) | 1.373 ± 11.079 | 1.014 | 0.314 |
| Wait-list group ($n = 67$) | −1.343 ± 9.019 | −1.219 | 0.227 |
| Overweight children | | | |
| Intervention group ($n = 28$) | 5.357 ± 14.095 | 2.011 | 0.054 |
| Wait-list group ($n = 27$) | 0.963 ± 9.382 | 0.533 | 0.598 |
| Obese children | | | |
| Intervention group ($n = 39$) | −1.487 ± 7.207 | −1.289 | 0.205 |
| Wait-list group ($n = 40$) | − 2.900 ± 8.533 | −2.149 | 0.038[b] |
| Percentage of total body fat | | | |
| Whole sample | | | |
| Intervention group ($n = 67$) | 0.912 ± 6.053 | 1.234 | 0.222 |
| Wait-list group ($n = 67$) | 0.655 ± 6.694 | 0.801 | 0.426 |
| Overweight children | | | |
| Intervention group ($n = 28$) | 2.451 ± 6.736 | 1.926 | 0.065 |
| Wait-list group ($n = 27$) | 1.963 ± 5.961 | 1.711 | 0.099 |
| Obese children | | | |
| Intervention group ($n = 39$) | −0.193 ± 5.330 | −0.226 | 0.822 |
| Wait-list group ($n = 40$) | −0.227 ± 7.083 | −0.203 | 0.840 |

[a]Using paired t-test; SD: standard deviation
[b]Significant at $p \leq 0.05$;
[c]This difference is baseline minus 6 month, with minus value depicting a higher measurement at 6-month post-training compared to baseline

mean waist circumference percentile at six-month follow-up (2.9 cm ± 8.5) compared to intervention group (1.5 cm ± 7.2). There was a higher reduction in within-group change for percentage of total body fat at six-month follow-up for overweight children in the intervention group (2.5% ± 6.7) compared to the wait-list group. However, this change was not significant ($p =$ 0.065).

Results from the mixed model analysis (Table 6) showed that at the end of 6 months, significantly higher proportion of children in the intervention group than in the wait-list group had reduced BMI z-score for all ($F(6, 517) = 2.817$, $p = 0.010$). Among obese children ($F(6, 297) = 6.072$, $p = < 0.001$), more children in the intervention group had reduced their waist circumference percentile ($F(6, 297) = 3.998$, $p = 0.001$) compared to the control group, while more overweight children in the intervention group had reduced their body fat percentage compared to the control group ($F(6, 201) = 2.526$, $p = 0.022$). Figure 2 shows changes in BMI z-scores, waist circumference percentile and body fat percentage from the mixed model analysis, between baseline and at 6 months ($p = 0.01$, $p = 0.001$ and $p = 0.022$ respectively).

We received positive feedback from parents regarding the use of social media. Parents felt social media was convenient to use and facilitated direct communication

**Table 6** Comparison of anthropometric measurements and body fat percentage between study groups, controlling for covariates

| Variable | Parameter | F | df1 | df2 | p-value[a] |
|---|---|---|---|---|---|
| BMI z-scores | | | | | |
| Whole sample | Group | 7.050 | 1 | 517 | 0.008[b] |
| ($n = 134$) | Group x Time | 2.817 | 6 | 517 | 0.010[b] |
| Overweight subgroup | Group | 9.341 | 1 | 201 | 0.003[b] |
| ($n = 55$) | Group x Time | 1.218 | 6 | 201 | 0.299 |
| Obese subgroup | Group | 0.033 | 1 | 297 | 0.855 |
| ($n = 79$) | Group x Time | 6.072 | 6 | 297 | < 0.001[b] |
| Waist circumference percentile | | | | | |
| Whole sample | Group | 13.935 | 1 | 517 | < 0.001[b] |
| ($n = 134$) | Group x Time | 1.410 | 6 | 517 | 0.209 |
| Overweight subgroup | Group | 30.245 | 1 | 201 | < 0.001[b] |
| ($n = 55$) | Group x Time | 1.683 | 6 | 201 | 0.127 |
| Obese subgroup | Group | 0.084 | 1 | 297 | 0.772 |
| ($n = 79$) | Group x Time | 3.998 | 6 | 297 | 0.001[b] |
| Body fat percentage | | | | | |
| Whole sample- | Group | 1.454 | 1 | 517 | 0.228 |
| ($n = 134$) | Group x Time | 0.802 | 6 | 517 | 0.569 |
| Overweight subgroup | Group | 0.575 | 1 | 201 | 0.449 |
| ($n = 55$) | Group x Time | 2.526 | 6 | 201 | 0.022[b] |
| Obese subgroup | Group | 0.093 | 1 | 297 | 0.760 |
| ($n = 79$) | Group x Time | 0.628 | 6 | 297 | 0.708 |

[a]Using generalized linear mixed model adjusted for child's age, child's gender, parents' body mass index, mother's education, father's education, family income, and child's baseline data (BMI z-score, waist circumference percentile and body fat percentage respectively)
[b]Significant at $p \leq 0.05$

with the researcher who provided the needed support. It also made possible discussion to solve problems that parents may face regarding the study, and enabled performance feedback to the parents.

## Discussion

In this randomized controlled field trial, our results suggest that the use of social media and face-to-face sessions in the family-based, theory-driven intervention for management of childhood obesity can decrease children's adiposity (BMI z-score, waist circumference percentile and percentage of body fat). No adverse events or unintended adverse consequences of the intervention were reported by the participants.

These results showed almost similar magnitude of decrease in BMI z-score found in Cochrane meta-analysis among 37 studies for children aged 6–12 years with mean effect of – 0.15 (95% CI: -0.23 to – 0.08) [37]. This difference is expected to have clinical benefits as a study by Kolsgaard et al. (2011) showed that even a modest reduction in BMI z-score (≥0.00 - < 0.1) was associated with significant improvement in several cardiovascular risk factors i.e. improved insulin and insulin resistance, total cholesterol, LDL cholesterol and total/HDL cholesterol ratio [38].

A recent systematic review and meta-analysis of eight studies examining the effectiveness of family-based eHealth intervention among overweight and obese children and adolescents found that the difference in BMI or BMI z-score between the intervention and control groups at post-intervention were not statistically significant [39]. The REDUCE intervention also produced a greater reduction in BMI z-scores than some of the face-to-face only interventions for parents of overweight and obese children [40–44] that measured similar outcomes. We postulate that a combination of social media and face-to-face intervention may have produced more favourable results compared with standalone intervention of either internet/social media or face-to-face intervention. The results of the REDUCE intervention compare favourably with a more intensive intervention [32] that involved 18 two-hour face-to-face sessions delivered over 9 weeks. There are, however, some face-to-face interventions that have produced larger group differences than the REDUCE intervention [12, 45]. Their interventions however, involved more sessions than the REDUCE intervention.

Subgroup analysis showed that in the intervention group, obese children had significantly lesser increment at the end of the 6-month post-training in waist circumference percentile whereas overweight children had significantly reduced percentage of total body fat compared to the wait-list group. The result of our study was comparable to those of a face-to-face intervention study by Sacher et al. [32]. Their intervention resulted in a – 4.1 cm significant difference in waist circumference between intervention (77.7 ± 7.2 cm) and control groups (82.0 ± 8.6 cm) over a six-month period. Our study showed a – 4.1 cm difference in waist circumference between intervention (71.49 ± 6.04 cm) and wait-list (75.63 ± 6.49 cm) groups for overweight children at six-month follow-up even though it was not significant, most likely due to insufficient power. The study by Reinehr et al. (2010) among overweight children also found a significant difference between the waist circumference of the intervention and control groups [46]. However, other conventional family-based behavioural treatment of childhood obesity found no difference in waist circumference between the intervention and control groups [41, 43].

The REDUCE intervention had a greater impact on percentage body fat than another Internet-based family intervention [47] and a conventional family intervention [32] both of which found no difference between intervention and wait-list groups after the same period of

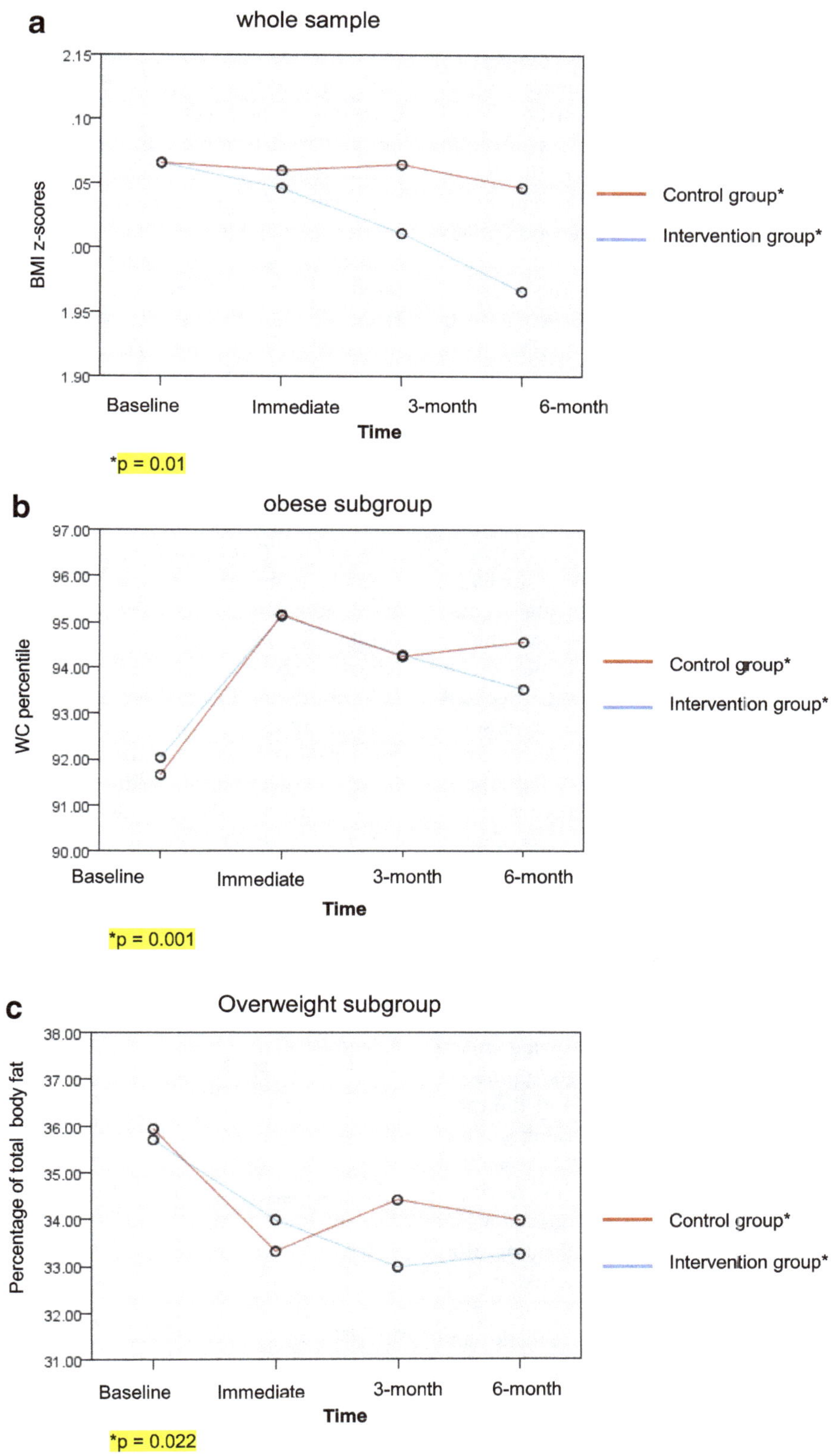


**Fig. 2** Changes in BMI z-scores, waist circumference percentile and body fat percentage from the mixed model analysis, between baseline and at 6 months

follow-up. However, they did not perform subgroup analysis based on obesity status (overweight or obese). The children in our study had high values of percentage body fat with a mean value of more than 35%. Yamashita et al. (2012) had suggested the cut-off point for cardiovascular risk for Asian adults to be 20.3% [48]. No cut-off point as yet has been developed for children but the values found in the current study are much higher compared with the adult values, putting these children potentially at elevated cardiovascular risk later in life.

Our study showed a high response rate in the intervention group, with higher rates of parents' participation in the WhatsApp and Facebook sessions compared to face-to-face sessions, indicating that the social media approach is better received than the face-to-face sessions. This is possibly due to the rigid nature of the face-to-face sessions where parents had to attend the sessions within the allocated time, making these sessions least attended. However, omitting the face-to-face approach could possibly have affected the results of this study. In comparing parents' participation in the two types of social media i.e. Facebook and WhatsApp, results showed a greater participation in WhatsApp. We postulate that this was due to the longer duration of contact with parents (3 months) in WhatsApp compared to Facebook (1 month). Facebook has been reported to be the most commonly used social medium in delivering health interventions compared to other social media [23]. However, the use of WhatsApp in health settings has not been widely established as yet. A study by Cheung et al. evaluated the effectiveness of using WhatsApp or Facebook to prevent smoking relapse in recent quitters and found that respondents were more likely to participate using WhatsApp (76%) than Facebook (42%) [49]. WhatsApp may be gaining greater acceptance than Facebook because its features are more convenient and easier to use without requiring logging in, or a username and password [49–51]. Apart from notifying smartphone users about incoming messages, WhatsApp allows them to make quick and simple responses and the messages were encrypted [50, 51]. During the training phase of this intervention, Facebook was used because at that time, WhatsApp did not support the uploading of documents. Even though this function was introduced when the booster phase began, nevertheless, downloading inordinately large documents via WhatsApp caused mobile phones to cease to respond.

The intervention incorporated setting realistic and achievable goals for the children. However, there are several limitations to this study. Generalizability is limited due to the sample being among urban, Malay and educated parents. The respondents could possibly have been highly motivated parents. Parents' BMI was self-reported with the possibility of recall bias being introduced. The poor attendance in face-to-face sessions could have affected the effectiveness of the intervention. To minimize this effect, the respective materials of the module were uploaded to Facebook, and the parents' adherence in Facebook was assessed by the number and percentage who accessed this module. However, we were not able to determine the association between adherence and outcomes as we did not measure individual adherence scores. Another limitation is that the effect of other influences outside the home environment was not controlled for. Lastly, this study was retrospectively registered. However, there was no element of selective reporting for this study, with the original protocol uploaded in its entirety. Future research should be conducted to have a longer follow-up with a cost-effectiveness study before implementing this programme in child obesity prevention programme.

## Conclusions

The REDUCE intervention programme shows that it is possible, in an urban Malay community, to reduce childhood adiposity in primary school children by using a combined face-to-face approach and social media in educating parents on child nutrition, physical activity, behaviour modification techniques and parenting skills. This study thus provides evidence of the potential usefulness of using face-to-face interaction and social media for a family-based intervention in urban community settings to help curb the epidemic of childhood obesity. However, a longer duration of study is needed to ascertain the sustainability of the intervention. A cost-effectiveness study is recommended before incorporating this intervention in a child obesity prevention programme.

#### Abbreviations

BM: Body mass index; REDUCE: Reorganise diet, unnecessary screen time and exercise; SCT: Social cognitive theory

#### Acknowledgements

The authors thank the Ministry of Education, school principals and teachers as well as parents and students who participated in this study.

#### Funding

The research was funded by Universiti Putra Malaysia, grant number GP-IPS/ 2013/9398400. The funding agency did not influence the planning and execution of this study.

#### Authors' contributions

NA was the principle researcher and was responsible for the data collection and performing the data analysis. NA, LMS, ZMS and FM contributed to the study design and supervision. LMS advised and supervised the analyses and edited the manuscript. All authors were involved in writing the paper and authorized final approval of the submitted and published versions.

### Competing interests

The authors declare that they have no competing interests.

### Author details

[1]Department of Community Health, Faculty of Medicine and Health Sciences, Universiti Putra Malaysia, Level 1, Block B (Academic), 43400 UPM, Serdang, Selangor, Malaysia. [2]Department of Nutrition, Faculty of Medicine and Health Sciences, Universiti Putra Malaysia, Serdang, Selangor, Malaysia. [3]Department of Psychiatry, Faculty of Medicine and Health Sciences, Universiti Putra Malaysia, Serdang, Selangor, Malaysia.

### References

1. World Heath Organization. New global estimates of child and adolescent obesity released on World Obesity Day. 2017. Available from: http://www.who.int/end-childhood-obesity/news/new-estimate-child-adolescent-obesity/en/. Accessed 17 Oct 2017.
2. Ng M, Fleming T, Robinson M, Thomson B, Graetz N, Margono C, et al. Global, regional, and national prevalence of overweight and obesity in children and adults during 1980-2013: a systematic analysis for the global burden of disease study 2013. Lancet. 2014;384(9945):766–81.
3. Institute of Public Health Malaysia. National Health and Morbidity Survey 2011. Non communicable diseases. Volume II. Institute of Public Health Malaysia. 2011. 192 p. Available from: http://www.iku.gov.my/images/IKU/AQ9Document/REPORT/NHMS2011-VolumeII.pdf. Accessed 21 Nov 2013.
4. Institute of Public Health Malaysia. National Health & Morbidity Survey 2015. Non-communicable diseases, risk factors & other health problems. [Internet]. Kuala Lumpur: Institute of Public Health Malaysia; 2015. Available from: http://www.iku.gov.my/images/IKU/Document/REPORT/nhmsreport2015vol2.pdf. Accessed 20 Apr 2016.
5. World Health Organization. Obesity and overweight [Internet]. Geneva: World Health Organization; 2018. Available from: http://www.who.int/news-room/fact-sheets/detail/obesity-and-overweight. Accessed 20 July 2018.
6. Department of Statistics Malaysia. Current population estimates, Malaysia, 2014–2016. 2017. Available from: https://www.dosm.gov.my/v1/index.php?r=column/cthemeByCat&cat=155&bul_id=OWlxdEVoYlJCS0hUZzJyRUcvZEYxZz09&menu_idL0pheU43NWJwRWVSZklWdzQ4TlhUUT09. Accessed 4 Jan 2016.
7. Mudd-martin G, Martinez MC, Rayens MK, Meininger JC. Sociocultural tailoring of a healthy lifestyle intervention to reduce cardiovascular disease and type 2 diabetes risk among Latinos. Prev Chronic Dis. 2013;10(E200):1–10.
8. Epstein LH. Family-based behavioural intervention for obese children. Int J Obes Relat Metab Disord. 1996;20(Suppl 1):S14–21.
9. Epstein LH, Valoski A, Wing RR, McCurley J. Ten-year outcomes of behavioral family-based treatment for childhood obesity. Health Psychol. 1994;13(5):373–83.
10. Gruber KJ, Haldeman LA. Using the family to combat childhood and adult obesity. Prev Chronic Dis. 2009;6(3):A106.
11. Moens E, Braet C. Training parents of overweight children in parenting skills: a 12-month evaluation. Behav Cogn Psychother. 2012;40(01):1–18.
12. Epstein LH, Paluch RA, Roemmich JN, Beecher MD. Family-based obesity treatment, then and now: twenty-five years of pediatric obesity treatment. Health Psychol. 2007;26(4):381–91.
13. Institute of Medicine. Parents can play a role in preventing childhood obesity. Fact sheet. 2004. Available from http://www.nationalacademies.org/hmd/ ~/media/Files/Report%20Files/2004/Preventing-Childhood-Obesity-Health-in-the-Balance/FactSheetHomeFINALBitticks.ashx. Accessed 31 May 2018.
14. Coppock JH, Ridolfi DR, Hayes JF, St. Paul M, Wilfley DE. Current approaches to the Management of Pediatric Overweight and Obesity. Curr Treat Options Cardiovasc Med. 2014;16(11):1–15.
15. Lindsay AC, Sussner KM, Kim JGS. The role of parents in preventing childhood obesity. Futur Child. 2006;16(1):169–86.
16. Jiang JX, Xia XL, Greiner T, Lian GL, Rosenqvist U. A two year family based behaviour treatment for obese children. Arch Dis Child. 2005;90(12):1235–8.
17. McGarvey E, Keller A, Forrester M, Williams E, Seward D, Suttle DE. Feasibility and benefits of a parent-focused preschool child obesity intervention. Am J Public Health. 2004;94(9):1490–5.
18. Golley RK, Perry RA, Magarey A, Daniels L. Family-focused weight management program for five- to nine-year-olds incorporating parenting skills training with healthy lifestyle information to support behaviour modification. Nutr Diet. 2007;64(3):144–50.
19. Marshall S, Golley R, Hendrie G. Expanding the understanding of how parenting influences the dietary intake and weight status of children: a cross-sectional study. Nutr Diet. 2011;68(2):127–33.
20. Skelton JA, Beech BM. Attrition in paediatric weight management: a review of the literature and new directions. Obes Rev. 2011;12(5):e273–81.
21. Statista. Most popular social networks worldwide as of April 2018, ranked by number of active users (in millions). 2018. Available from: https://www.statista.com/statistics/272014/global-social-networks-ranked-by-number-of-users/. Accessed 31 May 2018.
22. Malaysian Communications and Multimedia Commission. Internet users survey 2017. 2017 Available from: https://www.mcmc.gov.my/skmmgovmy/AQ16media/General/pdf/MCMC-Internet-Users-Survey-2017.pdf. Accessed 24 May 2018.
23. Maher C, Ryan J, Kernot J, Podsiadly J, Keenihan S. Social media and applications to health behavior. Curr Opin Psychol. 2016;9:50–5. Available from: https://doi.org/10.1016/j.copsyc.2015.10.021
24. Laranjo L, Arguel A, Neves AL, Gallagher AM, Kaplan R, Mortimer N, et al. The influence of social networking sites on health behavior change: a systematic review and meta-analysis. J Am Med Inform Assoc. 2015;22(1):243–56.
25. Dahl AA, Hales SB, Turner-McGrievy GM. Integrating social media into weight loss interventions. Curr Opin Psychol. 2016;9:11–5.
26. Herring SJ, Cruice JF, Bennett GG, Davey A, Foster GD. Using technology to promote postpartum weight loss in urban, low-income mothers: a pilot randomized controlled trial. J Nutr Educ Behav. 2014;46(6):610–5.
27. Napolitano M, Hayes S, Bennett G, Ives AK, Foster GD. Using Facebook and text messaging to deliver a weight loss program to college students. Obes J. 2013;21(1):25–31.
28. Patrick K, Marshall SJ, Davila EP, Kolodziejczyk JK, Fowler JH, Calfas KJ, et al. Design and implementation of a randomized controlled social and mobile weight loss trial for young adults (project SMART). Contemp Clin Trials. 2014;37(1):10–8.
29. Doub AE, Small M, Birch LL. A call for research exploring social media in fl uences on mothers ' child feeding practices and childhood obesity risk. Appetite. 2016;99:298–305.
30. Norliza A, Lye MS, Zalilah MS, Firdaus M. Harnessing social media in family-based intervention for childhood obesity: Study protocol fro randomised controlled field trial of REDUCE programme. 2016;3(5):95–109. Available from: http://publichealthmy.org/ejournal/ojs2/AQ17index.php/ijphcs/article/view/341.
31. Urbaniak GC, Plous S. Research randomizer [Internet]. 2007. 2007. Available from: https://www.randomizer.org/. Accessed 11 Feb 2015.
32. Sacher PM, Kolotourou M, Chadwick PM, Cole TJ, Lawson MS, Lucas A, et al. Randomized controlled trial of the MEND program: a family-based community intervention for childhood obesity. Obesity (Silver Spring). 2010;18(Suppl 1):S62–8.
33. Bandura A. Social foundations of thought and action: a social-cognitive theory. Prentice-hall. Englewood Cliffs, NJ: Prentice-Hall; 1986.
34. World Health Organization. WHO Anthroplus [Internet]. 2006. Available from: http://en.freedownloadmanager.org/Windows-PC/WHO-AnthroPlus-FREE.html. Accessed 6 Mar 2015.
35. World Health Organization. Waist Circumference and Waist-Hip Ratio: Report of a WHO Expert Consultation. Geneva: World Heal Organ; 2008. (December):8–11.
36. Poh BK, Nurul Jannah A, Chong LK, Ruzita AT, Mohd Noor I, McCarthy D. Waist circumference percentile curves for Malaysian children and

adolescents aged 6.0 – 16.9 years. Int J Pediatr Obes. 2011;6(3–4):229–35.
37. Waters E, de Silva-Sanigorski A, Hall BJ, Brown T, Campbell KJ, Gao Y, et al. Interventions for preventing obesity in children. Cochrane Database Syst Rev. 2011;(12):CD001871.
38. Kolsgaard MLP, Joner G, Brunborg C, Anderssen SA, Tonstad S, Andersen LF. Reduction in BMI z-score and improvement in cardiometabolic risk factors in obese children and adolescents. The Oslo adiposity intervention study - a hospital/public health nurse combined treatment. BMC PediatrBioMed Central Ltd. 2011;11(1):47.
39. Hammersley M, Jones R, Okely A. Parent-Focused Childhood and Adolescent overweight and obesity eHealth interventions: a systematic review and meta-analysis [internet]. J Med Internet Res. 2016;18(7).
40. Wilfley DE, Stein RI, Saelens BE, Matt GE, Hayden-wade HA, Welch RR, et al. Efficacy of Maintenance Treatment J Am Med Assoc. 2007;298(14):1661–73.
41. Croker H, Viner R, Nicholls D. Family-based Behavioural treatment of childhood obesity in a UK National Health Service setting : randomised controlled trial. J Obes. 2011;36(1):1–19.
42. McCallum Z, Wake M, Gerner B, Baur LA, Gibbons K, Gold L, et al. Outcome data from the LEAP (live, eat and play) trial: a randomized controlled trial of a primary care intervention for childhood overweight/mild obesity. Int J Obes. 2007;31(4):630–6.
43. Hughes AR, Stewart L, Chapple J, McColl JH, Donaldson MDC, Kelnar CJH, et al. Randomized, controlled trial of a best-practice individualized behavioral program for treatment of childhood overweight: Scottish childhood overweight treatment trial (SCOTT). Pediatrics. 2008;121(3):e539–46.
44. Boudreau ADA, Kurowski DS, Gonzalez WI, Dimond MA, Oreskovic NM. Latino families, primary care, and childhood obesity: A randomized controlled trial. Am J Prev Med. 2013;44(3 Suppl 3):S247-57.
45. Kalavainen M, Korppi M, Nuutinen O. Long-term efficacy of group-based treatment for childhood obesity compared with routinely given individual counselling. Int J Obes Nature Publishing Group. 2011;35(4):530–3.
46. Reinehr T, Schaefer A, Winkel K, Finne E, Toschke AM, Kolip P. An effective lifestyle intervention in overweight children: findings from a randomized controlled trial on ' Obeldicks light. Clin Nutr. 2010;29(3):331–6.
47. Chen JL, Weiss S, Heyman MB, Cooper B, Lustig RH. The efficacy of the web-based childhood obesity prevention program in Chinese American adolescents (web ABC study). J Adolesc Health. 2011;49(2):148–54.
48. Yamashita K, Kondo T, Osugi S, Shimokata K, Maeda K, Okumura N, et al. The significance of measuring body fat percentage determined by bioelectrical impedance analysis for detecting subjects with cardiovascular disease risk factors. Circ J. 2012;76(10):2435–42.
49. Derek Cheung YT, Helen Chan CH, Lai CKJ, Vivian Chan WF, Wang MP, William Li HC, et al. Using Whatsapp and Facebook online social groups for smoking relapse prevention for recent quitters: a pilot pragmatic cluster randomized controlled trial. J Med Internet Res. 2015;17(10):1–15.
50. Lingaraju VS. Why are people choosing WhatsApp Messenger over Facebook Messenger? [Internet]. 2013 [cited 2017 Jan 3]. Available from: https://www.quora.com/Why-are-people-choosing-WhatsApp-Messenger-over-Facebook-Messenger. Accessed 3 Jan 2017.
51. Amrita K. The pros and cons of Facebook Messenger and WhatsApp [Internet]. The Daily Dot. 2017 [cited 2018 May 31]. Available from: https://www.dailydot.com/debug/facebook-messenger-vs-whatsapp/. Accessed 31 May 2018.

# 9

# Severely malnourished children with a low weight-for-height have a higher mortality than those with a low mid-upper-arm-circumference: III. Effect of case-load on malnutrition related mortality– policy implications

Emmanuel Grellety[1*] and Michael H. Golden[2]

**Abstract**

**Background:** Severe acute malnutrition (SAM) is diagnosed when the weight-for-height Z-score (WHZ) is <−3Z of the $WHO_{2006}$ standards, or a mid-upper-arm circumference (MUAC) of < 115 mm or there is nutritional oedema. Although there has been a move to eliminate WHZ as a diagnostic criterion we have shown that children with a low WHZ have at least as high a mortality risk as those with a low MUAC. Here we take the estimated case fatality rates and published case-loads to estimate the proportion of total SAM related deaths occurring in children that would be excluded from treatment with a MUAC-only policy.

**Methods:** The effect of varying case-load and mortality rates on the proportion of all deaths that would occur in admitted children was examined. We used the same calculations to estimate the proportion of all SAM-related deaths that would be excluded with a MUAC-only policy in 48 countries with very different relative case loads for SAM by only MUAC, only WHZ and children with both deficits. The case fatality rates (CFR) are taken from simulations, empirical data and the literature.

**Results:** The relative number of cases of SAM by MUAC alone, WHZ alone and those with both criteria have a dominant effect on the proportion of all SAM-related deaths that would occur in children excluded from treatment by a MUAC-only program. Many countries, particularly in the Sahel, West Africa and South East Asia would fail to identify the majority of SAM-related deaths if a MUAC only program were to be implemented. Globally, the estimated minimum number of deaths that would occur among children excluded from treatment in our analyses is 300,000 annually.

**Conclusions:** The number, proportion or attributable fraction of children excluded from treatment with any change of current policy are the correct indicators to guide policy change. CRFs alone should not be used to guide policy in choosing whether or not to drop WHZ as a diagnostic for SAM. All the criteria for diagnosis of malnutrition need to be retained. It is critical that methods are found to identify those children with a low WHZ, but not a low MUAC, in the community so that they will not remain undetected.

(Continued on next page)

* Correspondence: Emmanuel.Grellety.Bosviel@ulb.ac.be
[1]Research Center Health Policy and Systems - International Health, School of Public Health, Université Libre de Bruxelles, Bruxelles, Belgium
Full list of author information is available at the end of the article

(Continued from previous page)
**Keywords:** Nutrition, Acute malnutrition, Severe acute malnutrition, SAM, Mid-upper-arm circumference, MUAC, Weight-for-height, WHZ, Mortality, Case fatality rate, Wasting, Oedema, Kwashiorkor, Diagnosis, Case load, Prognosis, Child, Human

## Background

Severe acute malnutrition (SAM) is a lethal condition accounting for about half to one million childhood deaths [1] annually for children with a weight-for-height/length (WHZ) below the recommended WHO cut-off. If children with the other WHO definitions of SAM are added the death toll is much larger. Identification and treatment of all children with any of the current definitions of SAM mandated by the World Health Organisation (WHO) is a public health priority.

The WHO defines SAM using three independent criteria, WHZ of <−3Z of the $WHO_{2006}$ growth standards, an absolute mid-upper-arm circumference (MUAC) of < 115 mm or the presence of nutritional oedema [2, 3]. Some children satisfy several of these criteria.

MUAC can be easily and quickly measured using a simple coloured tape around the upper arm and oedema can also be easily assessed in the field. On the other hand, assessment of WHZ requires the weight and height to be taken and the resulting numbers looked up in tables. There is no doubt that MUAC is much easier to assess than WHZ. For reasons of speed, convenience, cheapness and simplicity MUAC has been used for many years to assess malnutrition [4–8]. The ease of use makes community screening for SAM with MUAC practical and has been a great advance in identifying affected individuals in the community.

However, there has now arisen a concerted movement to stop the assessment of WHZ altogether, even in hospitals and clinics where it is routinely measured at present. The advocates for only using MUAC are adamant that any research to develop innovative methods to assess WHZ in the community is a "*waste of effort*" as MUAC is the only criterion that is needed [9–11]. We examined community based survey data from 48 countries and find that only 16.5% of children who fulfil the WHO definitions of SAM meet both the MUAC and WHZ criteria. If WHZ is abandoned as a criterion about 45% of children with SAM by WHZ alone will fail to be identified because their MUAC is above 115 mm. Which criterion identifies the majority of SAM children varies dramatically from country to country and the two criteria identify different individuals. For these reasons we advocated that both MUAC and WHZ continue to be routinely used to assess children for SAM and, critically, that convenient and simple ways to assess WHZ in the community to identify children with only a deficit in WHZ but not MUAC has to be a major research priority [12].

These suggestions met with a forceful criticism from a multi-authored paper [9] which appears to have widespread support by both agencies and donors [13]. The putative basis of the opinion that WHZ should not be used at all was that anything that diverts resources from the widespread use of MUAC to identify SAM would hinder its implementation and therefore WHZ assessment must be suppressed [9, 14]. The reasons given against the use of WHZ did not simply emphasise its inconvenience, with which we agree. The following were asserted: 1) children with a low WHZ are healthy; 2) their low WHZ is due entirely to their having longer legs so they do not require treatment; 3) WHZ is a poor predictor of mortality in children; 4) MUAC is a good predictor of mortality in children; 5) the two diagnostic parameters are not complementary; and 6) addition of WHZ does not improve the sensitivity or specificity of future all-cause mortality prediction with MUAC. These contentions were robustly refuted [15].

We have shown in the two preceding papers [16, 17], 1) that WHZ < −3Z carries as high, or higher, risk of death as MUAC < 115 mm; they are clearly not "healthy" and undeserving of treatment. 2) That the two parameters not only identify different children, and therefore different risks, but also children satisfying both criteria have a higher mortality showing the defects to be additive. 3) That "long legs" is an inadequate explanation for the regional difference in SAM by WHZ [12, 18, 19]. 4) That all the data previously analysed by comparison of ROC curves, and relied upon to make the assertions of MUAC's superiority are severely biased because of mathematical coupling [20, 21] as well as stochastic and other problems of interpretation [15]. 5) Despite the flaws the data actually show that WHZ carries a higher mortality risk than MUAC when appropriately analysed [16]. Indeed, there are abundant data to confirm that WHZ < −3Z carries a substantial risk of death [22–26], but these papers did not measure MUAC for comparison. Thus, all the criticisms asserted by Briend et al., and repeated [9, 14, 27, 28] are, in our opinion, incorrect. Nevertheless, their advocacy has led most humanitarian agencies and some Governments to abandon WHZ altogether.

We do agree that WHZ is more inconvenient and difficult to measure than MUAC; but this is the *only* legitimate criticism of widespread use of WHZ. The question arises as to the potential fate of the ≈45% of children who would not be identified if WHZ measurement was omitted completely.

Having shown that the case fatality rates (CFRs) are not lower in children with only a deficit in WHZ, this paper examines the practical programmatic differences between a MUAC-only program and a complete program.

The object of this study was to estimate the proportion and where possible the numbers of all SAM related deaths that would occur in children who would be excluded from treatment if a MUAC-only program replaced a complete program.

## Methods

### Effect of case-load

We used a simple excel spreadsheet to demonstrate the effect of variations of the proportions of the total case-load comprised of children with SAM by MUAC, WHZ and by both MUAC and WHZ with their corresponding CFRs on the proportion of SAM deaths that would occur in excluded children if a MUAC-only program was used.

The total SAM-related-deaths is given by:

$$(\mathbf{M}_{CL}\mathbf{x}\ \mathbf{M}_{CFR} + \mathbf{W}_{CL}\mathbf{x}\ \mathbf{W}_{CFR} + \mathbf{B}_{CL}\mathbf{x}\ \mathbf{B}_{CFR})$$

Where M = children with MUAC < 115 mm and WHZ > −3Z (S-muac): W = children with WHZ < −3Z and MUAC > 115 mm (S-whz): B = children with "Both" MUAC < 115 mm and WHZ < −3Z (S-both): subscript *CL* = the proportions of the total case load of SAM that are in categories M, W and B: subscript *CFR* = Case fatality rates for children with M, W and B. The case load always sums to 100% of SAM children (i.e. SAM due to oedema, kwashiorkor with or without wasting, is not considered in this calculation).

Then the proportion of total SAM-related-deaths that would occur in children that would **not** be eligible for admission and treatment if WHZ were to be dropped as an admission criterion is given by:

$$\mathbf{1} - (\mathbf{M}_{CL}\mathbf{x}\ \mathbf{M}_{CFR} + \mathbf{B}_{CL}\mathbf{x}\ \mathbf{B}_{CFR})/(\mathbf{M}_{CL}\mathbf{x}\ \mathbf{M}_{CFR} + \mathbf{W}_{CL}\mathbf{x}\ \mathbf{W}_{CFR} + \mathbf{B}_{CL}\mathbf{x}\ \mathbf{B}_{CFR}).$$

For the simulation, the relative case-loads were varied from zero children with S-muac to zero children with S-whz. The remainder of the children either had the alternative criterion or had S-Both. The proportion of children with S-both was varied from 10 to 30% (the limits we found in representative nutritional surveys [12]). The CFRs for S-muac, S-whz and S-both were examined by changing the ratio of S-muac to S-whz mortality from half to twice the mortality of the other to represent the likely limits of the variation in mortality risk. S-both's CFR was set at the sum of the CFRs of S-muac and S-whz in accordance with the empirical data and most of the literature reports [16, 17]. Variation of the overall CFR will affect the total number of deaths, but the proportions of SAM-related deaths which would be eligible or ineligible for treatment is not affected by the absolute CFRs, only by their ratios and relative case-loads. Thus, if the sizes of the three CFRs and the proportions of the three case loads do not change the percent of children that will become ineligible for treatment does not change when the total SAM-related death rate rises or falls.

### Proportion of all SAM-related-deaths that would occur in children ineligible for treatment with a MUAC-only program by country

The literature and patient data reported in the first and second papers [16, 17] were subject to ascertainment bias which made the proportions of the case load coming from the different categories unrepresentative of SAM in the community. In particular, the proportion of children in the S-both category was much higher than that found in the community. That is, the case load ratios of S-muac: S-whz: S-both differed significantly from that found in representative community surveys of malnourished children [9]. For that reason the case load ratios of S-muac, S-whz and S-both reported in papers I and II [16, 17] were not used in any calculation. To fairly represent the situation of SAM children in the community we used the data previously published from representative community surveys [12]. These ratios are derived from analysis of 48,697 SAM children out of a total surveyed population of 1,384,068 children, 6–59 months, (1832 surveys) from 48 countries.

The community-derived, proportionate case-load estimates were then used to estimate the proportion of the total deaths that would occur in SAM children with a MUAC-only program; the residue of S-whz would be excluded. As the mortality rates for S-muac, S-whz and S-both that would occur in untreated SAM-children in the communities are unknown we used mortality rates from 3 sources. First, those used in our theoretical simulation; second, those found in paper 1 [16]; third, the relative risks of death derived from the meta-analysis of the literature values where WHO criteria were used and oedematous cases excluded [17]. The forest plots from the meta-analyses comparing S-muac with S-whz and S-both, using adjustment for study quality, [17] are given in Additional file 1. The relative risks of death from S-muac, S-whz and S-both were 1.00: 1.14: 2.70 respectively.

The calculations were the same as for the theoretical simulation.

### How many are affected?

In order to estimate the number of children excluded by a MUAC-only program we examined data from a global estimate of SAM-related deaths [1] and from India [29]. These estimates are minimum estimates because they were based upon prevalence data rather than incidence data and only on WHZ data. We used case loads of S-muac, 39.5%, S-whz 44.0% and S-both 16.5% for the global SAM-deaths estimate and S-muac 15.5%, S-whz

61.6% and S-both 22.9% for India [12]. The CFRs were the same for the single deficits and double for S-both.

### Ethical statement

This analysis used published data only thus no formal ethical clearance was required.

## Results

### Theoretical considerations

Figure 1 illustrates the effect of variation of the case-loads of S-muac, S-whz and S-both and corresponding CFRs to derive the percent of deaths occurring in children excluded by a MUAC-only program. The three lines in each block show the effect of S-muac CFR being half, the same or twice the CFR of S-whz. These CFRs represent the likely relative risk and the outside limits. The three blocks show the effect of an increasing S-both percentages.

If a WHZ-only program was used the results would be the exact inverse of the percentage exclusion shown.

With a MUAC-only policy, if there are no children in the community with S-whz (col 1) then all the SAM children will be identified. If there are no children with S-muac (last col) the only deaths of MUAC children will be those who also have S-whz, i.e. those with S-both. There will be slightly more deaths than the proportion of overlap because of the higher mortality risk of S-both children.

A likely scenario is given in block two, second row. As the percentage of S-muac in the community decreases from 60 to 20% the deaths that occur in excluded children increases from 17 to 50%. To have 20% S-muac is frequently found in nutritional surveys from some regions [12]. Figure 1 also shows that the exclusion rate is reduced with more S-both children. For example, if 50% of the children have S-muac (column 5) as S-both increases from 10 to 20 to 30% the relative proportion of deaths of excluded children decreases from 36, to 33 to 31% respectively. As the proportion of S-muac decreases the effect of S-both on excluded cases increases; thus, were there is 20% of S-muac children (col 7) the percent of excluded children falls from 64 to 50% to 38%.

**Relative Case Load**

| Case fatality rates % S-muac | S-whz | S-both | | | | | | | | | |
|---|---|---|---|---|---|---|---|---|---|---|---|
| | | S-muac % | *90* | *80* | *70* | *60* | *50* | *30* | *20* | *10* | *0* |
| | | S-whz % | *0* | *10* | *20* | *30* | *40* | *60* | *70* | *80* | *90* |
| | | S-both % | *10* | *10* | *10* | *10* | *10* | *10* | *10* | *10* | *10* |
| **BOTH = 10%** | | | | | | | | | | | |
| 5.0 | 10.0 | 15.0 | 0 | 15 | 29 | 40 | 50 | 67 | 74 | 80 | 86 |
| 10.0 | 10.0 | 20.0 | 0 | 9 | **18** | **27** | **36** | **55** | **64** | 73 | 82 |
| 10.0 | 5.0 | 15.0 | 0 | 5 | 11 | 17 | 24 | 40 | 50 | 62 | 75 |
| **BOTH = 20%** | | | | | | | | | | | |
| | | S-muac | *80* | *70* | *60* | *50* | *40* | *30* | *20* | *10* | *0* |
| | | S-whz | *0* | *10* | *20* | *30* | *40* | *50* | *60* | *70* | *80* |
| | | S-both | *20* | *20* | *20* | *20* | *20* | *20* | *20* | *20* | *20* |
| 5.0 | 10.0 | 15.0 | 0 | 13 | 25 | 35 | 44 | 53 | 60 | 67 | 73 |
| **10.0** | **10.0** | **20.0** | 0 | 8 | **17** | **25** | **33** | **42** | **50** | 58 | 67 |
| 10.0 | 5.0 | 15.0 | 0 | 5 | 10 | 16 | 22 | 29 | 38 | 47 | 57 |
| **BOTH = 30%** | | | | | | | | | | | |
| | | S-muac | *70* | *60* | *50* | *40* | *30* | *30* | *20* | *10* | *0* |
| | | S-whz | *0* | *10* | *20* | *30* | *40* | *40* | *50* | *60* | *70* |
| | | S-both | *30* | *30* | *30* | *30* | *30* | *30* | *30* | *30* | *30* |
| 5.0 | 10.0 | 15.0 | 0 | 12 | 22 | 32 | 40 | 40 | 48 | 55 | 61 |
| 10.0 | 10.0 | 20.0 | 0 | 8 | **15** | **23** | **31** | **31** | **38** | 46 | 54 |
| 10.0 | 5.0 | 15.0 | 0 | 5 | 10 | 15 | 21 | 21 | 28 | 35 | 44 |

**Fig. 1** Percentage of SAM-related-deaths of children that would be excluded from treatment in a MUAC-only program. Simulation of the effect of various case loads and case fatality rates for children with SAM by MUAC-only, WHZ-only and Both criteria. The data gives the percent of total SAM-related-deaths that would occur in children excluded from treatment in a MUAC-only program. Case Loads and Case Fatality Rates for: S-muac = MUAC < 115 mm with WHZ > = −3Z: S-whz = WHZ < −3Z with MUAC > 115 mm: S-both = MUAC < 115 mm and WHZ < −3Z. The colours represent the percent of deaths occurring in cases that would be excluded from treatment in such a program: Red 75–100%: Pink 50–75%: Orange 25–50%: green 10–25%: Blue 0–10%

In contrast, a change of CFR ratios from half to twice has a relatively minor effect on the proportion of excluded children (compare the 3 rows vertically). Thus, a change of case-load ratio is more important than a change in CRFs ratio within the ranges reported [16, 17] in determining the extent of exclusion of S-whz children.

It should be emphasised that these simulations compares the deaths in excluded children (S-whz) with all the children that would be identified using a MUAC measurement (i.e. S-muac plus S-both). In papers [16, 17], CFRs from S-muac and S-whz were compared. Here, by combining S-both with S-muac in the calculations we replicate the actual effect of only measuring MUAC on the proportion of deaths related to SAM that would be excluded from treatment or considered in a coverage survey.

### Country data

Because the mortality ratios in nearly all communities is unknown, in Fig. 2 we have used the CFRs from the simulation and estimated from papers I and II [16, 17]. These CFRs are then combined with the actual country case-loads found in community nutrition surveys published previously [12].

In Fig. 2 we present, by country, the estimates of the percentage of deaths of SAM children that would occur in children excluded from treatment if only MUAC measurements are taken. There is reasonable agreement between the estimates based upon the different CFRs. For example, in Senegal the three main CFR estimates indicate that 82, 81 and 83% of deaths occur in excluded children; whereas, in Mozambique only 13, 12 and 15% of deaths occur in excluded children. Taking the average of the empirical and literature exclusion rates, 12 countries would exclude more than three quarters and 34 would exclude more than half of the SAM children that die. Only 3 of the 48 countries would include more than 80% of children who die with SAM.

The corresponding analysis using a WHZ-only program is given in Additional file 2. It is clear that a WHZ-only program would also fail to identify a large proportion of the children at high risk of death.

The countries are grouped by region in Fig. 3. If the countries of South & South East Asia and the Sahel were to adopt a MUAC-only policy then a substantial proportion of SAM children's deaths would occur in excluded children. The same applies in many of the countries in West Africa. Some of these countries are characterised by a dry Sahalian type interior and a wet, heavily populated coast. These ecologically different areas may have different levels of exclusion of S-whz so that the effect of only measuring MUAC may be more deleterious in some areas than others, and may give a within-country bias to nutritional surveys aimed at establishing the prevalence of SAM and the level of exclusion. The same conditions apply to some of the East African countries. On the other hand several countries in West, East and Central Africa as well as Asia and Latin America would exclude less than 25% of children that contribute to SAM mortality.

### Numbers of excluded SAM children who die

Conversion of relative case loads and CFRs into the number of deaths of SAM children who will be ineligible for any treatment under a MUAC-only program is shown in Table 1. Using Black et al.'s [1] estimate of global SAM deaths of 540,000 calculated from WHZ prevalence, the total deaths increases to over 800,000 when we include S-muac deaths. Of these over 300,000 children (38%) will die without the possibility of treatment if WHZ is not measured. In India, although Black et al. estimated that there would be 145,000 deaths, Mohan & Mohan [29] estimated the actual number of deaths due to SAM to be 270.000; of these, more than half, 155,000, would be excluded with a MUAC-only policy.

## Discussion

If the primary objective of treating children with SAM is to prevent death then it is logical to look at the percent of deaths that occur in SAM children that would be excluded from treatment with any change in policy. This should then determine whether or not a policy change is unacceptable. This information cannot be obtained from comparison of CFRs by regression or areas under ROC curves.

The CFRs estimated from our empirical data [16] and a meta-analysis of the literature [17] are consistent and show that the CFRs for S-muac and S-whz are not sufficiently different to affect the rate of exclusion when only MUAC is used for SAM diagnosis. The dominant factor is the case-load mix because even when the CFRs differ substantially the numbers of children that are excluded show relatively minor changes.

The present country data, by themselves, cannot be used to determine the absolute numbers of children calculated to die or that would be excluded because of a change in policy. This requires our data to be combined with the prevalence/incidence rates, population size and community mortality rate for at least one of the diagnostic groups. To then derive population attributable fractions also needs the relative risks of death from SAM children using the non-malnourished children in the same community as the reference [30, 31]. The results comparing Black et al. [1] and Mohan & Mohan [29] demonstrate the difficulties in arriving at accurate estimates. Nevertheless, the numbers of children who die with SAM who would be ignored, if only MUAC is used is massive. We estimate this to be about 40% of all SAM children's deaths globally; but this is variable by country and region as Fig. 3 shows. Ignoring these children and

| | CFR from | | | Sim | Limits | | Literature | All | OTP | IPF | SFC |
|---|---|---|---|---|---|---|---|---|---|---|---|
| | CFR S-muac % | | | 10 | 5 | 10 | 1.00 | 0.78 | 1.15 | 2.77 | 0.46 |
| | CFR S-whz % | | | 10 | 10 | 5 | 1.14 | 2.01 | 2.77 | 4.01 | 0.44 |
| | CFR S-Both % | | | 20 | 15 | 15 | 2.70 | 4.96 | 4.74 | 9.34 | 1.15 |
| **Country** | **% Case Load** | | | | | | | | | | |
| | S-muac | S-whz | S-both | | | | | | | | |
| Thailand* | 20.0 | 80.0 | 0.0 | 80 | 89 | 67 | 82 | 91 | 91 | 85 | 79 |
| Sri Lanka | 7.0 | 87.0 | 6.1 | 82 | 87 | 73 | 81 | 83 | 87 | 82 | 79 |
| Senegal | 5.7 | 87.7 | 6.6 | 82 | 87 | 74 | 81 | 83 | 86 | 82 | 79 |
| Philippines | 12.2 | 81.6 | 6.1 | 77 | 84 | 66 | 76 | 80 | 84 | 78 | 74 |
| Gambia | 8.3 | 81.5 | 10.2 | 74 | 81 | 63 | 72 | 74 | 80 | 73 | 70 |
| Kenya ** | 12.9 | 78.3 | 8.8 | 72 | 80 | 60 | 71 | 75 | 79 | 73 | 68 |
| Togo | 30.0 | 64.0 | 6.0 | 60 | 73 | 45 | 61 | 71 | 74 | 65 | 57 |
| Mauritania | 27.5 | 61.3 | 11.2 | 55 | 67 | 41 | 55 | 62 | 67 | 58 | 51 |
| Guinea-Bissau* | 31.8 | 59.1 | 9.1 | 54 | 67 | 39 | 54 | 63 | 67 | 58 | 51 |
| Mali | 23.9 | 61.5 | 14.6 | 54 | 65 | 40 | 53 | 58 | 64 | 55 | 49 |
| Benin | 25.8 | 59.1 | 15.1 | 51 | 63 | 38 | 50 | 56 | 62 | 53 | 47 |
| India | 16.2 | 62.5 | 21.3 | 51 | 61 | 39 | 49 | 51 | 59 | 51 | 46 |
| Cameroun | 25.5 | 57.4 | 17.0 | 49 | 60 | 36 | 48 | 53 | 59 | 50 | 44 |
| Burkina Faso | 23.3 | 58.4 | 18.3 | 49 | 60 | 37 | 48 | 52 | 59 | 50 | 44 |
| Sudan | 19.8 | 59.9 | 20.3 | 50 | 60 | 37 | 48 | 51 | 58 | 50 | 45 |
| Somalia | 31.1 | 54.8 | 14.1 | 48 | 60 | 34 | 47 | 54 | 60 | 50 | 44 |
| South Sudan | 26.8 | 55.2 | 17.9 | 47 | 58 | 34 | 46 | 50 | 57 | 48 | 42 |
| Eritrea | 45.2 | 45.2 | 9.5 | 41 | 55 | 28 | 42 | 52 | 56 | 46 | 38 |
| Bangladesh | 44.3 | 45.1 | 10.6 | 41 | 54 | 27 | 41 | 51 | 55 | 45 | 38 |
| Tchad | 26.4 | 51.4 | 22.2 | 42 | 52 | 30 | 40 | 44 | 51 | 42 | 37 |
| Nigeria | 32.4 | 48.5 | 19.1 | 41 | 52 | 28 | 40 | 45 | 51 | 42 | 36 |
| Niger | 25.5 | 49.6 | 24.9 | 40 | 50 | 28 | 38 | 41 | 48 | 40 | 35 |
| Ethiopia | 41.3 | 43.2 | 15.5 | 37 | 50 | 25 | 37 | 44 | 50 | 40 | 34 |
| Nepal | 36.8 | 42.7 | 20.5 | 35 | 47 | 24 | 35 | 40 | 46 | 37 | 31 |
| Zimbabwe | 47.4 | 36.8 | 15.8 | 32 | 44 | 21 | 32 | 39 | 44 | 35 | 29 |
| Myanmar | 37.4 | 39.8 | 22.8 | 32 | 43 | 22 | 31 | 36 | 42 | 34 | 29 |
| Liberia | 46.9 | 35.7 | 17.4 | 30 | 42 | 20 | 30 | 37 | 42 | 33 | 27 |
| Pakistan | 44.6 | 35.3 | 20.1 | 29 | 40 | 19 | 29 | 34 | 40 | 31 | 26 |
| DRC | 58.0 | 30.5 | 11.5 | 27 | 40 | 17 | 28 | 38 | 41 | 31 | 25 |
| Tanzania | 44.6 | 32.7 | 22.7 | 27 | 37 | 17 | 26 | 31 | 36 | 28 | 23 |
| Timor* | 32.5 | 35.0 | 32.5 | 26 | 35 | 18 | 25 | 27 | 34 | 26 | 23 |
| Guinea | 56.6 | 28.3 | 15.1 | 25 | 36 | 15 | 25 | 32 | 36 | 28 | 22 |
| CAR | 59.2 | 27.5 | 13.4 | 24 | 36 | 15 | 25 | 33 | 37 | 28 | 22 |
| Haiti | 62.8 | 25.9 | 11.3 | 23 | 35 | 14 | 24 | 33 | 36 | 27 | 21 |
| Angola | 56.5 | 26.1 | 17.4 | 22 | 32 | 14 | 22 | 29 | 33 | 25 | 20 |
| Afghanistan | 52.8 | 26.9 | 20.3 | 22 | 32 | 14 | 22 | 28 | 32 | 24 | 20 |
| Madagascar | 53.6 | 26.5 | 19.9 | 22 | 32 | 14 | 22 | 27 | 32 | 24 | 20 |
| Uganda | 65.2 | 23.3 | 11.6 | 21 | 32 | 12 | 22 | 30 | 33 | 24 | 19 |
| Burundi | 59.3 | 24.3 | 16.4 | 21 | 31 | 13 | 21 | 28 | 31 | 23 | 19 |
| Ivory Coast | 63.5 | 22.6 | 13.9 | 20 | 30 | 12 | 20 | 28 | 31 | 23 | 18 |
| Rwanda | 51.6 | 25.1 | 23.3 | 20 | 29 | 13 | 20 | 24 | 29 | 22 | 18 |
| Sierra Leone | 50.9 | 24.1 | 25.1 | 19 | 28 | 12 | 19 | 23 | 27 | 20 | 17 |
| Zambia | 75.6 | 17.1 | 7.3 | 16 | 26 | 9 | 17 | 26 | 28 | 20 | 15 |
| Tajikistan | 68.5 | 17.8 | 13.7 | 16 | 25 | 9 | 16 | 23 | 26 | 18 | 14 |
| Malawi | 74.7 | 16.4 | 8.8 | 15 | 25 | 9 | 16 | 24 | 26 | 19 | 14 |
| Zambia* | 77.3 | 15.9 | 6.8 | 15 | 25 | 8 | 16 | 25 | 27 | 19 | 14 |
| Mozambique | 53.0 | 16.8 | 30.3 | 13 | 19 | 8 | 12 | 15 | 18 | 14 | 11 |
| Guatemala* | 92.9 | 7.1 | 0.0 | 7 | 13 | 4 | 8 | 17 | 16 | 10 | 7 |

**Fig. 2** Percentage of SAM-related-deaths of children that would be excluded for treatment with a MUAC-only program by country. *Sim* simulation data from Fig. 1, representing the probable ratio of case fatality rates (CFRs) and likely extremes; *All, IPF, OPT, SFC* are the empirical case fatality rates of patients under different modes of treatment [16]; *Literature* mortality rates from Additional file 1 derived from the data in reference [17]; *Case Loads* S-muac = MUAC < 115 mm with WHZ > = −3Z: S-whz = WHZ < −3Z with MUAC > 115 mm: S-both = MUAC < 115 mm and WHZ < −3Z; *DRC* Democratic Republic of the Congo; *CAR* Central African Republic. The case loads per country are from reference [12]. The colours represent the percent of total SAM-related-deaths occurring in cases that would be excluded from treatment in a MUAC-only program: Red 75–100%: Pink 50–75%: Orange 25–50%: green 10–25%: Blue 0–10%. * These countries case load comes from a small sample size. ** The case load from Kenya comes from the North of Kenya (similar to Sahel)

their deaths is the real cost of promoting a MUAC-only program, and begs the question of "what is acceptable" from a humanitarian point of view. Reliable and appropriate estimates are essential if correct priorities and policies are to be set by Governments to address SAM. Death is not the only adverse effect of severe malnutrition. There are other major health and long term consequences of failing to identify and treat the very much larger number of children with SAM that do not die, estimated to be 10 million in India by WHZ [29].

| Case Load country | CFRs From Simulation | CFRs From Literature | CFRs From Empirical |
|---|---|---|---|
| **SE Asia** | | | |
| Thailand* | 80 | 82 | 91 |
| Philippines | 77 | 76 | 80 |
| Myanmar | 32 | 31 | 36 |
| Timor* | 26 | 25 | 27 |
| **S Asia** | | | |
| Sri Lanka | 82 | 81 | 83 |
| India | 51 | 49 | 51 |
| **Bangladesh** | 41 | 41 | 51 |
| Nepal | 35 | 35 | 40 |
| Pakistan | 29 | 29 | 34 |
| **West Africa** | | | |
| Gambia | 74 | 72 | 74 |
| Togo | 60 | 61 | 71 |
| Guinea-Bissau* | 54 | 54 | 63 |
| Benin | 51 | 50 | 56 |
| Cameroun | 49 | 48 | 53 |
| **Nigeria** | 41 | 40 | 45 |
| Liberia | 30 | 30 | 37 |
| Guinea | 25 | 25 | 32 |
| Ivory Coast | 20 | 20 | 28 |
| Sierra Leone | 19 | 19 | 23 |
| **Asia** | | | |
| Tajikistan | 16 | 16 | 23 |
| Afghanistan | 22 | 22 | 28 |
| **Latin America & Caribbean** | | | |
| Haiti | 23 | 24 | 33 |
| Guatemala* | 7 | 8 | 17 |

| Case Load country | CFRs from Simulation | CFRs from Literature | CFRs from Empirical |
|---|---|---|---|
| **Sahel** | | | |
| Senegal | 82 | 81 | 83 |
| Mauritania | 55 | 55 | 62 |
| Mali | 54 | 53 | 58 |
| Burkina Faso | 49 | 48 | 52 |
| Sudan | 50 | 48 | 51 |
| Somalia | 48 | 47 | 54 |
| **South Sudan** | 47 | 46 | 50 |
| Tchad | 42 | 40 | 44 |
| Niger | 40 | 38 | 41 |
| **East Africa** | | | |
| Kenya** | 72 | 71 | 75 |
| Eritrea* | 41 | 42 | 52 |
| Ethiopia | 37 | 37 | 44 |
| Zimbabwe* | 32 | 32 | 39 |
| Tanzania | 27 | 26 | 31 |
| Angola | 22 | 22 | 29 |
| Madagascar | 22 | 22 | 27 |
| Uganda | 21 | 22 | 30 |
| Malawi | 15 | 16 | 24 |
| Zambia | 15 | 16 | 25 |
| Mozambique | 13 | 12 | 15 |
| **Central Africa** | | | |
| DRC | 27 | 28 | 38 |
| CAR | 24 | 25 | 33 |
| Burundi | 21 | 21 | 28 |
| Rwanda | 20 | 20 | 24 |

**Fig. 3** Percentage of SAM-related-deaths of children that would be excluded for treatment with a MUAC-only program by Region. *Simulation* see Fig. 1; *Literature* data from [17]; *Empirical* data from [16]; *Case load* data from [12]; *CFRs* Case fatality rates; *SE Asia* South East Asia; *S Asia* South Asia; *DRC* Democratic Republic of the Congo; *CAR* Central African Republic. The colour code is the same as Figs. 1 and 2. * Case load ratios from these countries is based on a small sample size. ** For Kenya the case load data comes from the North of Kenya (could be counted with Sahel). In bold are some of the countries whose governments have officially adopted a MUAC-only program (2017)

One answer to the problem of excluded children could be to increase the MUAC cut-off point. This is a simplistic suggestion that is impractical as it would then include a very large proportion of the whole childhood population at a much lower risk of death [9, 13, 28, 32, 33] and divert and dilute the attention needed for the high risk children.

The paper from Uttar Pradesh, India, by Kapil et al. [34] is germane to addressing this suggestion. SAM in Uttar Pradesh by WHZ was 2.2%; when MUAC was added the prevalence increased to 2.5%. If the MUAC cut-off was increased to 135 mm then 17% of all the children in the population would need to be identified; however, 12% of the S-whz children would still be missed and the extra case load would only identify a further 15% of S-whz. Five in 6 of the extra children would be "false positives" for SAM. Our unpublished analysis from Africa is in agreement with these figures. The cost, logistics, staff time with inevitable disruption to other essential medical services, add-on costs for the parents, possible family guilt or stigma concerning the need to be checked for SAM and risk of bringing the program into disrepute all mitigate against this policy. Elsewhere evidence shows that

**Table 1** Estimation of the possible number of deaths from SAM that would be missed using a MUAC only program

| | WHZ deaths | Total deaths | WHZ only (S-whz) | MUAC only (S-muac) | Both criteria (S-both) | MUAC-only %missed | WHZ-only %missed |
|---|---|---|---|---|---|---|---|
| Global | 540,000[a] | 817,000 | 309,000 | 277,000 | 231,000 | 37.8 | 33.9 |
| India | 270, 000[b] | 309,000 | 155,000 | 39,000 | 115,000 | 50.2 | 12.6 |

The estimates of total deaths and proportions were derived as in methods. *WHZ deaths* deaths estimated by WHZ < −3Z (i.e. S-whz + S-both); *Total deaths* WHZ deaths plus MUAC-only deaths based on ratios found in reference [12] for Global and India (S-both = 16.5 and 22.9%). Equal mortality risk for S-whz < −3Z and S-muac < 115 mm and twice the mortality risk for S-both is assumed. [a] Data from reference [1]; [b] Data from reference [29] there are several major difficulties when a false positive rate exceeds the true positive rate [35, 36]. Furthermore, WHO now recommends *"not to provide formulated supplementary foods on a routine basis to children who are moderately wasted"* [37].

In view of the evidence, why has MUAC morphed from a simple and effective community screening program into a MUAC-only program? Is it really necessary for total suppression of WHZ as a diagnostic for SAM to legitimise the use of MUAC?

We suggest that there are several reasons. First, based upon the data presented in the first two papers of this series [16, 17] as well as the present paper it is clear that an inappropriate statistical strategy has been exclusively used in the past using ROC curve analysis of entire populations to compare the relative CFRs [15]; when the risks are suffered by different children entirely, the risks are also different, making comparisons for diagnostic purposes largely meaningless. Second, the exclusive focus on CFRs alone and the notion that MUAC is a "superior" test; it can only be superior if it identifies the same risk. Third, the neglect of case load in determining the numbers of excluded children or the calculation and use of further derived statistics such as population attributable fraction. Fourth, repeated assertions that it is safe to ignore S-whz children because they are healthy when there are no data to support this contention and abundant data to show that these children are at high risk of death combined with misquotation and criticism of any data that does not support the proposition [38]. Fifth, by forceful advocacy to donors, research funding agencies, UN agencies and many in the humanitarian organisations [13]. Sixth, because of an understandable desire to make everything as simple as possible whilst denying there is any cost of excluding SAM children [26]. Simplification beyond what is possible renders programs unworkable or unethical (try removing the cold chain from vaccination services). An effort to simplify SAM treatment by suppressing use of F75, the initial diet designed for the most critically ill of children [39] was dropped when the reasons for F75 were properly explained to the agencies. Only using MUAC is certainly simple, but it has a real cost, and that is measured in lives lost. Last, because of cognitive biases, particularly confirmation bias [40] among those subscribing to a MUAC-only policy and those providing "confirmatory" low quality evidence such as some of the papers reviewed in [17].

The ease of use of MUAC makes community screening to identify children in need to SAM treatment practical and has led to increasingly greater "coverage" rates for those children with MUAC < 115 mm. Our data does not question the utility of this, what is does demand is research to find ways that are sufficiently simple to be applied in the community so that children with WHZ < – 3 can also be included in treatment programs. Stereo-photography has been used for many years [41] but with modern technology this has become practical [42–44]. There are reports of low cost scanning attachments to smart-phones that give precise measures of height, head-circumference and MUAC [45]. Therefore, on the horizon are techniques that will make the assessment of WHZ simple to use in the community. Such studies must be properly funded, supported and then implemented and make it premature to cease considering WHZ as a proper diagnostic for SAM.

## Conclusions

Some within the nutritional community has been misled by replicated but flawed analyses and assertions. They are also attracted by the ease and low cost of MUAC screening; these practical aspects are clearly advantages to be considered. MUAC-only programs fail to identify enormous numbers of the most vulnerable children in many societies. It may be difficult to identify S-whz children, but that is not a reason to pretend these children do not exist or to justify ignoring them by making false claims such as that they are healthy. It is essential that they are included in any program that claims to address the scourge of SAM. In our opinion many of these programs should be considered as contravening the dictates of Hippocrates.

Both a WHZ < –3Z and MUAC < 115 mm must be retained and used wherever possible as diagnostic criteria for SAM. The research priority must be to develop innovative ways of assessing WHZ so that it can be extended to S-whz identification in the community.

## Additional files

**Additional file 1: Figure S1.** Forest plots of papers 1–7 of [17] to determine the CRFs of children with S-muac, S-whz and S-both. The meta-analyses were performed as in [17] using the quality of the study as weighting (QE); only reports that used the recommended WHO diagnostic criteria, and excluded oedematous (oed) cases were selected for this analysis. *IND* India; *NER* Niger; *SDN* South Sudan; *UGA* Uganda; *MWI* Malawi; *SEN* Senegal; *RR* relative risk; CI confidence intervals.

**Additional file 2: Figure S2.** Percentage of SAM-related-deaths of children that would be excluded from treatment by a WHZ-only program. *Sim* simulation data from Fig. 1, representing the likely extremes and probable ratio of case fatality rates (CFRs); *All, IPF, OPT, SFC* are the empirical case fatality rates of patients under different modes of treatment [16]; *Literature* mortality rates from Additional file S1, from reference [17]; *Case Loads* S-muac = MUAC < 115 mm with WHZ > = –3Z: S-whz = WHZ < –3Z with MUAC > 115 mm: S-both = MUAC < 115 mm and WHZ < –3Z; *DRC* Democratic Republic of the Congo; *CAR* Central African Republic. The case loads per country are from reference [12]. The colours represent the percent of total SAM-related-deaths occurring in cases that would be excluded from treatment in a MUAC-only program: Red 75–100%: Pink 50–75%: Orange 25–50%: green 10–25%: Blue 0–10%. * These countries case load comes from a small sample size. ** The case load from Kenya comes from the North of Kenya (similar to Sahel).

#### Abbreviations

CFR: Case fatality rate; IPFs: In-patient treatment facilities; MAM: Moderate acute malnutrition; MUAC: Mid-upper-arm-circumference; NGOs: Non-governmental organisations; OTPs: Out-patient treatment programs; ROC curve: Receiver operating characteristic curve; SAM: Severe acute malnutrition; SFCs: Supplementary feeding centres; WHO: the World Health Organisation; WHZ: Weight-for-height Z-score

**Funding**
Nutriset provided a PhD fellowship to Université Libre de Bruxelles in support of EG. Nutriset had no role in any aspect of this research including data collection, design, analysis, interpretation or writing the article. MHG received no support.

**Authors' contributions**
EG & MHG were involved in all stages from the conception and design, data acquisition, analysis and interpretation. Both authors approved the final version of the article.

**Competing interests**
The authors declare that they have no competing interests.

**Author details**
[1]Research Center Health Policy and Systems - International Health, School of Public Health, Université Libre de Bruxelles, Bruxelles, Belgium. [2]Department of Medicine and Therapeutics, University of Aberdeen, Aberdeen, Scotland.

**References**

1. Black RE, Victora CG, Walker SP, Bhutta ZA, Christian P, De Onis M, et al. Maternal and child undernutrition and overweight in low-income and middle-income countries. Lancet. 2013;382:427–51. http://www.sciencedirect.com/science/article/pii/S014067361360937X
2. WHO, Unicef. WHO child growth standards and the identification of severe acute malnutrition in infants and children: a joint statement by the World Health Organization and the United Nations Children's fund. 2009. http://www.who.int/nutrition/publications/severemalnutrition/9789241598163_eng.pdf
3. WHO. Guideline: Updates on the management of severe acute malnutrition in infants and children. Geneva, World Health Organization; 2013. http://www.who.int/nutrition/publications/guidelines/updates_management_SAM_infantandchildren/en/.
4. Jelliffe DB. The assessment of nutritional status of the community. Geneva: WHO; 1966. PMID: 4960818
5. Jelliffe EFP, Jelliffe DB. The arm circumference as a public health index of protein-calorie malnutrition of early childhood. J Trop Pediatr. 1969; 32:1527–30.
6. Jelliffe DB. Arm circumference in children. Lancet. 1970;1(7641):305–6.
7. Shakir A, Morley D. Measuring malnutrition. Lancet. 1974;1:758–9.
8. Shakir A. Arm circumference in the surveillance of protein-calorie malnutrition in Baghdad. Am J Clin Nutr. 1975;28:661–5.
9. Briend A, Alvarez JL, Avril N, Bahwere P, Bailey J, Berkley JA, et al. Low mid-upper arm circumference identifies children with a high risk of death who should be the priority target for treatment. BMC Nutr. 2016;2:63. https://bmcnutr.biomedcentral.com/articles/10.1186/s40795-016-0101-7
10. EN-Net. WFH versus MUAC. 2015. Emergency Nutrition Network. http://www.en-net.org/question/1915.aspx
11. EN-Net. Only MUAC for admission and discharge? 2015. Emergency Nutrition Network. http://www.en-net.org/question/1922.aspx
12. Grellety E, Golden MH. Weight-for-height and mid-upper-arm circumference should be used independently to diagnose acute malnutrition: policy implications. BMC Nutr 2016, 2: 10. https://bmcnutr.biomedcentral.com/articles/10.1186/s40795-016-0049-7
13. Bailey J, Chase R, Kerac M, Briend A, Manary M, Opondo C et al. Combined protocol for SAM/MAM treatment. The ComPAS study. Field exchange 2016, 53: 44. http://www.ennonline.net/fex/53/thecompasstudy
14. Hammond W, Badawi AE, Deconinck H. Detecting severe acute malnutrition in children under five at scale. The Challenges of Anthropometry to Reach the Missed Millions. Ann Nutr Disord Ther. 2016;3:1030. http://austinpublishinggroup.com/nutritional-disorders/fulltext/andt-v3-id1030.php
15. Grellety E, Golden MH. Response to Briend et al "low mid-upper-arm-circumference identifies children with a high risk of death and should be the priority target for treatment". BMC Nutr. 2016;2-63:1–12. https://bmcnutr.biomedcentral.com/articles/10.1186/s40795-016-0101-7
16. Grellety E, Golden MH. Severely malnourished children with a low weight-for-height have a higher mortality than those with a low mid-upper-arm-circumference: I. Empirical data demonstrates Simpson's paradox. Nutr J. 2018. https://doi.org/10.1186/s12937-018-0384-4
17. Grellety E, Golden MH. Severely malnourished children with a low weight-for-height have a higher mortality than those with a low mid-upper-arm-circumference: II. Systematic literature review and meta-analysis. Nutr J. 2018. https://doi.org/10.1186/s12937-018-0383-5
18. Post CL, Victora CG. The low prevalence of weight-for-height deficits in Brazilian children is related to body proportions. J Nutr 2001;131:1290–1296. http://jn.nutrition.org/content/131/4/1290.full
19. Roberfroid D, Huybregts L, Lachat C, Vrijens F, Kolsteren P, Guesdon B. Inconsistent diagnosis of acute malnutrition by weight-for-height and mid-upper arm circumference: contributors in 16 cross-sectional surveys from South Sudan, the Philippines, Chad, and Bangladesh. Nutr J. 2015;14:1. https://nutritionj.biomedcentral.com/articles/10.1186/s12937-015-0074-4
20. Archie JP Jr. Mathematic coupling of data: a common source of error. Ann Surg. 1981;193:296. http://journals.lww.com/annalsofsurgery/abstract/1981/03000/mathematic_coupling_of_data__a_common_source_of.8.aspx
21. Tu YK, Maddick IH, Griffiths GS, Gilthorpe MS. Mathematical coupling can undermine the statistical assessment of clinical research: illustration from the treatment of guided tissue regeneration. J Dent. 2004;32:133–42. https://doi.org/10.1016/j.jdent.2003.10.001
22. Puffer RR, Serrano CV. Patterns of mortality in childhood: report of the inter-American investigation of mortality in childhood, Paho scientific publication no. 262, 1–470. Washington: Pan American Health Organization; 1973. http://www.popline.org/node/518356
23. Puffer RR, Serano CV. The role of nutritional deficiency in mortality: findings of the inter-American investigation of mortality in childhood. Bol Ofic Sanit Panam. 1973;7:1–25.
24. Pelletier DL. The relationship between child anthropometry and mortality in developing countries: implications for policy, programs and future research. J Nutr. 1994;124(10 Suppl):2047S–81S.
25. O'Neill SM, Fitzgerald A, Briend A, Van Den Broeck J. Child mortality as predicted by nutritional status and recent weight velocity in children under two in rural Africa. J Nutr. 2012;142:520–5. https://doi.org/10.3945/jn.111.151878.
26. Olofin I, McDonald CM, Ezzati M, Flaxman S, Black RE, Fawzi WW, et al. Associations of suboptimal growth with all-cause and cause-specific mortality in children under five years: a pooled analysis of ten prospective studies. PLoS One. 2013;8:e64636.
27. Briend, A. Use of MUAC for severe acute malnutrition. CMAM forum 2012. http://citeseerx.ist.psu.edu/viewdoc/download?doi=10.1.1.662.303&rep=rep1&type=pdf
28. Briend A, Maire B, Fontaine O, Garenne M. Mid-upper arm circumference and weight-for-height to identify high-risk malnourished under-five children. Matern Child Nutr. 2012;8:130–3. http://onlinelibrary.wiley.com/doi/10.1111/j.1740-8709.2011.00340.x/full
29. Mohan P, Mohan SB. Management of Children with severe acute malnutrition in India: we know enough to act, and we should act now. Indian Pediatr. 2017;54(10):813–4. http://indianpediatrics.net/oct2017/813.pdf
30. Rockhill B, Newman B, Weinberg C. The use and misuse of population attributable fractions. Am J Public Health. 1998;98:2119–21.
31. Hanley JA. A heuristic approach to the formulas for population attributable fraction. J Epidemiol Community Health. 2001;55:508–14. http://jech.bmj.com/content/55/7/508.full
32. Shepherd S, Becquet R. Integrated Treatment Protocol for Acute Malnutrition: A Non Inferiority Trial in Burkina Faso (MUAC-Only). ClinicalTrials.gov 2017. https://clinicaltrials.gov/ct2/show/NCT03027505
33. Maust A, Koroma AS, Abla C, Molokwu N, Ryan KN, Singh L, et al. Severe and moderate acute malnutrition can be successfully managed with an integrated protocol in Sierra Leone. J Nutr. 2015;145(11):2604–9. https://doi.org/10.3945/jn.115.214957
34. Kapil U, Pandey RM, Bansal R, Pant B, Varshney AM, Yadav CP, et al. Mid-upper arm circumference in detection of weight-for-height Z-score below–3 in children aged 6–59 months. Public Health Nutr. 2018;5:1–6. https://doi.org/10.1017/S1368980017004165
35. Wald NJ, Hackshaw AK, Frost CD. When can a risk factor be used as a worthwhile screening test? BMJ: Br Med J. 1999;319:1562–5. https://doi.org/10.1136/bmj.319.7224.1562
36. Rosenblatt RA. The perinatal paradox: doing more and accomplishing less. Health Aff. 1989;8:158–68. https://doi.org/10.1377/hlthaff.8.3.158

37. World Health Organization. Guideline: assessing and managing children at primary health-care facilities to prevent overweight and obesity in the context of the double burden of malnutrition. Updates for the Integrated Management of Childhood Illness (IMCI) Geneva (Switzerland): World Health Organization; 2017. http://apps.who.int/iris/bitstream/10665/259133/1/9789241550123-eng.pdf
38. Murray C. How to accuse the other guy of lying with statistics. Stat Sci. 2005;20:239–41. http://www.jstor.org/stable/20061179
39. Briend A. Management of severe malnutrition: efficacious or effective? J Pediatr Gastroenterol Nutr. 2001;32:521–2. http://journals.lww.com/jpgn/Fulltext/2001/05000/Management_of_Severe_Malnutrition__Efficacious_or.5.aspx
40. Kahneman D. Thinking, Fast and Slow. Macmillan, 2011. http://www.math.chalmers.se/~ulfp/Review/fastslow.pdf
41. Piebson WR. Monophotogrammetric determination of body volume. Ergonomics. 1961;4:213–8. http://www.tandfonline.com/doi/abs/10.1080/00140136108930521
42. Wells JCK, Ruto A, Treleaven P. Whole-body three-dimensional photonic scanning: a new technique for obesity research and clinical practice. Int J Obes. 2008;32:232–8. http://www.nature.com/ijo/journal/v32/n2/abs/0803727a.html
43. Yu W. Development of a three-dimensional anthropometry system for human body composition assessment. The University of Texas at Austin; 2008. https://repositories.lib.utexas.edu/bitstream/handle/2152/17838/yuw.pdf%3Bjsessionid%3D61F89DE75AA927339A6A0909C615A7FE?sequence%3D2
44. Mikat RP. Chest, waist, and hip circumference estimations from stereo photographic digital topography. J Sports Med Phys Fitness. 2000;40:58.
45. Conkle J, Ramakrishnan U, Flores-Ayala R, Suchdev PS, Martorell R. Improving the quality of child anthropometry: manual anthropometry in the body imaging for nutritional assessment study (BINA). PLoS One. 2017;12(12):e0189332. http://journals.plos.org/plosone/article?id=10.1371/journal.pone.0189332

# 10

# Severely malnourished children with a low weight-for-height have similar mortality to those with a low mid-upper-arm-circumference

Emmanuel Grellety[1*] and Michael H. Golden[2]

**Abstract**

**Background:** The WHO recommended criteria for diagnosis of sever acute malnutrition (SAM) are weight-for-height/length Z-score (WHZ) of <− 3Z of the $WHO_{2006}$ standards, a mid-upper-arm circumference (MUAC) of < 115 mm, nutritional oedema or any combination of these parameters. A move to eliminate WHZ as a diagnostic criterion has been made on the assertion that children with a low WHZ are healthy, that MUAC is a "superior" prognostic indicator of mortality and that adding WHZ to the assessment does not improve the prediction of death. Our objective was to examine the literature comparing the risk of death of SAM children admitted by WHZ or MUAC criteria.

**Methods:** We conducted a systematic search for reports which examined the relationship of WHZ and MUAC to mortality for children less than 60 months. The WHZ, MUAC, outcome and programmatic variables were abstracted from the reports and examined. Individual study's case fatality rates were compared by chi-squared analysis and random effects meta-analyses for combined data.

**Results:** Twenty-one datasets were reviewed. All the patient studies had an ascertainment bias. Most were inadequate because they had insufficient deaths, used obsolete standards, combined oedematous and non-oedematous subjects, did not report the proportion of children with both deficits or the deaths occurred remotely after anthropometry. The meta-analyses showed that the mortality risks for children who have SAM by MUAC < 115 mm only and those with SAM by WHZ < −3Z only are not different.

**Conclusions:** As the diagnostic criteria identify different children, this analysis does not support the abandonment of WHZ as an important independent diagnostic criterion for the diagnosis of SAM. Failure to identify such children will result in their being denied treatment and unnecessary deaths from SAM.

**Keywords:** Nutrition, Acute malnutrition, Severe acute malnutrition, SAM, Mid-upper-arm circumference, MUAC, Weight-for-height, WHZ, Mortality, Case fatality rate, Wasting, Oedema, Kwashiorkor, Diagnosis, Meta-analysis, Systematic review, Simpson's paradox, Child, Human

* Correspondence: Emmanuel.Grellety.Bosviel@ulb.ac.be
[1]Research Center Health Policy and Systems - International Health, School of Public Health, Université Libre de Bruxelles, Bruxelles, Belgium
Full list of author information is available at the end of the article

## Background

Severe acute malnutrition (SAM) affects at least 19 million children at any one time [1]. Identification of all these children and admission to treatment programs is a public health priority. The World Health Organisation (WHO) has established three independent criteria for the diagnosis of children with SAM. These are a weight-for-height/weight-for-length Z-score (WHZ) of <−3Z or an absolute mid-upper-arm circumference (MUAC) of < 115 mm to assess marasmus, and bilateral nutritional oedema to include kwashiorkor and marasmic-kwashiorkor when both oedema and an anthropometric deficit are present.

Because of its simplicity, ease of use and relative cheapness as a screening tool MUAC has been readily taken up to identify and treat children with SAM in the community and elsewhere [2]. Thus, MUAC has been widely adopted by many agencies and several governments as the only anthropometric criterion for SAM; they consider WHZ cumbersome and difficult to assess. However, although the prevalence of SAM is about the same in representative community nutritional surveys, different children are identified by the two anthropometric criteria with a considerable discordance in individual countries [3–20]. Data from representative community samples of children from 47 countries [21] show that the overall overlap for anthropometric SAM (i.e. children fulfilling both the WHZ and MUAC criteria) was only 16.5%. About 45% of the children fulfil the WHZ definition for SAM but not the MUAC criterion. Where a MUAC only policy has been adopted children fulfilling WHO's WHZ criterion, but not the MUAC criterion, for SAM remain un-identified and un-treated.

Because the two diagnostic parameters select different children we proposed that both MUAC and WHZ have to be retained and continue to be used routinely to identify all those children who need to be treated for SAM and methods found to more easily identify those children with a low WHZ in the community [21]. These proposals led to forceful criticism from Briend et al. [22] who maintain that only MUAC should be used to identify severely malnourished children and that the use of WHZ can be safely dispensed with. This proposal appears to have widespread approval [23–28].

Briend et al. [22, 26] contend that children with a low WHZ do not need to be identified or treated on the grounds that, 1) MUAC has been repeatedly shown to be a "superior" diagnostic parameter to predict subsequent death of SAM children, 2) that children with a low WHZ are healthy and thus do not need treatment; 3) that they only have a low WHZ because their legs are relatively long, 4) that the two anthropometric criteria are proxies for each other, 5) that when children satisfy both criteria their mortality rate is not additive, but that MUAC mortality is universally higher than that with WHZ [22, 26, 29–31] and 6) that addition of WHZ to MUAC does not increase the prognostic sensitivity or specificity of future death prediction and is therefore redundant [31]. These repeated assertions have consequently led to failure to identify children with a WHZ < −3Z, but a normal MUAC, in many programs and officially by some governments who have abandoned the use of WHZ altogether. What started as a simple screening tool for the community identification and as an alternative to WHZ has changed into the primary tool to be used to diagnose SAM with advocacy to extend the suppression of WHZ assessment universally [22, 29, 30, 32].

This series of papers addresses the veracity of these assertions. As we consider whether all the criteria for SAM should be routinely used, or whether WHZ assessment can be omitted safely, the mortality risk of children who would be excluded from diagnosis and treatment as a result of such a policy must be the focus of consideration. As the fate of millions of SAM children is at stake, such a change of policy must be based upon unequivocal robust evidence. In paper I [33] we present empirical data to show that children under treatment for SAM have a higher mortality when admitted with the WHZ criterion, without fulfilling the MUAC criterion, than with the MUAC criterion without fulfilling the WHZ criterion. In paper III [34] we examine the influence of the relative case-load with each criterion on the potential avoidable deaths that would occur in excluded children.

The objective of this paper is to examine the evidence in the published literature that compares the risk of death of severely malnourished children who satisfy the WHZ with those that satisfy the MUAC criteria and to assess whether those that fulfil the WHZ criterion only can be safely omitted from treatment programs.

## Methods

We used the Preferred Reporting Items for Systematic Reviews and Meta-Analysis (PRISMA) statement to guide our review [35].

### Papers included in the analysis

In order to exhaustively include as much evidence as possible pertaining to mortality risk of SAM children by the two anthropometric criteria, all studies were eligible for inclusion if they contained the numbers of children, less than 60 months of age, that were alive and dead when they exited the study, and who had SAM by any WHZ and any MUAC criteria, in any language and at any time.

In February 2017 we searched Pubmed, Scopus and CABI- index for papers of relevance using the search terms: (Mortality or Death or Case Fatality) and (MUAC or mid-upper-arm circumference or arm-circumference or Perimeter Brachial) and (WHZ or weight-for-height or weight-for-length or poids pour taille or PPT). Google-Scholar was also regularly consulted, particularly for papers indexed after our initial search. The search strategy is shown in Fig. 1. Papers that did not provide the numbers of children with MUAC, WHZ and outcome were not considered. Papers relating to children with primary disease unrelated to nutrition were not considered (e.g. congenital heart disease, chronic renal failure, malignancies, cystic fibrosis, etc.). Where possible the original theses, reports and supplementary information from which the paper was written were obtained as these usually gave fuller information. The data presented in our companion paper [33] were not included. One conference presentation [36] was included in the analysis. From the final 20 reports (21 datasets) containing relevant information the following data were abstracted: authors and reference: date: place: type and purpose of study: study setting, in-patient facility (IPF), out-patient treatment program (OTP) or Community cohort: the length of time the children were observed: the standards used for diagnosis of SAM by MUAC and WHZ: the age range of the children included: whether oedematous children were included or excluded: the percent of overlap between the two parameters (i.e. those fulfilling both WHZ and MUAC criteria for SAM / total SAM): the percent of missing data: the default rate: the total number of children and the number that died in the WHZ and MUAC categories. Were possible the number of children fulfilling both diagnostic criteria was obtained and these reports then formed a separate category. It was not possible to estimate the proportions of overlap for those reports where this information was not given.

### Statistical analysis

The original authors analysed their data in a number of ways and some did not present results that directly compared the risk of death of SAM children diagnosed by MUAC, WHZ or both. Most analysed all-cause mortality in the whole childhood community or patient population, including children who did not have SAM by any definition. The area-under a ROC curve, logistic regression, life table, etc., including all available children, were then used in the analysis. For the present analysis the subjects that did not have SAM were not considered; this was because the objective was not to compare SAM children with non-SAM children, but to compare the relative mortality risks of children with SAM who fulfilled either the MUAC or the WHZ criterion. Therefore the original analyses were not considered. The actual

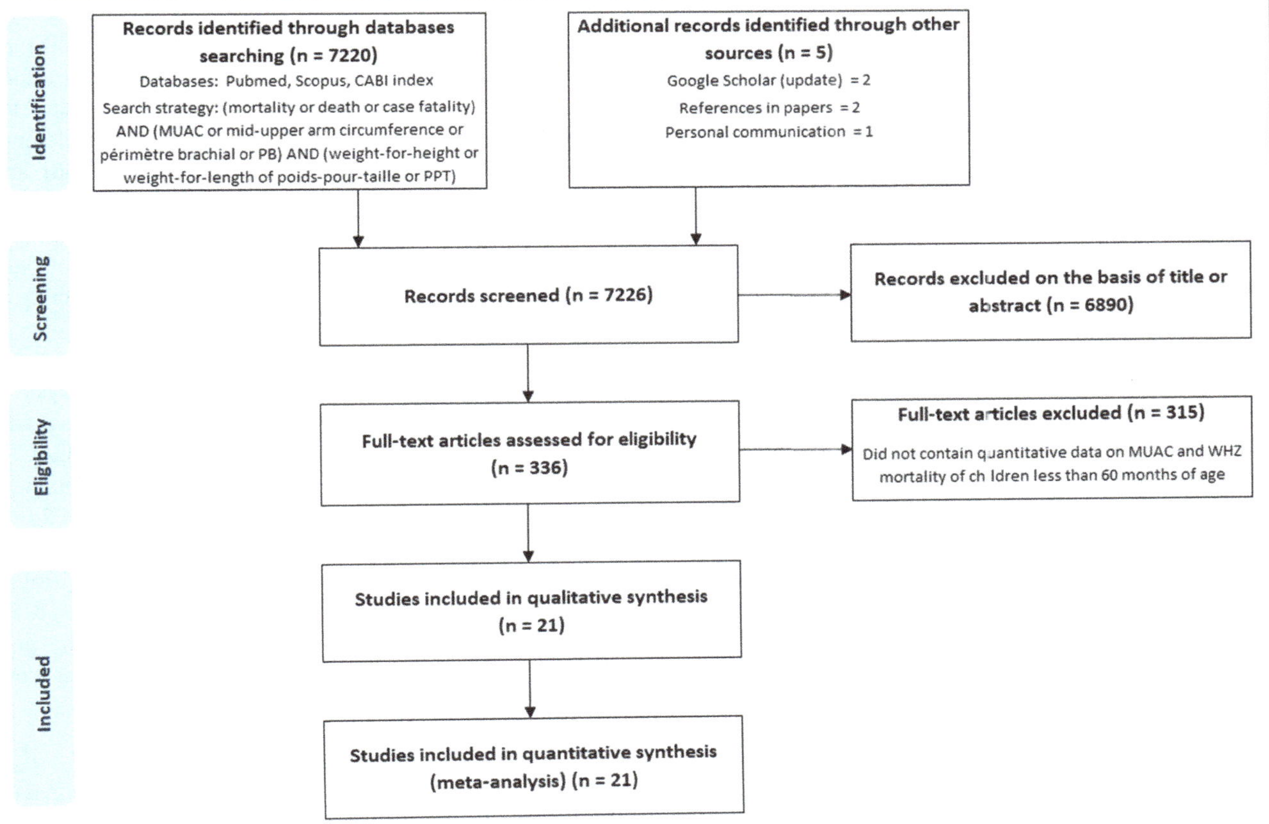


**Fig. 1** Flow of study selection

numbers of children who were below the cut-off points used in the paper to define SAM who survived and those who died were used to re-analyse the data. We directly compared the case fatality rates (CFR) and relative risk (RR) of death of children with SAM by MUAC with SAM by WHZ.

There were 10 datasets where children with SAM could be divided into the following groups:

SAM by MUAC but not by WHZ criteria – designated as "S-muac"

SAM by WHZ but not by MUAC criteria – designated as "S-whz"

SAM by both MUAC and WHZ criteria – designated as "S-both"

There were 11 datasets where children with SAM by both criteria were not separately reported from those children with SAM by one or the other criterion (i.e. S-both could not be determined). In these reports children with SAM by MUAC may, or may not, also have SAM by WHZ; they are designated as "All-muac". Similarly, those with SAM by WHZ may, or may not, also have SAM by MUAC; they are designated as "All-whz". These papers were potentially in error because of mathematical coupling (see companion paper I [33]) and are examined as a separate group. Mathematical coupling occurs where *"one variable directly or indirectly contains the whole or part of another, and the two variables are analysed using standard statistical techniques"* [37, 38]. Thus, S-muac, S-whz and S-both data are mutually exclusive, but All-muac and All-whz are not mutually exclusive. There were also papers where oedematous children were incorporated into the analysis, usually with an unknown proportion of oedematous children in each group; this is known to be a major confounder [33]. Thus, where oedematous children were included in the dataset, so that marasmus could not be differentiated from marasmic-kwashiorkor the reports were analysed in a sub-category.

The data from two studies were each reported using different standards (study from Senegal in datasets 18 & 19 [39, 40] and from Democratic Republic of Congo in datasets 20 & 21 [40, 41]). Each of the duplicate datasets were included in an initial analysis by subgroup comparing the effect of using different diagnostic cut-off points to analyse the data and demonstrate the effect of using different references on the derived outcomes. The duplicated data (18 to 21) were not used in the other analyses as report 7 had incorporated the same two datasets, combined with a study from Nepal, into their analysis. As report 7 used WHO criteria, separated children with both criteria (S-both) and as far as possible excluded oedematous children the data in this report was considered to be most reliable.

Individual datasets with S-muac vs, S-whz and All-muac vs All-whz were analysed by 2 × 2 chi-squared. Where there were fewer than 5 children in any expected category the analysis was by Fisher's exact test.

#### Meta-analyses

The data abstracted from the individual papers were examined by meta-analyses using MetaXL version 5.3 software [42]; the random effects model with relative risk (RR) output divided by subgroups, was used to compare the effects of potential bias. The quality effects model was used for the final analysis where the studies are grouped by whether S-both data were available or not [43]. Tests for heterogeneity were generated for each analysis by two methods (funnel plots and Doi plot). In the funnel plot, the ORs were plotted against the standard error, while in Doi plots, the ORs were plotted against z-score. To examine the potential effects of bias because of the differences in the study type, standards and inclusion criteria, the meta-analyses were repeated dividing the studies into the following sub-categories: 1) to test the biasing effect of oedema inclusion, S-muac v S-whz with and without oedematous case inclusion (i.e. omitting the 11 studies with only All-muac and All-whz information): 2) to test the effects of using different definitions of SAM, the datasets were divided by the standards and cut-off points for diagnosis: 3) to examine ascertainment and treatment bias, the studies were grouped by type of study (community cohort, in-patients treated for SAM, out-patients treated for SAM): and, 4) the difference between those that excluded children with S-both and those that incorporated them into their dataset. The assessment of study quality and potential for bias was assessed, using the criteria in table Additional file 1: Table S1. Confidence intervals are 95% for all reports and a probability of 0.05 is considered significant.

#### Effect of including or excluding "S-both" in the analyses

In order to examine the effects of including children suffering from both deficits (i.e. WHZ < −3Z and MUAC < 115 mm) in the comparison of mortality related to WHZ and MUAC, we calculated both the CFRs of S-whz and S-muac and for the same cohorts of SAM children when S-both was added to S-whz and S-muac to give the corresponding All-whz and All-muac CFR from the same study. This analysis could only be performed with the reports that differentiated S-both from the single deficit categories.

#### Ethical statement

This is a secondary analysis of published data in the public domain. As such no ethical clearance was required.

## Results

The 21 datasets' characteristics are shown in Table 1 and the derived mortality data in Table 2 [16, 36, 39–41, 44–58]. A brief description and comments on each study are given in Additional file 2. We have divided the datasets into: 1) those that reported the proportion of children fulfilling both anthropometric criteria (S-both) separately from those children with single deficits (S-muac and S-whz) and excluding oedema: 2) those that reported children with S-both separately, but also included an admixture of oedematous patients: and, 3) those that failed to differentiate those with both deficits from those with a single deficit as well as including oedematous cases in most of these reports.

As the current proposal is to cease using WHZ and implement MUAC-only programs, in deciding whether such a policy is ethical, the focus has to be on those children who would then be excluded; that is, children diagnosed by WHZ but have neither the MUAC nor the oedema criteria for SAM. The only studies which make this differentiation possible are those giving data for S-both. This is because the CFR for S-whz cannot be ascertained when the WHZ category also includes S-both children. These are shown in the first two categories (datasets 1 to 10). In order to examine the relative mortality statistically it is necessary to have sufficient deaths in each group. Reports 1 to 7, individually, have insufficient deaths to allow for meaningful differentiation of WHZ from MUAC mortality risk; none were statistically different using Fisher's exact test.

### The effect of oedema

From our empirical data [33] and other studies [59, 60] it is clear that children with oedema have a higher mortality than those that are oedema free, no matter their anthropometric status. However, the augmentation of oedema related mortality appears to be different in children who have wasting by MUAC or by WHZ.

Figure 2 shows a meta-analysis of papers 1 to 10 comparing those with and without admixture of oedematous cases. Although none of the pooled differences are significant, the first 7 studies that have excluded oedematous cases show that the RR of death is greater in S-whz than S-muac (RR, 1.12; CI, 0.75–1.68). For the 3 studies that included oedema the RR indicates that S-muac has a higher mortality risk than S-whz (RR, 0.59; CI, 0.28–1.21).

### Effect of the reference criteria

WHO recommends that only the $WHO_{2006}$ standards be used as the reference for WHZ and < 115 mm for MUAC diagnosis of SAM in children 6 to 59 months [61, 62]. Obsolete references were naturally used for studies published before 2006 and these have not, to our knowledge, been re-published using WHO criteria. References that are more stringent than the $WHO_{2006}$ standards, such as the NCHS reference, should have a higher case fatality rate (CFR) and a lower case load than would be the case if the WHO standards were used. This is because the children then diagnosed as SAM will have a lower mean WHZ and thus be more severely malnourished with a higher risk of death than those included with a less stringent reference. Fig. 3 shows the cut-off weights for given heights of the references used in the various studies. Where a more lenient reference, such as the $CDC_{2000}$ curves, is used to define SAM the additional children included in the SAM cohort will have an ameliorating effect on the CFR as they are at a lower mean risk of death, but the additional children will increase the case load. This effect can be quite profound because the absolute number of children included in the SAM category increases exponentially as the diagnostic criteria are relaxed. This is because the shape of the distribution curve of anthropometric parameters in the community is approximately Gaussian [63, 64]. Similarly, where a MUAC of < 110 mm has been used we expect a higher CFR and a lower case-load, than where < 115 mm has been used to define SAM. Thus, whether either the MUAC or WHZ criterion is more or less stringent the relative CFRs and case-loads will change reciprocally. The interpretation of the mortality rates must be judged by the references used. As shown in Fig. 3, the different reference slopes are non-linear. It is not possible to convert data obtained from one set of references to another or to properly amalgamate the data from studies that used obsolete standards.

Figure 4 shows the meta-analysis of all the datasets grouped by the standards that were used. None of the pooled differences showed a significant difference between the risk of death of children fulfilling the MUAC or the WHZ criteria. The studies that used the WHO recommended criteria have an equivalent mortality risk for WHZ and MUAC.

Unexpectedly, those studies that used the NCHS reference had the same RR as those that used the WHO standards with no difference between MUAC and WHZ. Theoretically, WHZ should have had a higher mortality because of the shape of the cut-off for NCHS -3Z; but, as the WHO and NCHS reference lines cross each other at about 73 cm height the net effect will depend upon the height (age) distribution of the children in the studies. The lack of difference between WHO and NCHS could also be due to confounding by inclusion of oedematous children in each of the NCHS studies as well as some of the WHO studies. Nevertheless, there is no net difference and for this reason we have included studies that used the NCHS reference in our main meta-analysis.

**Table 1** Characteristics of studies included in the analysis

| Ref | Study | Author & year | Country | Setting[a] | Study design | Prospect Retrosp | Date of data | MUAC stand | WHZ stand | Age range | Oed | Oed cases | "Both" in study | "Both" in survey | Time obs | Missing data | Default or lost | Original analysis |
|---|---|---|---|---|---|---|---|---|---|---|---|---|---|---|---|---|---|---|
| # | # | | | | | | year | mm | Z or % | month | | % | % | % | d.m | % | % | |
| Studies giving numbers of children fulfilling both WHZ and MUAC criteria | | | | | | | | | | | | | | | | | | |
| 41 | 1 | Aguayo 2015 | India | IPF | Case notes | Retrosp | 2009–11 | < 115 | <−3 WHO | 6–59 | excl | | 63.9 | 21.3 | 14 d | ng | 22.9 | Log reg |
| 42 | 2 | Grellety 2012 | Niger | Com | Com trial | Prospect | 2010 | < 115 | <−3 WHO | **6–23** | excl | | 35.1 | 24.9 | 5 m | 5.3 | 0.0 | Cox PH reg |
| 21 | 3 | Grellety 2015 | South Sudan | OTP | Case notes | Retrosp | 2008 | < 115 | <−3 WHO | 6–59 | excl | | 31.7 | 20.3 | 51 d | 8.6 | 15.0 | Binom reg |
| 43 | 4 | Isanaka 2015 | Niger | OTP | RCT | Prospect | 2012–3 | < 115 | <−3 WHO | 6–59 | excl | | 39.2 | 24.9 | 29.5 d | 0.0 | 1.0 | Log-binom |
| 44 | 5 | Lowlaavar 2016 | Uganda | IPF | Cohort | Prospect | 2012–3 | < 115 | <−3 WHO | 6–60 | excl | | 22.5 | 11.6 | 3 d | ng | 9.7 | Log reg |
| 45 | 6 | LaCourse 2014 | Malawi | IPF | Case notes | Prospect | 2011–2 | **< 110** | < 70% NCHS | 6–60 | excl | | 14.2 | 8.8 | ng | 0.5 | 0.0 | Chisq OR |
| 35 | 7 | Olofin 2016 | DRC,Senegal,Nepal | Com | Com cohort | Prospect | 1983–92 | < 115 | <−3 WHO | 6–59 | excl | | 21.9 | 20,12,7 | 2–6 m | ng | ng | Cox PH reg |
| Studies including oedema | | | | | | | | | | | | | | | | | | |
| 46 | 8 | Berkley 2005 | Kenya | IPF | Case notes | Prospect | 1999–02 | < 115 | <−3 NCHS | **12–59** | incl | 34.2 | 42.9 | 8.8[b] | ng | 3.6 | ng | ROC curve |
| 47 | 9 | Chiabi 2017 | Cameroun | IPF | Case notes | Retrosp | 2006–14 | < 115 | <− 3 WHO | 6–59 | incl | ng | 58.5 | 17.0 | ng | 30.7 | 10.1 | ROC curve |
| 48 | 10 | Sachdeva 2016 | India | IPF | Case notes | Prospect | 2012–3 | < 115 | <−3 WHO | 6–60 | incl | 3.8 | 32.2 | 21.3 | 3.7 d | ng | 15.0 | ROC curve |
| Studies where children fulfilling both criteria are incorporated into both the WHZ and MUAC categories | | | | | | | | | | | | | | | | | | |
| 49 | 11 | Burza 2016 | India | Com | Follow up | Prospect | 2009–11 | < 115 | <−3 WHO | 6–59 | ng | ng | ng | 21.3 | 18 m | 26.7 | ng | Log reg |
| 50 | 12 | Mogeni 2011 | Kenya | IPF | Case notes | Prospect | 2007–9 | < 115 | <−3 WHO | 6–60 | incl | 19.2 | ng | 8.8[b] | ng | 5.4 | ng | Chisq |
| 51 | 13 | Sylla 2015 | Senegal | IPF | Case notes | Retrosp | 2012 | < 115 | <− 3 WHO | **0–60** | ng | ng | ng | 6.6 | ng | ng | ng | Log reg |
| 52 | 14 | Vella 1990 | Uganda | Com | Com cohort | Prospect | 1988 | < 115 | <−3 NCHS | **0–60** | incl | ng | ng | 11.6 | ng | 13.0 | 10.0 | Log reg |
| 53 | 15 | Dramaix 1993 | DRC | IPF | Case notes | Prospect | 1986–8 | < 115 | < 70% NCHS | 0–60 | incl | 28.9 | ng | 11.5 | 60 d | 15.4 | ng | Log reg |
| 54 | 16 | Girum 2017 | Ethiopia | IPF | Case notes | Retrosp | 2013–5 | < 115 | **< 70% ng** | ng | incl | 66.6 | ng | 15.5 | 13 d | ng | 11.6 | Cox PH reg |
| 55 | 17 | Savadogo 2007 | BFA | IPF | Case notes | Retrosp | 1999–03 | **Tertile** | **<−3 NCHS** | 0-< 36 | excl | ng | ng | 18.3 | 19 d | ng | 18.3 | Cox PH reg |

**Table 1** Characteristics of studies included in the analysis *(Continued)*

| Ref | Study | Author & year | Country | Setting[a] | Study design | Prospect Retrosp | Date of data | MUAC stand | WHZ stand | Age range | Oed | Oed cases | "Both" in study | "Both" in survey | Time obs | Missing data | Default or lost | Original analysis |
|---|---|---|---|---|---|---|---|---|---|---|---|---|---|---|---|---|---|---|
| # | # | | | | | | year | mm | Z or % | month | | % | % | % | d.m | % | % | |
| 36 | 18 | Garenne1987 | Senegal | Com | Com cohort | Prospect | 1983–4 | < 115 | <–3 NCHS | **1–60** | incl | ng | ng | 6.6 | 3 m | ng | ng | Life table |
| 37 | 19 | Garenne 2009 | Senegal | Com | Com cohort | Prospect | 1983–4 | **< 110** | **CDC2000** | **1–60** | incl | ng | ng | 6.6 | 3 m | ng | ng | Life table |
| 37 | 20 | Garenne 2009 | DRC | Com | Com cohort | Prospect | 1989–92 | **< 110** | **CDC2000** | **1–60** | incl | ng | ng | 11.5 | 6 m | ng | ng | Life table |
| 38 | 21 | VD Broeck 1993 | DRC | Com | Com cohort | Prospect | 1989–92 | **<–4 SD** | <–3 NCHS | **0–60** | incl | ng | ng | 11.5 | 3 m | ng | ng | Life table |

[a] For brief description of each study and comments please see Additional File 2

[b] These studies were on the Kenya coast and the nutritional survey was from North Kenya

*DRC* Democratic Republic of Congo (COD), *BFA* Burkina Faso, *IPF* In-patient Facility, *Com* community study, *OTP* Out-patient treatment program, *RCT* randomized controlled trial, *Retrosp* retrospective, *Prospect* prospective, *stand* standards used to define SAM, *WHO* World Health Organisation 2006 WHZ standards, *NCHS* National Center for Health Statistics 1996 standards, *CDC2000* Centre for Disease Control 2000 standards, *Oed* oedematous cases (kwashiorkor and marasmic-kwashiorkor), *excl* excluded from analysis, *incl* included in analysis, *ng* not given in report, *"Both" in study* the proportion of all the SAM cases which had both WHZ < – 3Z and MUAC < 115 mm in the study's subjects, *"Both" in survey* the proportion of all SAM cases that had both WHZ < – 3Z and MUAC < 115 mm derived from a nutritional survey of a random sample of the community (see [21]), *obs* average time the subjects were observed to determine the outcome, *d.m* days or months, *log* logistic, *reg* regression, *Binom* binomial, *PH* Proportional Hazards, *Chisq* Chi-squared Test, *OR* odds ratio. Non-standard definitions of SAM and age ranges not within the 6-60 month age range are shown in bold script.

**Table 2** The numbers, mortality and significance of differences by criterion for studies analysed

| Ref | Study | Author & year | Kwash | | Total SAM | | S-whz | | S-muac | | S-both | | *S-whz* | *S-muac* | *S-both* | WHZ v MUAC | | | |
|---|---|---|---|---|---|---|---|---|---|---|---|---|---|---|---|---|---|---|---|
| | | | Total | dead | Total | dead | Total | dead | Total | dead | Total | dead | *CFR* | *CFR* | *CFR* | $\chi^2$ | $\chi^2$ | Fisher | Cramer |
| # | # | | # | # | # | # | # | # | # | # | # | # | *%* | *%* | *%* | value | p (2-tail) | p (1-tail) | V |
| Studies giving numbers of children fulfilling both WHZ and MUAC criteria | | | | | | | | | | | | | | | | | | | |
| 41 | 1 | Aguayo 2015 | 231 | 11 | 6076 | 32 | 1333 | 3 | 859 | 2 | 3884 | 27 | *0.23* | *0.23* | *0.70* | | | 0.65 | 0.00 |
| 42 | 2 | Grellety 2012 | 2 | 0 | 530 | 13 | 177 | 3 | 167 | 2 | 186 | 8 | ***1.69*** | *1.20* | *4.30* | | | 0.53 | 0.02 |
| 21 | 3 | Grellety 2015 | excl | excl | 2205 | 40 | 1486 | 13 | 21 | 1 | 698 | 26 | *0.87* | ***4.76*** | *3.72* | | | 0.22 | 0.12 |
| 43 | 4 | Isanaka 2015 | excl | excl | 2399 | 13 | 530 | 3 | 929 | 4 | 940 | 6 | ***0.57*** | *0.43* | *0.64* | | | 0.48 | 0.03 |
| 44 | 5 | Lowlaavar 2016 | excl | excl | 262 | 21 | 171 | 11 | 32 | 0 | 59 | 10 | ***6.43*** | *0.00* | *16.95* | | | 0.14 | 0.10 |
| 45 | 6 | LaCourse 2014 | 97 | 8 | 210 | 15 | 29 | 2 | 68 | 4 | 16 | 1 | ***6.90*** | *5.88* | *6.25* | | | 0.58 | 0.02 |
| 35 | 7 | Olofin 2016 | ng | ng | 767 | 145 | 116 | 18 | 483 | 64 | 168 | 63 | ***15.50*** | *13.25* | *37.50* | 0.41 | 0.52 | 0.31 | 0.03 |
| Studies including oedema | | | | | | | | | | | | | | | | | | | |
| 46 | 8 | Berkley 2005 | 390 | ng | 1140 | 193 | 267 | 27 | 384 | 42 | 489 | 124 | *10.11* | ***10.94*** | *25.36* | 0.11 | 0.74 | 0.42 | 0.01 |
| 47 | 9 | Chiabi 2017 | ng | ng | 106 | 22 | 23 | 1 | 21 | 3 | 62 | 18 | *4.35* | ***14.29*** | *29.03* | | | 0.27 | 0.17 |
| 48 | 10 | Sachdeva 2016 | ng | ng | 447 | 59 | 228 | 18 | 75 | 15 | 144 | 26 | *7.89* | ***20.00*** | *18.06* | 8.52 | **0.004** | **0.004** | 0.17 |
| Studies where children fulfilling both criteria are incorporated into both the WHZ and MUAC categories | | | | | | | | | | | | | | | | | | | |
| | | | | | | | All-whz | | All-muac | | | | *All-whz* | *All-muac* | | All-whz v All-muac | | | |
| 49 | 11 | Burza 2016 | ng | ng | 650 | 36 | 295 | 26 | 650 | 36 | | | ***8.81*** | *5.54* | | 3.55 | 0.06 | **0.042** | 0.06 |
| 50 | 12 | Mogeni 2011 | 392 | ng | 1768 | 217 | 966 | 101 | 802 | 116 | | | *10.46* | ***14.46*** | | 6.54 | **0.011** | | 0.06 |
| 51 | 13 | Sylla 2015 | ng | ng | 272 | 42 | 90 | 27 | 117 | 15 | | | ***30.00*** | *12.82* | | 9.28 | **0.002** | **0.002** | 0.21 |
| 52 | 14 | Vella 1990 | ng | ng | 118 | 22 | 34 | 3 | 96 | 18 | | | *8.82* | ***18.75*** | | | | 0.14 | 0.12 |
| 53 | 15 | Dramaix 1993 | 320 | 102 | 442 | 122 | 267 | 63 | 175 | 57 | | | *23.60* | ***32.57*** | | 4.31 | **0.038** | **0.025** | 0.10 |
| 54 | 16 | Girum 2017 | 363 | 25 | 545 | 51 | 130 | 26 | 277 | 41 | | | ***20.00*** | *14.80* | | 1.74 | 0.19 | 0.12 | 0.07 |
| 55 | 17 | Savadogo 2007 | excl | excl | 1322 | 212 | 930 | 168 | 387 | 95 | | | *18.03* | ***24.50*** | | 7.19 | **0.007** | | 0.01 |
| 36 | 18 | Garenne1987 | ng | ng | 622 | 63 | 92 | 14 | 569 | 54 | | | ***15.22*** | *9.49* | | 2.81 | 0.09 | 0.06 | 0.07 |
| 37 | 19 | Garenne 2009 | ng | ng | 281 | 44 | 183 | 23 | 98 | 21 | | | *12.57* | ***21.43*** | | 3.79 | 0.051 | **0.040** | 0.12 |
| 37 | 20 | Garenne 2009 | ng | ng | 388 | 25 | 150 | 9 | 238 | 16 | | | *6.00* | ***6.72*** | | 0.08 | 0.78 | 0.48 | 0.01 |
| 38 | 21 | Broeck 1993 | 56 | 8 | 652 | 13 | 113 | 3 | 539 | 6 | | | ***2.65*** | *1.11* | | | | 0.14 | 0.05 |

*S-whz* WHZ below cut off point with MUAC above cut-off point as defined in the paper, *S-muac* MUAC below cut off point with WHZ above cut-off point as defined in the paper, *S-both* MUAC and WHZ both below the cut-off point as defined in the paper, *All-whz* WHZ below the cut-off point, with MUAC either above or below the cut-off point as defined in the paper, *All-muac* MUAC below the cut-off point, WHZ either above or below the cut-off as defined in the paper, *excl* excluded from analysis, *ng* not given in report, *CFR* Case Fatality Rate in percentage, $\chi^2$ Pearson's chi squared test (two-way significance), *Fisher* Fisher's exact test (one-tailed test of significance), *Cramer* Cramer's V test of association between the groups. The higher CFR and significant differences are shown in bold script

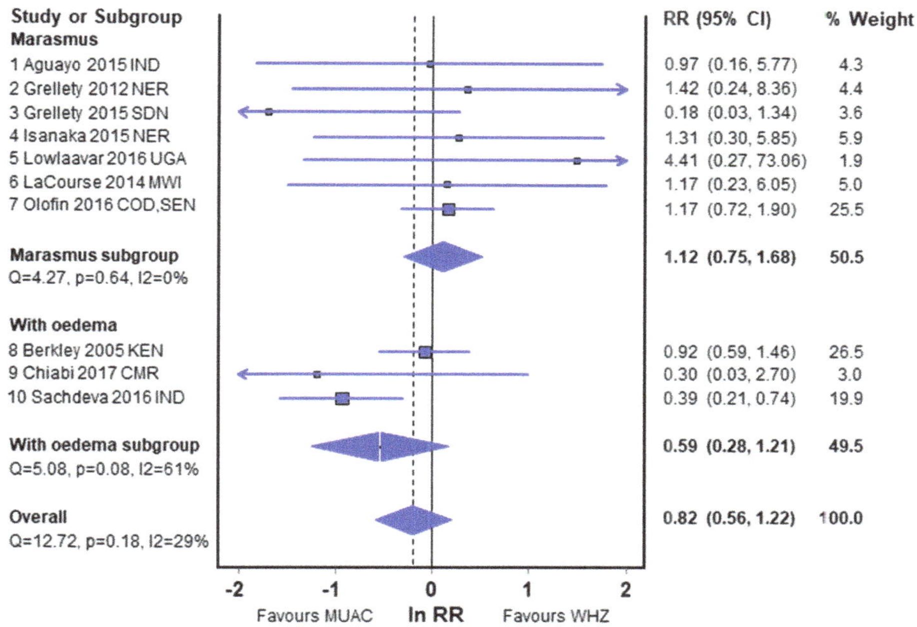


**Fig. 2** Forest plot of the RR in children diagnosed by WHZ-only relative to MUAC-only with and without oedema. Legend: *IND* India; NER Niger; *SDN* South Sudan; *UGA* Uganda; *MWI* Malawi; *COD* Democratic Republic of the Congo; *SEN* Senegal; *KEN* Kenya; *CMR* Cameroun; Ln *RR* natural log of relative risk; *CI* confidence intervals. In each of the forest plots "favours WHZ" indicates that the Relative Risk for death is higher in children with WHZ < − 3Z than with a MUAC of < 115 mm; "favours MUAC" indicates that the Relative Risk for death of children with a MUAC < 115 mm is higher than those with WHZ < − 3Z

The two datasets (a single report) that used the CDC2000 criteria [40] and reduced the cut-off for MUAC to < 110 mm (CDC2000/110) strongly favoured a higher risk of death for those admitted by MUAC; this was expected and almost reached significance. Report 18 and 19, from Senegal, used exactly the same original data, therefore these reports can be directly compared. When NCHS and MUAC< 115 mm (NCHS/115) was used All-whz has a much higher mortality than All-muac (RR, 1.60; CI, 0.93–2.77); whereas, when CDC2000/110 was used All-muac had a much higher risk than All-whz which just reaches significance (RR, 0.59; CI, 0.34–1.00). The

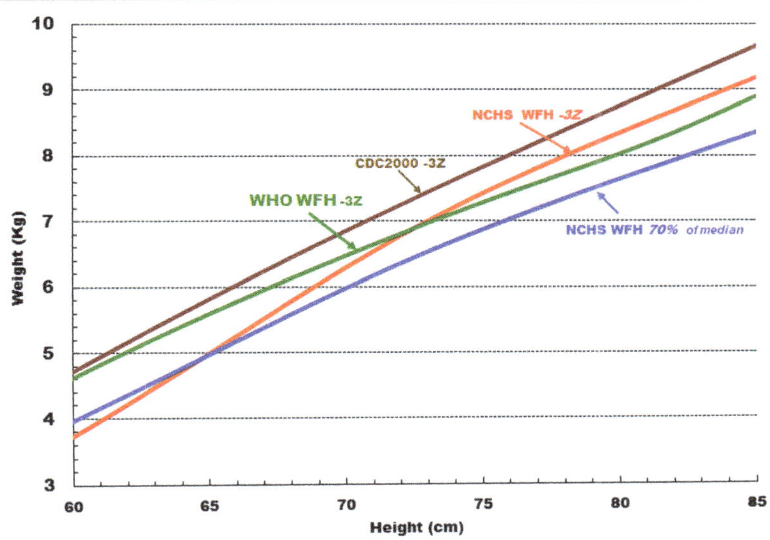


**Fig. 3** The cut-off weights for heights that define SAM by the different references in use in the studies reviewed. Legend: *WHO* World Health Organisation, 2006 standards; *NCHS* National Center for Health Statistics (USA) 1977; *CDC2000* Center for Disease control and Prevention, Atlanta, USA, 2000 reference

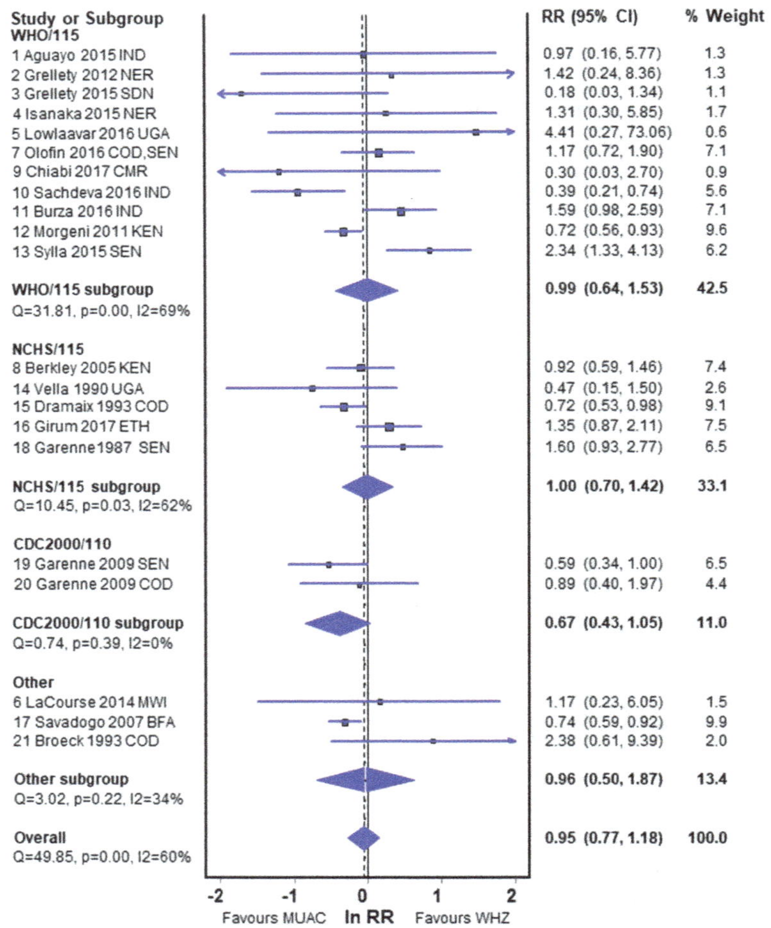


**Fig. 4** Forest plot of the RR in children diagnosed by WHZ relative to MUAC grouped by the standards used. Legend: *WHO/115* WHO criteria and MUAC< 115 mm; NCHS/115 NCHS criteria and MUAC< 115 mm; *CDC2000/110* CDC2000 criteria and MUAC< 110 mm; *IND* India; *NER* Niger; *SDN* South Sudan; *UGA* Uganda; *SEN* Senegal; *CMR* Cameroun; *KEN* Kenya; *COD* Democratic Republic of the Congo; *ETH* Ethiopia; *MWI* Malawi; *BFA* Burkina Faso; RR relative risk; CI confidence intervals

same data were also used in reports 20 and 21 from DRC; again there is a substantial difference between the RRs when using the two different anthropometric references. Savadogo et al. [58], in the "other" group, used an obsolete MUAC-for-age formula to calculate All-muac Z-scores [65] and then divided the results into tertiles for analysis; minus 4Z using this standard increases from 103 mm to 111 mm between 6 and 59 months of age. The mean Z score of Savadogo's children on admission was − 4.59Z which for a 12 to 24 month old child equates to about 100 mm. It is clear that the MUAC standard for these children was very low which would account for the RR of death being significantly greater for S-muac than S-whz (RR, 0.74; CI, 0.59–0.92).

In each of the other meta-analyses we have omitted these reports using CDC2000 reference and MUAC< 110 mm (# 19 & 20), the duplicated data from those reports (# 18 & 21) as well as Savadogo's report (# 17). The data from datasets 18 to 21 are incorporated into report #7.

### Effect of mode of treatment

In-patient cohort studies are often criticised on the basis that they do not represent the children in the community and are subject to ascertainment bias [22, 30]. In Fig. 5 we sub-divide the reports by mode of treatment to determine whether this has an effect on comparison of WHZ and MUAC deaths. The in-patients had about the same mortality risk with MUAC and WHZ (RR, 0.92; CI, 0.66–1.28).

The two OTP studies are dominated by a retrospective study from Sudan (study 3) where there were very few S-muac admissions (WHZ 1486 with 13 deaths; MUAC 21 with 1 death); there was no follow-up of defaulters to distinguish death from simple non-attendance. The other report (study 4) from a secondary analysis of a prospective RCT is much more reliable and shows

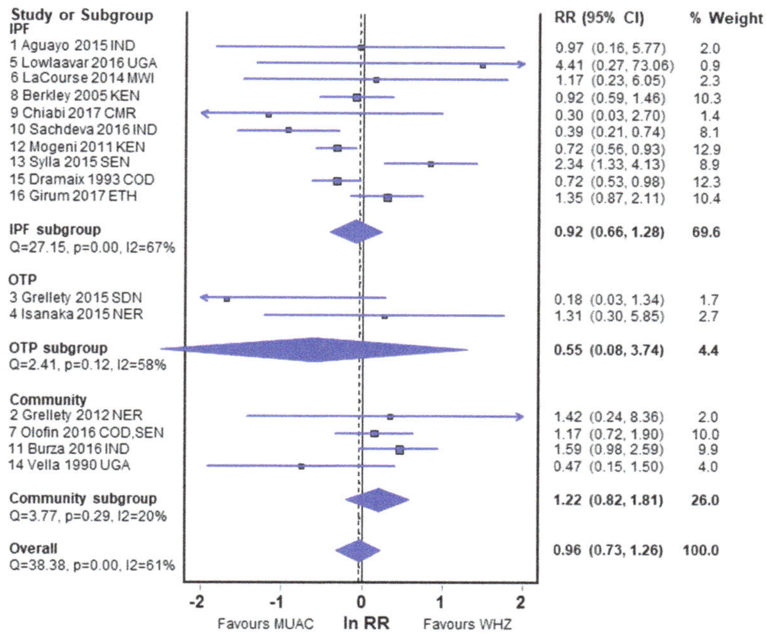


**Fig. 5** Relative Risk of mortality in children diagnosed by WHZ relative to MUAC by mode of treatment. Legend: *IPF* In-patient Facility (Hospital, Therapeutic Feeding Center); *OTP* Out-patient treatment program (Home treatment); *Com* community study; *IND* India; *NER* Niger; *SDN* South Sudan; *UGA* Uganda; *SEN* Senegal; *CMR* Cameroun; *KEN* Kenya; *COD* Democratic Republic of the Congo; *ETH* Ethiopia; *MWI* Malawi; *BFA* Burkina Faso; RR relative risk; CI confidence intervals

S-whz to have a greater, but non-significant, RR of death (RR, 1.31; CI, 0.30–5.8).

The community studies also showed a non-significant higher risk with WHZ than MUAC (RR, 1.22; CI, 0.82–1.81).

### Overall analysis

Figure 6 shows the overall analysis, omitting the duplicated studies found in the previous analyses. Here they are sub-grouped by whether S-both was incorporated or excluded from the analysis. There was no difference in the risk of death between those with a low MUAC and those with a low WHZ (RR, 0.99; CI, 0.73–1.35). The heterogeneity of the S-whz v S-muac group was low ($I^2$ = 23%) but high in the All-whz v All-muac group ($I^2$ = 80%). The statistics, sensitivity analysis, Doi and funnel plots are given in Additional file 3: Figure S1.

### Grouping of deficits

As there was no difference in the meta-analysis of children with single and double deficits (Fig. 6), and we had found in our empirical data that inclusion of both deficits into the S-whz and S-muac groups gave erroneous results due to mathematical coupling, we examined the difference this change in analytical procedures would cause using the studies where we had information on S-both.

The differences between CFRs of S-whz v S-muac and All-whz v All-muac in reports 1 to 10 are shown in Table 3. In two of the papers the All-whz/muac gave a larger difference in CFR than the S-whz/muac comparison; in 6 of the papers S-whz/muac CFR comparison was larger than the All-whz/muac comparison. In the other 2 papers by Lowlaavar et al. [47] and Berkley et al. [49] the direction of the difference was actually reversed (in opposite directions), so by inclusion of children with both deficits into each of the single groups contrary conclusions would have been reached. These latter studies are examples of Simpson's paradox, an extreme form of confounding [33, 66], but inclusion of S-both into the whz v muac comparison led to erroneous results in every study.

## Discussion

Most of the original analyses in the papers examined considered the whole population of children, either in the community or admitted to the IPF (hospital). They tested the diagnostic ability of MUAC and WHZ to predict the death of the children compared to those that did not fulfil any of the criteria for SAM and then compared statistics such as the areas under a ROC curve. They frequently proposed changes in the cut-off points to maximise the sensitivity and specificity (giving sensitivity and specificity equal importance) of the diagnosis to predict death. Comparison of SAM with non-SAM

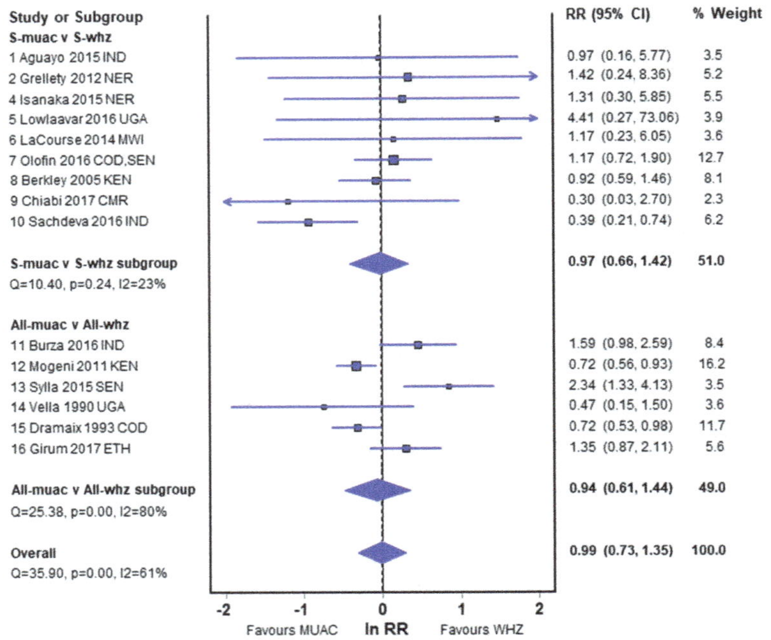


**Fig. 6** Relative Risk of mortality in children diagnosed by WHZ relative to MUAC omitting the duplicate data. Legend: *S-whz* WHZ below cut off point with MUAC above cut-off point as defined in the paper; *S-muac* MUAC below cut off point with WHZ above cut-off point as defined in the paper; *All-whz* WHZ below the cut-off point, with MUAC either above or below the cut-off point as defined in the paper; *All-muac* MUAC below the cut-off point, WHZ either above or below the cut-off as defined in the paper; *IND* India; *NER* Niger; *SDN* South Sudan; *UGA* Uganda; *SEN* Senegal; *CMR* Cameroun; *KEN* Kenya; *COD* Democratic Republic of the Congo; *ETH* Ethiopia; *MWI* Malawi; *BFA* Burkina Faso; RR relative risk; CI confidence intervals

**Table 3** The effect of mathematical coupling on the interpretation of CFR and possibility of Simpson's paradox

| Study | Author & year | Single deficits alone | | | | | Single and both deficits | | | | | Difference WHZ-MUAC | | |
|---|---|---|---|---|---|---|---|---|---|---|---|---|---|---|
| | | *S-whz* *CFR* | *S-muac* *CFR* | S-whz v S-muac $\chi^2$ | Fisher | Cramer | All-whz CFR | All-muac CFR | All-whz v All-muac $\chi^2$ | Fisher | Cramer | S-whz-S-muac | All-whz-All-muac | Effect on CFR |
| | | % | % | *p* | *p* | | % | % | p | p | | | | |
| 1 | Aguayo 2015 | 0.23 | 0.23 | *nc* | (0.96) | 0.00 | 0.58 | 0.61 | 0.81 | nc | 0.00 | −0.01 | −0.04 | >All |
| 2 | Grellety 2012 | 1.69 | 1.20 | *nc* | 0.73 | 0.02 | 3.03 | 2.83 | 0.88 | 0.880 | 0.01 | 0.50 | 0.20 | >S |
| 3 | Grellety 2015 | 0.87 | 4.76 | *nc* | (0.19) | 0.05 | 1.79 | 3.76 | 0.002 | nc | 0.06 | −3.89 | −1.97 | >S |
| 4 | Isanaka 2015 | 0.57 | 0.43 | *nc* | (0.68) | 0.01 | 0.61 | 0.54 | 0.77 | nc | 0.01 | 0.14 | 0.08 | >S |
| 5 | Lowlaavar 2016 | 6.43 | 0.00 | *nc* | 0.14 | 0.10 | 9.13 | 10.99 | 0.61 | 0.607 | 0.03 | 6.43 | −1.86 | Reverse |
| 6 | LaCourse 2014 | 6.90 | 5.88 | *nc* | 0.83 | 0.02 | 6.67 | 5.95 | nc | 0.860 | 0.01 | 1.01 | 0.71 | >S |
| 7 | Olofin 2016 | 15.52 | 13.25 | 0.52 | 0.52 | 0.03 | 28.52 | 19.51 | 0.002 | nc | 0.10 | 2.27 | 9.01 | >All |
| 8 | Berkley 2005 | 10.11 | 10.94 | 0.74 | 0.74 | 0.01 | 19.97 | 19.01 | 0.63 | nc | 0.01 | −0.83 | 0.96 | Reverse |
| 9 | Chiabi 2017 | 4.35 | 14.29 | *nc* | 0.31 | 0.17 | 22.35 | 25.30 | 0.65 | 0.659 | 0.03 | −9.94 | −2.95 | >S |
| 10 | Sachdeva 2016 | 7.89 | 20.00 | **0.004** | **0.005** | 0.17 | 11.83 | 18.72 | **0.021** | **0.023** | 0.09 | −12.11 | −6.89 | >S |

*S-whz* WHZ below cut off point with MUAC above cut-off point as defined in the paper, *S-muac* MUAC below cut off point with WHZ above cut-off point as defined in the paper, *All-whz* WHZ below the cut-off point, with MUAC either above or below the cut-off point as defined in the paper, *All-muac* MUAC below the cut-off point, WHZ either above or below the cut-off as defined in the paper, *S-whz–S-muac* (single deficit) WHZ minus MUAC CFR, *All-whz – All-muac* (combined deficits) WHZ minus MUAC CFR, *CFR* Case Fatality Rate in percentage; $\chi^2$ significance of Chi-squared analysis of MUAC against WHZ CFRs; *Fisher* Fisher's exact test, two-sided mid *P*-value (values in parentheses are approximate as one cell number too large); *Cramer* Cramer's V of association between variables; *">All"* the difference in CFRs between WHZ and MUAC is greater with All-whz/muac; *">S"* the difference is greater with S-whz/muac; *"Reverse"* the direction of the change is reversed (Simpson's paradox), negative numbers WHZ < MUAC, positive numbers WHZ > MUAC. Significant differences are shown in bold script children was not the objective of our analysis. The WHO has specified the standards and cut-off points that are used to define SAM; we are not examining how appropriate these cut-off points are to define SAM-related deaths or to see how a change is the MUAC cut-off would capture more children with WHZ < −3Z. Our objective was to compare the risk of death of SAM children identified by either the WHO specified MUAC or WHZ criteria directly. Thus, unlike the reported studies, the children who did not have SAM were not considered relevant in our analysis. This is the first review of SAM-related mortality data to be examined in this way.

The most reliable of the meta-analyses is probably the first subgroup shown in Fig. 2. These 7 reports are the only reports where children with S-whz and S-muac were separated in the analyses to eliminate the effect of mathematical coupling [37, 38], oedematous children were excluded, the age range of the children was from 6 to 60 months and the WHO recommended criteria for diagnosis of SAM were used. However, 6 of the 7 studies were under-powered. The pooled result showed no significant difference between the risk of death for those admitted that fulfilled the WHZ criterion and those that fulfilled the MUAC criterion. Nevertheless, the combined data showed that WHZ had a slightly higher mortality risk (RR, 1.12; CI, 0.75–1.68) than children fulfilling the MUAC criterion. The group of studies from the community in Fig. 5, although old and subject to mathematical coupling, should not have an ascertainment bias; they also showed a higher risk with a low WHZ (RR, 1.22; CI, 0.82–1.81). These two groups are probably more reliable than the other studies and are both in agreement with our empirical data showing a higher risk of death for children with WHZ < −3Z than MUAC < 115 mm. These latter community studies are the class of study that is most frequently quoted in favour of a MUAC only program.

When the other studies that are potentially subject to more severe bias are included there was no difference in the relative mortality risks between children admitted by MUAC and those admitted by WHZ (RR 0.99). It is clear that 6–60 month old children with WHZ < −3Z or MUAC < 115 mm both have a substantial risk of death and that children with WHZ < −3Z are at an equivalent or higher risk than those with a low MUAC. There is no justification in labelling children with a WHZ < −3Z and a MUAC > 115 mm as healthy and denying then treatment [22, 23, 25–30] in preference to children with a MUAC < 115 mm, although it is acknowledged pragmatically that MUAC is a much easier and more convenient measure at the present time.

### Potential sources of Bias

The data from the studies included in this review are all subject to bias, some sufficiently severs to render the studies of little value in setting policy. The major problems with some of the studies are outlined in Additional file 2.

### Confounding

#### *Oedema*

Oedema is clearly a major confounder in some studies. The paper by Girum et al. [57] had 67% of oedematous children in their analysis, and in the paper by Berkley et al. [49], which is very widely quoted, 38% of the children fulfilling the S-muac criterion and 14% of those with S-whz had oedema. It is unclear which way oedema affects the relative mortality of S-muac and S-whz children. In paper I [33] oedematous children had a much higher mortality when associated with WHZ < −3Z, whereas in our meta-analysis oedematous children with a low MUAC had the higher risk of death. We do not have an explanation for this discrepancy.

In the report by LaCourse [48], infants with a low MUAC and oedema had a 21% CFR, compared to 6% in those with only a low MUAC. This large difference may indicate a different prognostic impact of oedema in infants, possibly because sodium homeostasis appears to be different in malnourished children less than 12 months of age from older children [67]. However, oedematous malnutrition normally has a higher incidence in older children. The degree of oedema may also affect the increase in mortality risk [60]. It is thus difficult to predict the relative magnitude of the increase in mortality risks due to oedema in different groups of patients.

The community based studies, which are quoted extensively in support of MUAC-only programs [40, 68–78] did not exclude oedematous cases. As oedematous malnutrition usually has a short history before death (a few days), it will not have been recorded during the antecedent anthropometric measurements and oedema is not usually observed by parents unless it is gross and accompanied by other signs of kwashiorkor. This problem does not arise with the patient based studies.

#### *Other co-morbidity bias*

Most of the studies do not report signs and symptoms, investigations, infections, complications or other characteristics of their children and how they differ between groups. They rarely report the putative causes of death. Where such data are reported there are always significant differences in the characteristics of the children admitted with S-muac and S-whz apart from age and oedema status. For example, Berkley et al. [49] report significant differences between their groups in degree of stunting, skin/hair signs of kwashiorkor, and gender. Sachdeva et al. [51] report differences in age, fast breathing and duration of illness. But they do not report statistical comparisons between the anthropometric groups, only between those that survived and died.

When the putative causes of death are recorded, it appears that many of the deaths were due to conditions that are not normally associated with SAM and would not be alleviated by treatment with the standard protocols for the management of SAM. For example, in the reports by Sachdeva and Berkley, 30 and 10% of the SAM children had convulsions respectively; these were of unreported/undetermined aetiologies, but are not normally a feature of malnutrition per se [79]. As the proportion with convulsions varied with diagnostic group there is a potential co-morbidity bias in these studies, and also in the studies that did not report the prevalence of complications in the respective groups.

One of the problems of interpreting the community studies is that death occurs remotely in time to the antecedent anthropometry so it is unknown whether and how the children were malnourished, or not, at the time of death, their relative WHZ and MUAC status, whether their deaths were confounded by oedema and whether the death was from non-nutrition related illness. It is noteworthy in reading the reports that a relatively small proportion of all deaths occurred in malnourished children in the community cohorts. For example, the very careful report by Van den Broeck et al. record 87% of deaths as miscellaneous or unknown [41]. The causes of death vary by age and thus are likely to have different MUAC and WHZ profiles. Non-nutritional mortality requires different strategies to prevent death: for example, immunisation, sanitation, maternal services, HIV prevention, etc. The extent to which nutritional treatment would affect non-nutrition related mortality is unknown, but this and many other studies were conducted in malaria hyper-endemic areas. The potentiating effect of malnutrition on malarial mortality is controversial [1, 80, 81].

#### *Diagnostic bias (references used)*

The use of obsolete standards also has a profound effect. The reports by Garenne [40], Van den Broeck [41] and Savadogo [58] each used very stringent diagnostic cut-offs for MUAC and Garenne's report a very lenient WHZ reference. This makes these reports unreliable for setting policy. Of course, as we show in paper III [34] the importance of the CFR has to be judged in relation to the case-load. It is noteworthy that by choosing to use obsolete standards in Garenne et al's 2009 Senegal report they generated a CRF that is much greater with MUAC than with WHZ. Nevertheless, the attributable risk percentage for severe wasting to cause death was 12.1% for WHZ and only 5.7% for MUAC. Attributable risk is a much more important statistic for setting policy than CFR. By their choice of diagnostic criteria the case load changed in a reciprocal fashion to the CFR. The CFR quoted in Garenne et al's 2009 paper must not continue to be used to advocate for a MUAC-only policy. Despite this, papers which used obsolete criteria for both WHZ and MUAC, and other biases, are misleadingly quoted as evidence in favour of a MUAC only program [39–41, 48, 49, 55, 56].

#### *Ascertainment bias*

When focusing upon SAM, the whole community is not relevant. What is relevant is the extent to which the children in the study represent the children *with SAM* in the community. The least biased sample of such children should come from those children with SAM in a large random sample of the community. Although with demographic, social and nutritional change, historical cohorts may not represent SAM in present day circumstances or in other countries, apart from Senegal and the Democratic Republic of Congo, as the diagnosis of SAM by the two criteria differs markedly from place to place [21].

The patients selected in IPFs and OTPs that satisfy both the WHZ and the MUAC criteria are more at risk and are less representative of SAM in the community than those that satisfy a single criterion. We include in Table 2 and Additional file 1: Table S1 a measure of this discordance between the ratios of S-both to total SAM found in the study and in representative samples of SAM in the community [21]; we consider this as an indication of the extent of ascertainment bias. This bias will be much greater if the severest children (those with both criteria) are included in the analysis of patients. We maintain that one reason for splitting the children into those with single deficits is that the S-whz is more likely to be representative of the S-whz children in the community than total SAM in a patient cohort is to total SAM in the community. This is because children with S-both are common in the patient groups and much less common in the community.

The reports from patient cohorts in both IPFs and OTPs have been criticised because they "do not represent the community" and have been dismissed as valid evidence by some [22, 30]. When we eliminate the studies using inappropriate criteria, it is noteworthy that the community derived cohorts have a higher risk of death for WHZ than MUAC diagnosed children (Fig. 5), and not the reverse as those advocating MUAC-only programs speculate [29, 30].

### Verification bias

#### *Length of observation*

Two of the studies, Lowlaavar [47] and Sachdeva [51], had extremely short observation periods for children in hospital before they died or were discharged. They also have a very high mortality which calls into question the severity of SAM, the admission criteria and the quality of treatment given. It is likely that only children brought directly for clinical care by the parents because of severe complications, and were admitted in extremis, form the bases for these two reports. Such children may not be appropriate to guide admission policy for less critically ill children from the community or elsewhere. This is because it is unknown whether children who die with a low MUAC or WHZ have a different time course to death after presentation to the health services. Varied time of observation for each child at risk is a potential source of verification bias.

#### *Missing data and defaulting*

Missing data is a potential source of bias. Two studies [50, 52] had over one quarter of their data missing. Unfortunately, 9 of the other 18 reports did not give any indication of the extent of missing data.

Defaulting is another source of verification bias. In IPF this is less serious as children that die from SAM usually die early after admission (about 70% of deaths occur in the first week), and most defaults occur later when the caretakers themselves consider that the child has sufficiently recovered, that they are not making any progress or competing priorities at home mount and demand the mother's attention.

Of more concern is defaulting as outpatients (OTP). There is very rarely any follow up to determine the outcome of children who simply do not return for treatment, so it is not known what proportion of these children "default" because they are actually dead. The CFR for the OTP studies must be seen as a minimum and not an actual death rate. This can lead to very substantial verification bias. OTP study number 4, by Isanaka et al. [46] did not suffer from this defect.

### Mathematical coupling

From our empirical data [33] it is clear that, in judging MUAC and WHZ as independent criteria for diagnosis of SAM, the children with both deficits have a significantly augmented mortality risk. This is confirmed by most of the studies which report the outcome of children with both deficits and have sufficient events (Table 2). Many studies only counted children with a low MUAC and added to that group those that also had a low WHZ (S-both), and their deaths, without separating those with double defects (datasets 11 to 21).

This incorporation of exactly the same data into both groups, and then comparing the groups, results in a phenomenon termed mathematical coupling [37, 38] that causes the analytical results to be in error. In other words some of the children were compared with themselves. The meta-analysis did not show any difference between these two types of selection of children to include in an analysis. We therefore examined the papers where we could assess the extent to which this may have affected the data (Table 3) and found that CFRs were different in each case, some with greater augmentation of WHZ and others of MUAC; two of the studies even reversed the relative magnitude of the WHZ and MUAC mortality rates, a phenomenon termed Simpson's paradox [66]. The degree and direction of the changes depend upon the relative mortality in the data common to both groups and the relative size of the three groups. These factors were different in each of the studies shown in Table 3.

The report by Lowlaavar [47] is particularly illustrative of the errors that can occur. There were no deaths at all in the children with S-muac and a CFR in the S-whz children of over 6%. When the children with both a low MUAC and WHZ who have a high CFR (17%) are added to the analysis of both groups there is a dramatic reversal so that All-muac now appears to have a higher CFR than All-whz. This analytical error affected most of the studies reported, including those where single defects were also reported, because, in every report the combined data was used in their life tables, logistic (or other) regressions and generated ROC curves. As Tu et al. [66] state: "Incorrect use of statistical models might produce consistent, replicable, yet erroneous results" this seems to be the case with all the original analyses in the literature reviewed.

### Limitations

All the studies reviewed have limitations that are presented in the discussion and in Additional file 2. Community representative samples of children 6–59 months show that only an average of 16.5% of the children meeting the criteria for SAM have both a MUAC and WHZ below the WHO cut-off points; the rest of the SAM children have either one or the other criterion making them eligible for treatment [21]. The studies reviewed all have a higher proportion of children satisfying both criteria than are present in the community. In Table 1 we show the overlap (S-both) of children in the study, and that found in recent representative samples of the community.

The heterogeneity of the standards, the admixture of oedematous cases and the failure to account for confounding, such as TB, HIV, and non-nutrition related conditions, makes simple amalgamation of data from the different study populations problematic. Similarly, there are major co-morbidity, temporal and stochastic biases with the community studies [82]. The community studies were performed at a time when most countries had a much higher prevalence of malnutrition, all-cause mortality, and poor coverage of other public health programs such as measles vaccination, vitamin A capsule distribution, salt iodisation, insecticide impregnated bed-nets and HIV services. It is perhaps for this reason that the community studies also have a higher proportion of children satisfying both criteria than are found with recent surveys in the same areas. It is also probably the reason why the attributable fraction of death due to SAM in these older community studies was lower than expected. It is estimated that SAM and moderate acute malnutrition underlie up to half of all paediatric deaths [80].

The meta-analyses are only as good as the studies that are incorporated into the analysis. We have eliminated the most egregious of the studies, but it must be acknowledged that none of the studies are without potential bias. Therefore, unfortunately, there are no definitive unflawed data upon which to rely in order to unequivocally inform public health policy.

## Conclusions

None of the datasets reviewed, with the possible exception of our empirical data [33] were large enough to have sufficient power to distinguish between the CFRs associated with the WHO criteria for SAM by MUAC and WHZ. They used inappropriate standards, included children outside the age range used by WHO's SAM treatment protocols [83], included children with oedema or entered individuals with both defects into each of the groups being compared. All the patient studies have an ascertainment bias. None of these studies provide sufficient evidence to support the assertions made by those seeking to drop WHZ as a routine diagnostic criterion for SAM.

The assertions of Briend et al. [22, 26, 31], in particular, that MUAC is consistently "superior" to WHZ as a prognostic indicator, that children with a low WHZ are healthy and do not have an independent mortality risk, and that the two parameters are not additive are all incorrect. Although papers, with completely inadequate data, have been heavily criticised [84], they are still being used to justify a MUAC-only policy [85]; these papers are reviewed here and are found sufficiently problematic that they should not be used to guide policy decisions.

The conclusions drawn from our empirical data [33] are supported by the published reports comparing the prognostic value of WHZ and MUAC. That is that children with a WHZ of <−3Z have about the same or higher risk of death as children with a MUAC < 115 mm. They both are at substantial risk of death, and neither should be omitted from protocols aimed at diagnosis and treatment of all SAM cases.

The relative case loads not only differ between countries, but also determine the absolute number of deaths that occur in each of the diagnostic groups. This is explored in detail in paper III [34]; it has not been sufficiently considered by those advocating for abandonment of WHZ as a diagnostic criterion for SAM.

#### Abbreviations

CFR: Case fatality rate; IPFs: In-patient treatment facilities; MAM: Moderate acute malnutrition; MUAC: Mid-upper-arm-circumference; OTPs: Out-patient treatment programs; ROC curve: Receiver operating characteristic curve; RR: relative risk; SAM: Severe acute malnutrition; SFCs: Supplementary feeding centres; WHO: the World Health Organisation; WHZ: Weight-for-height Z-score

#### Acknowledgements

We would like to acknowledge the contribution made by the reviewers of our initial submission of this article.

#### Funding

Nutriset provided a PhD fellowship to Université Libre de Bruxelles in support of EG. Nutriset had no role in any aspect of this research including data collection, design, analysis, interpretation or writing the article. MHG received no support.

#### Authors' contributions

EG & MHG were involved in all stages from the conception and design, data acquisition, analysis and interpretation. Both authors approved the final version of the article.

#### Competing interests

The authors declare that they have no competing interests.

#### Author details

[1]Research Center Health Policy and Systems - International Health, School of Public Health, Université Libre de Bruxelles, Bruxelles, Belgium. [2]Department of Medicine and Therapeutics, University of Aberdeen, Aberdeen, Scotland, UK.

#### References

1. Black RE, Victora CG, Walker SP, Bhutta ZA, Christian P, De Onis M, et al. Maternal and child undernutrition and overweight in low-income and middle-income countries. Lancet. 2013;382:427–51. http://www.sciencedirect.com/science/article/pii/S014067361360937X.
2. Myatt M, Khara T, Collins S. A review of methods to detect cases of severely malnourished children in the community for their admission into community-based therapeutic care programs. Food Nutr Bull. 2006;27:S7–23. http://archive.unu.edu/unupress/food/FNB_v27n3_suppl.pdf#page=7.
3. John C, Ocheke IE, Diala U, Adah RO, Envuladu EA. Does mid upper arm circumference identify all acute malnourished 6-59 month old children, in field and clinical settings in Nigeria? S Afr J Clin Nutr. 2016;1–5. http://www.tandfonline.com/doi/abs/10.1080/16070658.2016.1255486.

4. Manyike PC, Chinawa JM, Ubesie A, Obu HA, Odetunde OI, Chinawa AT. Prevalence of malnutrition among pre-school children in, South-east Nigeria. Italian J Pediatrics. 2014;40:75. https://ijponline.biomedcentral.com/articles/10.1186/s13052-014-0075-5.
5. Gayle HD, Binkin NJ, Staehling NW, Trowbridge FL. Arm circumference v. weight-for-height in nutritional assessment: are the findings comparable? J Trop Pediatr. 1988;34:213–7. https://academic.oup.com/tropej/article-abstract/34/5/213/1632459/Arm-Circumference-v-Weight-for-Height-in.
6. Ross DA, Taylor N, Hayes R, McLean M. Measuring malnutrition in famines: are weight-for-height and arm circumference interchangeable? Int J Epidemiol. 1990;19:636–45. https://academic.oup.com/ije/article-abstract/19/3/636/760605/Measuring-Malnutrition-in-Famines-Are-Weight-for.
7. Bern C, Nathanail L. Is mid-upper-arm circumference a useful tool for screening in emergency settings? Lancet. 1995;345:631–3. http://www.sciencedirect.com/science/article/pii/S0140673695905278.
8. Rees DG, Henry CJK, Diskett P, Shears P. Measures of nutritional status: survey of young children in north-East Brazil. Lancet. 1987;329:87–9. http://www.sciencedirect.com/science/article/pii/S0140673687919209.
9. Hop LT, Gross R, Sastroamidjojo S, Giay T, Schultink W. Mid-upper-arm circumference development and its validity in assessment of undernutrition. Asia Pac J Clin Nutr 1998, 7: 65–69. apjcn.nhri.org.tw/server/apjcn/7/1/65.pdf.
10. Tripathy JP, Sharma A, Prinja S. Is mid-upper arm circumference alone sufficient to identify severe acute malnutrition correctly. Indian Pediatr. 2016;53:166–7. http://indianpediatrics.net/feb2016/166.pdf.
11. Roberfroid D, Huybregts L, Lachat C, Vrijens F, Kolsteren P, Guesdon B. Inconsistent diagnosis of acute malnutrition by weight-for-height and mid-upper arm circumference: contributors in 16 cross-sectional surveys from South Sudan, the Philippines, Chad, and Bangladesh. Nutr J. 2015;14:1. https://nutritionj.biomedcentral.com/articles/10.1186/s12937-015-0074-4.
12. Dasgupta R, Sinha D, Jain SK, Prasad V. Screening for SAM in the community: is MUAC a simple tool? Indian Pediatr 2013, 50: 154–155. http://link.springer.com/article/10.1007/s13312-013-0032-1
13. Fernandez MA, Delchevalerie P, Van HM. Accuracy of MUAC in the detection of severe wasting with the new WHO growth standards. Pediatrics. 2010;126:e195–201. http://citeseerx.ist.psu.edu/viewdoc/download?doi=10.1.1.919.6180&rep=rep1&type=pdf.
14. Carter EP. Comparison of weight: height ratio and arm circumference in assessment of acute malnutrition. Arch Dis Child. 1987;62:833–5. https://adc.bmj.com/content/62/8/833.short.
15. Laillou A, Prak S, de Groot R, Whitney S, Conkle J, Horton L et al. Optimal screening of children with acute malnutrition requires a change in current WHO guidelines as MUAC and WHZ identify different patient groups. PLoS ONE 2014, 9: e101159. https://bmcnutr.biomedcentral.com/articles/10.1186/s40795-016-0049-7.
16. Grellety E, Krause LK, Shams EM, Porten K, Isanaka S. Comparison of weight-for-height and mid-upper arm circumference (MUAC) in a therapeutic feeding programme in South Sudan: is MUAC alone a sufficient criterion for admission of children at high risk of mortality? Public Health Nutr. 2015;18: 2575–81. http://www.epicentre.msf.org/sites/preprod.epicentre.actency.fr/files/661_Comparison%20of%20weight-for-height.pdf.
17. Talapalliwar MR, Garg BS. Diagnostic accuracy of mid-upper arm circumference (MUAC) for detection of severe and moderate acute malnutrition among tribal children in Central India. Int J Med Sci Public Health. 2016;5:1317–21. http://www.ejmanager.com/mnstemps/67/67-1441365239.pdf.
18. Dukhi N, Sartorius B, Taylor M. Mid-upper arm circumference (MUAC) performance versus weight for height in south African children (0-59 months) with acute malnutrition. S Afr J Clin Nutr. 2017;1–6. http://www.tandfonline.com/doi/abs/10.1080/16070658.2016.1255483.
19. Fiorentino M, Sophonneary P, Laillou A, Whitney S, de Groot R, Perignon M et al. Current MUAC Cut-Offs to Screen for Acute Malnutrition Need to Be Adapted to Gender and Age: The Example of Cambodia. PLoS ONE. 2016; 11:e0146442. http://journals.plos.org/plosone/article/file?id=10.1371/journal.pone.0146442&type=printable.
20. Tadesse AW, Tadesse E, Berhane Y, Ekstrom EC. Comparison of mid-upper arm circumference and weight-for-height to diagnose severe acute malnutrition: a study in southern Ethiopia. Nutrients. 2017;9:267. http://www.mdpi.com/2072-6643/9/3/267/htm.
21. Grellety E, Golden MH. Weight-for-height and mid-upper-arm circumference should be used independently to diagnose acute malnutrition: policy implications. BMC Nutr. 2016;2:10. https://bmcnutr.biomedcentral.com/articles/10.1186/s40795-016-0049-7.
22. Briend A, Alvarez JL, Avril N, Bahwere P, Bailey J, Berkley JA et al. Low mid-upper arm circumference identifies children with a high risk of death who should be the priority target for treatment. BMC Nutrition. 2016;2:63. https://bmcnutr.biomedcentral.com/articles/10.1186/s40795-016-0101-7.
23. Hammond W, Badawi AE, Deconinck H. Detecting severe acute malnutrition in children under five at scale. The Challenges of Anthropometry to Reach the Missed Millions. Ann Nutr Disord & Ther. 2016;3:1030. http://austinpublishinggroup.com/nutritional-disorders/fulltext/andt-v3-id1030.php#Top.
24. Bailey J, Chase R, Kerac M, Briend A, Manary M, Opondo C, et al. Combined protocol for SAM/MAM treatment. The ComPAS study. Field exchange. 2016;53:44. http://www.ennonline.net/fex/53/thecompasstudy.
25. Garenne M, Maire B, Fontaine O, Briend A. Adequacy of child anthropometric indicators for measuring nutritional stress at population level: a study from Niakhar, Senegal. Public Health Nutr. 2013;16:1533–9. https://www.cambridge.org/core/services/aop-cambridge-core/content/view/S136898001200448X.
26. Briend A. Use of MUAC for severe acute malnutrition. CMAM forum. 2012; http://citeseerx.ist.psu.edu/viewdoc/download?doi=10.1.1.662.303&rep=rep1&type=pdf.
27. Taren D, de Pee S. The Spectrum of Malnutrition. In: Nutrition and Health in a Developing World. New York: Springer International Publishing; 2017. p. 91–117.
28. Deconinck H. Understanding pathways of integrating severe acute malnutrition interventions into national health systems in low-income countries: Doctoral dissertation. Université catholique de Louvain; 2017. https://dial.uclouvain.be/pr/boreal/object/boreal%3A183112/datastream/PDF_02/view.
29. EN-Net. WFH versus MUAC. 2015. Emergency Nutrition Network. http://www.en-net.org/question/1915.aspx.
30. EN-Net. Only MUAC for admission and discharge? 2015. Emergency Nutrition Network. http://www.en-net.org/question/1922.aspx.
31. Briend A, Maire B, Fontaine O, Garenne M. Mid-upper arm circumference and weight-for-height to identify high-risk malnourished under-five children. Maternal & child nutrition 2012, 8: 130–133. http://onlinelibrary.wiley.com/doi/10.1111/j.1740-8709.2011.00340.x/full.
32. The Council of Research & Technical Advice on Acute Malnutrition (CORTASAM). No Wasted Lives 2017. https://www.nowastedlives.org/advisory-group/.
33. Grellety E, Golden MH. Severely malnourished children with a low weight-for-height have a higher mortality than those with a low mid-upper-arm-circumference: I. Empirical data demonstrates Simpson's paradox. Nutr J. 2018. https://doi.org/10.1186/s12937-018-0384-4.
34. Grellety E, Golden MH. Severely malnourished children with a low weight-for-height have a higher mortality than those with a low mid-upper-arm-circumference: III. Effect of case-load on malnutrition related mortality: policy implications. Nutr J. 2018. https://doi.org/10.1186/s12937-018-0382-6.
35. Moher D, Liberati A, Tetzlaff J, Altman DG. Preferred reporting items for systematic reviews and meta-analyses: the PRISMA statement. Ann Intern Med. 2009;151:264–9. https://doi.org/10.7326/0003-4819-151-4-200908180-00135.
36. Olofin I, Guesdon B, Roberfroid D. Associations of suboptimal MUAC and WHZ combinations with child mortality: a pooled analysis: Action Against Hunger, Research for Nutrition Conference; 2016. http://files.ennonline.net/attachments/2604/ACF-conference-special-section.pdf.
37. Archie JP Jr. Mathematic coupling of data: a common source of error. Ann Surg. 1981;193:296. http://journals.lww.com/annalsofsurgery/abstract/1981/03000/mathematic_coupling_of_data__a_common_source_of.8.aspx.
38. Tu YK, Maddick IH, Griffiths GS, Gilthorpe MS. Mathematical coupling can undermine the statistical assessment of clinical research: illustration from the treatment of guided tissue regeneration. J Dentistry 32: 133–142. http://dx.doi.org/10.1016/j.jdent.2003.10.001
39. Garenne M, Maire B, Fontaine O, Dieng K, Briend A. Risques de décès associés à différents états nutritionnels chez l'enfant d'âge préscolaire: étude réalisée à Niakhar (Sénégal), 1983–1986. ORSTOM Dakar; 1987. http://horizon.documentation.ird.fr/exl-doc/pleins_textes/divers11-10/24687.pdf.
40. Garenne M, Willie D, Maire B, Fontaine O, Eeckels R, Briend A, et al. Incidence and duration of severe wasting in two African populations. Public Health Nutr. 2009;12:1974. https://www.cambridge.org/core/services/aop-cambridge-core/content/view/S1368980009004972.

41. Van Den Broeck J, Eeckels R, Vuylsteke J. Influence of nutritional status on child mortality in rural Zaire. Lancet. 1993;341:1491–5. http://www.sciencedirect.com/science/article/pii/014067369390632Q.
42. Barendregt JJ, Doi SA. Meta XL. 5.32 [computer program]. Queensland: EpiGear International Pty Ltd; 2016. https://www.epigear.com/index_files/metaxl.html
43. Doi SAR, Barendregt JJ, Khan S, Thalib S, Williams GM. Advances in the meta-analysis of heterogeneous clinical trials II: The quality effects model. Contemp Clin Trials 2015; 45 (Pt A):123–129. https://doi.org/10.1016/j.cct.2015.05.010.
44. Aguayo VM, Aneja S, Badgaiyan N, Singh K. Mid upper-arm circumference is an effective tool to identify infants and young children with severe acute malnutrition in India. Public Health Nutr. 2015;18:3244–8. https://www.cambridge.org/core/services/aop-cambridge-core/content/view/S1368980015000543.
45. Grellety E, Shepherd S, Roederer T, Manzo ML, Doyon S, Ategbo EA, et al. Effect of mass supplementation with ready-to-use supplementary food during an anticipated nutritional emergency. PLoS One. 2012;7:e44549. http://www.ncbi.nlm.nih.gov/pmc/articles/PMC3440398/pdf/pone.0044549.pdf.
46. Isanaka S, Guesdon B, Labar AS, Hanson K, Langendorf C, Grais RF. Comparison of clinical characteristics and treatment outcomes of children selected for treatment of severe acute malnutrition using mid upper arm circumference and/or weight-for-height Z-score. PLoS One. 2015;10: e0137606. http://journals.plos.org/plosone/article?id=10.1371/journal.pone.0137606.
47. Lowlaavar N, Larson CP, Kumbakumba E, Zhou G, Ansermino JM, Singer J, et al. Pediatric in-hospital death from infectious disease in Uganda: derivation of clinical prediction models. PLoS One. 2016;11:e0150683. http://journals.plos.org/plosone/article?id=10.1371/journal.pone.0150683.
48. LaCourse S, Chester FM, Preidis G, McCrary LM, Maliwichi M, McCollum ED, et al. Lay-screeners and use of WHO growth standards increase case finding of hospitalized Malawian children with severe acute malnutrition. J Trop Pediatr. 2014;61:44–53. https://doi.org/10.1093/tropej/fmu065.
49. Berkley J, Mwangi I, Griffiths K, Ahmed I, Mithwani S, English M, et al. Assessment of severe malnutrition among hospitalized children in rural Kenya: comparison of weight for height and mid upper arm circumference. Jama. 2005;294:591–7. http://jamanetwork.com/journals/jama/fullarticle/201328.
50. Chiabi A, Mbanga C, Mah E, Nguefack DF, Nguefack S, Fru F, et al. Weight-for-Height Z Score and Mid-Upper Arm Circumference as Predictors of Mortality in Children with Severe Acute Malnutrition. J Trop Pediatr. 2017; https://academic.oup.com/tropej/article-abstract/63/4/260/2671088.
51. Sachdeva S, Dewan P, Shah D, Malhotra RK, Gupta P. Mid-upper arm circumference v. weight-for-height Z-score for predicting mortality in hospitalized children under 5 years of age. Public Health Nutr. 2016:1–8. https://www.cambridge.org/core/services/aop-cambridge-core/content/view/S1368980016000719.
52. Burza S, Mahajan R, Marino E, Sunyoto T, Shandilya C, Tabrez M, et al. Seasonal effect and long-term nutritional status following exit from a community-based Management of Severe Acute Malnutrition program in Bihar, India. Eur J Clin Nutr. 2015; http://www.nature.com/ejcn/journal/v70/n4/full/ejcn2015140a.html.
53. Mogeni P, Twahir H, Bandika V, Mwalekwa L, Thitiri J, Ngari M, et al. Diagnostic performance of visible severe wasting for identifying severe acute malnutrition in children admitted to hospital in Kenya. Bull WHO. 2011;89:900–6. http://www.who.int/bulletin/volumes/89/12/11-091280/en/.
54. Sylla A, Gueye M, Keita Y, Seck N, Seck A, Mbow F, et al. Dehydration and malnutrition as two independent risk factors of death in a Senegalese pediatric hospital. Archives de pediatrie: organe officiel de la Societe francaise de pediatrie. 2015;22:235–40. https://doi.org/10.1016/j.arcped.2014.11.024.
55. Vella V. An epidemiological analysis of the determinants of childhood malnutrition and mortality in southwest Uganda. PhD thesis London School of Hygiene & Tropical Medicine; 1990. http://researchonline.lshtm.ac.uk/682267/1/296416.pdf.
56. Dramaix M, Hennart P, Brasseur D, Bahwere P, Mudjene O, Tonglet R et al. Serum albumin concentration, arm circumference, and oedema and subsequent risk of dying in children in central Africa. Bmj. 1993;307:710–3. https://doi.org/10.1136/bmj.307.6906.710.
57. Girum T, Kote M, Tariku B, Bekele H. Survival status and predictors of mortality among severely acute malnourished children< 5 years of age admitted to stabilization centers in Gedeo zone: a retrospective cohort study. Ther Clin Risk Manag. 2017;13:101. https://doi.org/10.2147/TCRM.S119826.
58. Savadogo L, Zoetaba I, Donnen P, Hennart P, Sondo BK, Dramaix M. Management of severe acute malnutrition in an urban nutritional rehabilitation center in Burkina Faso. Revue d'epidemiologie et de sante publique. 2007;55:265–74. https://doi.org/10.1016/j.respe.2007.05.006.
59. Nhampossa T, Sigauque B, Machevo S, Macete E, Alonso P, Bassat Q, Menendez C, Fumado V. Severe malnutrition among children under the age of 5 years admitted to a rural district hospital in southern Mozambique. Public Health Nutr. 2013;16(9):1565–74. https://doi.org/10.1017/S1368980013001080.
60. Acevedo P, Esteban MTG, Lopez-Ejeda N, Gómez A, Marrodán MD. Influence of malnutrition upon all-cause mortality among children in Swaziland. Endocrinología, Diabetes y Nutrición. 2017;64(4):204–10. https://doi.org/10.1016/j.endinu.2017.01.008.
61. WHO, Unicef. WHO child growth standards and the identification of severe acute malnutrition in infants and children: a joint statement by the World Health Organization and the United Nations Children's fund. 2009. http://www.who.int/nutrition/publications/severemalnutrition/9789241598163_eng.pdf.
62. WHO. Guideline: Updates on the management of severe acute malnutrition in infants and children. Geneva, World Health Organization; 2013. http://www.who.int/nutrition/publications/guidelines/updates_management_SAM_infantandchildren/en/ infantandchildren/en/.
63. Golden MH, Grellety Y. Population nutritional status during famine. 2002. http://www.nutrisurvey.de/ena_beta/Golden_Population_nutritional_status_during_famile_surveywhzdis.pdf.
64. Frison S, Checchi F, Kerac M, Nicholas J. Is middle-upper arm circumference "normally" distributed? Secondary data analysis of 852 nutrition surveys. Emerg Themes Epidemiol. 2016;13:7.
65. De Onis M, Yip R, Mei Z. The development of MUAC-for-age reference data recommended by a WHO expert committee. Bull World Health Organ. 1997;75:11–8.
66. Tu YK, Gunnell D, Gilthorpe MS. Simpson's paradox, Lord's paradox, and suppression effects are the same phenomenon - the reversal paradox. Emerging Themes in Epidemiology. 2008;5:2. https://ete-online.biomedcentral.com/articles/10.1186/1742-7622-5-2.
67. Willis JS, Golden MH. Active and passive transport of sodium and potassium ions in erythrocytes of severely malnourished Jamaican children. Eur J Clin Nutr. 1988;42:635–45.
68. Bairagi R. On validity of some anthropometric indicators as predictors of mortality. Am J Clin Nutr. 1981;34(11):2592–4.
69. Briend A, Dykewicz C, Graven K, Mazumder RN, Wojtyniak B, Bennish M. Usefulness of nutritional indices and classifications in predicting death of malnourished children. Br Med J. 1986;293(6543):373–5. https://doi.org/10.1136/bmj.293.6543.373.
70. Alam N, Wojtyniak B, Rahaman MM. Anthropometric indicators and risk of death. Am J Clin Nutr. 1989;49(5):884–8.
71. Briend A, Garenne M, Maire B, Fontaine O, Dieng K. Nutritional status, age and survival: the muscle mass hypothesis. Eur J Clin Nutr. 1989;43(10):715–26.
72. Vella V, Tomkins A, Borghesi A, Migliori GB, Ndiku J, Adriko BC. Anthropometry and childhood mortality in northwest and Southwest Uganda. Am J Public Health. 1993;83(11):1616–8. https://doi.org/10.2105/AJPH.83.11.1616.
73. Pelletier DL, Low JW, Johnson FC, Msukwa LA. Child anthropometry and mortality in Malawi: testing for effect modification by age and length of follow-up and confounding by socioeconomic factors. J Nutr. 1994;124:2082S–105S.
74. Pelletier DL. The relationship between child anthropometry and mortality in developing countries: implications for policy, programs and future research. J Nutr. 1994;124(10 Suppl):2047S–81S.
75. Vella V, Tomkins A, Ndiku J, Marshal T, Cortinovis I. Anthropometry as a predictor for mortality among Ugandan children, allowing for socio-economic variables. Eur J Clin Nutr. 1994;48(3):189–97.
76. Van den Broeck J, Eeckels R, Massa G. Validity of single-weight measurements to predict current malnutrition and mortality in children. J Nutr. 1996;126(1):113–20.
77. Garenne M, Maire B, Fontaine O, Briend A. Distributions of mortality risk attributable to low nutritional status in Niakhar, Senegal. J Nutr. 2006;136:2893–900.
78. Mwangome MK, Fegan G, Fulford T, Prentice AM, Berkley JA. Mid-upper arm circumference at age of routine infant vaccination to identify infants at

elevated risk of death: a retrospective cohort study in the Gambia. Bull WHO. 2012;90(12):887–94. https://doi.org/10.2471/BLT.12.109009.
79. Waterlow JC, Tomkins A, Grantham-McGregor SM. Protein energy malnutrition. London: Edward Arnold; 1992.
80. Rice AL, Sacco L, Hyder A, Black RE. Malnutrition as an underlying cause of childhood deaths associated with infectious diseases in developing countries. Bull WHO. 2000;78:1207–21.
81. Muller O, Garenne M, Kouyate B, Becher H. The association between protein-energy malnutrition, malaria morbidity and all-cause mortality in west African children. Tropical Med Int Health. 2003;8:507–11. https://doi.org/10.1186/1475-2875-5-47.
82. Grellety E, Golden MH. Response to Briend et al "low mid-upper-arm-circumference identifies children with a high risk of death and should be the priority target for treatment". BMC Nutrition. 2016;2-63:1–12. https://bmcnutr.biomedcentral.com/articles/10.1186/s40795-016-0101-7.
83. WHO. Management of severe malnutrition: a manual for physicians and other senior health workers: World Health Organization; 1999. http://apps.who.int/iris/handle/10665/41999.
84. Golden MH. Comment on WHZ and MUAC for diagnosis of severe malnutrition by Chiabi A et al. J Trop Pediatr. 2017;0:1–2. https://doi.org/10.1093/tropej/fmx008.
85. Heikens GT, Manary MJ, Trehan I. African children with severe pneumonia remain at high risk for death even after discharge. Paediatr Perinat Epidemiol. 2017. http://onlinelibrary.wiley.com/doi/10.1111/ppe.12350/full.

# Ethnic disparities of beverage consumption in infants and children 0–5 years of age: National Health and Nutrition Examination Survey 2011 to 2014

Elieke Demmer[1*], Christopher J. Cifelli[1], Jenny A. Houchins[1] and Victor L. Fulgoni III[2]

## Abstract

**Background:** Dietary patterns, including beverage consumption, that are developed during a child's first few years of life have been shown to impact dietary choices made later in life. Authoritative sources provide beverage recommendations for infants and children; however, it is unclear if these guidelines are followed and what, if any, the differences are among races/ethnicities. The objective of this study was to examine beverage consumption to recommendations among children 0–5 months, 6–11 months, 12–23 months, 2–3 years, and 4–5 years. Additionally, examine how these beverage patterns associate with nutrient intake and to determine if differences exist in beverage consumption among race/ethnic groups (Non-Hispanic White, Non-Hispanic Black, Hispanic, and Asian) in children aged 0–23 months, 2–3 years, and 4–5 years.

**Methods:** Data from the 2011–2014 National Health and Nutrition Examination Survey (NHANES) for children 0–5 years were analyzed ($n = 2445$). Beverages were classified as follows; milk, 100% juice, diet beverages, sugar sweetened beverages (SSB), and water.

**Results:** Our results show that regardless of race/ethnicity, dietary recommendation were not always followed. Prior to 6 months, 10% of infants consumed any amount of 100% juice; from 6 to 11 months, 17% of young children were drinking any amount of milk. SSB consumption rapidly increased with age, whereas intake of milk and 100% juice declined after 2 to 3 years of age. Non-Hispanic Black young children consumed the most 100% juice from 2 to 3 years and up, exceeding recommended amounts, and throughout all age groups they consumed the least milk and most SSBs. The decreased intake of nutrient-rich beverages with age was associated with lower intakes of under-consumed nutrients of public health concern. By 4–5 years, 32.7% and 93.8% of children were consuming <EAR for calcium and vitamin D, respectively.

**Conclusions:** Dietary recommendations for both the introduction of beverages and amounts consumed were not consistently followed for American infants and children 0–5 years. Race/ethnic disparities exist in beverage consumption with Non-Hispanic Black children consuming the least amount of milk and most SSBs. Improving beverage consumption patterns could help improve overall diet quality which directly contributes to overall childhood health.

**Keywords:** Infants, Children, Beverage, Recommendations, Ethnic disparities, Milk, 100% juice, Sugar sweetened beverage, Nutrient intake

* Correspondence: eliekedemmer@gmail.com
[1]National Dairy Council, 10255 West Higgins Road, Suite 900, Rosemont, IL 60018-5616, USA
Full list of author information is available at the end of the article

## Background

Infancy and early childhood are periods of rapid growth and development, which requires adequate consumption of essential macro- and micronutrients. Dietary patterns developed during these early life stages can form the basis for future food and beverage preferences [1, 2], thus potentially impacting early- and later-life development. Beverages provide a substantial amount of kilocalories (kcals) and nutrients to the diets of children [3–5]. While some beverages are nutrient rich, others can be a source of nutrients to limit, such as added sugar. For this reason, the U.S. Department of Agriculture (USDA) and Health and Human Services (HHS) have asked for additional information to better understand beverage patterns among infants and children, as the 2020–2025 Dietary Guidelines for American (DGA) will include recommendations for the 0–2 years age range for the first time [6, 7].

Currently, the American Academy of Pediatrics (AAP) provides recommendations for the introduction of beverages to infants and children. Exclusive breastfeeding is recommended for approximately 6 months and continued breastfeeding for at least 12 months [8]. This recommendation is in part due to evidence suggesting that breastfeeding has a positive impact on the development of a child's later eating behavior [9, 10]. The AAP also recommends that 100% juice not be introduced to the diet before 1 year of age and, once introduced, consumption should be limited to 4 oz (oz) per day for children 1 to 3 years and 4–6 oz. per day for children 4 to 6 years [11]. These recently updated juice recommendations reflect the research showing that prolonged exposure of the teeth to the sugars in juice is a major contributing factor to dental caries, as well as the fact that fruit juices lack protein and fiber which can predispose children to inappropriate weight gain [11]. Cow's milk is not recommended for the first year of life as it provides inadequate iron, vitamin E, zinc, and essential fatty acids and excessive amounts of sodium, potassium, chloride, and protein for infants [12]. The introduction of plain whole milk is recommended at 1 year and the AAP suggests 16–24 oz. of milk per day [12]. According to experts, no restriction of fat or cholesterol is recommended for children younger than 2 years, as this is a period of rapid growth and neurologic development with high energy requirements, unless a concern for obesity or family history of cardiovascular disease exists [12]. The Institute of Medicine (IOM) has set Adequate Intakes (AI) for water consumption for 0–5 yrs. While the water AI for infants 7–12 mo of age is 0.8 l/day, it should be noted that all beverages and moisture in foods is included in this AI [13]. See Table 1 for a summary of all beverage recommendations for children 0–5 yrs. of age.

Starting at 2 years, the 2015–2020 DGA recommends low-fat or fat-free milk, in addition to 100% juice and water, as primary beverages of choice [3]. It should be noted that the DGA recommends no more than half of the fruit group be consumed as 100% juice [3]. The Academy of Nutrition and Dietetics (AND) does not recommend beverages with added sugars for infants and suggests that if toddlers consume sugar sweetened beverages (SSBs), they should be considered treats and potentially eliminated from the diet [14]. If SSB are consumed, overall amounts should be within overall kcal limits [3].

Several recent reports indicate that these recommendations for beverage intake in children are not consistently followed. In a 2004 to 2005 Oregon based population survey of nearly 2000 mothers, more than half (59.9%) of the mothers reported that their 2 year-old child drank a SSB at least 1 day per week [15]. Similarly, among a sample of 1189 parents participating in the 2005–2007 Infant Feeding Practices Study II and who were followed up with when their child was 6 years old, a quarter (25.9%) reported that their children consumed SSBs during infancy [16]. Additionally, these data showed that the prevalence of childhood obesity at 6 years was highest among children who either were introduced to SSBs before 6 months of age or who consumed SSBs more than 3 times per week during age 10–12 months [16]. Additionally, research has shown that higher SSB consumption is associated with decreased milk consumption, which could impact the ability of children to meet nutrient recommendations [17]. These observed beverage consumption patterns among infants and children are of concern as early dietary choices have

**Table 1** Beverage recommendations for children

| | 0–5 months[1] | 6–11 months[2] | 12–23 months[3] | 2–3 years[4] | 4–5 years[5] |
|---|---|---|---|---|---|
| 100% Juice | 0 | 0 | 4 oz | 4 oz | 4-6 oz |
| Water[6] | 0 | 0.8 Liters/day | 1.3 Liters/day | 1.3 Liters/day | 1.7 Liters/day |
| Milk | 0 | 0 | 16–24 oz. (whole milk) | 2 cups (low fat, fat free) | 2.5 cups (low fat, fat free) |
| Sweetened Beverages | 0 | 0 | Treats only, ideally eliminated | Within kcal limit | Within kcal limit |

1) *0–5 months* 100% Juice (11, 12, 27), water (12, 27), milk (12, 27), sweetened beverages (12, 14, 27); 2) *6–11 months* 100% Juice (11), water (13), milk (12), sweetened beverages (14); 3) *12–23 months* 100% Juice (11), water (13), milk, (12), sweetened beverages (14); 4) *2–3 years* 100% Juice (11), water (13), milk (3), sweetened beverages (3); 5) *4–5 years* 100% Juice (11), water (13), milk (3), sweetened beverages (3); 6) The adequate intake (AI) is listed for children 6 months to 5 years as recommended by the IOM, these AI's include water from all beverages and moisture in foods

been shown to influence diet choices made later in life and thus can influence diet quality and nutrient adequacy which are important modifiable risk factors for non-communicable diseases [18].

Few studies have researched beverage consumption in children by race/ethnicity, especially during the first 2 years of life. A trend analysis among children 2 to 11 years from 2003 to 2009 reported a decrease in consumption of 2 or more servings of 100% juice per day among Non-Hispanic White children and an increase among Hispanics [19]. Results from 2007 to 2010 National Health and Nutrition Examination Survey (NHANES) analysis showed that 100% fruit juice consumption was significantly higher among Non-Hispanic Black and Hispanic children compared to Non-Hispanic White children [20]. Marked differences among race/ethnic groups were reported for milk consumption for 2 to 18-year-old children and adolescents based on 2001 to 2004 NHANES data. Only 15% of Non-Hispanic Black children met the recommended servings for milk compared to 42% of Non-Hispanic White children and 49% of Hispanic children [21].

Nutrient rich beverages provide a significant percentage of essential nutrients to the diet of infants and young children [22]. The purpose of this analysis was to examine beverage patterns among American infants and young children (0–5 years); specifically, to determine the proportion of children who consume different beverage types across age groups, examine the impact of these beverage consumption patterns on nutrient adequacy for nutrients of public health concern, and determine if beverage recommendations are followed among varying age and race/ethnic groups.

## Methods

### Subjects

Using data from NHANES 2011–2014, we conducted separate analyses for various young age groups in the U.S. population (males and females combined; total *n* = 2445). Age groups were chosen to align with beverage recommendations from authoritative sources: 0–5 months (*n* = 233), 6–11 months (*n* = 301), 12–23 months (*n* = 397), 2–3 years, (*n* = 839) and 4–5 years (*n* = 675). Analyses were also run to determine if there were any differences among race/ethnic groups; Non-Hispanic White (*n* = 591), Non-Hispanic Black (*n* = 643), Hispanic (*n* = 833), Asians (*n* = 222), and other (*n* = 156). Due to smaller sample sizes for race/ethnic groups, within these race/ethnic analyses the following age breakdowns were used 0–23 months (*n* = 931), 2–3 years, (n = 839) and 4–5 years (*n* = 675) (Table 2). Subjects with other race/ethnicity designations were not studied as they were not representative of the national population. Only subjects with reliable 24-h recall interviews who met minimum criteria as established by the United States Department of Agriculture (USDA) were included in the analyses [22, 23]; additionally, given lack of quantification of intake, those consuming human milk were also excluded (*n* = 260).

**Table 2** Sample sizes by age and race/ethnicty

| Ethnicity | Age Group | | | |
|---|---|---|---|---|
| | 0-23 Months | 2-3 Years | 4-5 Years | All |
| Hispanic | 328 (39%) | 265 (32%) | 240 (29%) | 833 |
| Non-Hispanic White | 250 (42%) | 202 (34%) | 139 (24%) | 591 |
| Non-Hispanic Black | 233 (36%) | 242 (38%) | 168 (26%) | 643 |
| Asian | 62 (28%) | 80 (36%) | 80 (36%) | 222 |
| Other | 58 (37%) | 50 (32%) | 48 (31%) | 156 |
| All | 931 (38%) | 839 (34%) | 675 (28%) | 2,445 |

### Beverage and nutrient intakes

Day 1 24-h dietary recalls (provided by parents/caretakers) were used to assess intake of specific beverages on any given day using definitions in the USDA food category system used for NHANES [24]. The day 1 recall was collected via an in-person interview and used the validated Automated Multi Pass Method and is the best estimate of consumption on any given day. The beverage groups examined were as follows; 1) 100% Juice: citrus, apple, other fruit, vegetable, baby juice. 2) Water: tap, bottled, flavored, carbonated, enhanced, fortified, baby water. 3) Milk: milk, flavored milk, milk shakes, dairy drinks, milk substitutes. 4) Diet Beverages: diet soft drinks, diet sport drinks, diet energy drinks, other diet drinks. 5) Sugar Sweetened Beverages: soft drinks, fruit drinks, sport drinks, energy drinks, nutritional beverages. 6) Coffee and Tea: coffee, tea. Data representing the percent of children who consumed each beverage (any amount), the amount of beverage consumed, and energy from beverages are presented as mean ± standard error (SE) for each age group. For comparative purposes the percentage of kcals from each beverage was determined along with percent kcals from other foods. The intake of milk and flavored milk based on fat type using USDA defined categories were also determined (i.e., whole, reduced fat, low fat, and nonfat).

### Statistical analyses

The distribution of usual intake including percentiles and percentages meeting cutoffs was estimated using version 2.1 of the National Cancer Institute (NCI) usual intake programs [25]. The estimates are generated with 2 days of dietary data (second day recall was gathered via the telephone 3–10 days after the in-person interview; this second day data are used to help define intra- and inter-person variation) with day 1 dietary weights used in all stages of the estimation process. Balanced repeated replicates (BRR) were used which equal the smallest multiple of 4 that is greater than the number of NHANES strata in the input dataset for the usual intake. A non-response adjustment based on age, gender and race/ethnicity was made to BRR weights for each replication. The covariates used in the usual intake models were dietary recall number (1 or 2), and day of recall coded as weekday or weekend (Friday, Saturday, and Sunday). Nutrients reported included: calcium, iron, magnesium, phosphorus, potassium, zinc and vitamins A, C, and D. Race/ethnicity information came from NHANES demographic files based on responses during the in home questionnaire [26]. SAS 9.2 (SAS Institute, Cary, NC) was used with NHANES design aspects (primary sampling units and strata) and appropriate sampling weights to ensure estimates are nationally representative. Mean amounts, percentages and SEs were determined with "Proc Surveymeans" procedure and differences in means by age and or race/ethnicity were determined by t-tests with $p < 0.01$ as significant.

## Results

### Beverage choices

For the total sample of children, 20.5% of total kcals were from beverages evaluated (289 kcal) and 79.5% of kcals were from food (1100 kcal). The caloric contribution to the overall diet by beverage type were plain milk (10.7%), 100% juice (4.3%), SSBs (3.4%) and flavored milk (2.2%).

Reported beverage consumption on any given day by age among infants and children are presented in Table 3. Regardless of race/ethnicity, over 10% of infants younger than 6 months reported consuming 100% juice and more than 24% consumed small amounts of water despite recommendations to exclusively consume human milk, or in the absence of human milk, iron-fortified infant formula. The IOM recommends no supplementation of water, juice, nonhuman milk, or foods prior to 6 months of age [27]. For infants 6 to 11 months, over 17% consumed milk and 5% drank SSBs. Milk consumption was highest among 1 to 2 years where only 10% did not consume milk. Milk intake declined after the second year of life. More than 12% of 2 to 3-year olds did not consume milk and this number increased to over 17% in 4 to 5 years. While milk consumption decreased with age, consumption of SSBs significantly increased with age. For children 12–23 months, nearly 31% consumed SSBs, which significantly increased to 40% for children 2 to 3 years and to more than 51% for children 4 to 5 years.

Since milk recommendations vary by milk fat level as children get older, Table 4 presents the amount of milk consumed on any given day by type for each age group. Whole milk was the predominant type consumed by children 2 years and younger. For children 2 to 5 years reduced fat (2%) milk was the predominant type consumed. The mean amount of milk consumed was lower than recommendations for all age groups.

The amounts of milk, 100% juice and SSBs consumed on any given day by age and race/ethnicity are presented in Table 5. Milk consumption was highest among Non-Hispanic White children from 0 to 23 months, among Hispanic children from 2 to 3 years, and Asian children consumed the most milk from 4 to 5 years. Milk consumption was consistently the lowest among Non-Hispanic Black children after 2 years of age. Non-Hispanic Black children consumed the most 100% juice during the first 3 years of life, while Asian children consumed significantly less 100% juice from 4 to 5 years than all other races/ethnicities. 100% juice consumption decreased after 3 years across all the race/ethnic groups. Non-Hispanic Black children consumed the highest amount of SSBs among all age groups. In comparison, Asian children consumed the least amount of SSBs during the first 5 years of life.

The kcal contribution of the reported beverage choices on any given day is presented in Table 6. Regardless of

**Table 3** Percent of children consuming different beverage types on a given day, NHANES 2011–2014

| | 0–5 months ($n = 233$) | 6–11 months ($n = 301$) | 12–23 months ($n = 397$) | 2–3 years ($n = 839$) | 4–5 years ($n = 675$) |
|---|---|---|---|---|---|
| | Mean ± SEM | Mean ± SEM | Mean ± SEM | Mean ± SEM | Mean ± SEM |
| 100% Juice[1] | $10.13^{a} \pm 1.96$ | $38.78^{b} \pm 3.68$ | $58.23^{c} \pm 3.48$ | $53.97^{c} \pm 2.37$ | $49.05^{c} \pm 3.26$ |
| Water[2] | $24.69^{a} \pm 4.45$ | $61.88^{b} \pm 2.92$ | $77.46^{c} \pm 2.83$ | $82.18^{c} \pm 1.55$ | $79.23^{c} \pm 2.30$ |
| Milk[3] | $0.73^{a} \pm 0.54$ | $17.47^{b} \pm 3.09$ | $90.86^{c} \pm 1.97$ | $87.49^{c} \pm 1.47$ | $82.74^{c} \pm 2.13$ |
| Diet Beverages[4] | $0^{a} \pm 0$ | $0^{a} \pm 0$ | $2.11^{ab} \pm 1.08$ | $3.51^{b} \pm 0.93$ | $5.07^{b} \pm 0.79$ |
| Sweetened Beverages[5] | $0.66^{a} \pm 0.52$ | $5.05^{b} \pm 1.00$ | $30.97^{c} \pm 3.73$ | $40.19^{cd} \pm 3.04$ | $51.32^{d} \pm 3.83$ |
| Coffee and Tea[6] | $0^{a} \pm 0$ | $0.55^{a} \pm 0.56$ | $7.25^{b} \pm 1.70$ | $8.94^{b} \pm 1.41$ | $8.37^{b} \pm 1.35$ |

Data based on Day 1 dietary recalls
SEM, Standard Error of the Mean. 1) 100% Juice includes: citrus, apple, other fruit, vegetable, baby juice. 2) Water includes: tap, bottled, flavored, carbonated, enhanced, fortified, baby water. 3) Milk includes: milk, flavored milk, milk shakes, dairy drinks, milk substitutes. 4) Diet Beverages includes: diet soft drinks, diet sport drinks, diet energy drinks, other diet drinks. 5) Sugar Sweetened Beverages includes: soft drinks, fruit drinks, sport drinks, energy drinks, nutritional beverages. 6) Coffee and Tea includes: coffee, tea. [a,b,c,d] Means sharing the same superscripts are not significantly different across ages, $p < 0.01$

**Table 4** Amount of milk consumed on a given day by milk-type and age, NHANES 2011–2014

| | 0–5 months (*n* = 233) | 6–11 months (*n* = 301) | 12–23 months (*n* = 397) | 2–3 years (*n* = 839) | 4–5 years (*n* = 675) |
|---|---|---|---|---|---|
| | Grams[1] ± SEM | Grams[1] ± SEM | Grams[1] ± SEM | Grams[1] ± SEM | Grams[1] ± SEM |
| Milk, whole | $3.15^{a}$ ± 3.12 | $53.90^{b}$ ± 11.80 | $345.60^{c}$ ± 26.68 | $99.12^{d}$ ± 12.66 | $57.16^{b}$ ± 12.68 |
| Milk, reduced fat | $0.11^{a}$ ± 0.11 | $11.79^{b}$ ± 3.32 | $90.49^{c}$ ± 13.00 | $150.07^{d}$ ± 12.46 | $105.44^{c}$ ± 8.19 |
| Milk, lowfat | $0^{a}$ ± 0 | $3.56^{ab}$ ± 1.98 | $15.35^{bc}$ ± 5.14 | $34.12^{c}$ ± 6.51 | $45.46^{bc}$ ± 15.51 |
| Milk, nonfat | $0^{a}$ ± 0 | $0.02^{a}$ ± 0.02 | $2.25^{ab}$ ± 1.28 | $19.58^{b}$ ± 6.98 | $17.98^{b}$ ± 5.74 |
| Flavored Milk, whole | $0^{a}$ ± 0 | $0.34^{a}$ ± 0.34 | $8.23^{ab}$ ± 4.08 | $10.79^{b}$ ± 2.77 | $20.85^{b}$ ± 5.88 |
| Flavored Milk, reduced fat | $0^{a}$ ± 0 | $1.29^{a}$ ± 1.23 | $1.07^{a}$ ± 0.76 | $31.36^{b}$ ± 7.71 | $28.89^{b}$ ± 5.22 |
| Flavored Milk, lowfat | $0^{a}$ ± 0 | $0^{a}$ ± 0 | $0^{a}$ ± 0 | $11.96^{b}$ ± 3.06 | $8.53^{b}$ ± 2.49 |
| Flavored Milk, nonfat | $0^{a}$ ± 0 | $0^{a}$ ± 0 | $0^{a}$ ± 0 | $4.97^{b}$ ± 1.60 | $8.69^{b}$ ± 2.66 |
| Dairy Drinks and Substitutes | $0^{a}$ ± 0 | $5.35^{ab}$ ± 5.14 | $22.22^{b}$ ± 6.44 | $13.87^{b}$ ± 3.32 | $11.22^{b}$ ± 3.72 |

Data based on Day 1 dietary recalls
*SEM* Standard Error of the Mean. 1). One cup of milk is equivalent to 244 g. [a,b,c,d] Means sharing the same superscripts are not significantly different across ages, $p < 0.01$. Dairy drinks and substitutes includes milk substitutes, milk shakes, and other dairy drinks

race/ethnicity, milk and 100% juice contributed the most kcals for children across most age groups. The contribution of kcals from SSBs significantly increased with age. By 4 to 5 years, SSBs contributed 75 kcals to daily intake compared to 59 kcals from 100% juice.

### Nutrient intakes

Table 7 shows the percent of children below the Estimated Average Requirement (EAR) or above the AI for under-consumed nutrients that pose a public health concern by age. Over 90% of all children 2–3 and 4–5 years of age consumed less than the EAR for vitamin D. From 1 to 5 years our data showed the percent of children who consumed calcium amounts below the EAR consistently increased. Nearly 33% of children 4 to 5 years had calcium intakes below the EAR. Like calcium and vitamin D, potassium intake also decreased with age, particularly after the first year. Less than 1% of children had potassium intakes above the AI by 4 to 5 years of age.

**Table 5** Amount of Total Milk, 100% Juice, and Sugar Sweetened Beverages consumed on a given day by age and race/ethnicity, NHANES 2011–2014

| | 0–23 Months | 2–3 Years | 4–5 Years |
|---|---|---|---|
| | Mean ± SEM | Mean ± SEM | Mean ± SEM |
| Milk[1] *(cups eq.)* | | | |
| Non-Hispanic White (*n = 591*) | $1.31^{a}$ ± 0.12 | $1.50^{ab}$ ± 0.10 | $1.30^{ab}$ ± 0.18 |
| Non-Hispanic Black (*n = 643*) | $0.83^{b}$ ± 0.08 | $1.14^{a}$ ± 0.12 | $0.83^{a}$ ± 0.10 |
| Hispanic (*n = 833*) | $1.21^{a}$ ± 0.09 | $1.65^{b}$ ± 0.10 | $1.33^{b}$ ± 0.09 |
| Asian (*n = 222*) | $1.06^{ab}$ ± 0.24 | $1.61^{ab}$ ± 0.34 | $1.43^{b}$ ± 0.14 |
| 100% Juice[2] *(cups eq.)* | | | |
| Non-Hispanic White | 0.35 ± 0.06 | 0.57 ± 0.08 | $0.47^{b}$ ± 0.05 |
| Non-Hispanic Black | 0.44 ± 0.07 | 0.80 ± 0.11 | $0.44^{ab}$ ± 0.06 |
| Hispanic | 0.41 ± 0.04 | 0.51 ± 0.06 | $0.47^{b}$ ± 0.06 |
| Asian | 0.31 ± 0.07 | 0.62 ± 0.09 | $0.21^{a}$ ± 0.07 |
| Sugar Sweetened Beverages[3] *(oz)* | | | |
| Non-Hispanic White | $1.37^{ab}$ ± 0.38 | $3.76^{ab}$ ± 0.57 | $5.74^{b}$ ± 0.92 |
| Non-Hispanic Black | $3.54^{b}$ ± 0.82 | $5.63^{b}$ ± 0.70 | $9.12^{b}$ ± 1.01 |
| Hispanic | $2.28^{ab}$ ± 0.53 | $5.21^{ab}$ ± 0.76 | $6.79^{b}$ ± 0.95 |
| Asian | $0.63^{a}$ ± 0.42 | $2.82^{a}$ ± 0.75 | $2.19^{a}$ ± 0.65 |

Data based on Day 1 dietary recalls
*SEM* Standard Error of the Mean. 1) Milk includes: milk, flavored milk, milk shakes, dairy drinks, milk substitutes. 2) 100% Juice includes: citrus, apple, other fruit, vegetable, baby juice. 3) Sugar Sweetened Beverages includes: soft drinks, fruit drinks, sport drinks, energy drinks, nutritional beverages. [a,b] Means sharing the same superscripts are not significantly different by race/ethnicity within age groups, $p < 0.01$

**Table 6** Daily kilocalorie (kcal) contribution of beverage choice on a given day by age, NHANES 2011–2014

| | 0–5 Months n = 233 | | | 6–11 months n = 301 | | | 12–23 months n = 397 | | | 2–3 years n = 839 | | | 4–5 years n = 675 | | |
|---|---|---|---|---|---|---|---|---|---|---|---|---|---|---|---|
| | Mean (% total kcal) | | SEM | Mean (% total kcal) | | SEM | Mean (% total kcal) | | SEM | Mean (% total kcal) | | SEM | Mean (% total kcal) | | SEM |
| 100% Juice[1] | 5.44 | ± | 1.38 | 28.49 | ± | 3.31 | 65.72 | ± | 7.37 | 72.20 | ± | 5.10 | 59.21 | ± | 6.15 |
| | (0.08 | ± | 0.20) | (3.26 | ± | 0.38) | (5.31 | ± | .60) | (4.94 | ± | 0.35) | (3.66 | ± | 0.38) |
| Water[2] | 0.00 | ± | 0.00 | 0.00 | ± | 0.00 | 0.03 | ± | 0.03 | 0.57 | ± | 0.27 | 0.57 | ± | 0.40 |
| | (0 | ± | 0) | (0 | ± | 0) | (0 | ± | 0) | (0.04 | ± | 0.02) | (0.04 | ± | 0.02) |
| Milk[3] | 2.22 | ± | 2.15 | 43.78 | ± | 8.25 | 281.53 | ± | 14.67 | 211.15 | ± | 9.80 | 169.79 | ± | 12.49 |
| | (0.33 | ± | 0.32) | (5.01 | ± | 0.94) | (22.77 | ± | 1.19) | (14.45 | ± | 0.67) | (10.49 | ± | 0.77) |
| Diet Beverages[4] | 0.00 | ± | 0.00 | 0.00 | ± | 0.00 | 0.04 | ± | 0.02 | 0.23 | ± | 0.11 | 0.32 | ± | 0.20 |
| | (0 | ± | 0) | (0 | ± | 0) | (0 | ± | 0) | (0.02 | ± | 0.01) | (0.02 | ± | 0.01) |
| Sugar Sweetened Beverages[5] | 0.04 | ± | 0.03 | 2.40 | ± | 0.64 | 41.79 | ± | 7.29 | 49.92 | ± | 4.75 | 74.56 | ± | 7.62 |
| | (0.01 | ± | 0) | (0.27 | ± | 0.07) | (3.38 | ± | 0.59) | (3.42 | ± | 0.32) | (4.61 | ± | 0.47) |
| Coffee and Tea[6] | 0.00 | ± | 0.00 | 0.16 | ± | 0.16 | 3.21 | ± | 1.29 | 3.37 | ± | 0.61 | 3.20 | ± | 0.73 |
| | (0 | ± | 0) | (0.02 | ± | 0.02) | (0.26 | ± | 0.10) | (0.23 | ± | 0.04) | (0.20 | ± | 0.05) |

Data based on Day 1 dietary recalls
SEM, Standard Error of the Mean. 1) 100% Juice includes: citrus, apple, other fruit, vegetable, baby juice. 2) Water includes: tap, bottled, flavored, carbonated, enhanced, fortified, baby water. 3) Milk includes: milk, flavored milk, milk shakes, dairy drinks, milk substitutes. 4) Diet Beverages includes: diet soft drinks, diet sport drinks, diet energy drinks, other diet beverages. 5) Sugar Sweetened Beverages includes: soft drinks, fruit drinks, sport drinks, energy drinks, nutritional beverages. 6) Coffee and Tea includes: coffee, tea

## Discussion

Authoritative sources have put forward dietary recommendations, including for beverages, to help populations maintain health and reduce the risk for disease [3, 12, 14]. Traditionally the DGAs have only provided dietary recommendations for Americans ages 2 years and older; however, the 2020–2025 DGAs will include recommendations for infants and children from birth to 2 years [7]. As such, the USDA and HHS have asked for additional data on dietary and beverage patterns for this young age group [6]. Our study utilized NHANES data to determine if beverage recommendations were followed for American children during their first 5 years of life. Our results indicate that beverage recommendations were generally not followed across early childhood, despite providing significant amounts of kcals to the diet.

From birth to 6 months the AAP recommends exclusive breastfeeding or formula feeding [12], which the IOM explains as no supplementation of water, juice,

**Table 7** Percent of children below the Estimated Average Requirement (EAR) or above the Adequate Intake (AI) by age, NHANES 2011–2014

| | 12–23 months (n = 397) | | | | 2–3 years (n = 839) | | | | 4–5 years (n = 675) | | | |
|---|---|---|---|---|---|---|---|---|---|---|---|---|
| | % > AI | % < EAR | | SEM | % > AI | % < EAR | | SEM | % > AI | % < EAR | | SEM |
| Calcium (mg) | | 2.22[a] | ± | 0.75 | | 2.90[a] | ± | 0.76 | | 32.74[b] | ± | 3.13 |
| Iron (mg) | | 1.67[a] | ± | 0.58 | | 0.75[a] | ± | 0.19 | | 2.37[ab] | ± | 0.45 |
| Magnesium (mg) | | 0.02[a] | ± | 0.03 | | 0.004[a] | ± | 0.01 | | 1.15[b] | ± | 0.36 |
| Phosphorus (mg) | | 0.03 | ± | 0.05 | | 0.01 | ± | 0.01 | | 0.02 | ± | 0.02 |
| Vitamin A, (mcg) | | 0.69[a] | ± | 0.34 | | 0.63[a] | ± | 0.28 | | 3.88[b] | ± | 1.06 |
| Vitamin C (mg) | | 0.39 | ± | 0.21 | | 0.16 | ± | 0.09 | | 1.96 | ± | 0.73 |
| Vitamin D (mcg) | | 76.53[a] | ± | 3.51 | | 90.01[b] | ± | 1.96 | | 93.78[b] | ± | 1.67 |
| Zinc (mg) | | 0.02 | ± | 0.02 | | 0.00 | ± | 0.02 | | 0.45 | ± | 0.32 |
| Potassium (mg) | 1.67 | | ± | 0.70 | 2.82 | | ± | 0.68 | 0.13 | | ± | 0.12 |

Data from usual intake using the National Cancer Institute method with two days of dietary recalls. Nutrients from breast milk are not be included in these analyses
EAR, Estimated Average Requirement; AI, Adequate Intake; SEM, Standard Error of the Mean. [a,b] Means sharing the same superscripts for EAR percentages after 1 year are not significantly different across ages, $p < 0.01$

nonhuman milk, or foods [27]. However, our analysis showed that on any given day nearly 12% of infants under 6 months consumed 100% juice and over 21% consumed water. Early introduction of water to infants less than 6 months may be of concern since it can displace consumption of nutrient-rich human milk or infant formula.

### Milk

Our results show that milk was introduced earlier than recommended. On any given day, nearly 22% of children 6 to 11 months already consumed cow's milk in quantities ranging from 0.2 to 0.4 cups per day. The mean amount of milk consumed on any given day decreased after 2 years for each of the race/ethnic groups analyzed. All groups consumed less than 2 cups of milk per day among children 2 to 5 years, with Non-Hispanic Black children consuming the least. A decrease in milk consumption as children age has been reported previously in population, survey, and clinical trial studies [22, 28, 29]. Differences among race/ethnic groups have been reported for milk consumption among children and adolescents (2–18 years) based on 2001–2004 NHANES data [21]. These results, along with our current data, highlight that across all ages a very small proportion of Non-Hispanic Black children consume sufficient amounts of milk. Cross-sectional data indicate that diet quality can be related to socioeconomic status [30]; however, factors such as income and education level were not included in in this study. Additionally, NHANES 2013–2014 data show that total dairy and milk consumption do not vary by family income [31]. Differences in milk consumption might be explained by genetic predisposition of Non-Hispanic Blacks toward lactose intolerance, as well as cultural beliefs and perceptions about consumption of dairy products [32, 33]. Previous research indicates that approximately 20% of Hispanic, Asian, and Non-Hispanic Black children younger than 5 years of age have evidence of lactase deficiency and lactose malabsorption [34]. Nevertheless, the AAP encourages children with lactose intolerance to keep dairy foods in the diet to help meet nutrient needs [35]. Thus, personalized management strategies can help, such as consuming small amounts of dairy foods at a time, consuming milk with meals, and opting for lactose-free or reduced-lactose cow's milk to help ensure children meet nutrient recommendations [36]. Our results show that the Asian population, who is believed to have a high prevalence of lactase deficiency as well [35], has seemingly overcome these barriers as statistically Asian children consumed the same amount of milk as Non-Hispanic White and Hispanic children from 2 to 5 years.

### 100% juice

Our results show that 100% juice consumption decreased after 2 to 3 years, similar to milk consumption. The DGA recognizes 100% juice as a beverage that can contribute beneficial nutrients to the diet, but states that juice should not provide more than half of the recommended fruit intake [3]. One-hundred percent juice can provide substantial amounts of vitamin C and potassium, but lacks the dietary fiber found in whole fruits or vegetables [20]. Thus, the AAP recommends that juice should not be introduced into the diet of infants before 12 months of age, and the intake of juice should be limited to 4 oz. or 4–6 oz. per day for children 1 to 3 years and 4 to 6 years, respectively [11]. Based on these recommendations, our results indicate that on any given day, children consumed 100% juice too early (over 10% of infants 0–5 months and nearly 40% of 6–11 month old infants) and that Non-Hispanic Black children consumed the most 100% juice under 2 years of age. Non-Hispanic White, Non-Hispanic Black, Hispanic, and Asian children 2 to 3 years all consumed amounts of 100% juice that exceeded the AAP recommendations [11]. Higher 100% juice consumption for Non-Hispanic Black children has been reported previously [20]. Experts caution that excessive juice consumption may be associated with malnutrition, tooth decay, excessive weight gain, or gastrointestinal discomfort [11, 37–39].

### Sugar sweetened beverages

SSB consumption steadily increased over time, consistent with prior research [29]. Regardless of race/ethnicity, we found an increase in consumption of SSBs as children got older and by 4 to 5 years, on any given day, over 51% of all children consumed SSBs. Increased consumption of SSBs by children is of concern due to their contribution to empty kcals and added sugar intake as well as displacement of more nutrient-rich beverages such as milk and 100% juice in the diet. Prior research showed increased consumption of SSBs in children was associated with an overall decrease in children's diet quality [17], an increase in childhood obesity [40], and increased risk for development of non-communicable diseases [18]. A recent scientific statement by the American Heart Association indicates that there is strong evidence that added sugar intake among children is associated with increased cardiovascular disease risk through increased energy intake, increased adiposity, and dyslipidemia. It was also recognized that when added sugars are consumed within energy limits, it is better if the sugars are consumed as part of nutrient-rich foods [18].

Consumption of SSB in this sample varied by race/ethnicity. Non-Hispanic Black children consumed the most SSBs during 0–23 months. During these first 2 years of life, Non-Hispanic Black children consumed nearly 2, 3, and 6 times more SSB than Hispanic, Non-Hispanic White, and Asian children, respectively. These results align with previously reported data [15, 41]. Garnett et al. surveyed parents on their child's beverage intake and found that Non-Hispanic Black children had the highest consumption of SSBs for all age groups. Moreover, Hispanic and Non-Hispanic Black mothers were more likely to report that their 2 yr. old children consumed a SSB at least once a week [15].

### Nutrients

After 1 year, milk provided the most kcals of the beverages examined. This is appropriate as milk a nutrient rich food providing essential nutrients associated with proper growth [12], and its consumption has been associated with improved diet quality and bone health among children [42]. Milk is the number one food source of nine essential nutrients for children; protein, calcium, potassium, phosphorus, vitamins A, D, B12, riboflavin and niacin as niacin equivalents [5]. Among beverages consumed by American infants and children 0 to 5 years of age, our results show milk provided the largest nutrient contribution.

Non-Hispanic Black children consumed the least amounts of calcium and vitamin D from 1 to 5 years. Over 25% and 95% of Non-Hispanic Black children 1–5 years of age had inadequate intakes of calcium and vitamin D, respectively, as compared to 8.2 and 83.2% of Hispanics and 12.9 and 88.5% for Non-Hispanic White children (data not shown). Non-Hispanic Black children were the only race/ethnic group who consumed more SSBs than milk at 4 to 5 years of age. Regardless of race/ethnicity, our data showed that the decreased consumption of nutrient-rich beverages, such as milk, as children got older was reflected in decreased intakes of the nutrients of public health concern. For children 4 to 5 years, nearly 94% had vitamin D intakes below the EAR, over 32% had calcium intakes below the EAR and less than 1 % had potassium intakes above the AI. These low intakes for the under-consumed nutrients of public health concern among young American children are alarming as they are necessary for normal growth and development [36].

### Strengths and limitations

One of the strengths of this study was the use of a sample representative of the U. S population. A second strength was the inclusion of infants and children 0 to 24 months age group as many previous reports have focused only on children 2+ years. Finally, we utilized the National Cancer Institute method for estimating usual intake to estimate percentage of the population meeting or below dietary recommendations. This study was limited by the fact that we were not able to analyze race/ethnic data in smaller age sub-groups due to the small sample sizes among young infants (0–12 months). Additionally, due to the fact that NHANES data dietary information may be subject to over- or under-reporting and the accuracy of parents/caregivers reporting of their children's food intake is unknown.

## Conclusions

Beverage consumption among American infants and children 0 to 5 years, as reported in NHANES 2011 to 2014, did not consistently follow recommendations from authoritative sources. Consumption of milk and 100% juice decreased with age, particularly after 2 years, while consumption of SSBs steadily increased. Simultaneously, as children got older they had lower intakes of under-consumed nutrients of public health concern; calcium, vitamin D and potassium. Differences in beverage intakes exists when comparing various race/ethnic groups. Non-Hispanic Black children consumed the most 100% juice from 2 to 3 years, exceeding recommended amounts, and throughout all age groups they consumed the least milk and most SSBs. These results highlight that improving beverage consumption patterns, particularly for Non-Hispanic Black children, could help improve overall diet quality that can reduce risk for obesity and other diet-related chronic diseases.

#### Abbreviations

AAP: American Academy of Pediatrics; AI: Adequate Intake; AND: Academy of Nutrition and Dietetics; BBR: Balanced repeated replicates; DGA: Dietary Guidelines for Americans; EAR: Estimated Average Requirement; HHS: Health and Human Services; IOM: Institute of Medicine; kcals: Kilocalories; NCI: National Cancer Institute; NHANES: National Health and Nutrition Examination Survey; oz: Ounces; SE: Standard error; SSB: Sugar sweetened beverages; USDA: United States Department of Agriculture

#### Acknowledgements

The study and the writing of the manuscript were supported by National Dairy Council. The Authors would like to thank Carla McGill, PhD, RD, Principle at Healthy Science Communications for assistance with manuscript preparation.

#### Funding

National Dairy Council/Dairy Management Inc.

#### Authors' contributions

The authors' responsibilities were as follows- ED/CJC/JH/VLF: project conception, designed research, developed overall research plan, determined content for manuscript and collaborated on the writing; VLF: analyzed data and performed statistical analysis; All authors read and approved the final manuscript.

#### Competing interests

ED, CJC, and JAH are employees of National Dairy Council/Dairy Management Inc., Rosemont, Illinois, USA VLF as Senior Vice President of Nutrition Impact, LLC performs consulting and database analyses for various food and beverage companies and related entities.

**Author details**
[1]National Dairy Council, 10255 West Higgins Road, Suite 900, Rosemont, IL 60018-5616, USA. [2]Nutrition Impact, LLC, Battle Creek, MI 49014, USA.

**References**

1. Birch L, Arbor A, Savage JS, Ventura A. Influences on the development of Children's eating Behaviours: from infancy to adolescence. Can J Diet Pr Res. 2009;68:1–11.
2. Savage JS, Fisher JO, Birch LL. Parental influence on eating behavior. J Law Med Ethics. 2008;35:22–34.
3. U.S. Department of Health and Human Services and U.S. Department of Agriculture. Dietary Guidelines for Americans. 2015–2020.
4. Popkin BM. Patterns of beverage use across the lifecycle. Physiol Behav. 2010;100:4–9.
5. Keast D, Fulgoni V 3rd, Nicklas T, O'Neil CE. Food sources of energy and nutrients among children in the United States: National Health and Nutrition Examination Survey 2003–2006. Nutrients. 2013;5:283–301.
6. Federal Register. Dietary Guidelines for Americans: Request for Comments on Topics and Questions. National Archives. USA. 2018;83(40).
7. Agricultural Act of 2014. H.R.2642-113th Congress. 2014.
8. Moretti M. Breastfeeding and the use of antidepressants. J Popul Ther Clin Pharmacol. 2012;19:e387–90.
9. Kramer MS. Do breast-feeding and delayed introduction of solid foods protect against subsequent obesity? J Pediatr. 1981;98:883–7.
10. Owen CG, Martin RM, Whincup PH, Smith GD, Cook DG. Effect of infant feeding on the risk of obesity across the life course: a quantitative review of published evidence. Pediatrics. 2005;115:1367–77. https://doi.org/10.1542/peds.2004-1176.
11. Heyman MB, Abrams SA. Fruit juice in infants, children, and adolescents: current recommendations. Pediatrics. 2017;139:e20170967.
12. American Academy of Pediatrics Committee on Nutrition. In: Kleinmen, RE, Greer, FR, eds. Pediatric Nutrition. 7th ed. Elk Grove Village, IL: American Academy of Pediatrics; 2014.
13. The National Academies. Dietary Reference Intakes for Water, Potassium, Sodium, Chloride, and Sulfate. 2004. https://www.nap.edu/read/10925/chapter/1. Accessed Oct 2017.
14. Academy of Nutrition and Dietetics. Pediatric Nutrition Care Manual. http://www.nutritioncaremanual.org. Accessed Oct 2017.
15. Garnett BR, Rosenberg KD, Morris DS. Consumption of soda and other sugar-sweetened beverages by 2-year-olds: findings from a population-based survey. Public Health Nutr. 2013;16:1760–7.
16. Pan L, Li R, Park S, Galuska DA, Sherry B, Freedman DS. A longitudinal analysis of sugar-sweetened beverage intake in infancy and obesity at 6 years. World Rev Nutr Diet. 2016;114:34–5.
17. Marshall TA, Eichenberger Gilmore JM, Broffitt B, Stumbo PJ, Levy SM. Diet quality in young children is influenced by beverage consumption. J Am Coll Nutr. 2005;24:65–75.
18. Vos MB, Kaar JL, Welsh JA, van Horn LV, Feig DI, Anderson CAM, et al. Added sugars and cardiovascular disease risk in children: a scientific statement from the American Heart Association. Circulation. 2017;135(19):e1017–e1034.
19. Beck AL, Patel A, Madsen K. Trends in sugar-sweetened beverage and 100% fruit juice consumption among California children. Acad Pediatr. 2013;13:364–70.
20. Drewnowski A, Rehm CD. Socioeconomic gradient in consumption of whole fruit and 100% fruit juice among US children and adults. Nutr J. 2015;14:1–9.
21. Kirkpatrick SI, Dodd KW, Reedy J, Krebs-Smith SM. Income and race/ethnicity are associated with adherence to food-based dietary guidance among US adults and children. J Acad Nutr Diet. 2012;112:624–35.
22. Fulgoni VL, Quann EE. National trends in beverage consumption in children from birth to 5 years: analysis of NHANES across three decades. Nutr J. 2012;11:92.
23. Centers for Disease Control and Prevention. National Health and Nutrition Examination Survey (NHANES). Dietary Interview - Total Nutrient Intakes, First Day. 2016. https://wwwn.cdc.gov/Nchs/Nhanes/2013-2014/DR1TOT_H.htm.
24. U.S. Department of Agriculture, Agricultural Research Service. What We Eat in America Food Categories 2011-2012. https://www.ars.usda.gov/ARSUserFiles/80400530/pdf/1112/food_category_list.pdf. Accessed Oct 2017.
25. National Cancer Institute. Usual Dietary Intakes: SAS Macros for Analysis of a Single Dietary Component. USA. https://epi.grants.cancer.gov/diet/usualintakes/macros_single.html. Accessed Oct 2017.
26. CDC/National Center for Health Statistics. About the National Health and Nutrition Examination Survey. https://www.cdc.gov/nchs/nhanes/about_nhanes.htm. Accessed Oct 2017.
27. Institute of Medicine. Nutrition during lactation. Washington, D.C.: National Academies Press; 1991.
28. Wang YC, Bleich SN, Gortmaker SL. Increasing caloric contribution from sugar-sweetened beverages and 100% fruit juices among US children and adolescents, 1988-2004. Pediatrics. 2008;121:e1604–14.
29. Keller KL, Ph D, Kirzner J, Pietrobelli A, Faith MS. Increased sweetened beverage intake is associated with reduced milk and calcium intake in 3- to 7-yr old children at multi-item laboratory lunches. J Am Diet Assoc. 2010;109:497–501.
30. Darmon N, Drewnowski A. Does social class predict diet quality? Am J Clin Nutr. 2008;87:1107–17.
31. Centers for Disease Control and Prevention (CDC). National Center for Health Statistics (NCHS). National Health and Nutrition Examination Survey Data. Hyattsville, MD: U.S. Department of Health and Human Services, Centers for Disease Control and Prevention; 2013–2014.
32. National Medical Association. Lactose intolerance and African Americans: implications for the consumption of appropriate intake levels of key nutrients. J Natl Med Assoc. 2009;101:S5–23.
33. Bailey RK, Fileti CP, Keith J, Price W, Allison-ottey SD. Lactose intolerance and health disparities among African Americans and Hispanic Americans: an updated consensus statement. J Natl Med Assoc. 2013;105:112–27. https://doi.org/10.1016/S0027-9684(15)30113-9.
34. Woteki CE, Weser E, Young EA. Lactose malabsorption in Mexican-American children. Am J Clin Nutr. 1976;29:19–24.
35. Heyman MB, others. Lactose intolerance in infants, children, and adolescents. Pediatrics. 2006;118:1279–86.
36. Suchy FJ, Brannon PM, Carpenter TO, Fernandez JR, Gilsanz V, Gould JB, et al. National Institutes of Health consensus development conference: lactose intolerance and health. Ann Intern Med. 2010;152:792.
37. AAP. Committee on Nutrition The Use and Misuse of Fruit Juice in Pediatrics. Pediatrics. 2001;107:1210–3.
38. Frantsve-Hawley J, Bader J, Welsh J, Wright J. A systematic review of the association between consumption of sugar-containing beverages and excess weight gain among children under age 12. J Public Heal Dent. 2017;77(Supplement 1):S43–66.
39. Sonneville K, Long M, Rifas-Shiman S, Kleinman K, Gillman M, Taveras E. Juice and water intake in infancy and later beverage intake and adiposity: could juice be a gateway drink? Obesity. 2015;23:170–6.
40. Dubois L, Farmer A, Girard M, Peterson K. Regular sugar-sweetened beverage consumption between meals increases risk of overweight among preschool-aged children. J Am Diet Assoc. 2007;107:924–34.
41. Han E, Powell L. Consupmtion patterns of sugar sweetened beverages in the united state. J Acad Nutr Diet. 2014;113:43–53.
42. Lee WT, Leung SS, Lui SS, Lau J. Relationship between long-term calcium intake and bone mineral content of children aged from birth to 5 years. Br J Nutr. 1993;70:235–48.

12

# A health facility based case-control study on determinants of low birth weight in Dassie town, Northeast Ethiopia: the role of nutritional factors

Semira Ahmed[1†], Kalkidan Hassen[2] and Tolassa Wakayo[2*†]

**Abstract**

**Background:** Low birth weight remains a major public health problem affecting developing countries. Evidence shows that low birth weight has long lasting negative health consequences through its contribution to stunting, mental impairment and non-communicable chronic diseases in later life. Thus, it is worth investigating the role of nutritional factors as determinants of low birth weight to suggest nutritional interventions to curb its negative health outcomes. This study aimed to investigate the determinants of low birth weight with main focus on the role of nutritional factors in Ethiopia.

**Methods:** A facility-based case-control study was conducted from 3 February to 29 April, 2017. The data were collected using structured, pretested interviewer-administered questionnaire in all public health facilities of Dessie Town. Anthropometric measurements were made following standard procedures for both mothers and their newborns. Consecutive live births of < 2500 g and two succeeding normal weight babies were selected as cases and controls, respectively. Data were entered in to Epi-data software version 3.1, and exported to SPSS version 21, and analyzed using frequency, mean and percentage. Factors with $p < 0.25$ during bivariate analyses were entered into a multivariable logistic regression model to determine significant determinants of LBW. Statistical significance was considered at $p < 0.05$. Results were reported with odds ratio and 95% CI.

**Results:** Mean ± SD of birth weight (g) was 2138 ± 207 for cases and 3145 ± 415 for controls. After adjusting for potential confounders using multivariable logistic regression analysis, the absence of iron and folate supplementation, receiving no nutritional counseling and consuming no additional meal, maternal undernutrition, maternal anemia and inadequate dietary diversity during the current pregnancy were found to be significant determinants of low birth weight in our study.

**Conclusion:** Lack of nutritional counseling, absence of additional meal intake and iron and folate supplementation during pregnancy, and maternal undernutrition, maternal anemia and inadequate maternal dietary diversity were significant determinants of low birth weight. The importance of nutritional counseling, improving iron and folate supplementation during pregnancy, and nutritional status of pregnant women need to be strengthened to reduce the incidence of LBW in Ethiopia. In addition, behavioral change communications targeting pregnant women to improve women dietary diversity and their extra meal intake practice need to be enhanced in Ethiopia.

**Keywords:** Low birth weight, Maternal nutritional status, Determinants, Ethiopia

* Correspondence: wakayotolassa@yahoo.com
[†]Semira Ahmed and Tolassa Wakayo contributed equally to this work.
[2]Jimma University, Faculty of Public Health, Jimma, Ethiopia
Full list of author information is available at the end of the article

## Background

Low birth weight (LBW) is defined by the World Health Organization (WHO) as weight at birth less than 2500 g. Low birth weight is more common in developing countries and contributes to a range of poor health outcomes in later life [1].

Most of the LBW infants are born either preterm or have intrauterine growth retardation (IUGR). While most of the LBW newborns in developed countries are preterm, these are full-term infants who are small for gestational age (SGA) in developing nations. The causes of SGA include poor maternal nutritional status at conception, low gestational weight gain due to inadequate dietary intake or due to excess expenditure of calories (hard work), and short maternal stature resulting from early childhood undernutrition. Infections, malaria, anemia, acute and chronic infections that could result in maternal undernutrition can lead to SGA baby and subsequent LBW infant [2–4]. The incidence of LBW is estimated to be 15% to 20% worldwide, representing more than 20 million births a year [5]. The great majority of low birth weight occurs in low- and middle-income countries and especially in the most vulnerable populations accounting for 28% in south Asia, 13% in sub-Saharan Africa and 9% in Latin America [6]. Among children born with a reported birth weight in Ethiopia, 13% were LBW babies [7].

LBW has many negative health consequences for the infants. It contributes to 60% to 80% of all neonatal mortality and morbidity [3, 8]. LBW infants are many times more likely to end up with long-term handicapping conditions [8]. They are also at higher risk of infection, poor mental development, stunting and developing non-communicable chronic diseases in later life [2, 3, 9–11]. These consequences are more pronounced when LBW coincides with poor maternal nutritional status thereby adversely affecting the optimum fetal and child nutrition and development, cognitive function, motor and socio-emotional development and economic productivity being adult [12, 13]. Contrary to its known negative health consequences, studies have identified common prevalence and incidence of LBW in many developing countries; possible risk factors have also been reported. In India maternal age (< 19 years), rural residence, maternal weight (< 45 kg), gestational age (< 37 week), bad obstetric history and pregnancy induced hypertension had a strong association with LBW [14]. Low socio-economic status, anemia, primiparity, short maternal height and less than average weight had also strong association with LBW in Pakistan [15]. Other studies in developing countries have shown correlations of maternal nutritional status, young maternal age, bad maternal obstetric history, maternal anemia, rural residence of mothers, absence of maternal antennal care (ANC) follow up, prematurity, and birth interval with occurrence of LBW [13, 16–21]

In Ethiopia, maternal and environmental factors [22], inadequate ANC follow-up, unwanted pregnancy, sex of the neonate and pregnancy type [23], lower socioeconomic status, not attending ANC, maternal undernutrition, and experience of physical violence during the index pregnancy and longer time to walk to health facility [22, 24], urban residence, prematurity, having weight loss and receiving no additional diet during pregnancy, and multiple gestations [25, 26], marital status, monthly family income, and maternal HIV status were predictors of LBW babies [26]. The most recent study in northern Ethiopia also reported some non-nutritional factors predicting LBW [27].

Though there are some studies undertaken in Ethiopia aiming at determining predictors of LBW [22, 23, 25, 28–34], these studies considered only environmental, socioeconomic, demographic, maternal, and newborns characteristics and the majority of these studies used cross-sectional design. Few studies [24, 35] have been conducted with regard to maternal nutritional status and dietary practices towards contributing to the incidence of LBW in Ethiopia. However, these studies overlooked some important nutritional factors that may contribute to LBW babies in Ethiopia. Therefore, the aim of this study was to investigate nutritional determinants of LBW among newborns delivered at public health facilities in Dessie Town, Northeast Ethiopia.

## Method and material

### Study design and subjects

A facility based unmatched case-control study was conducted from 3 February to 29 April 2017 in all public health facilities in Dessie Town, Northeast Ethiopia. Dessie Town, located in Amhara regional state of Ethiopia, is located at 401 km from Addis Ababa, the capital of Ethiopia and 523 km from Bahir Dar, the capital of the region. The town is situated at a latitude and longitude of 11°8′N 39°38′E, with an elevation between 2470 and 2550 m above sea level. It has ten sub-cities and six rural kebeles. According to the 2007 National Censes, the total population of the town was about 151,174; of whom 72,932 were men and 78,242 were women; 79.44% were urban inhabitants living in the town, the rest of the population was living in rural kebeles surrounding the town. All neonates delivered in all public health facilities of Dessie Town were considered the source population of the study. Cases were those neonates delivered with birth weight of < 2500 g while controls were those neonates delivered with birth weight of ≥2500 g in each health facility of the town.

### Sample size determination

The sample size was determined using a proportional difference approach for case-control study using Epi-Info statistical software package (Version-7) taking into account maternal anemia as main exposure variable and considering 95% confidence level, 80% power of the study and control to case ratio of 2:1 for estimating low birth weight. As such, we considered that the percent of controls exposed (having anemic mothers) among the controls was 11.6% [36]. Assuming a 15% difference (increase) in cases that was assumed in advance, proportion of cases with exposure became 26.6% producing the least extreme Odds Ratio of 2.76 to be detected. Accordingly, after adding 10% non-response rate to each, 95 cases and 191 controls were estimated making a total sample size 286 subjects to be included in the study.

### Sampling procedure

All of ten public health facilities in the Dessie Town (Two hospitals: Dessie Referral Hospital, and Borumeda Hospital, and eight health centers: Bwanbwawua, Dessie, Segno Gebya, Gerado, Tita, Kurkur and Boruslasie health centres) were included in this study to compensate for short data collection period to acquire the required number of cases. The allocation of the required number of study subjects to each health facility was based on the proportion of number of deliveries during same time interval of the preceding year (from records) in each health facility. After allocating the total sample size to each health facility using population proportional to size approach, consecutive live births (< 2500 g) each health facility were selected as cases and two babies with normal birth weight (≥2500 g) succeeding each case were selected as controls. Neonates with major congenital anomalies such as macrocephaly, neural tube defect and limb reduction, whose mothers are known diabetic, and those whose mothers didn't know their last menstrual period (LMP) were excluded from the study while cases and controls with term singleton live-births were included in the study. Few deaths were reported with in 1 h of delivery and they were also included in the study.

### Ethical consideration

Ethical clearance letter was obtained from Jimma University Institute of Health, Research and Community Service Office. Then, written letter of support to conduct the research was obtained from Ethical Review Board of Dessie Town Health Administration Department and presented to respective public health facilities in the town. The interviewers discuss the issue of confidentiality and obtained verbal consent before the actual interview was administered.

### Data collection

Data were collected by trained nurses using face to face interview and structured and pretested questionnaire was used to collect data. The interviews were conducted at each health facility after the mother had given birth and the neonate weight was measured within 1 h of delivery. Ten data collectors, six midwives and four nurses were recruited to accommodate the wide range of health facilities. Four first degree nurses supervised data collection in all health facilities while the principal investigator had overall role of facilitating research works during data collection.

### Anthropometric measurement

Anthropometric measurements were measured following standardized techniques. Weights of the newborns were taken within 1 h after delivery using a balanced digital Seca scale (Germany). The scales were always calibrated using a material with standard weight and the reading on each scale was taken to zero level before weighing each newborn. Height of the mother was measured using height board while the mother was in standing position. Each height was taken to the nearest 0.1 cm. Mothers were asked to stand without shoes in front of the height board, with the head erect and the arms hanging naturally at the sides. The mid-upper arm circumference (MUAC) of the mother was measured after delivery using flexible non-stretchable standard tape measure. The circumference was measured at the mid-point between the tip of the acromion process of the scapula and olecranon process of the ulna. Measurements were taken while the right arm was hanging relaxed, to the nearest 0.1 cm.

### Dietary assessment

The minimum dietary diversity for women (MDD-W) was collected using 24-h recall method by using MDD-W tool [37]. Briefly, the pregnant women were asked to recall the foods they had consumed in the previous 24 h, first spontaneously followed by probes to ascertain that no meal or snack was left out. A detailed list of all the ingredients of the dishes, snacks, or other foods consumed was generated to enable better classification of mixed dishes. The foods were then categorized into 10 food groups. Then, tabulation of the MDD-W was done using SPSS and a pregnant woman was assigned in the adequate dietary diversity group if her MDD-W ≥ 5 food groups or in the inadequate group if her MDD-W < 5 food groups.

### Micronutrient intake and hemoglobin level

Iron and folic acid (IFA) supplementation along with history of ANC (how many times did the mother visit health facility during pregnancy to receive routine ANC services) were asked for each mother. The hemoglobin level of each mother was taken from her health card as hemoglobin is routinely done for each mother receiving delivery services in each public health facility. WHO recommends four ANC visits during pregnancy and visits less than four were considered inadequate.

#### Data quality control

Data were collected by trained data collectors after full understanding the objectives of the study, contents of the questionnaire and method of data collection. The questionnaire was prepared in English and translated to Amharic and back translated to English to keep the consistency of the questions and increase understanding with respondents. Both supervisors and principal investigator were closely following the data collection process. The questionnaire was pretested on 5% of the sample size in another health facility out of the study area before the actual data collection was implemented. The collected data were checked for completeness and consistency on daily basis by principal investigator and supervisors.

#### Wealth index

Socioeconomic index was developed as follows: first all study participants were asked about the ownership of fixed assets by their household with a score 1 given to those who own the asset and score of "0" given to those who did not own. Then all items asked were assessed for internal consistency and showed to be reliable with a cronbach's alpha value of 0.82 (> 0.7 is considered as reliable). Then principal component analysis was used to develop the wealth index. The first factors were taken and rank ordered into tertiles.

#### Statistical analysis

Data were checked for completeness and consistencies, and then edited, coded and entered using Epi-data version 3.1, and then exported to SPSS version 21 for further analysis. Variables were checked for missing values before analysis. Descriptive statistics were computed for all variables according to their type. Means, medians and standard deviations were computed for continuous variables. The categorical variables were described by their frequencies. Normality of continues variables was checked using the Kolmogorov–Smirnov test. Bivariate analyses were done to identify the candidate variables for multivariable logistic regression model to determine risk factors of LBW. Accordingly, any variable having $p \leq 0.25$ was considered as a candidate variable for multivariable analysis and entered into multivariable logistic regression model using backward elimination stepwise likelihood ratio method. All tests were two-sided and $p < 0.05$ was considered statistically significant. The results were reported as Odds Ratio (OR) and 95% Confidence Interval (CI).

### Results

#### Socio demographic characteristics

A total of 279 mothers with their respective newborns (93 cases and 186 controls) were included in the study making the response rate of 97.6%. The mean ± SD of birth weight was 2138 ± 206 g for cases and 3145 ± 415 g for controls. A higher proportion of newborns were males both in cases (52.7%) and controls (62.9%). The mean ± SD of maternal age among the cases was 27.3 ± 5.5 years and it was 26.2 ± 4.7 years among controls. The majority, 82.8% vs. 79.6%, of mothers among the cases and the controls were in the age group of 21–35 years, respectively. The largest proportion, 82.8% vs. 90.3%, of mothers among cases and controls were Amhara, while 74.2% of mothers among cases and 75.3% among controls were Muslim in religion. Among the mothers of the cases and the controls, 34.4% and 17.2% respectively, had informal education. Overall, most of the mothers in both cases and control groups were married (93.5% and 92.5%, respectively). Fifty-eight (62.4%) of the mothers among the cases and 54.3% of the mothers among controls were in lower wealth index category. Moreover, 44.1% of mothers among cases and 40.3% among controls were living in rural setting. The higher number of mothers in both cases (69.9%) and controls (48.9%) were housewives followed by employed (18.3% and 33.9%, respectively) (Table 1).

#### Nutritional, anthropometric characteristics and substance abuse

The mean ± SD of maternal height for cases and controls was 155 ± 0.1 cm and 159 ± 0.1 cm, respectively. The percentage of mothers having height of < 150 cm was twice as high among cases compared to controls (23.7% vs 12.4%). Undernutrition in mothers as defined by MUAC < 23 cm was 52.7% and 13.4% among cases and controls, respectively. Mothers who did not receive iron and folate supplementation during pregnancy were 31.2% and 10.8% among cases and controls, respectively. The largest proportion of mothers, 93.5% among cases and 62.9% among controls, had inadequate MDD-W. Nutritional counselling and extra meal consumption during pregnancy were less practiced in mothers from cases. Maternal anemia among cases was 32.3% while it was 9.1% among controls. Maternal khat chewing habit during pregnancy was 35.5% among cases compared to 26.9% among controls. Likewise, mothers who had history of alcohol consumption during pregnancy were 5.4% and 8.1% among cases and controls, respectively (Table 2).

#### Medical and obstetrics characteristics

Proportions of ANC follow up among cases and controls were 89.2% and 96.8%, respectively indicating the majority of mothers in both group had access to maternal care during pregnancy. Mothers who described their pregnancy as unplanned but wanted were 24.7% and 17.2% among cases and controls, respectively. Maternal chronic disease among cases was 14.0% while controls had 15.1%. Maternal pregnancy induced hypertension was 9.7% and 6.5% among cases and controls, respectively. Few mothers among cases and controls, had

**Table 1** Distribution of socio-economic and demographic characteristics among mothers of cases and controls in public health facilities of Dessie Town, Northeast Ethiopia, 2017

| Variables | Cases N (%) | Controls N (%) | Total N (%) |
|---|---|---|---|
| Infant sex | | | |
| Male | 49 (52.7) | 117 (62.9) | 166 (59.5) |
| Female | 44 (47.3) | 69 (37.1) | 113 (40.5) |
| Maternal age (year) | | | |
| ≤ 20 | 9 (9.7) | 32 (17.2) | 41 (14.7) |
| 21–35 | 77 (82.8) | 147 (79.6) | 225 (80.6) |
| > 35 | 7 (7.5) | 6 (3.2) | 13 (4.7) |
| Residence | | | |
| Rural | 41 (44.1) | 75 (40.3) | 116 (41.6) |
| Urban | 52 (55.9) | 111 (59.7) | 163 (58.4) |
| Religion | | | |
| Muslim | 69 (74.2) | 140 (75.3) | 209 (74.9) |
| Orthodox | 20 (21.5) | 42 (22.6) | 62 (22.2) |
| Others | 4 (4.3) | 4 (2.2) | 8 (2.9) |
| Ethnicity | | | |
| Amhara | 77 (82.8) | 168 (90.3) | 245 (87.8) |
| Oromo | 10 (10.8) | 7 (3.8) | 17 (6.1) |
| Gurage or Tigrae | 6 (6.5) | 11 (5.9) | 17 (6.1) |
| Marital status | | | |
| Married | 87 (93.5) | 172 (92.5) | 259 (92.8) |
| single, separated or divorced | 6 (6.5) | 14 (7.5) | 20 (7.2) |
| Maternal Educational | | | |
| Informal education | 32 (34.4) | 32 (17.2) | 64 (23.0) |
| Formal education | 61 (65.6) | 154 (82.8) | 214 (77.0) |
| Maternal Occupation | | | |
| Employed | 17 (18.3) | 63 (33.9) | 80 (28.7) |
| Merchant | 5 (5.4) | 24 (12.9) | 29 (10.4) |
| Housewife | 65 (69.9) | 91 (48.9) | 156 (55.9) |
| Others | 6 (6.5) | 8 (4.3) | 14 (5.0) |
| Wealth index | | | |
| Lower | 58 (62.4) | 101 (54.3) | 159 (57.0) |
| Middle | 16 (17.2) | 49 (26.3) | 65 (23.3) |
| Upper | 19 (20.4) | 36 (19.4) | 55 (19.7) |

**Table 2** Distribution of nutritional characteristics among mothers of cases and controls in public health facilities of Dessie Town, Northeast Ethiopia, 2017

| Variables | Cases N (%) | Controls N (%) | Total N (%) |
|---|---|---|---|
| Height (cm) | | | |
| < 150 | 22 (23.7) | 23 (12.4) | 45 (16.1) |
| > =150 | 71 (76.3) | 163 (87.6) | 234 (83.9) |
| MUAC (cm) | | | |
| < 23 | 49 (52.7) | 25 (13.4) | 74 (26.5) |
| > =23 | 44 (47.3) | 161 (86.6) | 205 (73.5) |
| Iron and folate supplementation | | | |
| Yes | 64 (68.8) | 166 (89.2) | 230 (82.4) |
| No | 29 (31.2) | 20 (10.8) | 49 (17.6) |
| Any multivitamin use | | | |
| Yes | 9 (9.7) | 36 (19.4) | 45 (16.1) |
| No | 84 (90.3) | 150 (80.6) | 234 (83.9) |
| Nutritional counseling during pregnancy | | | |
| Yes | 40 (43.0) | 153 (82.3) | 193 (69.2) |
| No | 53 (57.0) | 33 (17.7) | 86 (30.8) |
| Additional food intake during pregnancy | | | |
| Yes | 34 (36.6) | 134 (72) | 168 (60.2) |
| No | 59 (63.4) | 52 (28) | 111 (39.8) |
| MDD-W[a] | | | |
| inadequate | 87 (93.5) | 117 (62.9) | 204 (73.1) |
| adequate | 6 (6.5) | 69 (37.1) | 75 (26.9) |
| Anemia present | | | |
| Yes (Hb < 11 g/dl) | 30 (32.3) | 17 (9.1) | 47 (16.8) |
| No (Hb ≥11 g/dl) | 63 (67.7) | 169 (90.9) | 232 (83.2) |
| Eating out of home | | | |
| Yes | 81 (87.1) | 167 (89.8) | 248 (88.9) |
| No | 12 (12.9) | 19 (10.2) | 31 (11.1) |
| Khat chewing | | | |
| Yes | 33 (35.5) | 50 (26.9) | 83 (29.7) |
| No | 60 (64.5) | 136 (73.1) | 196 (70.3) |
| Alcohol consumption | | | |
| Yes | 5 (5.4) | 15 (8.1) | 20 (7.2) |
| No | 88 (94.6) | 171 (91.9) | 259 (92.8) |

[a]MDD-W indicates minimum dietary diversity for women

history of preterm delivery and reactive for HIV test. History of abortion was observed among 23.7% of mothers of cases and 11.8% of mothers of controls. Majority of mothers both in cases and controls were primi-gravida (Table 3).

### Determinants of low birth weight

In bivariate analyses performed to identify candidate variables for multivariable analysis, variables having $p < 0.25$ were considered candidates for the final multivariable logistic regression model in investigating significant determinants of LBW among study subjects (Table 4).

In multivariable analysis, selected covariates with $p < 0.25$ in bivariate analyses were entered into the multivariable logistic regression model to control for potential confounders in determining the independent determinants of LBW using backward elimination stepwise likelihood ratio

**Table 3** Distribution of medical and obstetrics characteristics among mothers of cases and controls in public health facilities of Dessie Town, Northeast Ethiopia, 2017

| Variables | Cases N (%) | Controls N (%) | Total N (%) |
|---|---|---|---|
| Parity | | | |
| Primigravida | 50 (53.8) | 100 (53.8) | 150 (53.8) |
| Multipara | 43 (46.2) | 86 (46.2) | 129 (46.2) |
| History of abortion | | | |
| Yes | 22 (23.7) | 22 (11.8) | 44 (15.8) |
| No | 71 (76.3) | 164 (88.2) | 235 (84.2) |
| History of preterm delivery | | | |
| Yes | 10 (10.8) | 5 (2.7) | 15 (5.4) |
| No | 83 (89.2) | 181 (97.3) | 264 (94.6) |
| ANC follow up | | | |
| Yes | 83 (89.2) | 180 (96.8) | 263 (94.3) |
| No | 10 (10.8) | 6 (3.2) | 16 (5.7) |
| HIV status | | | |
| Reactive | 5 (5.4) | 4 (2.2) | 9 (3.2) |
| Non- reactive | 88 (94.6) | 182 (97.8) | 270 (96.8) |
| Pregnancy induced hypertension (PIH) | | | |
| Yes | 9 (9.7) | 12 (6.5) | 21 (7.5) |
| No | 84 (90.3) | 174 (93.5) | 258 (92.5) |
| Type of pregnancy | | | |
| Planned and wanted | 66 (71.0) | 149 (80.1) | 215 (77.1) |
| Unplanned but wanted | 23 (24.7) | 32 (17.2) | 55 (19.7) |
| Unplanned and unwanted | 4 (4.3) | 5 (2.7) | 9 (3.2) |

method. Accordingly, absence of iron and folate supplementation, receiving no nutritional counseling and consuming no additional meal during the current pregnancy, and maternal undernutrition, maternal anemia and inadequate MDD-W were found to be significant determinants of low birth weight (Table 5).

The study showed that mothers who did not take iron and folate supplementation were about three times more likely to deliver LBW babies compared to mothers who did take iron and folate supplementation during current pregnancy [AOR = 2.84: CI (1.15,7.03)]. Mothers who did not receive nutrition counseling during current pregnancy were about four times more likely to deliver LBW babies compared to their counterparts [AOR = 4.05: CI (1.95, 8.38)]. Similarly, mothers who did not take additional meal during current pregnancy were three times more likely to have babies with LBW compared to those mothers who had additional meal during pregnancy [AOR = 3.25: CI (1.64, 6.44)]. Likewise, the odds of giving birth to LBW babies among undernourished mothers compared to their well-nourished counterparts were nearly six fold [AOR = 5.62: CI (2.64, 11.97)]. Anemic mothers had odds of nearly four times to give birth to LBW babies compared to non-anemic mothers [AOR = 3.54: CI (1.46, 8.61)]. Furthermore, mothers who had inadequate dietary diversity had about seven times higher odds of giving birth to LBW babies compared to mothers with adequate dietary diversity [AOR = 6.65: CI(2.31, 19.16)].

## Discussion

The present study revealed that mothers who did not receive nutritional counseling during current pregnancy had higher odds for giving birth to LBW babies in comparison to mothers who did receive nutritional counseling. This might be due to the fact that nutritional counseling might improve women's food intake and hence, their nutritional status and therefore decrease the risk of delivering LBW babies. This finding was consistent with a study conducted in Gondar University Hospital where mothers who did not have ANC follow up had higher odds of giving LBW babies while this might be ascribed to the routine provision of nutritional counseling during ANC visits [36].

The risk of LBW was higher among mothers who did not receive an additional daily meal during current pregnancy as compared to mothers who did receive an additional meal. This finding was consistent with other similar studies done in Ethiopia [36] and Ghana [38]. Mothers who consumed more food during pregnancy period were 88% less likely to give birth to a LBW infants than those who consumed the same as before pregnancy [38]. Controlled trials have shown that improving meal intakes during pregnancy effectively reduces the risk of giving LBW babies [9]. Likewise, intake of iron and folate supplements during pregnancy had significant association with LBW in our study. Mothers who did not take iron and folate supplementation were more likely to deliver LBW babies than mothers who did take iron and folate supplementation during pregnancy. This finding is in agreement with a study done in Bangladesh that showed intake of iron and folate supplements during pregnancy was found to have a protective effect against LBW [39]. These findings were also consistent with studies done in rural Ethiopia [35], Pakistan [40] and a study from developed country [41]. Iron supplementation during pregnancy protects women from becoming anemic and subsequent increased risk of giving LBW babies, because the required amounts may not be supplied from dietary intake alone during this period [40]. A randomized controlled trial that compared standard iron supplementation with multiple micronutrients during pregnancy on birth size found that women in iron supplementation group had babies with higher birth weight [42]. Furthermore, review of controlled trials suggested 41% reduction in the incidence of IUGR when

**Table 4** Bivariate analyses to identify candidate variables for multivariable logistic regression to identify determinants of LBW, Dessie Town, Ethiopia, 2017

| Variables | Cases No % | Controls No % | Crude OR (95%CI) | *p*-value |
|---|---|---|---|---|
| Maternal age (year) | | | | |
| ≤ 20 | 9 (9.7) | 32 (17.2) | 0.54 (0.25,1.19) | 0.127* |
| 21–35 | 77 (82.8) | 147 (79.6) | 1 | |
| > 35 | 7 (7.5) | 6 (3.2) | 2.24 (0.73,6.91) | 0.159* |
| Residence | | | | |
| Urban | 52 (55.9) | 111 (59.7) | 1 | |
| Rural | 41 (44.1) | 75 (40.3) | 1.17 (0.71,1.93) | 0.548 |
| Educational status of mothers | | | | |
| Informal | 32 (34.4) | 32 (17.2) | 2.53 (1.42,4.48) | 0.002* |
| Formal | 61 (65.6) | 154 (82.8) | 1 | |
| Occupation of mothers | | | | |
| Employed | 17 (18.3) | 63 (33.9) | 1 | |
| Merchant | 5 (5.4) | 24 (12.9) | 0.77 (0.26,2.33) | 0.646 |
| Housewife | 65 (69.9) | 91 (48.9) | 2.65 (1.42,4.94) | 0.002* |
| Others | 6 (6.5) | 8 (4.3) | 2.78 0.85,9.1) | 0.091 |
| Wealth index | | | | |
| Lower | 58 (62.4) | 101 (54.3) | 1.09 (0.57,2.07) | 0.797 |
| Middle | 16 (17.2) | 49 (26.3) | 0.62 (0.28,1.37) | 0.235* |
| Upper | 19 (20.4) | 36 (19.4) | 1 | |
| Height (cm) | | | | |
| < 150 | 22 (23.7) | 23 (12.4) | 2.21 (1.15,4.21) | 0.017* |
| > =150 | 71 (76.3) | 163 (87.6) | 1 | |
| MUAC | | | | |
| < 23 | 49 (52.7) | 25 (13.4) | 7.17 (3.99,12.88) | < 0.0001** |
| > =23 | 44 (47.3) | 161 (86.6) | 1 | |
| Any multivitamin | | | | |
| Yes | 9 (9.7) | 36 (19.4) | 1 | |
| No | 84 (90.3) | 150 (80.6) | 2.24 (1.03,4.88) | 0.042* |
| Iron and folate supplementation | | | | |
| Yes | 64 (68.8) | 166 (89.2) | 1 | |
| No | 29 (31.2) | 20 (10.8) | 3.76 (1.99,7.12) | < 0.0001** |
| Anemia | | | | |
| Yes | 30 (32.3) | 17 (9.1) | 4.73 (2.44, 9.17) | < 0.0001** |
| No | 63 (67.7) | 169 (90.9) | 1 | |
| ANC follow up | | | | |
| Yes | 83 (89.2) | 180 (96.8) | 1 | |
| No | 10 (10.8) | 6 (3.2) | 3.61 (1.27, 10.28) | 0.016* |
| Nutritional counseling | | | | |
| Yes | 40 (43.0) | 153 (82.3) | 1 | |
| No | 53 (57.0) | 33 (17.7) | 6.14 (3.52,10.72) | < 0.0001** |
| Additional food intake during pregnancy | | | | |
| Yes | 34 (36.6) | 134 (72) | 1 | |
| No | 59 (63.4) | 52 (28) | 4.47 (2.63, 7.61) | < 0.0001** |

**Table 4** Bivariate analyses to identify candidate variables for multivariable logistic regression to identify determinants of LBW, Dessie Town, Ethiopia, 2017 *(Continued)*

| Variables | Cases<br>No % | Controls<br>No % | Crude OR (95%CI) | *p*-value |
|---|---|---|---|---|
| MDD-W | | | | |
| inadequate | 87 (93.5) | 117 (62.9) | 8.55 (3.55, 20.61) | < 0.0001** |
| adequate | 6 (6.5) | 69 (37.1) | 1 | |
| Khat chewing | | | | |
| Yes | 33 (35.5) | 50 (26.9) | 1.51 (0.88, 2.55) | 0.14* |
| No | 60 (64.5) | 136 (73.1) | 1 | |
| History of abortion | | | | |
| Yes | 22 (23.7) | 22 (11.8) | 2.31 (1.20, 4.44) | 0.012* |
| No | 71 (76.3) | 164 (88.2) | 1 | |
| History of preterm delivery | | | | |
| Yes | 10 (10.8) | 5 (2.7) | 4.36 (1.45, 13.16) | 0.009* |
| No | 83 (89.2) | 181 (97.3) | 1 | |
| HIV status | | | | |
| Reactive | 5 (5.4) | 4 (2.2) | 2.59 (0.68, 9.87) | 0.164* |
| Non-reactive | 88 (94.6) | 182 (97.8) | 1 | |
| Type of pregnancy | | | | |
| Planned and wanted | 66 (71.0) | 149 (80.1) | 1 | |
| Unplanned but wanted | 23 (24.7) | 32 (17.2) | 1.62 (0.88, 2.98) | 0.119* |
| Unplanned and wanted | 4 (4.3) | 5 (2.7) | 1.81 (0.47, 6.94) | 0.389 |
| Infant sex | | | | |
| Male | 49 (52.7) | 117 (62.9) | 1 | |
| Female | 44 (47.3) | 69 (37.1) | 1.52 (0.92, 2.52) | 0.102* |

$^{**}P < 0.0001$ $^{*}p < 0.25$

pregnant mothers had folic acid supplementation, suggesting folate added to antenatal iron could independently affect birth weight of newborns [43]. This is further supported by larger cohort study undertaken in China indicating maternal daily intake of 400 μg of folic acid alone significantly reduced the risks of LBW and SGA status of infants [44].

Moreover, our study showed that anemic mothers had higher odds of delivering LBW neonates compared to non-anemic mothers. This finding was consistent with other studies [13, 39, 45]. Maternal anemia during pregnancy was found to increase odds of giving LBW babies in Yemen [13]. In Bangladesh [41] and India [45, 46] as well as in other settings [15, 18, 20] micronutrients deficiencies during pregnancy had been shown to have serious health implications on the developing fetus and hence, birth size [47]. Anemia could impair oxygen delivery to the fetus and thus interfere with normal intrauterine growth which possibly leads to LBW [19].

Inadequate dietary diversity and undernutrition during pregnancy independently and significantly affected LBW in our study. Mothers having inadequate MDD-W had significantly higher odds of giving birth to LBW babies. This finding was consistent with a study done in rural Ethiopia [35]. Similarly, a study from Ghana showed that women dietary diversity score and dietary patterns had protective effect against LBW [38]. However, recent randomized controlled trial in India reported that an intervention that increased consumption of dairy, fruits, and green leafy vegetables before and during pregnancy through a specially formulated snack had no effect on birth weight, but per-protocol and subgroup analyses showed that there was a possible increase in birth weight if the mother was supplemented for greater than or equal to 3 months before conception and was not underweight [48]. Malshani et al. (2017) showed that second trimester maternal carbohydrate intake had a significant impact on both total gestational weight gain and neonatal birth weight [49].

Undernutrition among mothers as measured by maternal MUAC of less than 23 cm significantly increased the maternal odds of having LBW babies in the present study. This is in agreement with study conducted in Eastern Ethiopia [24] and other countries; Yemen [13] and India [44]. The observed findings might be because anthropometric measurements relate to nutritional

**Table 5** Determinants of LBW in multivariable logistic regression analysis for newborns delivered in public health facilities in Dessie Town, Ethiopia, 2017

| Variables | Cases N(%) | Controls N(%) | COR (95%CI) | AOR [95% CI] |
|---|---|---|---|---|
| Iron and folate supplementation | | | | |
| Yes | 64 (68.8) | 166 (89.2) | 1 | 1 |
| No | 29 (31.2) | 20 (10.8) | 3.76 (1.99,7.12) | 2.84 (1.15,7.03) |
| Nutritional counseling | | | | |
| Yes | 40 (43.0) | 153 (82.3) | 1 | 1 |
| No | 53 (57.0) | 33 (17.7) | 6.14 (3.52, 10.72) | 4.05 (1.95, 8.38) |
| Additional meal | | | | |
| Yes | 34 (36.6) | 134 (72) | 1 | 1 |
| No | 59 (63.4) | 52 (28) | 4.47 (2.63, 7.61) | 3.25 (1.64, 6.44) |
| Nutritional status | | | | |
| MUAC < 23 | 49 (52.7) | 25 (13.4) | 7.17 (3.99,12.88) | 5.62 (2.64,11.97) |
| MUAC ≥23 | 44 (47.3) | 161 (86.6) | 1 | 1 |
| Anemia | | | | |
| Yes | 30 (32.3) | 17 (9.1) | 4.73 (2.44, 9.17) | 3.54 (1.46,8.61) |
| No | 63 (67.7) | 169 (90.9) | 1 | 1 |
| MDD-W | | | | |
| Inadequate | 87 (93.5) | 117 (62.9) | 8.55 (3.55, 20.61) | 6.65 (2.31,19.16) |
| Adequate | 6 (6.5) | 69 (37.1) | 1 | 1 |

**P*-value< 0.0001 ***p* < 0.05

status. Even though either acute or chronic maternal malnutrition has direct effect on the birth weight of a baby, acute maternal malnutrition has a more pronounced effect [24].

### Strength and limitation of the study

The present study has some strengths including conducting the study in all public health facilities in the study area, and taking new born weight within 1 h of delivery. Further, using case-control study design can be considered as another important strength of the current study. However, our study has limitations such as not including private health facilities. Also, the completed gestational age was taken from verbal response of respondents. There might be recall bias as respondents had to remember their last date of menstruation, provide intake data for dietary diversity, recall the number of ANC visits, and provide the number of IFA tablet taken. In addition, our study was able to determine the adherence of mothers who were taking iron, folate or multivitamin supplements.

## Conclusion

Lack of iron and folate supplementation, absence of nutritional counseling during pregnancy, lack of additional food during pregnancy, maternal undernutrition (MUAC < 23 cm), maternal anemia and inadequate MDD-W were identified as significant determinants of LBW among newborns included in our study. The importance of nutritional counseling, iron and folate supplementation and additional meal intake during pregnancy, and screening pregnant women for risk of malnutrition and proper identification of high risk-mother needs to be strengthened to reduce the incidence of LBW babies in Ethiopia. In addition, behavioral change communications targeting pregnant women in improving women's dietary diversity needs to be enhanced by health extension workers and health professionals in each health facility working at ANC clinics. Observational cohort studies and randomized controlled trials with larger sample size are required to confirm the observed associations.

**Acknowledgments**

The authors acknowledge Prof. Susan J Whiting for reviewing the manuscript for editorials and language problems.

**Funding**

This research was supported by Jimma University to support graduate students as the first author was MSc student in Jimma University. The funding body had no role in the design of the study and collection, analysis, and interpretation of data and in writing the manuscript.

**Authors' contributions**

SA, TW, and KH designed research; SA and TW conducted research; SA and TW analyzed data, interpreted the results and TW wrote the manuscript. All authors read and approved the final manuscript.

**Competing interests**

The authors declare that they have no competing interests.

**Author details**

[1]Gambella Regional State Health Bureau, Gambella, Ethiopia. [2]Jimma University, Faculty of Public Health, Jimma, Ethiopia.

**References**

1. United Nations Children's Fund and World Health Organization. Low Birthweight: Country, regional and global estimates. New York: UNICEF; 2004.
2. Strategies to promote optimal fetal growth and minimize the prevalence of LBW in Sri Lanka: Health sector response Family Health Bureau, Ministry of Health, 2013.
3. World Health Organization. Guidelines on optimal feeding of low birth weight in low and middle income countries. Geneva: WHO; 2011.
4. Kiess W, Chernausek SD, ACS H-K, editors. Small for Gestational Age. Causes and Consequences. Pediatr Adolesc Med. Basel, Karger. 2009;13:148–62.
5. World Health Organization. Global Nutrition Targets 2025: Low Birth Weight Policy Brief, 2014.

6. Kim D, Saada A. The social determinants of infant mortality and birth outcomes in western developed nations: across-country systematic review. Int J Environ Res Public Health. 2013;10:2296–35.
7. Ethiopian Demographic and Health Survey 2016. Central statistical agency. Addis Ababa; 2017.
8. Goldenberg RL, Culhane JF. Low birth weight in the United States. Am J Clin Nutr. 2007;85:584S–90S.
9. Ramakrishnan U. Nutrition and low birth weight: from research to practice. Am J Clin Nutr. 2004;79:17–21.
10. Barker DJP, Godfrey KM. Maternal nutrition, fetal programming and adult chronic disease. In: Gibney MJ, Margetts BM, Kearney JM, Arab L, editors. Public health nutrition. Oxford: Blackwell Science; 2004.
11. Torres-Arreola LP, Constantino-Casas P, Flores-Hernández S, Villa-Barragán JP, Rendón-Macías E. Socioeconomic factors and low birth weight in Mexico. BMC Public Health. 2005;5:20.
12. Muftah S. Maternal under-nutrition and anemia factors associated with low birth weight babies in Yemen. Int J Community Med Public Health. 2016;3: 2749–56.
13. Kramer MS. Determinants of low birth weight: methodological assessment and meta-analysis. Bull World Health Organ. 1987;65:663–37.
14. Ghimire R, Phalke DB, Phalke VD, Banjade B, Singh AK. Determinants of low birth weight: a case control study in Pravara rural Hospital in Western Maharashtra. India IJSR. 2014;3:243–5.
15. Khan A, Nasrullah FD, Jaleel R. Frequency and risk factors of low birth weight in term pregnancy. Pak J Med Sci. 2016;32:138–42.
16. Abubakari A, Kynast-Wolf G, Jahn A. Maternal determinants of birth weight in northern Ghana. PLoS One. 2015. https://doi.org/10.1371/ journal.pone.0135641.
17. Shakya KL, Shrestha N, Poudyal AK, Koju RP, Oyloe P, Onta SR. Key factors associated with low birth weight at term in Nepal. A case control study. Int J Clin and Biomed Res. 2015;1:62–9.
18. Sharma SR, Giri S, Timalsina U, Bhandari SS, Basyal B, Wagle K, et al. Low birth weight at term and its determinants in a tertiary Hospital of Nepal: a case-control study. PLoS One. 2015. https://doi.org/10.1371/journal.pone.0123962.
19. Muchemi OM, Echoka E, Makokh A. Factors associated with low birth weight among neonates born at Olkalou District hospital, central region, Kenya. Pan Afr Med J. 2015. https://doi.org/10.11604/pamj.2015.20.108.4831.
20. Sutan R, Mohtar M, Mahat AN, Tamil AM. Determinant of low birth weight infants: a matched case control study in Malaysia. Open J Prev Med. 2014;4:91–9.
21. Kayode GA, Amoakoh-Coleman M, Agyepong IA, Ansah E, Grobbee DE, et al. Contextual risk factors for low birth weight: a multilevel analysis. PLoS One. 2014. https://doi.org/10.1371/journal.pone.0109333.
22. Demelash H, Motbainor A, Nigatu D, Gashaw K, Melese A. Risk factors for low birth weight in bale zone hospitals, South-East Ethiopia. BMC Pregnancy and Childbirth. 2015;15:264.
23. Negassi T, Tesfaye H, Huruy A. Prevalence and factors associated with low birth weight in Axum and Laelay Miche districts, North Ethiopia: a comparative cross sectional study. IJNFS. 2014;3:560–6.
24. Assefa N, Berhane Y, Worku A. Wealth status, mid upper arm circumference (MUAC) and antenatal care (ANC) are determinants for low birth weight in Kersa, Ethiopia. PLoS One. 2012. https://doi.org/10.1371/journal.pone.0039957.
25. Tema T. Prevalence and determinants of low birth weight in Jimma zone, Southwest Ethiopia. East Afr Med J. 2006;83:366–71.
26. Eshete A, Birhanu D, Wassie B. Birth outcomes among laboring mothers in selected health facilities of north Wollo zone, Northeast Ethiopia: a facility based cross-sectional study. Health. 2013;5:1141–50.
27. Hailu LD, Kebede DL. Determinants of low birth weight among deliveries at a referral Hospital in Northern Ethiopia. Biomed Res Int. 2018;2018:8169615.
28. Zeleke BM, Zelalem M, Mohammed N. Incidence and correlates of low birth weight at a referral hospital in Northwest Ethiopia. Pan Afr Med J. 2012;12:4.
29. Gebremariam A. Factors predisposing to low birth weight in Jimma hospital south western Ethiopia. East Afr Med J. 2005;82:554–8.
30. Getachew G, Teumay A, Belaynew W, Berhe D. Incidence of low birth weight babies and associated factors among post-partum mothers who gave birth at Felege hiwot referral hospital, Bahirdar, Ethiopia. World J Pharm Pharm Sci. 2015;4:152–65.
31. Alemu T, Umeta M. Prevalence and predictors of "small size" babies in Ethiopia: in-depth analysis of the Ethiopian demographic and health survey, 2011. Ethiop J Health Sci. 2016;26:243–50.
32. Bugssa G, Dimtsu B, Alemayehu M. Socio demographic and maternal determinants of low birth weight at Mekelle hospital, Northern Ethiopia: A Cross Sectional Study. Am J Advn Drug Deliv. 2014;2:609–18.
33. Gebremedhin M, Ambaw F, Admassu E, Berhane H. Maternal associated factors of low birth weight: a hospital based cross-sectional mixed study in Tigray, northern Ethiopia. BMC Pregnancy and Childbirth. 2015;15:222.
34. Kahsay Z, Tadese A, Nigusie B. Low birth weight and associated factors among newborns in Gondar town, North West Ethiopia: Institutional Based Cross Sectional Study. Indo Global J Pharm Sci. 2014;4:74–80.
35. Zerfu TA, Umeta M, Baye K. Dietary diversity during pregnancy is associated with reduced risk of maternal anemia, preterm delivery, and low birth weight in a prospective cohort study in rural Ethiopia. Am J Clin Nutr. 2016;103:1482–8.
36. Food and Agriculture Organization and Food History Inventory. Minimum dietary Dieversity for women: a guide for measurement. Rome: FAO; 2016.
37. Adane AA, Ayele TA, Ararsa LG, Bitew BD, Zeleke BM. Adverse birth out comes among deliveries at Gondar University hospital, Northwest Ethiopia. BMC pregnancy and childbirth. 2014;14:90.
38. Abubakari A, Jahn A. Maternal dietary patterns and practices and birth weight in northern Ghana. PLoS One. 2016. https://doi.org/10.1371/journal.pone.0162285.
39. Matin A, Azimul SK, Matiur AKM, Shamianaz S, Shabnam JH, Islam T. Maternal socioeconomic and nutritional determinants of low birth weight in urban area of Bangladesh. J Dhaka Med Coll. 2008;17:83–7.
40. Rizvi SA, Hatcher J, Jehan I, Qureshi R. Maternal risk factors associated with low birth weight in Karachi: a case control study. East Mediterr Health J. 2007;13:1343–52.
41. Mitchell EA, Robinson E, Clark PM, Becroft DMO, Glavish N, Pattison NS, Pryor JE, Thompson JMD, Wild CJ. Maternal nutritional risk factors for small for gestational age babies in a developed country. Arch Dis Child Fetal Neonatal Ed. 2004;89:F431–5.
42. Ramakrishnan U, González-Cossío T, Neufeld LM, Rivera J, Martorell R. Multiple micronutrient supplementation during pregnancy does not lead to greater infant birth size than does iron-only supplementation: a randomized controlled trial in a semirural community in Mexico. Am J Clin Nutr. 2003;77:720–5.
43. Christian P, West KP, Khatry SK, Leclerq SC, Pradhan EK, Katz J, et al. Effects of maternal micronutrient supplementation on fetal loss and infant mortality: a cluster-randomized trial in Nepal. Am J Clin Nutr. 2003;78(6):1194–202.
44. Nan L, Zhiwen L, Rongwei Y, Jianmeng L, Aiguo R. Impact of Periconceptional folic acid supplementation on low birth weight and small-for-gestational-age infants in China: a large prospective cohort study. J Pediatr. 2017;187:105–10.
45. Dubey DK, Nath DC. An epidemiological model investigating the association between mothers nutritional status and low birth weight in India. Health. 2016;8:251–61.
46. Dharmalingam A, Navaneetham K, Krishnakumar CK. Nutritional status of mothers and low birth weight in India. Matern Child Health J. 2010;14:290–8.
47. Muthayya S. Maternal nutrition & low birth weight-what is really important? Indian J Med Res. 2009;130:600–8.
48. Potdar RD, Sahariah SA, Gandhi M, Kehoe SH, Brown N, Sane H, et al. Improving women's diet quality preconceptionally and during gestation: effects on birth weight and prevalence of low birth weight—a randomized controlled efficacy trial in India (Mumbai maternal nutrition project). Am J Clin Nutr. 2014;100:1257–68.
49. Pathirathna ML, Sekijima K, Sadakata M, Fujiwara N, Muramatsu Y, Wimalasiri KMS. Impact of second trimester maternal dietary intake on gestational weight gain and neonatal birth weight. Nutrients. 2017. https://doi.org/10.3390/nu9060627.

# 13

# Development and validation of a quantitative choline food frequency questionnaire for use with drinking and non-drinking pregnant women in Cape Town, South Africa

R. Colin Carter[1*], Sandra W. Jacobson[2,3,4], Sharmilah Booley[4], Baheya Najaar[4], Neil C. Dodge[2], Lori J. Bechard[5], Ernesta M. Meintjes[4], Christopher D. Molteno[3], Christopher P. Duggan[5], Joseph L. Jacobson[3,4] and Marjanne Senekal[4]

**Abstract**

**Background:** Although animal and human studies have demonstrated interactions between dietary choline and fetal alcohol spectrum disorders, dietary choline deficiency in pregnancy is common in the US and worldwide. We sought to develop and validate a quantitative food frequency questionnaire (QFFQ) to estimate usual daily choline intake in pregnant mothers.

**Methods:** A panel of nutrition experts developed a Choline-QFFQ food item list, including sources with high choline content and the most commonly consumed choline-containing foods in the target population. A data base for choline content of each item was compiled. For reliability and validity testing in a prospective longitudinal cohort, 123 heavy drinking Cape Coloured pregnant women and 83 abstaining/light-drinking controls were recruited at their first antenatal clinic visit. At 3 prenatal study visits, each gravida was interviewed about alcohol, smoking, and drug use, and administered a 24-hour recall interview and the Choline-QFFQ.

**Results:** Across all visits and assessments, > 78% of heavy drinkers and controls reported choline intake below the Dietary Reference Intakes adequate intake level (450 mg/day). Women reported a decrease in choline intake over time on the QFFQ. Reliability of the QFFQ across visits was good-to-acceptable for 2 of 4 group-level tests and 4 of 5 individual-level tests for both drinkers and controls. When compared with 24-hr recall data, validity of the QFFQ was good-to-acceptable for 3 of 4 individual-level tests and 3 of 5 group-level tests. For controls, validity was good-to-acceptable for all 4 individual-level tests and all 5 group-level tests.

**Conclusions:** To our knowledge, this is the first quantitative choline food frequency screening questionnaire to be developed and validated for use with both heavy and non-drinking pregnant women and the first to be used in the Cape Coloured community in South Africa. Given the high prevalence of inadequate choline intake and the growing evidence that maternal choline supplementation can mitigate some of the adverse effects of prenatal alcohol exposure, this tool may be useful for both research and future clinical outreach programs.

**Keywords:** Choline, Food frequency questionnaire, Nutrition, Alcohol consumption during pregnancy, Diet, Fetal alcohol spectrum disorders, Prenatal alcohol exposure

* Correspondence: rcolincarter@gmail.com
[1]Institute for Human Nutrition and Departments of Emergency Medicine and Pediatrics, Columbia University Medical Center, 3959 Broadway, CHN-1-116, New York, NY 10032, USA
Full list of author information is available at the end of the article

## Background

Fetal alcohol spectrum disorders (FASD) comprise a continuum of alcohol-related neurodevelopmental disorders ranging from the most severely affected children with fetal alcohol syndrome (FAS) to nonsyndromal children who also exhibit neurocognitive and/or behavioral deficits but may lack the facial features or growth deficits seen with FAS [1, 2]. Worldwide, a significant number of women drink heavily during pregnancy despite public health advisories and psychosocial interventions [3–5]. In the Western Cape Province of South Africa, where rates of heavy drinking during pregnancy are endemically high among women from the Cape Coloured (mixed ancestry) community [6–8], the prevalence of FAS is as high as 80 per 1000 [9].

A growing body of studies in FASD animal models has demonstrated that optimal maternal choline status can mitigate some of the teratogenic effects of alcohol [7, 10–16]. Thomas and colleagues have shown protective effects of pre- and postnatal choline supplementation on hippocampal development and related neurobehavioral outcomes in rats [10, 11], including reversal of alcohol-related deficits in eyeblink conditioning, which we have also shown to be profoundly affected in children prenatally exposed to alcohol [7, 12, 13]. We have recently extended these findings to humans in an exploratory randomized, double-blind, controlled trial, which demonstrated that high-dose choline supplementation initiated early in pregnancy can mitigate adverse effects of heavy drinking on infant eyeblink conditioning, cognition, and post-natal growth [14, 15].

Choline is an essential nutrient that is a constituent of the neurotransmitter acetylcholine and a precursor to phosphatidylcholine and sphingomyelin, which are major components of cell membranes and play an important role in cell membrane integrity, trans-membrane signaling, and triglyceride turnover from the liver and blood [16]. In addition, it serves as a methyl-group donor needed for homocysteine metabolism and DNA methylation, a critical mechanism in epigenetic processes that has been implicated in alcohol teratogenesis. Despite the fact that choline can be produced endogenously, it is classified as an essential nutrient [17, 18], and dietary intake, principally from eggs, liver, wheat germ, and milk, is imperative to meet physiological needs. The demand for choline is especially high during pregnancy, when it is actively transported to the fetus against a concentration gradient [19] and depletes maternal stores [20, 21]. In a recent randomized, double-blind, controlled trial comparing two 3$^{rd}$-trimester dietary regimens – 480 mg choline/day (just above the adequate intake level of 450 mg/day [19]) vs. 930 mg/day (just over twice adequate intake level), the higher choline intake arm was associated with faster infant processing speed through age 13 mo [22].

We have recently demonstrated that, although the diet and body composition of heavy drinking pregnant women is similar to that of abstaining/light-drinking pregnant women in socio-economically disadvantaged areas in Cape Town, South Africa, in repeated 24-hr dietary recall interviews, almost 90% of the women reported inadequate intake of choline [23]. High rates of inadequate choline intake during pregnancy have also been reported in the U.S. (90%) [24, 25], Canada (77%) [26], and New Zealand (84%) [27]. These studies emphasize the importance of assessment of dietary choline intake in groups at risk for inadequate intake, such as pregnant women, to inform dietary choline interventions, as well as the use of choline supplements. The use of repeated 24-hour recall interviews to assess usual daily intake of micronutrients has been validated in the U.S. and in resource-poor settings but is both labor and time-intensive [28]. One alternative is to use a dietary intake assessment method that focuses specifically on quantification of choline content using a quantitative nutrient-indicated food frequency questionnaire (QFFQ). This methodology is increasingly applied in assessment of usual intake of single nutrients (e.g., vitamin D [29], iron [30], and vitamin K [31].

We developed a quantitative choline food frequency questionnaire (Choline-QFFQ) to estimate usual dietary choline intake (mg/day) by participants in our Cape Town randomized clinical trial conducted to assess feasibility and efficacy of a maternal choline supplementation intervention conducted with heavy drinking women during pregnancy [14, 15]. The current study combines data from this trial and from our larger prospective longitudinal cohort on the effects of prenatal alcohol exposure on development that included both heavy drinking and abstaining/light-drinking pregnant women from the same community as the women in the trial [8, 32]. Our aims were (1) to develop a Choline-QFFQ that can be used to estimate usual daily intake of dietary choline and (2) to test its reliability and validity in both heavy drinkers and abstainers/light-drinkers.

## Methods

### Development of the Choline-QFFQ

The Choline-QFFQ food item list was developed by a panel of three nutrition experts in the Division of Human Nutrition, University of Cape Town, including M.S, S.B, and B.N., in which food sources with high choline content, as well as the most commonly consumed foods in the target population were included. The food sources list was derived from Nel and Steyn [33] and multiple unpublished field studies completed by post-graduate students in dietetics in Cape Town, South Africa. In addition to high choline-content foods, commonly consumed food sources with moderate or low-choline content were included in the final food list, as frequent consumption of such foods may also make a considerable contribution to choline intake. Lewis et al. [26] demonstrated that vegetables, baked products and fruits that are moderate to low sources of choline provided 8.5%, 7.7% and 6.6%, respectively, of total choline intake versus 12.2% provided by eggs and 11.1% by meat, which contain high levels of choline. The final food list was comprised of 10 groups, including beef (organ, mince, patty, chops and braised beef), lamb (chops and stew), chicken (fried or roasted in different cuts, giblets and liver), processed meats (salami, ham, polony, viennas and frankfurters), fish (canned sardines and canned pilchards), eggs (boiled or fried), legumes (baked beans, lentils, sugar beans, soy beans), vegetables (cauliflower, broccoli, corn/mealies, peas, mixed vegetables, spinach, gem squash, pumpkin, potatoes – fried or mashed with added milk), fruit (banana), dairy (milk drink, milk added to cereal or in tea/coffee and yoghurt) and other items (beer, chocolate cake, tomato sauce/ketchup and peanut butter). Participants were requested to report the number of times a particular food item had been consumed during the past week, either number of times per day, if consumed daily, or otherwise number of times in the past week.

The picture sort method was used for administration of the Choline-QFFQ, whereby participants were asked to sort picture cards of food items included in the food list into two piles, those consumed during the past week and those not consumed during the past week. Interviewers, either a registered dietician or a research assistant with extensive training in dietary interviewing by M.S., then proceeded to quantify the frequency of intake and typical portion size for items that had been consumed during the past week. Portion size estimation was conducted using pictures and portion size props (Fig. 1) included in the Dietary Assessment and Education Kit (DAEK) [34]. The Choline-QFFQ was pilot-tested with 24 women of child-bearing age from the same community as the main cohort in this study. Ease of procedure, face validity, and acceptability among subjects were excellent.

#### Study Participants for Reliability and Validity Testing

This study included pregnant women from the Cape Coloured (mixed ancestry) community who were recruited to participate in the choline clinical trial [14, 15] or the prospective longitudinal study [23] between October 2011 and December 2015. Women were recruited at their first visit to one of three antenatal midwife obstetric units that serve socioeconomically-disadvantaged communities in Cape Town (see [15, 16, 27] for further subject eligibility, recruitment, retention, and sample size calculation details). Each mother was interviewed at screening ($M$ = 21.1 weeks gestation, SD = 6.1) regarding her alcohol consumption both at time of conception and recruitment and again at 4 and 12 weeks after recruitment, by a research nurse using the timeline follow-back interview (TLFB; [35]) adapted for use with women in this community [7, 32]. Any woman averaging at least 1.0 oz absolute alcohol (AA)/day (1 oz AA~2 standard drinks) or reporting binge drinking (≥2.0 oz AA/drinking occasion) was invited to participate in the study. Women initiating antenatal care who drank only minimally and did not binge drink were invited to participate as abstainers/light drinkers. Exclusion criteria included age <18 years, HIV infection, and pharmacologic treatment for medical conditions, including diabetes, hypertension, epilepsy, or cardiac problems. All women who reported drinking during pregnancy were advised to stop or reduce their intake, and women were offered a referral for substance abuse treatment programs. Consent and interviews were conducted in Afrikaans or English, depending on the mother's preference.

#### Reliability and validity testing of the Choline-QFFQ

Study visits occurred at recruitment and again 4 and 12 weeks later. Both the test method (Choline-QFFQ) and reference method (24-hr recall) were administered at each visit, with the reference method given first. The reliability of the Choline-QFFQ was tested by comparing the results of three administrations of the questionnaire. The validity of the Choline-QFFQ was tested using a dietary reference method (three repeated 24-hour recalls). 24-hr dietary recall interviews were administered using the multiple-pass method [28] and pictures and portion size props provided by the DAEK (Steyn & Senekal 2004). Hand-written dietary records were reviewed by a U.S. registered dietician/research scientist (L.B.) who entered these data into the FoodFinder3® software program. The two interviewers and L.B. held regular Skype® meetings to discuss the interviews, questions that arose, and any outliers found.

Since FoodFinder3® does not provide values for choline content, a database was created to estimate the choline content of foods consumed by the women in the study. All foods reported by women in 24-hr dietary recall interviews and any additional foods included in the Choline-QFFQ (total = 382 foods) were matched to preparation-specific food items in the USDA Database for the Choline Content of Common Foods (Release 2 [36]). Choline content was calculated by linking the nutrient database number used in the USDA choline database with that used in the USDA National Nutrient Database for Standard Reference. For 16 reported foods that were not listed in the USDA choline database and consisted of multiple food items, recipes were constructed and used to calculate choline content based on

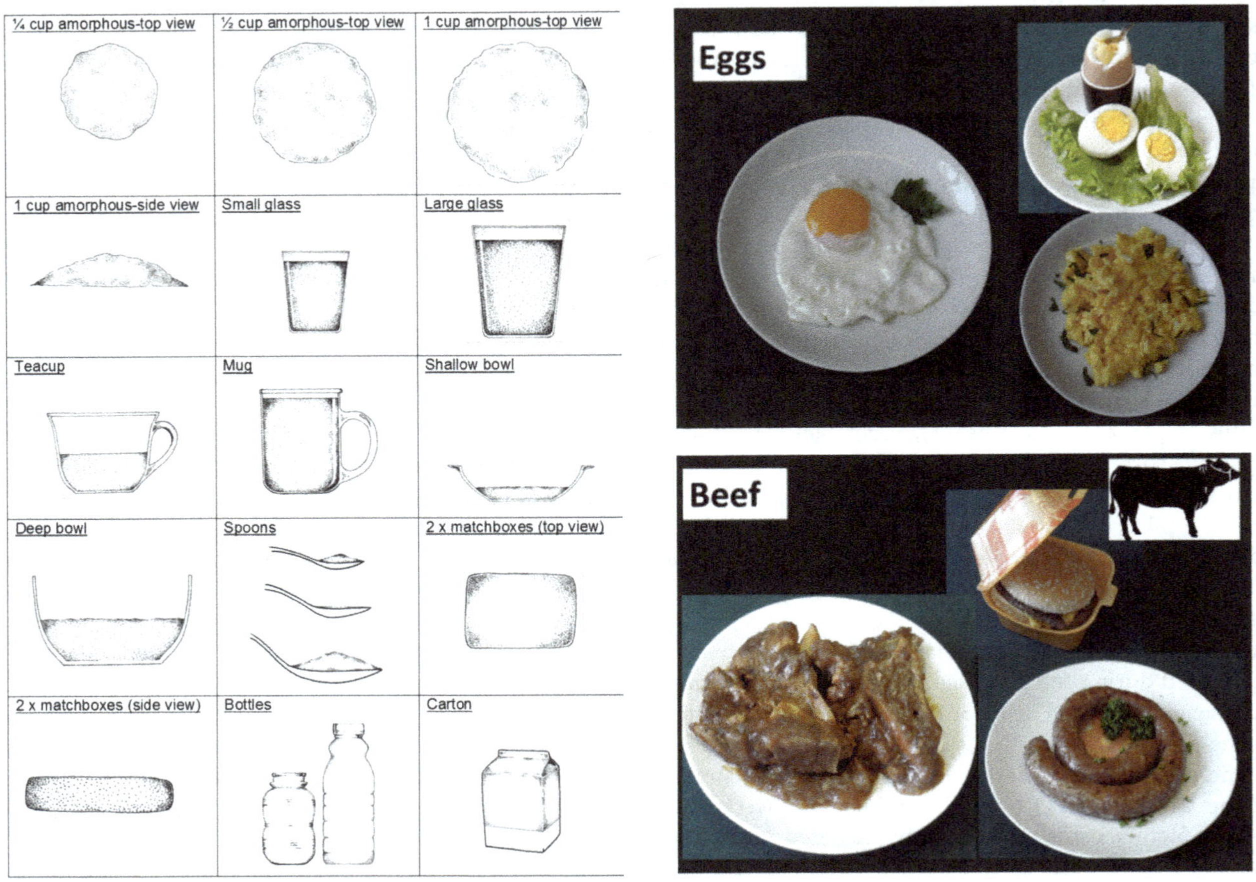


**Fig. 1** Pictures and portion size props used from the Dietary Assessment and Education Kit [34]

the quantity and content of individual ingredients. An additional 21 foods not listed in the USDA choline database were matched with nutritionally comparable foods, chosen by M.S. and R.C. based on similar content, energy, and appearance. One food, Maltabella (reported in two 24-hr recall interviews), was not included, as no appropriate substitution could be found. Total choline content was calculated for each 24-hr recall interview and each Choline-QFFQ. Values from the three 24-hr recall interviews for a given woman were then averaged to calculate usual daily intake, which was used as the reference method value [32]. Inadequate dietary choline intake was defined as average daily intake below the Adequate Intake level (AI) per the Dietary Reference Intake [19].

### Statistical analyses

Statistical analyses were performed using SPSS v.23 software (IBM, Chicago, IL, USA). Reliability and validity analyses were conducted separately for drinkers and abstainers/light-drinkers. Reliability of the Choline-QFFQ was assessed by comparing the daily dietary choline intake values between visits 1 and 2; visits 2 and 3; and visits 1 and 3, adapting the validity analyses and interpretations suggested by Lombard et al. [37]. Validity was assessed by comparing daily choline intake from the reference method (average of the woman's three 24-hr recall interviews) with daily dietary intake from the QFFQ at visit 1, the average of visits 1-2, and the average of visits 1-3; the latter two comparisons were conducted to evaluate whether validity is better with repeated administration of the QFFQ. Group-level agreement was examined using the Wilcoxon signed-rank test and by examining the mean difference between intake values from repeated QFFQ applications as a percentage of the recall value. To assess potential bias, Spearman correlation coefficients were calculated between the mean of the intake values for the repeated QFFQ applications and the mean difference of the two values (from Bland-Altman analyses). As suggested by Kowalkowska et al. [38], we also calculated the Bland Altman Index, the percentage of subjects with values outside of the limits of agreement (LOA; defined as mean ± 1.96 SD), with < 5% being acceptable. Individual agreement was examined by calculating the percentage of individuals placed in the same tertile by each measure and the percentage placed in opposite tertiles (i.e., lowest tertile for one and highest tertile for the other) and by calculating a weighted kappa statistic. A kappa statistic was also calculated to assess agreement on whether a woman reported intake below the choline AI. Spearman correlation was used to assess the strength of agreement between visits at the individual level. Intraclass correlations and within-subject coefficients of variation for [39] dietary nutrient intakes were calculated using the method developed by Hertzmark and Spiegelman (https://www.hsph.harvard.edu/donna-spiegelman/software/icc9/).

## Results

### Sample characteristics

The majority of the mothers (89.8%) were 20-40 years of age, and drinkers were 2 years older than abstainers/light--drinkers on average (Table 1). Three-fourths (76.1%) of the women had attended high school, but only 12.2% completed high school. Drinkers had attended school almost 1 year less than abstainers/light-drinkers. Average daily energy intake was similar between drinkers and abstainers/light-drinkers and was below the 2400 kcal/day recommended during pregnancy. As we have previously reported, the majority of the women received prenatal iron/folic acid supplementation and reported good adherence, taking the supplement on most days [23]. Almost three-quarters (72.5%) had full-term pregnancies. Almost all women (94.7%) completed at least two interviews, and 64.6% completed three interviews. Heavy drinkers and abstainers/light-drinkers did not differ in number of visits. As expected, alcohol use was heavy among drinkers, who averaged 9.4 standard drinks per occasion on 2.4 days per week around time of conception and 8.4 standard drinks on 1.3 days per week across pregnancy. All but 8 controls (9.6%) abstained from alcohol use: 4 reported drinking < 2 drinks per occasion (three of these reported 3 or fewer occasions, one 1-2 occasions per week); 2 drank < 3 drinks per occasion 1-2 times per month; and 2 reported a single binge episode that occured following recruitment into the study.

### Dietary choline intake

A large majority of women in both the heavy drinking and abstaining/light-drinking groups reported choline intake below the AI (Table 2). Both heavy drinkers and abstainers/light-drinkers in the cohort reported a lower choline intake at each consecutive visit on both the 24-hr recall interviews and the QFFQs, but this decrease over time was only statistically significant on the QFFQ. We have previously reported that average daily choline intake and the prevalence of inadequate intake were similar between heavy drinkers and abstainers/light-drinkers [23].

### Reliability of the Choline-QFFQ

When examining the group-level reliability of the Choline-QFFQ among heavy drinkers between visits, results for percentage difference pointed to good agreement, while agreement reflected by the Wilcoxon signed rank test was poor (Table 3). In Bland-Altman analyses, 5% or fewer of values fell outside of the limit of agreement (LOA) when comparing visits 1 and 2 and visits 2 and 3, but just above the 5% cutoff when comparing visits 1 and 3. Bias was evident in the Bland Altman Spearman correlation analyses with a positive correlation between the difference in reported intake between the two visits and the mean choline intake value for the 2 visits. Results for individual-level tests showed that percentage classified in the same tertiles and opposite tertiles (agreement including chance) was good for all comparisons with the exception of visit 1 vs. visit 3, which was poor. Agreement excluding chance, as reflected by the weighted kappa statistic, and strength of agreement, reflected by the Spearman correlation coefficient, was acceptable-to-good for all comparisons. Results were almost identical among abstainers/light--drinkers for group- and individual-level tests. Values for the QFFQ within-subject coefficient of variation (.53) and the ratio of within- to between-subject variance (2.2) were similar to those for 24-hr recall interviews (.58 and 2.1, respectively).

### Validity of the Choline-QFFQ

Among drinkers, agreement was good-to-acceptable on most group-level tests, with the exception of percentage difference between QFFQ values at visit 1 and the mean of the 24-hr recall interviews (reference method) and the LOA index when averaging QFFQ values from visits 1-2 (Table 4). Individual-level tests among drinkers were good for the Spearman correlation, acceptable for the weighted kappa test, and poor for both tertile classification methods (46.6% vs. ≥ 50% cutoff and 10.3% vs. ≤10% cutoff). Among abstainers/light-drinkers, all group-level tests were acceptable-to-good except for Bland-Altman Spearman correlation when using only visit 1 QFFQ values, with a weak, positive bias seen. At the individual-level, all tests were acceptable-to-good except for same-tertile classification when using the mean of visits 1-3, which was poor.

## Discussion

In this prospective longitudinal cohort of heavy drinking pregnant women and abstainers/light-drinkers, we developed and demonstrated reliability and validity of a QFFQ that assesses average daily choline intake and requires minimal time (~10-15 minutes) and resources (food

**Table 1** Sample characteristics

| | Heavy drinkers | | | | | Abstainers/light drinkers | | | | | $p^a$ |
|---|---|---|---|---|---|---|---|---|---|---|---|
| | *N* | *M* | SD | *n* | % | *N* | *M* | SD | *n* | % | |
| Maternal age at conception (yr) | 122 | 27.7 | 5.7 | | | 83 | 25.5 | 4.8 | | | .004 |
| Gravidity (no.) | 122 | 2.9 | 1.7 | | | 83 | 2.5 | 1.3 | | | .109 |
| Marital status (no. married) | 122 | | | 34 | 27.6 | 83 | | | 34 | 41.0 | .046 |
| Education (yr school completed) | 122 | 9.3 | 1.7 | | | 83 | 10.0 | 1.6 | | | .005 |
| Average daily energy intake (kilocalories/day) | 122 | 2247.9 | 810.1 | | | 83 | 2343.0 | 857.7 | | | .421 |
| Received prenatal iron/folic acid supplementation | 119 | | | 104 | 87.4 | 80 | | | 69 | 86.3 | .814 |
| Takes supplements most days (supplemented only) | | | | 104 | 90.4 | | | | 65 | 93.2 | .367 |
| Number of visits | 122 | 2.6 | 0.7 | | | 83 | 2.5 | 0.7 | | | .110 |
| Weeks gestation | | | | | | | | | | | |
| Initiation of antenatal care | 122 | 17.3 | 5.9 | | | 83 | 18.7 | 6.0 | | | .111 |
| Visit 1 | 122 | 22.9 | 5.8 | | | 83 | 25.5 | 5.0 | | | .001 |
| Visit 2 | 116 | 27.0 | 5.6 | | | 78 | 29.9 | 5.0 | | | <.001 |
| Visit 3 | 78 | 32.5 | 4.0 | | | 46 | 34.0 | 3.9 | | | .050 |
| Delivery | 122 | 38.8 | 2.1 | | | 83 | 39.0 | 2.2 | | | .626 |
| Alcohol and drug use | | | | | | | | | | | |
| AA/day (oz) | 122 | 0.9 | 1.2 | | | 83 | 0.0 | 0.0 | | | <.001 |
| AA/drinking day (oz) | 122 | 4.2 | 2.4 | | | 83 | 0.2 | 0.5 | | | <.001 |
| Drinking days/wk (days) | 122 | 1.3 | 1.1 | | | 83 | 0.0 | 0.1 | | | <.001 |
| No. reporting cigarette smoking | 122 | | | 106 | 86.2 | 83 | | | 57 | 68.7 | .002 |
| Cigarettes/day (smokers only) | | 6.8 | 4.1 | | | | 6.1 | 5.9 | | | .435 |
| No. reporting marijuana use | 122 | | | 29 | 23.6 | 83 | | | 8 | 9.6 | .011 |
| Marijuana use (users only; days/mo) | | 9.7 | 9.4 | | | | 4.0 | 4.7 | | | .026 |
| No. reporting methamphetamine use | 122 | | | 12 | 9.8 | 83 | | | 15 | 18.1 | .083 |
| Methamphetamine use (users only; days/mo) | | 4.5 | 5.4 | | | | 8.8 | 8.0 | | | .119 |

AA = absolute alcohol; 1 oz AA ≈ 2 standard drinks

[a]From $\chi 2$ for categorical variables and *t*-tests for all continuous variables except for weight, BMI, triceps and biceps skinfolds, and MUAC, for which values from repeated measures regression models are presented; weight, BMI and MUAC models include control for weeks gestation at time of measurement

identification cards and portion estimation props) to administer. To our knowledge, this is the first Choline-QFFQ to be developed and validated for use with pregnant women and the first to be used in the Cape Coloured community in South Africa. While this choline quantitative FFQ presented is specific to the Cape Coloured population, the development and validation steps we employed may be used to develop population-specific choline quantitative screening FFQs in other populations. Furthermore, the Choline-QFFQ performed well in our study population, suggesting that a Choline-QFFQ (and the development and validations steps we employed) can be used even in populations in which education is poor and/or socioeconomic status low. Despite extensive prevention efforts and guidelines (ACOG, 2011) and 4 decades of scientific research demonstrating teratogenic effects of prenatal alcohol exposure, women worldwide continue to drink during pregnancy. FASD comprise the most common preventable cause of neurodevelopmental disabilities, with prevalence estimates of 1.1-5.0% in the US and Western Europe [40, 41] and 13.6-20.9% in South Africa [9]. Evidence from both animal [10, 11, 42, 43] and human [14, 15] studies has demonstrated that high-dose choline supplementation can mitigate many of the teratogenic effects of alcohol. It is thus of concern that over 80% of the both heavy drinkers and abstainers/light-drinkers in this study reported choline intake below the AI in all assessments, as has been reported in other populations such as the U.S. [25], Canada [26], and New Zealand [27]. Given our reliability and validity findings, the QFFQ developed in this study may be used to screen alcohol-using pregnant mothers in Cape Town to identify women who may benefit from choline interventions, whether they be dietary counseling or choline supplementation programs. Given our finding that abstaining/light-drinking women in this cohort had similarly high rates of dietary choline inadequacy, this QFFQ may also be used to identify non-drinking pregnant women at risk for choline

**Table 2** Daily choline intake values by 24-hr recall interviews and semi-quantitative food frequency questionnaire (QFFQ)

| | Intake below AI | Average daily intake (mg) | |
|---|---|---|---|
| | *n* (%) | Mean (SD) | Median (IQR) |
| Heavy drinkers | | | |
| 24-hr recall[a] | | | |
| Visit 1 (*n* = 122) | 95 (77.9) | 338.6 (257.1) | 275.4 (156.7 – 410.5) |
| Visit 2 (*n* = 116) | 96 (82.8) | 310.8 (221.0) | 257.6 (176.1 – 359.4) |
| Visit 3 (*n* = 86) | 73 (84.9) | 279.8 (185.8) | 229.1 (141.3 – 370.0) |
| Visits 1-2 (mean; *n* = 116) | 94 (81.0) | 327.5 (200.0) | 274.7 (194.6 – 409.5) |
| Visits 1-3 (mean; *n* = 86) | 73 (84.9) | 304.6 (147.6) | 273.9 (195.7 – 379.3) |
| QFFQ[b] | | | |
| Visit 1 (*n* = 121) | 97 (80.2) | 340.4 (205.1) | 293.0 (208.2 – 436.0) |
| Visit 2 (*n* = 112) | 100 (89.3) | 286.0 (160.5) | 267.9 (176.7 – 352.0) |
| Visit 3 (*n* = 78) | 67 (85.9) | 259.1 (160.5) | 259.1 (175.9 – 337.4) |
| Visits 1-2 (mean; *n* = 112) | 97 (86.6) | 312.1 (152.1) | 301.8 (203.3 – 386.9) |
| Visits 1-3 (mean; *n* = 78) | 70 (89.7) | 322.8 (180.5) | 288.8 (186.3 – 410.5) |
| Abstainers/light drinkers | | | |
| 24-hr recall[a] | | | |
| Visit 1 (*n* = 83) | 70 (84.3) | 336.8 (255.9) | 279.7 (182.5 – 406.1) |
| Visit 2 (*n* = 78) | 61 (78.2) | 305.7 (179.7) | 267.1 (151.8 – 416.7) |
| Visit 3 (*n* = 47) | 39 (83.0) | 285.9 (175.7) | 232.2 (164.6 – 348.3) |
| Visits 1-2 (mean; *n* = 78) | 66 (84.6) | 318.1 (178.1) | 282.6 (186.8 – 386.4) |
| Visits 1-3 (mean; *n* =47 ) | 39 (83.0) | 303.1 (171.1) | 247.6 (196.5 – 364.1) |
| QFFQ[b] | | | |
| Visit 1 (*n* = 83) | 68 (81.9) | 316.4 (215.1) | 277.8 (166.5 – 378.5) |
| Visit 2 (*n* = 72) | 62 (86.1) | 275.3 (162.2) | 279.0 (149.0 – 356.7) |
| Visit 3 (*n* = 42) | 39 (92.9) | 199.6 (113.5) | 164.3 (125.1 – 211.9) |
| Visits 1-2 (mean; *n* = 72) | 64 (77.1) | 304.9 (178.0) | 279.1 (175.7 – 402.9) |
| Visits 1-3 (mean; *n* = 42) | 37 (88.1) | 290.7 (169.6) | 266.5 (161.6 – 371.2) |

AI = adequate intake (450 mg choline/day)
[a]Paired t-test comparing values between visits: Drinkers: $p = .191$ for visits 1-2, .607 for visits 2-3, and .055 for visits 1-3; Abstainers/light-drinkers: $p = .380$ for visits 1-2, .702 for visits 2-3, and .318 for visits 1-3.
[b]Paired t-test comparing values between visits: Drinkers: $p = .006$ for visits 1-2, .921 for visits 2-3, and .019 for visits 1-3; Abstainers/light-drinkers: $p = .224$ for visits 1-2, .001 for visits 2-3, and .009 for visits 1-3.

deficiency, which poses its own potential harms to the mother and developing fetus, including neural tube and craniofacial defects, as well as possible effects on neurocognitive development [18, 24, 44, 45].

The steps of development and validation we employed can be used to develop population-specific choline quantitative screening FFQs in other populations. Development and validation of a nutrient-specific screening QFFQ involved several steps, including 1) development of the local food list; 2) determining the most appropriate recall period, frequency options and portion size estimation method(s), based on the aim of the dietary intake assessment, the target population, and time available for the administration; 3) identifying an appropriate reference method; and 4) identification of interpretable statistical tests for examining the reliability and validity of the newly developed QFFQ. The food list for our Choline-QFFQ was developed based on the integration of the best known dietary sources of choline and knowledge of commonly consumed foods in the Cape Coloured community in Cape Town by a panel of nutrition researchers with expertise on the dietary patterns of the target population. The recall period was set at the previous week based on recommendations by Willett [28]. Portion size estimation was based on portions used in the FoodFinder program, which was developed for use in this population, and modified based on pilot interviews with women from this community. Administration of the Choline-QFFQ using the picture sort method proved to be simple and quick (~10-15 minutes), which is ideal for implementation as a screening procedure in a community healthcare setting. The dietary reference method used was three 24-hour

**Table 3** Reliability tests comparing dietary choline intake between quantitative food frequency questionnaire interviews

| | Group-level | | | | Individual-level | | | | | Summary | |
|---|---|---|---|---|---|---|---|---|---|---|---|
| | Agreement | Agreement | Agreement | Bias | Strength of association | Agreement including chance | | Agreement excluding chance | | | |
| | Wilcoxon signed rank test $p$ | Percentage difference | Bland-Altman LOA index | Bland-Altman Spearman correlation $p$ | Spearman correlation[2] | Tertile classification | | Kappa statistic | | Group-level tests at "Good" or "Acceptable" (of 4 tests) | Individual-level tests at "Good" or "Acceptable" (of 5 tests) |
| | | | | | | Same tertile | Opposite tertile | Weighted for tertiles | Above vs. below AI | | |
| Heavy drinkers: | | | | | | | | | | | |
| Visit 1 vs. 2 ($n$ = 112) | .001 | M -0.4% | 4.5% | < .001 | .52 | 54.5% | 9.8% | .44 | < .001 | | |
| Interpretation[1] | Poor | Good | Good | Poor | Good | Good | Good | Acceptable | Poor | 2 | 4 |
| Visit 1 vs. 3 ($n$ = 78) | .026 | M -2.8% | 7.7% | < .001 | .43 | 47.4% | 14.1% | .28 | < .001 | | |
| Interpretation[1] | Poor | Good | Poor | Poor | Acceptable | Poor | Poor | Acceptable | Poor | 1 | 2 |
| Visit 2 vs. 3 ($n$ = 78) | .606 | M -18.4% | 5.1% | < .001 | .56 | 50.0% | 9.0% | .41 | < .001 | | |
| Interpretation[1] | Good | Acceptable | Good | Poor | Good | Good | Good | Acceptable | Poor | 2 | 4 |
| Abstainers/light-drinkers: | | | | | | | | | | | |
| Visit 1 vs. 2 ($n$ = 72) | .522 | M -7.1% | 4.2% | .001 | .42 | 56.9% | 2.8% | .50 | .001 | | |
| Interpretation[1] | Good | Good | Good | Poor | Acceptable | Good | Good | Acceptable | Poor | 3 | 4 |
| Visit 1 vs. 3 ($n$ = 42) | < .001 | M 9.1% | 4.8% | < .001 | .37 | 47.6% | 2.4% | .49 | < .001 | | |
| Interpretation[1] | Poor | Good | Good | Poor | Acceptable | Poor | Good | Acceptable | Poor | 2 | 3 |
| Visit 2 vs. 3 ($n$ = 42) | .014 | M 16.2% | 2.4% | < .001 | .50 | 50.0% | 4.8% | .47 | < .001 | | |
| Interpretation[1] | Poor | Acceptable | Good | Poor | Good | Good | Good | Acceptable | Poor | 2 | 4 |

[1]Interpretation criteria [37]:
Wilcoxon signed rank test: Good: $p > 0.05$; Poor: $p \leq 0.05$
Percentage difference: Good: 0.0 – < 11%; Acceptable: 11 - 20.0%; Poor: > 20%
Bland-Altman LOA index (% outside of limit of agreement): Good: ≤ 5%; Poor: > 5%
Bland-Altman Spearman correlation coefficient: Good: $p > 0.05$; Poor: $p \leq 0.05$
Spearman correlation coefficient: Good: ≥ 0.50; Acceptable: 0.20 – 0.49; Poor < 0.20
Tertile classification (% in same tertile): Good: ≥ 50%; Poor: < 50%
Tertile classification (% in opposite tertile): Good: ≤ 10%, Poor: > 10%
Weighted Kappa statistic: Good: ≥ 0.60; Acceptable: 0.20 – 0.59; Poor: < 0.20
[2]$p < .001$ for all Spearman values

**Table 4** Validation tests comparing dietary choline intake between the semiquantitative food frequency questionnaire and 24-hour recall interviews

| | Group-level agreement | | | | Individual-level agreement | | | | | Summary | |
|---|---|---|---|---|---|---|---|---|---|---|---|
| | Agreement | Agreement | Agreement | Bias | Strength of association | Agreement including chance | | Agreement excluding chance | | | |
| | | | | | | Tertile classification | | Kappa statistic | | | |
| | Wilcoxon signed rank test $p$ | Percentage difference | Bland-Altman LOA index | Bland-Altman Spearman correlation $p$ | Spearman correlation[2] | Same tertile | Opposite tertile | Weighted for tertiles | Above vs. below AI | Group-level tests at "Good" or "Acceptable" (of 4 tests) | Individual-level tests at "Good" or "Acceptable" (of 5 tests) |
| Heavy drinkers: | | | | | | | | | | | |
| Visit 1 ($n$ = 121) | .258 | M 30.8% | 5.0% | .11 | .39 | 48.8% | 14.9% | .26 | .21 | 3 | 3 |
| Interpretation[1] | Good | Poor | Good | Good | Acceptable | Poor | Poor | Acceptable | Acceptable | | |
| Visits 1-2 (mean) ($n$ = 116) | .976 | M 16.6% | 8.0% | .552 | .39 | 46.6% | 10.3% | .31 | .20 | 3 | 3 |
| Interpretation[1] | Good | Acceptable | Poor | Good | Acceptable | Poor | Poor | Acceptable | Acceptable | | |
| Visits 1-3 (mean) ($n$ = 78) | 1.00 | M -9.5% | 5.1% | .148 | .43 | 47.4% | 7.7% | .40 | .18 | 4 | 2 |
| Interpretation[1] | Good | Good | Good | Good | Acceptable | Poor | Poor | Acceptable | Poor | | |
| Abstainers/light-drinkers: | | | | | | | | | | | |
| Visit 1 ($n$ = 83) | .440 | M 7.2% | 4.8% | .04 (.23) | .51 | 50.6% | 9.9% | .39 | .35 | 4 | 5 |
| Interpretation[1] | Good | Good | Good | Poor | Good | Good | Good | Acceptable | Good | | |
| Visits 1-2 (mean) ($n$ = 68) | .366 | M 0.0% | 4.2% | .269 | .52 | 50.0% | 8.8% | .42 | .35 | 4 | 5 |
| Interpretation[1] | Good | Good | Good | Good | Good | Good | Good | Acceptable | Acceptable | | |
| Visits 1-3 (mean) ($n$ = 42) | 1.00 | M 5.2% | 2.4% | .171 | .56 | 45.0% | 10.0% | .33 | .63 | 4 | 4 |
| Interpretation[1] | Good | Good | Good | Good | Good | Poor | Good | Acceptable | Good | | |

[1]Interpretation criteria [37]:
Wilcoxon signed rank test: Good: $p > 0.05$; Poor: $p \leq 0.05$
Percentage difference: Good: 0.0 – < 11%; Acceptable: 11 - 20.0%; Poor: > 20%
Bland-Altman LOA index (% outside of limit of agreement): Good: ≤ 5%; Poor: > 5%
Bland-Altman Spearman correlation coefficient: Good: $p > 0.05$; Poor: $p \leq 0.05$
Spearman correlation coefficient: Good: ≥ 0.50; Acceptable: 0.20 – 0.49; Poor < 0.20
Tertile classification (% in same tertile): Good: ≥ 50%; Poor: < 50%
Tertile classification (% in opposite tertile): Good: ≤ 10%, Poor: > 10%
Weighted Kappa statistic: Good: ≥ 0.60; Acceptable: 0.20 – 0.59; Poor: < 0.20
[2]$p < .001$ for all Spearman values

recall interviews, the method most strongly recommended for validation of food frequency questionnaires [32], especially in communities where literacy and education issues may preclude the use of food diaries, such as this socioeconomically disadvantaged community in Cape Town.

We used the statistical tests and interpretations recommended by Lombard et al. [37] to assess different features of reliability and validity. Lombard recommends three group-level comparison tests (comparison of means using the Wilcoxon signed rank test, percentage difference, and Bland Altman Spearman test for bias) and four individual-level tests (Spearman correlation coefficient, same- and opposite-tertile classification, and the weighted kappa statistic for tertile classification). We added a fourth group-level test, the Bland Altman limit of agreement index (as recommended by Kowalkowska et al. [38]), and a fifth individual-level test, a kappa statistic examining the classification agreement for whether a woman reported intake below the choline AI, to provide a measure of clinical relevance. Group level tests are most relevant for research studies, where errors for a single woman are less important as long as group-level associations are acceptable-to-good, and individual-level tests are most relevant for clinical practice, in which a woman's reported values will guide targeted recommendations and/or interventions. The majority of the five individual level statistical tests indicated acceptable to good reliability of the QFFQ for all comparisons conducted for both heavy drinkers and abstainers/light--drinkers, except for comparisons of visits 1 and 3 among drinkers, suggesting that reliability may decline over time. At the group level, reliability was good-to-acceptable for 2 of 4 tests, namely percentage difference in reported values between visits (≤ 20% = acceptable) and the Bland Altman limit of agreement index, a measure of how many outliers are present. Reliability was poor for the Wilcoxon signed rank test, a measure of how similarly ranked women are between visits, and the Bland Altman test for bias, which demonstrated a greater difference between reported intake between visits if the reported intake was higher. When examining the validity of the Choline-QFFQ compared with the mean of three 24-hour recalls, all group-level tests were acceptable-to-good, as were all individual level test results, except for classification into tertiles for the alcohol users for all comparisons conducted. Of note, the weighted kappa statistic for tertile classification was acceptable across almost all comparisons. The weighted kappa assesses agreement excluding chance and thus may provide a more accurate measure of agreement than the raw tertile agreement % measures.

Reliability and validity are measured separately, but results of the tests should be interpreted in light of each other. Although the QFFQ demonstrated both reliability and validity, tests of validity were more consistently acceptable-to-good than tests of reliability, particularly at the group level, as reflected in the Wilcoxon and Bland Altman bias tests, and the individual-level, when examining agreement as to whether a woman had inadequate intake. The relatively poorer reliability seen in these tests is likely due to the fact that women reported lower choline intake at each visit. This trend may reflect interview fatigue, as has been reported in several other studies [46]; after familiarization with the procedure, women may have chosen fewer cards from the QFFQ card sorting as a result of fatigue and/or a conscious attempt to shorten the interview. Indeed, reliability was better from visits 1-2 than 2-3, but this difference may also reflect the longer time period between interviews (8 weeks for visits 2-3 vs. 4 weeks for visits 1-2). An actual reduction in food and thus choline intake towards the end of the pregnancy must, however, also be considered. The mean energy intake per day decreased somewhat from each visit to the next (2294 kcal/day at visit 1, 2280 kcal/day at visit 2, 2194 kcal/day visit 3). As repeated administration of the QFFQ did not significantly improve validity the Choline-QFFQ screener could be used as a single-visit screener.

This study had limitations common to other longitudinal studies of nutrition. 24-hr dietary recall interviews can yield inaccurate estimates of usual intake due to recall errors. However, we have previously reported that intraclass correlations and within-subject coefficients of variation for dietary nutrient intakes in this cohort, including choline, were similar to those of NHANES and other peer-reviewed epidemiologic studies in the U.S. [23], indicating that random error in this study did not exceed levels generally accepted in the nutritional epidemiology community. Furthermore, we found that energy intake predicted gestational weight gain, further supporting the validity of the 24-hr recall data. Where possible, the method of triads, in which two dietary assessment methods and a biochemical marker of nutritional status for a given nutrient are compared, is recommended for validation of FFQs [46]. We did not employ this method because free choline and other choline metabolites are tightly regulated and relatively unresponsive to dietary changes, as homeostatic mechanisms, such as estrogen-induced endogenous choline production by the PEMT enzyme during pregnancy act to keep plasma choline values in the normal range; lack of correlation between diet and biochemical values is thus common, particularly in cohorts without high rates of severe choline deficiency [47, 48]. Differences between true and estimated levels of maternal alcohol consumption are likely small, given the validity of the interviewing techniques demonstrated in this community in relation to meconium levels of fatty acid ethyl ester metabolites of alcohol [49], infant and child behavior [7, 35, 50], somatic growth [51], and brain structure [52–54] and function [55].

## Conclusions

To our knowledge, this is the first quantitative choline food frequency screening questionnaire to be developed and validated for use in both heavy and non-drinking pregnant women and the first to be used in the Cape Coloured community in South Africa. Given the high prevalence of inadequate choline intake in this and other communities worldwide and the growing evidence that maternal choline supplementation may benefit infant neurodevelopment and can mitigate adverse effects of prenatal alcohol exposure, this tool may be useful for both research and for future clinical outreach programs aimed at identifying pregnant women at risk for choline deficiency. The Choline-QFFQ development and validation methodology we employed can be used in other communities as well, which may be of significant public health utility given the widespread public health burdens of dietary choline inadequacy and maternal alcohol consumption during pregnancy. Our findings demonstrating validity of the QFFQ for use in this highly disadvantaged, poorly educated population supports its potential utility for use in a broad range of social contexts.

### Abbreviations

AA: Absolute alcohol; FAS: Fetal alcohol syndrome; FASD: Fetal alcohol spectrum disorders; QFFQ: Quantitative food frequency questionnaire

### Acknowledgments

We thank Susan Fawcus, Head of Department of Obstetrics, Mowbray Maternity Hospital and the nursing and records department staff at the Hanover Park and Retreat Midwife Obstetric Units, Mowbray Maternity Hospital, Somerset Hospital, and Groote Schuur Hospital, where the women were recruited. We thank our research nurses Maggie September, Beverly Arendse, and Patricia O'Leary, and our research driver Patricia Solomon for their dedicated work on cohort recruitment, scheduling, and retention; our dietary interviewers Catherine Day, Monika Uys, and Nicola Cooper; and Renee Sun and our UCT and WSU research staff for their contributions to data collection and management. We also extend our deep appreciation to the mothers in the study for their participation and contributions to this study.

### Funding

This study was funded by grants from NIH/National Institute on Alcohol Abuse and Alcoholism (R01 AA016781, R21AA020332, K23 AA020516), NIH/National Institute of Diabetes and Digestive and Kidney Diseases (K24DK104676 and 2P30 DK040561), and the Lycaki-Young Fund from the State of Michigan.

### Authors' contributions

SWJ, JLJ, CPD, RCC, and CDM, conceptualized the original maternal choline supplementation study. RCC, MS, SWJ, and JLJ then designed the QFFQ study to document and quantify the dietary intake of choline by the pregnant women. MS, SB, and BN developed the QFFQ, and LJB reviewed the dietary records and held regular meetings with the dietary interviewers to address questions that arose. CDM and EMM coordinated and supervised data collection. RCC and MS conducted the data analyses and wrote the initial draft of the manuscript. NCD coordinated data management and assisted with statistical analyses. All of the authors reviewed, revised, edited, and approved the manuscript.

### Competing interests

The authors declare that they have no competing interests..

### Author details

[1]Institute for Human Nutrition and Departments of Emergency Medicine and Pediatrics, Columbia University Medical Center, 3959 Broadway, CHN-1-116, New York, NY 10032, USA. [2]Department of Psychiatry and Behavioral Neurosciences, Wayne State University School of Medicine, Detroit, USA. [3]Department of Psychiatry and Mental Health, University of Cape Town Faculty of Health Sciences, Cape Town, South Africa. [4]Department of Human Biology, University of Cape Town Faculty of Health Sciences, Cape Town, South Africa. [5]Division of Gastroenterology, Hepatology, and Nutrition, Boston Children's Hospital, Boston, USA.

### References

1. Hoyme HE, May PA, Kalberg WO, Kodituwakku P, Gossage JP, Trujillo PM, Buckley DG, Miller JH, Aragon AS, Khaole N, et al. A practical clinical approach to diagnosis of fetal alcohol spectrum disorders: clarification of the 1996 Institute of Medicine criteria. Pediatrics. 2005;115:39–47.
2. Hoyme HE, Kalberg WO, Elliott AJ, Blankenship J, Buckley D, Marais A-S, Manning MA, Robinson LK, Adam MP, Abdul-Rahman O, et al. Updated clinical guidelines for diagnosing fetal alcohol spectrum disorders. Pediatrics. 2016;138:e20154256.
3. ACOG. Committee opinion no. 496: At-risk drinking and alcohol dependence: obstetric and gynecologic implications. Obstet Gynecol. 2011;118:383–8.
4. Warren KR, Calhoun FJ, May PA, Viljoen DL, Li TK, Tanaka H, Marinicheva GS, Robinson LK, Mundle G. Fetal alcohol syndrome: an international perspective. Alcohol Clin Exp Res. 2001;**25**:202S–6S.
5. SAMHSA: Results from the 2009 National Survey on Drug Use and Health. Volume 1. Edited by SAMHSA. Rockville: Health and Human Services; 2010
6. Croxford J, Viljoen D. Alcohol consumption by pregnant women in the Western Cape. S Afr Med J. 1999;89:962–5.
7. Jacobson SW, Stanton ME, Molteno CD, Burden MJ, Fuller DS, Hoyme HE, Robinson LK, Khaole N, Jacobson JL. Impaired eyeblink conditioning in children with fetal alcohol syndrome. Alcohol Clin Exp Res. 2008;32:365–72.
8. Carter RC, Wainwright H, Molteno CD, Georgieff MK, Dodge NC, Warton F, Meintjes EM, Jacobson JL, Jacobson SW. Alcohol, methamphetamine, and marijuana exposure have distinct effects on the human placenta. Alc Clin Exp Res. 2016;40:753–64.
9. May PA, Blankenship J, Marais A-S, Gossage JP, Kalberg WO, Barnard R, De Vries M, Robinson LK, Adnams CM, Buckley D, et al. Approaching the prevalence of the full spectrum of fetal alcohol spectrum disorders in a South African population-based study. Alcohol Clin Exp Res. 2013;37:818–30.
10. Tran TD, Thomas JD. Perinatal choline supplementation mitigates trace eyeblink conditioning deficits associated with 3rd trimester alcohol exposure in rodents. San Diego: Society for Neuroscience; 2007.
11. Thomas JD, Abou EJ, Dominguez HD. Prenatal choline supplementation mitigates the adverse effects of prenatal alcohol exposure on development in rats. Neurotoxicol Teratol. 2009;31:303–11.

12. Jacobson SW, Stanton ME, Dodge NC, Pienaar M, Fuller DS, Molteno CD, Meintjes EM, Hoyme HE, Robinson LK, Khaole N, Jacobson JL. Impaired delay and trace eyeblink conditioning in school-age children with fetal alcohol syndrome. Alcohol Clin Exp Res. 2011;35:250–64.
13. Cheng DT, Meintjes EM, Stanton ME, Dodge NC, Pienaar M, Warton CMR, Desmond JE, Molteno CD, Peterson BS, Jacobson JL, Jacobson SW. Functional MRI of Human Eyeblink Classical Conditioning in Children with Fetal Alcohol Spectrum Disorders. Cereb Cortex. 2017;**27**:3752–67.
14. Jacobson SW, Carter RC, Molteno CD, Stanton ME, Herbert J, Lindinger NM, Lewis CE, Dodge NC, Hoyme HE, Zeisel SH, et al. Efficacy of maternal choline supplementation during pregnancy in mitigating adverse effects of prenatal alcohol exposure on growth and cognitive function: A randomized, double-blind, placebo-controlled clinical trial. Alcohol Clin Exp Res. 2018;42:1327–41.
15. Jacobson SW, Carter RC, Molteno CD, Meintjes EM, Senekal M, Lindinger NM, Dodge NC, Zeisel SH, Duggan CP, Jacobson JL. Feasibility and acceptability of maternal choline supplementation in heavy drinking pregnant women: A randomized, double-blind, placebo-controlled clinical trial. Alcohol Clin Exp Res. 2018;42:1315–26.
16. Zeisel SH, Niculescu MD. Perinatal choline influences brain structure and function. Nutr Rev. 2006;64:197–203.
17. Medicine Io. Choline. In: Dietary reference intakes for folate, thiamin, riboflavin, niacin, vitamin B12, panthothenic acid, biotin, and choline. Washington DC: National Academy Press; 2006.
18. Strupp BJ, Powers BE, Velazquez R, Ash JA, Kelley CM, Alldred MJ, Strawderman M, Caudill MA, Mufson EJ, Ginsberg SD. Maternal Choline Supplementation: A Potential Prenatal Treatment for Down Syndrome and Alzheimer's Disease. Curr Alzheimer Res. 2016;13:97–106.
19. Sweiry JH, Page KR, Dacke CG, Abramovich DR, Yudilevich DL. Evidence of saturable uptake mechanisms at maternal and fetal sides of the perfused human placenta by rapid paired-tracer dilution: studies with calcium and choline. J Dev Physiol. 1986;**8**:435–45.
20. Zeisel SH, Mar M-H, Zhou Z-W, da Costa K-A. Pregnancy and lactation are associated with diminished concentrations of choline and its metabolites in rat liver. J Nutr. 1995;125:3049–54.
21. McMahon KE, Farrell PM. Measurement of free choline concentrations in maternal and neonatal blood by micropyrolysis gas chromatography. Clin Chim Acta. 1985;149:1–12.
22. Caudill MA, Strupp BJ, Muscalu L, Nevins JEH, Canfield RL. Maternal choline supplementation during the third trimester of pregnancy improves infant information processing speed: a randomized, double-blind, controlled feeding study. FASEB J. 2018;32:2172–80.
23. Carter RC, Senekal M, Dodge NC, Bechard L, Meintjes EM, Molteno CD, Duggan C, Jacobson JL, Jacobson SW. Maternal alcohol use and nutrition during pregnancy: diet and anthropometry. Alcohol Clin Exp Res. 2017;41:2114–27.
24. Shaw GM, Carmichael SL, Yang W, Selvin S, Schaffer DM. Periconceptional dietary intake of choline and betaine and neural tube defects in offspring. Am J Epidemiol. 2004;160:102–9.
25. Jensen H, Batres-Marquez S, Carriquiry A, Schalinske K. Choline in the diets of the U.S. population: NHANES, 2003–2004. FASEB J. 2007;21:219.
26. Lewis ED, Subhan FB, Bell RC, McCargar LJ, Curtis JM, Jacobs RL, Field CJ, team AP. Estimation of choline intake from 24 h dietary intake recalls and contribution of egg and milk consumption to intake among pregnant and lactating women in Alberta. Br J Nutr. 2014;112:112–21.
27. Mygind VL, Evans SE, Peddie MC, Miller JC, Houghton LA. Estimation of usual intake and food sources of choline and betaine in New Zealand reproductive age women. Asia Pac J Clin Nutr. 2013;22:319–24.
28. Baranowski T. 24-hour recall and diet record methods. In: Willett WC, editor. Nutritional Epidemiology. 3rd ed. New York: Oxford University Press; 2013.
29. Glabska D, Guzek D, Sidor P, Wlodarek D. Vitamin D Dietary Intake Questionnaire Validation Conducted among Young Polish Women. Nutrients. 2016;8:E36.
30. Glabska D, Guzek D, Slazak J, Wlodarek D. Assessing the Validity and Reproducibility of an Iron Dietary Intake Questionnaire Conducted in a Group of Young Polish Women. Nutrients. 2017;9:E199.
31. Kim E, Kim M, Sohn C. Validity and Reliability of a Self-administered Food Frequency Questionnaire to Assess Vitamin K Intake in Korean Adults. Clin Nutr Res. 2016;5:153–60.
32. Jacobson SW, Jacobson JL, Molteno CD, Warton CMR, Wintermark P, Hoyme HE, De Jong G, Taylor P, Warton F, Lindinger NM, et al. Heavy prenatal alcohol exposure is related to smaller corpus callosum in newborn MRI scans. Alcohol Clin Exp Res. 2017;41:965–75.
33. Nel JH, Steyn NP. Report on South African food consumption studies undertaken amongst different population groups (1983 - 2000): average intakes of foods most commonly consumed. Pretoria: Republic of South Africa, Department of Health; 2002.
34. Steyn N, Senekal M. Dietary Assessment and Education Kit (DAEK) Photo Cards. Chronic Diseases of Lifestyle Unit, Medical Research Council: Tygerberg; 2004.
35. Jacobson SW, Chiodo LM, Sokol RJ, Jacobson JL. Validity of maternal report of prenatal alcohol, cocaine, and smoking in relation to neurobehavioral outcome. Pediatrics. 2002;109:815–25.
36. Agriculture UDo, Service AR, Laboratory ND. USDA National Nutrient Database for Standard Reference. Release 28 edition. Washington DC: USDA; 2016.
37. Lombard MJ, Steyn NP, Charlton KE, Senekal M. Application and interpretation of multiple statistical tests to evaluate validity of dietary intake assessment methods. Nutr J. 2015;14:40.
38. Kowalkowska J, Slowinska MA, Slowinski D, Dlugosz A, Niedzwiedzka E, Wadolowska L. Comparison of a full food-frequency questionnaire with the three-day unweighted food records in young Polish adult women: implications for dietary assessment. Nutrients. 2013;5:2747–76.
39. Hankinson SE, Manson JE, Spiegelman D, Willett WC, Longcope C, Speizer FE. Reproducibility of plasma hormone levels in postmenopausal women over a 2-3-year period. Cancer Epidemiol Biomarkers Prev. 1995;4:649–54.
40. May PA, Gossage JP, Kalberg WO, Robinson LK, Buckley D, Manning M, Hoyme HE. Prevalence and epidemiologic characteristics of FASD from various research methods with an emphasis on recent in-school studies. Dev Dis Res Rev. 2009;15:176–92.
41. May PA, Chambers CD, Kalberg WO, Zellner J, Feldman H, Buckley D, Kopald D, Hasken JM, Xu R, Honerkamp-Smith G, et al. Prevalence of Fetal Alcohol Spectrum Disorders in 4 US Communities. JAMA. 2018;319:474–82.
42. Otero NKH, Thomas JD, Saski CA, Xia X, Kelly SJ. Choline supplementation and DNA methylation in the hippocampus and prefrontal cortex of rats exposed to alcohol during development. Alcohol Clin Exp Res. 2012;36:1701–9.
43. Idrus NM, Breit KR, Thomas JD. Dietary choline levels modify the effects of prenatal alcohol exposure in rats. Neurotoxicol Teratol. 2017;59:43–52.
44. Shaw GM, Carmichael SL, Laurent C, Rasmussen SA. Maternal nutrient intakes and risk of orofacial clefts. Epidemiology. 2006;17:285–91.
45. Boeke CE, Gillman MW, Hughes MD, Rifas-Shiman SL, Villamor E, Oken E. Choline intake during pregnancy and child cognition at age 7 years. Am J Epidemiol. 2013;177:1338–47.
46. Willett WC, Lenart E. Reproducibility and validity of food-frequency questionnaires. In: Willett WC, editor. Nutritional Epidemiology. 3rd ed. New York: Oxford University Press; 2013.
47. Abratte CM, Wang W, Li R, Axume J, Moriarty DJ, Caudill MA. Choline status is not a reliable indicator of moderate changes in dietary choline consumption in premenopausal women. J Nutr Biochem. 2009;20:62–9.
48. Yan J, Jiang X, West AA, Perry CA, Malysheva OV, Brenna JT, Stabler SP, Allen RH, Gregory JF 3rd, Caudill MA. Pregnancy alters choline dynamics: results of a randomized trial using stable isotope methodology in pregnant and nonpregnant women. Am J Clin Nutr. 2013;98:1459–67.
49. Bearer CF, Jacobson JL, Jacobson SW, Barr D, Croxford J, Molteno CD, Viljoen DL, Marais AS, Chiodo LM, Cwik AS. Validation of a new biomarker of fetal exposure to alcohol. J Pediatr. 2003;143:463–9.
50. Lindinger NM, Malcolm-Smith S, Dodge NC, Molteno CD, Thomas KGF, Meintjes EM, Jacobson JL, Jacobson SW. Theory of mind in children with fetal alcohol spectrum disorders. Alcohol Clin Exp Res. 2016;40:367–76.
51. Carter RC, Jacobson JL, Molteno CD, Dodge NC, Meintjes EM, Jacobson SW. Fetal alcohol growth restriction and cognitive impairment. Pediatrics. 2016;138:e20160775.
52. De Guio F, Mangin J-F, Rivière D, Perrot M, Molteno CD, Jacobson SW, Meintjes EM, Jacobson JL. A study of cortical morphology in children with fetal alcohol spectrum disorders. Hum Brain Mapp. 2014;35:2285–96.

53. Fan J, Jacobson SW, Taylor PA, Molteno CD, Dodge NC, Stanton ME, Jacobson JL, Meintjes EM. White matter deficits mediate effects of prenatal alcohol exposure on cognitive development in childhood. Hum Brain Mapp. 2016;37:2943–58.
54. Meintjes EM, Narr KL, van der Kouwe AJW, Molteno CD, Pirnia T, Gutman B, Woods RP, Thompson PM, Jacobson JL, Jacobson SW. A tensor-based morphometry analysis of regional differences in brain volume in relation to prenatal alcohol exposure. NeuroImage: Clinical. 2014;5:152–60.
55. Woods KJ, Meintjes EM, Molteno CD, Jacobson SW, Jacobson JL. Parietal dysfunction during number processing in children with fetal alcohol spectrum disorders. Neuroimage Clin. 2015;8:594–605.

# 14

# Dairy intake revisited – associations between dairy intake and lifestyle related cardio-metabolic risk factors in a high milk consuming population

Ingegerd Johansson[1,2*], Lena Maria Nilsson[1], Anders Esberg[2], Jan-Håkan Jansson[3] and Anna Winkvist[4]

**Abstract**

**Background:** The association between milk and dairy intake and the incidence of cardiometabolic diseases, cancer and mortality has been evaluated in many studies, but these studies have had conflicting results with no clear conclusion on causal or confounding associations. The present study aims to further address this association by cross-sectional and longitudinal evaluation of the associations between exposure to various types of dairy products and metabolic risk markers among inhabitants in northern Sweden while taking other lifestyle factors into account.

**Methods:** Respondents in the Västerbotten Intervention Programme with complete and plausible diet data between 1991 and 2016 were included, yielding 124,934 observations from 90,512 unique subjects. For longitudinal analysis, 27,682 participants with a visit 8–12 years after the first visit were identified. All participants completed a validated Food Frequency Questionnaire. Metabolic risk markers, including body mass index (BMI), blood pressure, serum (S) cholesterol and triglycerides, and blood glucose, were measured. Participants were categorized into quintiles by intake of dairy products, and risk (odds ratios, OR) of undesirable levels of metabolic risk markers was assessed in multivariable logistic regression analyses. In longitudinal analyses, intake quintiles were related to desirable levels of metabolic risk markers at both visits or deterioration at follow-up using Cox regression analyses.

**Results:** The OR of being classified with an undesirable BMI decreased with increasing quintiles of total dairy, cheese and butter intake but increased with increasing non-fermented milk intake. The OR of being classified with an undesirable S-cholesterol level increased with increasing intake of total dairy, butter and high fat (3%) non-fermented milk, whereas an undesirable S-triglyceride level was inversely associated with cheese and butter intake in women. In longitudinal analyses, increasing butter intake was associated with deterioration of S-cholesterol and blood glucose levels, whereas increasing cheese intake was associated with a lower risk of deterioration of S-triglycerides.

**Conclusions:** Confounding factors likely contribute to the demonstrated association between dairy intake and mortality, and other medical conditions and analyses should be stratified by dairy type.

**Keywords:** Dairy products, Milk, Cheese, Butter, Fermented milk, Non-fermented milk, BMI, Serum lipids, Blood glucose, Blood pressure

* Correspondence: ingegerd.johansson@umu.se
[1]Department of Nutritional Research, Umeå University, Umeå, Sweden
[2]Department of Odontology, Umeå University, Umeå, Sweden
Full list of author information is available at the end of the article

## Introduction

The association between milk and dairy intake and the incidence of cardiometabolic diseases, cancer and mortality has been evaluated in a large number of observational studies, meta-analyses and gene based Mendelian randomization studies [1–3]. Many, but not all, of these studies showed a null or protective effect of dairy intake. However, most studies were carried out in countries with low milk consumption concurrent with a high prevalence of lactose intolerance. In this respect, Sweden represents contrasting environmental and genetic exposure. Here, milk consumption is frequent, and only 5–7% of inhabitants carry the lactose intolerant associated C/C allele of C/T-13910 (rs4988235) or G/A-22018 (rs182549) in the MCM6 gene, which regulates lactase production by the lactase-phlorizin hydrolase (LCT) gene [4, 5]. According to FAO food balance sheets, Sweden had the fourth highest per capita milk supply worldwide in 2013 with an average of 341.2 kg per year [6]. Consequently, Sweden offers a suitable setting for research on the impact of dairy intake on human health.

To date, nine observational studies on dairy intake and health have been carried out in Sweden [7–15]. Of these, five evaluated their association with cardiovascular diseases and confirmed the null or protective effect pattern for intake of total dairy foods, specific type of dairy products or fatty acid biomarkers 15:0 and 17:0 [7–11]. In contrast, recent studies in Sweden [12–15] found an association between increasing non-fermented milk intake and total mortality. In our study [14], we also demonstrated significantly higher total mortality in subjects with high butter intake, whereas high cheese intake was associated with lower total mortality.

Importantly, the dairy types non-fermented milk, fermented milk and cheese differ in fat, lactose and bioactive peptide content with potential health effects. The deleterious health effects of high fat diets have long been known; hence, low fat milk and dairy products have been promoted as healthy and nutritious by the Nordic Nutrition Recommendations and by international recommendations [16, 17]. Accordingly, intake of high fat milk dropped markedly in favour of medium fat options from 1986 to 1991 in Sweden [18]. However, in recent years, fat intake from milk and other dairy products has increased again in Sweden, likely reflecting the strong promotion of high fat diets in Swedish media for a period [19]. Further, lactose is degraded to free galactose in the intestine, and this degradation has been associated with oxidative stress and chronic inflammation in animals [20]. Notably, bacterial scavenging of galactose in the intestine is low as galactose metabolism is not favoured in the presence of glucose, which is the case after lactose degradation. Finally, bioactive peptides have effects on the microbiota in the gastrointestinal canal, inflammatory responses and cell signalling in the host [21]. In short, the effects on health-associated events likely differ by dairy type and fat content, which has been addressed in only a few studies comparing these factors to total dairy intake [22].

Does increased all-cause mortality concurrent with the consumption of non-fermented milk and butter represent a causal association or simply residual confounding by associated lifestyle factors? The present study aims to address this question by cross-sectional and longitudinal evaluations of the associations between exposure to different types of dairy products and risk markers for cardiovascular diseases in a large cohort of inhabitants in northern Sweden while taking other lifestyle factors into account.

## Subjects and methods

### Data source and study participants

Respondents in the Västerbotten Intervention Programme (VIP) and included in the Northern Sweden Diet Database (NSDD; http://www.biobank.umu.se/biobank/northern-sweden-diet-database/?languageId=1) were eligible for the present study. The VIP runs in the county of Västerbotten in Northern Sweden with approximately 260,000 inhabitants, out of which close to 121,000 live in the main city of Umeå. Residents are invited to receive a health examination at 40, 50 and 60 years of age and, for a period, some communities also invited 30-year-olds. Thus, 10- and 20-year follow-up data are available for a subgroup. Participants in the VIP undergo an extensive health examination, including anthropometric measurements, blood pressure, serum lipid profiles, and oral glucose levels before and after a glucose tolerance test, and they answer an extensive questionnaire on diet, lifestyle, health and life conditions. The average recruitment rate has been approximately 60% of available participants. Only very limited evidence of selection bias in relation to income, age and unemployment has been reported [23], and no difference was observed in cancer incidence in the VIP cohort versus in the general population of Västerbotten [24].

The basic database included 166,496 observations (51.3% women) from Jan 1st, 1991, to December 31, 2016. For the present study, observations were excluded if (*i*) the food intake recording was incomplete, i.e., ≥10% missing data and/or a missing portion indication, extreme (highest and lowest 1%) food intake levels (FIL; [18]), and extreme energy intake (lowest 1% and > 5000 kCal); (*ii*) age < 29 years or > 65 years, implausible height (< 130 or > 210 cm) or weight (< 35 kg) values, or BMI < 15. In addition, subjects who reported intake of serum lipid, blood glucose or blood pressure lowering medication, who have diabetes or who had been hospitalized for a myocardial infarction were excluded. The final study group included 124,934 observations, 90,512 of which were unique subjects (51.3% women and 48.7% men) from the first screening event between 1991 and 2016. The flow chart is shown in Fig. 1.

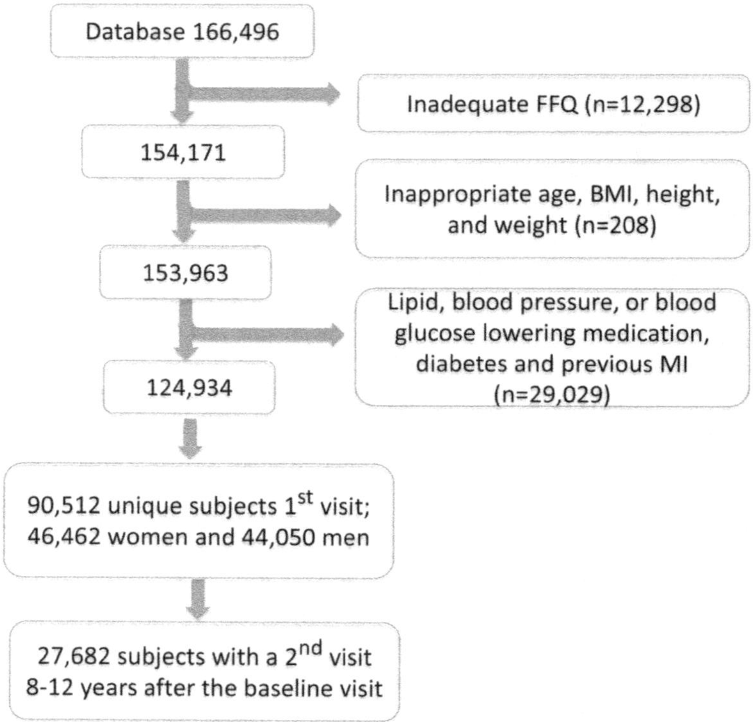


**Fig. 1** Study flow chart

### Dietary assessments

All participants completed a Food Frequency Questionnaire (FFQ) targeting their dietary habits, including beer, wine and spirits in the most recent year. Over the study period, two versions of the FFQ were used: a longer version (84 food items/aggregates) and a shortened version (64–66 food items/aggregates). The longer version, which was used until 1996, was completed by 31%, and the shorter version was completed by 69% of the participants at their first visit and 100% at follow-up visits. The shorter version was created by deleting and merging a few related food items. The questions about dairy products and beer, wine and spirits remained unchanged over the study period. In the FFQ, intake was reported on a fixed 9-level scale. Meal-time portion sizes were estimated with the support of four colour pictures of a plate containing increasing amounts of staple foods (potato/rice/pasta), main protein sources (meat/fish), and vegetables. For other foods, either sex- and age-specific portion sizes or fixed sizes, such as an apple or egg, were applied. Total estimated daily intake of energy (excluding energy from alcohol) and nutrients was calculated by weighting reported intake frequencies by food composition provided by the National Food Agency (https://www.livsmedelsverket.se/en/food-and--content/naringsamnen/livsmedelsdatabasen). Estimated intake of energy, nutrients, vitamins and minerals was previously validated against repeated 24-h dietary records and biological markers [25–28].

A diet score reflecting healthy eating habits was calculated based on rankings by sex and 10-year age groups of daily intake frequencies of four favourable food groups (fish, fruits, vegetables and whole grain foods) and four unfavourable food/beverage groups (red or processed meats, desserts and sweets, sugar-sweetened beverages and fried potatoes). The sum of all quartile ranks represents the Healthy Diet Score, which has a minimum of 0 and a maximum of 24 with higher ranks indicating healthier food and beverage choices [29].

Further, a Dietary Inflammatory Index (DII) was calculated as suggested by Shivappa and colleagues [30], but modified to fit the examined population [31]. The modified index was described previously [32].

### Assessment of metabolic markers

Body weight (kg) and height (m) were measured in participants wearing light clothes and no shoes, and BMI was calculated (body weight/height$^2$). Total cholesterol (S-cholesterol) and triglycerides (S-triglycerides) were analysed in serum at the health centres using a Reflotron bench-top analyser (Boerhinger Mannheim GmbH Diagnostica, Germany) in the earliest years and using an enzymatic routine method at the Clinical Chemistry Department at the nearest local hospital after Sep 1st, 2009. Measures by the Reflotron bench-top analyser were calibrated to measures by the enzymatic routine method using algorithms created from a calibration sub-study. In addition, high density lipoprotein (S-HDL, determined enzymatically after precipitation of other lipoproteins), and low density lipoprotein (S-LDL, estimated indirectly with the Friedewald equation) were determined for all participants from 2010 onward. An oral glucose tolerance test (OGTT) following WHO standards was performed with a 75 g oral glucose load [33], and blood glucose levels (B-glucose) were analysed before and 2 h after the test using a bench-top analyser. Systolic and diastolic blood pressures were measured after 5 min of rest.

Subjects were categorized as having normal weight or not (cut-off BMI ≤ 25), optimal total cholesterol levels or not (< 5.2 mmol/l), optimal triglyceride levels or not (< 1.7 mmol/l), optimal HDL levels or not (≥1 mmol/l), optimal LDL levels or not (≤3 mmol/l), or optimal fasting blood glucose levels or not (< 6.1 mmol/l), and optimal blood pressure levels or not (systolic blood pressure < 130 mmHg or diastolic blood pressure < 80 mmHg) [34].

### Assessment of potential confounding factors

Information on tobacco use (smoking and Swedish snus (snuff)), highest level of education, and physical activity in leisure time was collected from the questionnaires. Smoking and use of Swedish snus were categorized as never used, past daily or occasional use, or present daily or occasional use. For education, participants were categorized into four levels with academic education as the highest level, and for physical activity into five levels reflecting from inactive to active. Intakes of alcohol (gram/day), fruit and vegetables (servings/day), and non-alcohol energy were estimated from the FFQ.

### Statistical analyses

Respondents were categorized into quintile groups based on their reported intake (servings/day) of total dairy products, non-fermented milk, fermented milk, cheese and butter by ranking within sex and 10-year age strata.

Quantitative measures are presented as the means [95% confidence limits (CI)] after confirmation of normality by the Kolmogorov-Smirnov test. Means were adjusted for sex, age, BMI and screening year using general lineal modelling (GLM). Discrete variables are presented as frequencies and percentages. Differences between group means/numbers were not tested since large groups led to statistically significant differences even when the differences were interpreted as biologically irrelevant.

Bivariable logistic regression was used to calculate odds ratios (OR) and corresponding 95% confidence limits (CI) of having undesirable values for total S-cholesterol, S-triglycerides, S-HDL, S-LDL, fasting B-glucose levels and blood pressure using the cut-off values described above. These models were run separately for men and women. The crude model included dairy quintile and age (and for cholesterol and triglycerides, period of analyses, i.e., before or after Sept 1st, 2009). In the full model, education, physical activity, smoking, BMI (except models with weight-associated outcome), reported alcohol, fruit and vegetable and energy intake, and screening year were added.

Participants with a follow-up screening 8–12 years after the baseline visit and with data that met the quality criteria were identified ($n = 27{,}682$; Fig. 1). Subjects with a desirable value for total S-cholesterol, S-triglycerides, S-HDL, S-LDL, fasting B-glucose or blood pressure at baseline and whose levels remained desirable over the follow-up period and patients who had a desirable level at baseline and were classified with an undesirable level at follow-up were included for prospective risk analysis by Cox proportional hazards regression models. Time between visits was the underlying time metric to estimate hazard ratios (HR) with 95% CI for the associations between total dairy intake/dairy type and an impairment of the medical variables, i.e., having a desirable level at baseline and an undesirable level 8–12 years later. The models included quintiles of dairy intake, sex, age at follow-up, education, smoking, year at follow-up, BMI at follow-up, physical activity at baseline and follow-up, and mean intake of alcohol, fruits and vegetables and energy over the follow-up period. All baseline measures were made before Sept 1st, 2009, but follow-up partly occurred later and therefore models on impairments of cholesterol and triglyceride status included period of analysis as a covariate. Dairy product exposure corresponded to the mean reported intake over the follow-up period to account for eventual changes over the follow-up period. The proportional hazards assumption was assured by the Schoenfeld test [35].

Partial least square multivariate modelling (PLS) was used to characterize subjects who reported the highest versus lowest intake of butter products and subjects who reported exclusive consumption of high (3%), medium (1.5%) or low (0.5%) fat non-fermented milk. The models included all 66 FFQ items (except items used for calculating the respective dependent variables) as the block of independent variables. Circos plots were used to illustrate the food selection pattern for the respective butter and milk groups based on standardized mean intake of foods with a PLS loading value (VIP) > 1.00.

Statistical analyses were performed with SPSS version 25 (IBM; SPSS Software), SAS version 9.4 and SIMCA P+ (Umetrics, Sartorius Stedim Biotech). All tests were two-sided, and $P < 0.05$ was considered statistically significant.

## Results

### Characteristics of study participants by sex and age

Characteristics of the study participants (46,462 women and 44,050 men) are presented in Table 1. Every third to more than every second participant had an undesirable (untreated) blood pressure, S-cholesterol, S-LDL or BMI, whereas every 10th participant had an undesirable (untreated) fasting blood glucose level. A higher proportion of men than women had undesirable levels of serum lipids and blood pressure.

Generally, the intake of all dairy products increased by 10-year age groups and was higher in men than in women (Additional file 1). The difference was mainly driven by differences in high fat non-fermented milk and butter intake, whereas intake of other dairy products was more stable between the sexes and 10-year age groups (Additional file 1).

### Cross-sectional associations between dairy intake and cardiovascular risk factors

The OR to be classified with undesirable BMI, S-cholesterol, or S-triglycerides by dairy product intake are presented in Table 2 and are presented in Additional files 2, 3, 4 and 5 for blood glucose, blood pressure, S-HDL and S-LDL. In both women and men, the OR to be classified with undesirable BMI accounting for potential confounders decreased with increasing intake quintiles of total dairy product, cheese and butter, whereas it increased with increasing intake quintiles of non-fermented milk. The OR to be classified with undesirable S-cholesterol increased with increasing intake quintile of butter and total dairy products. Further, in women, the OR to be classified with undesirable S-triglyceride was inversely associated with intake quintiles of butter in women and men and cheese in women (Table 2).

Having an undesirable level of fasting B-glucose was inversely associated with intake quintiles of butter for men and cheese for women (Additional file 2). In both women and men, the OR for an undesirable blood pressure decreased with increasing intake quintiles of fermented milk (Additional file 3). Concurrently, the OR for an undesirable low level of S-HDL decreased with increasing intake quintiles of total dairy products, cheese and butter in men (Additional file 4). Finally, the OR to have undesirably

**Table 1** Characteristics for the 29–65 year old women ($n = 46{,}462$) and men ($n = 44{,}050$) at recruitment to the study

| | Women | | | Men | | |
|---|---|---|---|---|---|---|
| | N | mean (95% CI) or proportion (%) | % classified as undesirable | N | mean (95% CI) or proportion (%) | % classified as undesirable |
| BMI, kg/m$^2$ | 46,462[a] | 25.2 (25.2, 25.2) | 42.9% (BMI > 25) | 44,050 | 26.2 (26.1, 26.2) | 59.2% (BMI > 25) |
| S-Cholesterol, mmol/l | 46,293[a] | 5.55 (5.54, 5.56) | 60.8% (≥5.2 mmol/l) | 43,900 | 5.72 (5.71, 5.73) | 68.4% (≥5.2 mmol/l) |
| S-Triglycerides, mmol/l | 43,938[a] | 1.05 (1.04,1.05) | 2.0% (≥1.7 mmol/l) | 38,230 | 1.19 (1.18, 1.19) | 7.1% (≥1.7 mmol/l) |
| S-HDL, mmol/l[b] | 8,398[b] | 1.55 (1.54, 1.56) | 4.6% (< 1.0 mmol/l) | 8496 | 1.29 (1.28, 1.30) | 18.8% (< 1.0 mmol/l) |
| S-LDL, mmol/l[b] | 8,369[b] | 3.13 (3.11, 3.15) | 48.3% (> 3.0 mmol/l) | 8287 | 3.54 (3.52, 3.56) | 70.0% (> 3.0 mmol/l) |
| B-Glucose 0 h, mmol/l | 46,294[a] | 5.32 (5.31, 5.33) | 10.4% (≥6.1 mmol/l) | 43,899 | 5.40 (5.39, 5.40) | 13.2% (≥6.1 mm9 l/l) |
| Systolic blood pressure, mmHg | 46,101[a] | 121.2 (121.0, 121.3) | 21.8% (≥130 mmHg) | 43,783 | 126.6 (126.5, 126.7) | 30.2% (≥130 mmHg) |
| Diastolic blood pressure, mmHg | 46,082[a] | 75.5 (75.5, 75.6) | 24.7% (≥80 mmHg) | 43,766 | 79.5 (79.4, 79.6) | 37.8% (≥80 mmHg) |
| High blood pressure | 44,082[a] | | 31.1% (dbp or sbt ↑) | 43,766 | | 44.9% (dbp or sbt ↑) |
| Education, academic level, % | 46,195[a] | 35.7 | | 43,858 | 26.2 | |
| Smoking, present smoker, % | 46,105[a] | 21.0 | | 43,447 | 19.1 | |
| Swedish snuff, present user, % | 43,908[a] | 7.9 | | 42,631 | 27.8 | |
| Inactive at leisure time, % | 45,846[a] | 17.0 | | 43,433 | 17.7 | |
| Total fat intake, E% | 46,462[a] | 34.3 (34.2, 34.3) | | 44,050 | 37.8 (37.8, 37.9) | |
| Saturated fat intake, E% | 46,462[a] | 14.3 (14.2, 14.3) | | 44,050 | 16.0 (15.9, 16.0) | |
| Protein intake, E% | 46,462[a] | 15.2 (15.2, 15.2) | | 44,050 | 14.6 (14.6, 14.7) | |
| Carbohydrate intake, E% | 46,462[a] | 49.8 (49.8, 49.9) | | 44,050 | 46.5 (46.4, 46.6) | |
| Sucrose, E% | 46,462[a] | 6.56 (6.53, 6.59) | | 44,050 | 6.39 (6.36, 6.42) | |

Age adjusted means (95% CI limits) are presented for continuous variables and percent for categorical variables. Proportions (%) classified with undesirable levels are given with cut-off limits in parentheses

*Abbreviations*: *BMI* body mass index, *LDL* low density lipoprotein, *HDL* high density lipoprotein, *E%* energy in per cent of total energy

[a]Data were collected from 1991 through 2016 and represent subjects without serum lipid, blood pressure or blood glucose lowering medication and no self-reported diabetes or myocardial infarction

[b]Data are from 2010 to 2016 when HDL and LDL were estimated in all participants. Before 2010 HDL and LDL were performed at risk indications. In total, HDL was measured in 18,240 women and 18,915 men, and LDL in 11,520 women and 11,978 men. The differences between all measurements and those after 2010 in mean values or proportions with undesirable values were modest

**Table 2** Odds ratio (95% CI) from multivariable logistic regression by dairy food type

| | Sex | Crude model[a] | | | | Adjusted model[b] | | | |
|---|---|---|---|---|---|---|---|---|---|
| | | Q2 | Q3 | Q4 | Q5 | Q2 | Q3 | Q4 | Q5 |
| BMI | | | | | | | | | |
| Dairy products | W | 0.87 (0.82, 0.92)$^{<0.001}$ | 0.83 (0.78, 0.88)$^{<0.001}$ | 0.75 (0.71,0.80)$^{<0.001}$ | 0.70 (0.66, 0.74)$^{<0.001}$ | 0.89 (0.82, 0.95)$^{0.001}$ | 0.0.85 (0.79, 0.92)$^{<0.001}$ | 0.71 (0.66, 0.77)$^{<0.001}$ | 0.66 (0.61, 0.72)$^{<0.001}$ |
| | M | 0.87 (0.82, 0.93)$^{<0.001}$ | 0.80 (0.75, 0.85)$^{<0.001}$ | 0.71 (0.67, 0.76)$^{<0.001}$ | 0.71 (0.67, 0.75)$^{<0.001}$ | 0.87 (0.81, 0.94)$^{<0.001}$ | 0.0.82 (0.76, 0,89)$^{<0.001}$ | 0.73 (0.67, 0.79)$^{<0.001}$ | 0.72 (0.66, 0.79)$^{<0.001}$ |
| Non-fermented milk | W | 1.06 (1.00, 1.13)$^{0.044}$ | 1.03 (0.97,1.09) | 1.05 (0.99, 1.12) | 1.15 (1.08, 1.21)$^{<0.001}$ | 1.14 (1.06, 1.23)$^{0.001}$ | 1.06 (0.98, 1.14) | 1.20 (1.11, 1.30)$^{<0.001}$ | 1.25 (1.15,1.35)$^{<0.001}$ |
| | M | 1.08 (1.01, 1.14)$^{0.019}$ | 1.01 (0.95, 1.07) | 0.98 (0.92, 1.04) | 1.07 (1.01, 1.14)$^{0.028}$ | 1.11 (1.03, 1.20)$^{0.006}$ | 1.06 (0.98, 1.14) | 1.11 (1.03, 1.19)$^{0.008}$ | 1.20 (1.11,1.30)$^{<0.001}$ |
| Fermented milk | W | 1.05 (0.99, 1.12) | 0.98 (0.92, 1.04) | 0.91 (0.85, 0.96)$^{<0.001}$ | 0.91 (0.86, 0.97)$^{0.002}$ | 1.09 (1.02, 1.18)$^{0.017}$ | 1.08 (1.00, 1.17)$^{0.043}$ | 1.03 (0.96, 1.11) | 0.98 (0.91, 1.06) |
| | M | 1.04 (0.98, 1.10) | 0.98 (0.92, 1.04) | 0.87 (0.82, 0.93)$^{<0.001}$ | 0.78 (0.73, 0.83)$^{<0.001}$ | 1.04 (0.96, 1.12) | 1.07 (0.99, 1.15) | 0.96 (0.89, 1.04) | 0.92 (0.85, 0.99)$^{0.035}$ |
| Cheese | W | 1.00 (0.95, 1.06) | 0.84 (0.79, 0.88)$^{<0.001}$ | 0.81 (0.76, 0.86)$^{<0.001}$ | 0.69 (0.65, 0.73)$^{<0.001}$ | 1.04 (0.97, 1.11) | 0.88 (0.82, 0.95)$^{0.001}$ | 0.88 (0.82, 0.95)$^{0.001}$ | 0.71 (0.65, 0.77)$^{<0.001}$ |
| | M | 1.03 (0.97, 1.09) | 0.94 (0.89, 1.00)$^{0.059}$ | 0.83 (0.78, 0.88)$^{<0.001}$ | 0.80 (0.75, 0.85)$^{<0.001}$ | 1.03 (0.96, 1.11) | 0.93 (0.86, 1,00) | 0.87 (0.80, 0.94)$^{<0.001}$ | 0.90 (0.83, 0.98)$^{0.013}$ |
| Butter | W | 0.88 (0.83, 0.93)$^{<0.001}$ | 0.91 (0.86, 0.97)$^{0.002}$ | 0.82 (0.78, 0.87)$^{<0.001}$ | 0.68 (0.64, 0.72)$^{<0.001}$ | 0.82 (0.76, 0.89)$^{<0.001}$ | 0.84 (0.78, 0.90)$^{<0.001}$ | 0.75 (0.70, 0.81)$^{<0.001}$ | 0.60 (0.57, 0.65)$^{<0.001}$ |
| | M | 1.06 (1.00, 1.13)$^{0.060}$ | 0.99 (0.93, 1.05) | 0.78 (0.73, 0.82)$^{<0.001}$ | 0.80 (0.75, 0.85)$^{<0.001}$ | 1.03 (0.93, 1.08) | 0.85 (0.79, 0.92)$^{<0.001}$ | 0.71 (0.65, 0.77)$^{<0.001}$ | 0.72 (0.67, 0.78)$^{<0.001}$ |
| S-CHOLESTEROL | | | | | | | | | |
| Dairy products | W | 0.99 (0.93, 1.05) | 1.04 (0.98, 1.11) | 1.07 (1.00, 1.13)$^{0.045}$ | 1.12 (1.05, 1.19)$^{<0.001}$ | 1.05 (0.97, 1.14) | 1.10 (1.02, 1.19)$^{0.020}$ | 1.11 (1.03, 1.21)$^{0.011}$ | 1.20 (1.09, 1.31)$^{<0.001}$ |
| | M | 1.02 (0.96, 1.09) | 1.06 (0.99, 1.13) | 1.11 (1.04, 1.18)$^{0.001}$ | 1.07 (1.01, 1.14)$^{0.032}$ | 1.06 (0.98, 1.14) | 1.11 (1.03, 1.20)$^{0.007}$ | 1.16 (1.06, 1.25)$^{0.001}$ | 1.22 (1.11, 1.34)$^{<0.001}$ |
| Non-fermented milk | W | 0.99 (0.93, 1.06) | 1.01 (0.95, 1.07) | 0.95 (0.89, 1.01) | 1.01 (0.95, 1.07) | 1.02 (0.94, 1.10) | 1.00 (0.93, 1.08) | 0.98 (0.90, 1.07) | 1.00 (0.92, 1.09) |
| | M | 1.03 (0.97, 1.10) | 1.06 (0.99, 1.12) | 1.02 (0.96, 1.09) | 1.05 (0.98, 1.11) | 1.04 (0.97, 1.12) | 1.09 (1.01, 1.18)$^{0.029}$ | 1.10 (1.02, 1.19)$^{0.012}$ | 1.05 (0.96, 1.14) |
| Fermented milk | W | 1.01 (0.95, 1.08) | 1.01 (0.95, 1.08) | 0.92 (0.86, 0.98)$^{0.006}$ | 0.86 (0.81, 0.91)$^{<0.001}$ | 1.02 (0.95, 1.11) | 1.07 (0.99, 1.16) | 0.99 (0.92, 1.08) | 0.96 (0.88, 1.04) |
| | M | 1.07 (1.01, 1.14)$^{0.030}$ | 1.00 (0.94, 1.06) | 0.92 (0.87, 0.98)$^{0.015}$ | 0.81 (0.76, 0.86)$^{<0.001}$ | 1.12 (1.04, 1.21)$^{0.004}$ | 1.05 (0.97, 1.13) | 1.03 (0.95, 1.12) | 0.95 (0.88, 1.03) |
| Cheese | W | 1.00 (0.94, 1.06) | 1.05 (0.98, 1.11) | 1.11 (1.05, 1.19)$^{0.001}$ | 1.10 (1.03, 1.17)$^{0.004}$ | 1.01 (0.94, 1.09) | 1.04 (0.96, 1.12) | 1.09 (1.00, 1.18)$^{0.044}$ | 1.02 (0.94, 1.12) |
| | M | 1.11 (1.04, 1.18)$^{<0.001}$ | 1.07 (1.00, 1.14)$^{0.042}$ | 1.04 (0.98, 1.11) | 1.04 (0.98, 1.11) | 1.11 (1.03, 1.19)$^{0.008}$ | 1.05 (0.97, 1.13) | 1.02 (0.94, 1.10) | 1.01 (0.93, 1.09) |

**Table 2** Odds ratio (95% CI) from multivariable logistic regression by dairy food type *(Continued)*

| | Sex | Crude model[a] | | | | Adjusted model[b] | | | |
|---|---|---|---|---|---|---|---|---|---|
| | | Q2 | Q3 | Q4 | Q5 | Q2 | Q3 | Q4 | Q5 |
| Butter | W | 1.03 (0.97, 1.09) | 1.07 (1.01, 1.14)$^{0.024}$ | 1.16 (1.09, 1.23)$^{<0.001}$ | 1.21 (1.14, 1.29)$^{<0.001}$ | 1.09 (1.00, 1.18)$^{0.047}$ | 1.14 (1.05, 1.23)$^{0.001}$ | 1.20 (1.11, 1.30)$^{<0.001}$ | 1.31 (1.21, 1.43)$^{<0.001}$ |
| | M | 0.99 (0.93, 1.06) | 1.13 (1.06, 1.20)$^{<0.001}$ | 1.20 (1.13, 1.27)$^{<0.001}$ | 1.15 (1.08, 1.23)$^{<0.001}$ | 1.05 (0.97, 1.13) | 1.18 (1.10, 1.28)$^{<0.001}$ | 1.23 (1.14, 1.34)$^{<0.001}$ | 1.27 (1.17, 1.38)$^{<0.001}$ |
| S-TRIGLYCERIDES | | | | | | | | | |
| Dairy products | W | 1.01 (0.92, 1.10) | 0.95 (0.87, 1.04) | 0.93 (0.85, 1.02) | 0.93 (0.85, 1.02) | 1.07 (0.96, 1.20) | 0.96 (0.85, 1.08) | 0.85 (0.75, 0.97)$^{0.013}$ | 0.92 (0.79, 1.06) |
| | M | 0.96 (0.90, 1.03) | 0.94 (0.88, 1.01) | 0.89 (0.83, 0.95)$^{0.001}$ | 0.86 (0.81, 0.93)$^{<0.001}$ | 1.04 (0.96, 1.14) | 1.05 (0.96, 1.15) | 0.99 (0.90, 1.09) | 0.99 (0.89, 1.10) |
| Non-fermented milk | W | 1.00 (0.91, 1.10) | 1.03 (0.94, 1.13) | 1.02 (0.92, 1.12) | 1.19 (1.09, 1.30)$^{<0.001}$ | 1.06 (0.94, 1.19) | 0.98 (0.87, 1.11) | 1.00 (0.87, 1.14) | 1.06 (0.94, 1.20) |
| | M | 1.04 (0.97, 1.11) | 0.96 (0.89, 1.03) | 1.00 (0.93, 1.07) | 1.08 (1.00, 1.16)$^{0.039}$ | 1.05 (0.96, 1.14) | 1.04 (0.95, 1.14) | 1.09 (1.00, 1.19) | 1.11 (1.00, 1.22) |
| Fermented milk | W | 0.91 (0.84, 1.00)$^{0.041}$ | 0.88 (0.81, 0.96)$^{0.005}$ | 0.77 (0.71, 0.85)$^{<0.001}$ | 0.85 (0.78, 0.92)$^{<0.001}$ | 0.97 (0.86, 1.09) | 1.01 (0.90, 1.14) | 0.87 (0.77, 0.99)$^{0.031}$ | 0.97 (0.85, 1.09) |
| | M | 0.99 (0.93, 1.06) | 0.92 (0.86, 0.99)$^{0.028}$ | 0.84 (0.78, 0.90)$^{<0.001}$ | 0.72 (0.67, 0.77)$^{<0.001}$ | 1.04 (0.95, 1.13) | 1.04 (0.95, 1.14) | 1.03 (0.94, 1.13) | 0.95 (0.86, 1.04) |
| Cheese | W | 0.88 (0.81, 0.96)$^{0.003}$ | 0.86 (0.79, 0.94)$^{0.001}$ | 0.85 (0.78, 0.93)$^{<0.001}$ | 0.81 (0.75, 0.89)$^{<0.001}$ | 0.85 (0.76, 0.95)$^{0.003}$ | 0.91 (0.81, 1.02) | 0.87 (0.77, 0.98)$^{0.026}$ | 0.77 (0.67, 0.89)$^{<0.001}$ |
| | M | 1.01 (0.94, 1.08) | 0.96 (0.90, 1.04) | 0.85 (0.79, 0.91)$^{<0.001}$ | 0.87 (0.81, 0.94)$^{<0.001}$ | 1.04 (0.96, 1.14) | 1.00 (0.92, 1.09) | 0.93 (0.85, 1.02) | 0.93 (0.85, 1.03) |
| Butter | W | 0.84 (0.77, 0.92)$^{<0.001}$ | 0.82 (0.76, 0.90)$^{<0.001}$ | 0.83 (0.76, 0.91)$^{<0.001}$ | 0.80 (0.73, 0.87)$^{<0.001}$ | 0.88 (0.78, 0.99)$^{0.031}$ | 0.88 (0.78, 0.98)$^{0.025}$ | 0.86 (0.76, 0.97)$^{0.012}$ | 0.81 (0.71, 0.92)$^{0.001}$ |
| | M | 0.93 (0.86, 1.00)$^{0.038}$ | 0.98 (0.91, 1.05) | 0.90 (0.84, 0.97)$^{0.005}$ | 0.85 (0.79, 0.92)$^{<0.001}$ | 0.95 (0.87, 1.03) | 1.00 (0.92, 1.09) | 0.92 (0.84, 1.01) | 0.89 (0.81, 0.98)$^{0.017}$ |

*Abbreviations*: *W* women, *M* men

Odds ratio (95% CI) are from multivariable logistic regression for being classified with an undesirable level of BMI, cholesterol or triglycerides and increasing quintile groups (Q1 to Q5) for intake of dairy products. Q1, lowest intake, is the reference category. Statistically significant *p*-values are in superscript

[a]The crude models included age and dairy type

[b]The adjusted models also included screening year, education, BMI, physical activity, smoking, intakes of fruits and vegetables, alcohol and non-alcohol energy. The models with overweight did not include BMI, and models including S-cholesterol or S-triglyceride were also adjusted for if the analyses were performed before or after the change of analyses methods

**Table 3** Multivariable logistic regression by fat content of consumed non-fermented milk

| | Non-fermented milk | | | p-value |
|---|---|---|---|---|
| | 0.5% fat<br>n = 5237 | 1.5% fat<br>n = 25,667 | 3% fat<br>n = 5352 | ANOVA |
| OR (95% CI)[a] | | | | |
| BMI | 1.00 | 0.63 (0.58, 0.69)$^{< 0.001}$ | 0.52 (0.47, 0.57)$^{< 0.001}$ | |
| S-Cholesterol | 1.00 | 1.10 (1.01, 1.20)$^{0.025}$ | 1.13 (1.02 1.26)$^{0.026}$ | |
| S-Triglycerides | 1.00 | 0.96 (0.87, 1.08) | 0.90 (0.79 1.04) | |
| S-HDL[b] | 1.00 | 1.13 (0.84, 1.53) | 1.30 (0.92 1.83) | |
| S-LDL[b] | 1.00 | 1.22 (1.01, 1.46)$^{0.039}$ | 1.40 (1.12 1.74)$^{0.003}$ | |
| B-Glucose | 1.00 | 0.89 (0.79, 1.00)$^{0.042}$ | 0.96 (0.83, 1.11) | |
| Blood pressure | 1.00 | 1.04 (0.96, 1.14) | 0.92 (0.82, 1.03) | |
| Adjusted mean (95% CI) | | | | |
| BMI | 26.8 (26.7, 30.0) | 25.8 (25.8, 25.9) | 25.3 (25.2, 25.5) | < 0.001 |
| S-Cholesterol | 5.36 (5.32, 5.39) | 5.42 (5.41, 5.44) | 5.47 (5.44, 5.52) | < 0.001 |
| S-Triglycerides | 1.27 (1.25, 1.30) | 1.27 (1.26, 1.28) | 1.26 (1.24, 1.29) | 0.841 |
| S-HDL[b] | 1.42 (1.40, 1.45) | 1.43 (1.42, 1.44) | 1.43 (1.41, 1.45) | 0.872 |
| S-LDL[b] | 3.26 (3.19, 3.33) | 3.33 (3.31, 3.36) | 3.43 (3.38, 3.48) | < 0.001 |
| B-Glucose | 5.43 (5.40, 5.46) | 5.39 (5.37, 5.40) | 5.40 (5.38, 5.43) | 0.013 |
| Systolic blood pressure | 123 (123, 124) | 124 (123, 124) | 124 (123, 124) | 0.964 |
| Diastolic blood pressure | 77.7 (77.3, 78,0) | 77.7 (77.5, 77.8) | 77.4 (77.[illegible], 77.7) | 0.316 |
| Healthy Diet Score | 13.0 (12.9, 13.1) | 11.8 (11.7, 11.8) | 11.4 (11.3, 11.5) | < 0.001 |
| DII-score | 0.79 (0.75, 0.84) | 1.15 (1.13, 1.17) | 1.38 (1.33, 1.43) | < 0.001 |

*Abbreviations*: *BMI* body mass index, *LDL* low density lipoprotein, *HDL* high density lipoprotein, *DII* dietary inflammation index
OR (95% CI with statistically significant *p*-values in superscript) from multivariable logistic regression for being categorized with an undesirable level of BMI, cholesterol (total, HDL or LDL) or triglycerides and increasing intake of non-fermented milk of different fat content in subjects reporting exclusive consumption of one milk type. Low fat milk is the reference category. The lower section shows sex and age adjusted means for the same variables and scores for the Healthy Diet Score and the DII-score. S-cholesterol and S-triglycerides were also adjusted for if the analyses were performed before or after the change of analyses methods
[a]Fully adjusted models, including cheese type, sex, age, screening year, education, BMI, physical activity, smoking, intakes of fruits and vegetables, alcohol and non-alcohol energy, are presented. The models with overweight did not include BMI. Models including S-cholesterol or S-triglyceride were also adjusted for whether the analyses were performed before or after the change of laboratory analysis method. Interactions with gender was tested and found non-significant
[b]Subjects participating 2010 and later; n = 651, 5185 and 1141, respectively

high levels of S-LDL increased with increasing intake quintiles of butter in both women and men (Additional file 5).

### Cross-sectional associations between non-fermented milk types and cardiovascular risk factors

As a next step, we identified individuals who reported that they only consumed one type of non-fermented milk, i.e., milk with low (0.5%, $n = 5237$), medium (1.5%, $n = 25{,}667$) or high (3%, $n = 5352$) fat content. These individuals were categorized into regular consumers (≥1/day) or non-regular consumers (< 1/day but excluding those who never consumed the milk type). The OR to be overweight was significantly lower among both middle and high fat non-fermented milk consumers than among low fat non-fermented milk consumers. In contrast, consumers of middle and high fat non-fermented milk had significantly higher OR to have undesirable serum levels of total S-cholesterol and S-LDL than the low fat non-fermented milk consumers (Table 3).

In line with the results from the logistic regression, consumers of low fat non-fermented milk had the highest BMI but the lowest total S-cholesterol and S-LDL, and more favourable healthy diet and DII scores than the other consumers (Table 3).

### Cross-sectional associations between cheese types and cardiovascular risk factors

Individuals who reported consuming 28% or more fat containing cheese only ($n = 6805$) exhibited lower OR to have undesirable BMI, S-triglycerides but higher OR to have undesirable fasting blood glucose levels, than those who reported consuming cheese with 10–17% fat ($n = 9476$) only (Tables 4). Though statistically significant for most cardio-metabolic risk factors and the Healthy Diet Score, the differences for the adjusted means in consumers of 10–17% fat cheese versus 28% + fat cheese were moderate (Table 4). The exception was the higher score for the inflammatory index in high fat cheese consumers (Table 4).

**Table 4** Multivariable logistic regression by fat content of consumed cheese

| | Cheese | | p-value |
|---|---|---|---|
| | 10–17% fat<br>n = 9476 | ≥28% fat<br>n = 6805 | t-test |
| OR (95% CI)[a] | | | |
| BMI | 1.00 | 0.87 (0.84, 0.90)$^{< 0.001}$ | |
| S-Cholesterol | 1.00 | 0.99 (0.95, 1.03) | |
| S-Triglycerides | 1.00 | 0.95 (0.90, 1.00)$^{0.047}$ | |
| S-HDL[b] | 1.00 | 0.99 (0.89, 1.10) | |
| S-LDL[b] | 1.00 | 1.05 (0.98, 1.12) | |
| B-Glucose | 1.00 | 1.07 (1.01, 1.13)$^{0.030}$ | |
| Blood pressure | 1.00 | 0.97 (0.93, 1.02) | |
| Adjusted mean (95% CI) | | | |
| BMI | 25.7 (25.7, 25.8) | 25.4 (25.4, 25.5) | 0.001 |
| S-Cholesterol | 5.49 (5.48, 5.50) | 5.46 (5.44, 5.47) | < 0.001 |
| S-Triglycerides | 1.31 (1.30, 1.31) | 1.29 (1.28, 1.30) | < 0.001 |
| S-HDL[b] | 1.41 (1.41, 1.42) | 1.43 (1.42, 1.44) | 0.001 |
| S-LDL[b] | 3.33 (3.31, 3.35) | 3.35 (3.33, 3.36)7 | < 0.001 |
| B-Glucose | 5.36 (5.35, 5.36) | 5.34 (5.33, 5.36) | < 0.001 |
| Systolic blood pressure | 123.9 (123.8, 124.0) | 123.6 (123.5, 123.9) | < 0.001 |
| Diastolic blood pressure | 77.4 (77.3, 77.5) | 77.5 (77.4, 77.6) | 0.141 |
| Healthy Diet Score | 12.0 (12.0, 12.1) | 11.8 (11.7, 11.8) | 0.001 |
| DII-score | 0.87 (0.85, 0.88) | 1.19 (1.16, 1.21) | 0.006 |

*Abbreviations*: *BMI* body mass index, *LDL* low density lipoprotein, *HDL* high density lipoprotein, *DII* dietary inflammation index
OR (95% CI with statistically significant *p*-values in superscript) from multivariable logistic regression for being categorized with an undesirable level of BMI, cholesterol (total, HDL or LDL) or triglycerides and increasing intake of cheese of different fat content in subjects reporting exclusive consumption of one cheese type. Low fat cheese is the reference category. The lower section shows sex and age adjusted means for the same variables and scores for the Healthy Diet Score and the DII-score. S-cholesterol and S-triglycerides were also adjusted for if the analyses were performed before or after the change of analyses methods
[a]Fully adjusted models, including cheese type, sex, age, screening year, education, BMI, physical activity, smoking, intakes of fruits and vegetables, alcohol and non-alcohol energy, are presented. The models with overweight did not include BMI. Models including S-cholesterol or S-triglyceride were also adjusted for whether the analyses were performed before or after the change of laboratory analysis method. Interactions with gender was tested and found non-significant
[b]Subjects participating 2010 and later; *n* = 651, 5185 and 1141, respectively

#### Prospective associations between dairy intake and cardiovascular risk factor deterioration

Individuals with desirable BMI, S-cholesterol, or S-triglycerides, fasting B-glucose or blood pressure at their first VIP visit and who maintained or deteriorated their status to an undesirable level over the follow-up period were identified from the subgroup of 27,682 individuals with a follow-up visit after 8–12 years (Fig. 1). In this prospective evaluation, increasing butter intake was associated with a deterioration of S-cholesterol from less than to above 5.2 mmol/l and of B-glucose from less than to above 6.1 mmol/l (Table 5). Compared to the reference group (Q1, i.e., lowest quintile for butter intake), the adjusted HR (95% CI) increased consecutively up to Q4 (1.16 (1.03, 1.30), $p = 0.012$) with stagnation for Q5 (1.12, (0.99, 1.26), $p = 0.064$). The HR for having an undesirable B-glucose at follow-up was 1.24 ((1.03, 1.50), $p = 0.027$) in Q4 and slightly higher in Q5 than in Q1 (Table 4). Further, increasing cheese intake was associated with a reduced risk of having undesirable S-triglyceride values at follow-up than at baseline. Thus, the HR (95% CI) for the Q5 group with the highest cheese intake was 0.66 ((0.52, 0.83), $p = 0.001$) compared to the Q1 group (Table 4). No associations were found for non-fermented or fermented milk or total dairy product intake.

#### Characterization of subjects by reported dairy intake

To better understand the characteristics of the groups with different dairy intake, we evaluated their association with the scores from two diet indices that have been associated with health in other studies [29, 30]. These were the Healthy Diet Score with higher scores reflecting a healthier diet and an index reflecting the inflammatory potential of the diet (DII) with low scores reflecting a healthier diet. Overall, general linear modelling of sex, age, BMI and screening year adjusted means of the Healthy Diet Score increased with increasing intake of fermented milk and decreased for butter intake groups, whereas the DII score decreased consecutively with increasing dairy

**Table 5** Hazard ratio (95% CI) for developing an undesirable level of metabolic risk markers by dairy food type

| | Hazard ratios of adjusted model[a,b] | | | |
|---|---|---|---|---|
| | Q2 | Q3 | Q4 | Q5 |
| BMI | | | | |
| Dairy products | 0.86 (0.75, 0.99)$^{0.037}$ | 1.01 (0.88, 1.16) | 0.97 (0.84, 1.13) | 0.90 (0.76, 1.07) |
| Non-fermented milk | 0.92 (0.80, 1.05) | 0.95 (0.83, 1.09) | 1.00 (0.87, 1.15) | 0.92 (0.79, 1.07) |
| Fermented milk | 1.03 (0.90. 1.18) | 0.93 (0.81, 1.07) | 0.91 (0.79, 1.05) | 0.95 (0.82, 1.10 |
| Cheese | 1.01 (0.89, 1.15) | 1.04 (0.91, 1.19) | 0.98 (0.85, 1.13) | 1.00 (0.68, 1.16) |
| Butter | 0.99 (0.86, 1.15) | 0.97 (0.84, 1.12) | 1.00 (0.86, 1.16) | 1.06 (0.91, 1.23) |
| S-Cholesterol | | | | |
| Dairy products | 1.04 (0.93, 1.16) | 1.00 (0.90, 1.12) | 1.01 (0.90, 1.14) | 0.98 (0.86, 1.12) |
| Non-fermented milk | 0.99 (0.89, 1.09) | 1.01 (0.91, 1.12) | 0.96 (0.86, 1.07) | 0.92 (0.82, 1.03) |
| Fermented milk | 1.01 (0.91, 1.13) | 1.00 (0.90, 1.11) | 1.00 (0.89, 1.11) | 0.96 (0.87, 1.09) |
| Cheese | 1.01 (0.91, 1.12) | 1.03 (0.93, 1.14) | 0.97 (0.87, 1.09) | 0.92 (0.81, 1.03) |
| Butter | 1.08 (0.96, 1.21) | 1.13 (1.01, 1.26)$^{0.042}$ | 1.16 (1.03, 1.30)$^{0.012}$ | 1.12 (0.99, 1.26)$^{0.064}$ |
| S-Triglycerides | | | | |
| Dairy products | 0.93 (0.76, 1.14) | 0.93 (0.76, 1.14) | 0.85 (0.68, 1.06) | 0.93 (0.72, 1.19) |
| Non-fermented milk | 0.92 (0.75, 1.13) | 1.02 (0.83, 1.25) | 1.03 (0.84, 1.26) | 1.06 (0.86, 1.32) |
| Fermented milk | 1.19 (0.96, 1.45) | 0.97 (0.79, 1.20) | 0.96 (0.77, 1.19) | 1.01 (0.81, 1.25) |
| Cheese | 0.82 (0.68, 0.99)$^{0.034}$ | 0.95 (0.79, 1.15) | 0.85 (0.70, 1.04) | 0.66 (0.52, 0.83)$^{0.001}$ |
| Butter | 1.07 (0.86, 1.34) | 1.07 (0.86, 1.33) | 0.95 (0.76, 1.19) | 0.98 (0.77, 1.23) |
| B-Glucose | | | | |
| Dairy products | 1.10 (0.93, 1.30) | 0.85 (0.70, 1.02) | 1.02 (0.84, 1.23) | 1.11 (0.89, 1.37) |
| Non-fermented milk | 0.90 (0.75, 1.06) | 0.98 (0.82, 1.16) | 0.98 (0.82, 1.16) | 0.87 (0.72, 1.06) |
| Fermented milk | 0.92 (0.77, 1.09) | 0.90 (0.76, 1.08) | 0.89 (0.75, 1.06) | 0.87 (0.72, 1.05) |
| Cheese | 1.00 (0.85, 1.17) | 0.96 (0.81, 1.14) | 0.87 (0.73, 1.05) | 0.90 (0.74, 1.09) |
| Butter | 1.26 (1.04, 1.52) | 1.11 (0.92, 1.34) | 1.24 (1.03, 1.50)$^{0.027}$ | 1.28 (1.04, 1.56)$^{0.018}$ |
| Blood pressure | | | | |
| Dairy products | 1.03 (0.92, 1.15) | 1.03 (0.92, 1.15) | 0.98 (0.87, 1.11) | 0.99 (0.86, 1.14) |
| Non-fermented milk | 1.04 (0.93, 1.15) | 1.03 (0.93, 1.15) | 0.93 (0.83, 1.05) | 0.93 (0.82, 1.05) |
| Fermented milk | 1.06 (0.95, 1.19) | 1.07 (0.96, 1.19) | 0.99 (0.88, 1.11) | 0.93 (0.82, 1.04) |
| Cheese | 1.00 (0.90, 1.11) | 1.06 (0.95, 1.18) | 1.08 (0.96, 1.21) | 1.05 (0.93, 1.19) |
| Butter | 0.91 (0.81, 1.02) | 1.01 (0.90, 1.13) | 0.99 (0.88, 1.11) | 1.00 (0.88, 1.13) |

Hazard ratio (95% CI) for developing an undesirable level of BMI, cholesterol, triglycerides, blood glucose, or blood pressure over the 8–12 year follow-up period and increasing quintile groups (Q1 to Q5) for intake of dairy products. Q1, lowest intake, is the reference category. Statistically significant *p*-values are in superscript

[a]Crude models with sex, age and dairy quintiles were tested and HRs were not statistically significant. The adjusted models included sex, age at follow-up, education, year at follow-up, BMI at follow up, physical activity at baseline and follow-up, mean intake of fruits and vegetables and energy over the follow-up period and dairy group. The models with overweight did not include BMI, and models including S-cholesterol or S-triglyceride were also adjusted for if the analyses were performed before or after the change of laboratory analyses methods

[b]Q1, Q2, Q3, Q4, Q5 median values (servings/day) are for all dairy products 1.6, 2.8, 3.9, 5.1, 7.1; for non-fermented milk 0.08, 0.53, 1.0, 1.4, 2.5; for fermented milk 0.006, 0.16, 0.36, 0.78, 1.1; for cheese 0.14, 0.36, 0.78, 1.0, 2.5; and for butter 0.003, 0.15, 1.0, 2.5, 3.2

intake for all products except butter as shown in box plots for the quintile groups of dairy products (Figs. 2 and 3).

We also compared the food selection patterns by PLS modelling as illustrated in Circos plots for subjects who reported exclusive intake, illustrating that high fat (3% fat) non-fermented milk consumers choose saturated fat or sugar products, whereas low (0.5% fat) fat non-fermented milk consumers choose foods that are considered health associated (Fig. 4). A similar pattern was seen when comparing those with the highest versus lowest butter intake (Fig. 5).

## Discussion

The present study follows three independent cohort studies from Sweden in which a positive association between non-fermented milk intake and all-cause mortality was reported [12, 14, 15] with an unclear nature of the association, i.e., causal or due to confounding bias. Here, a

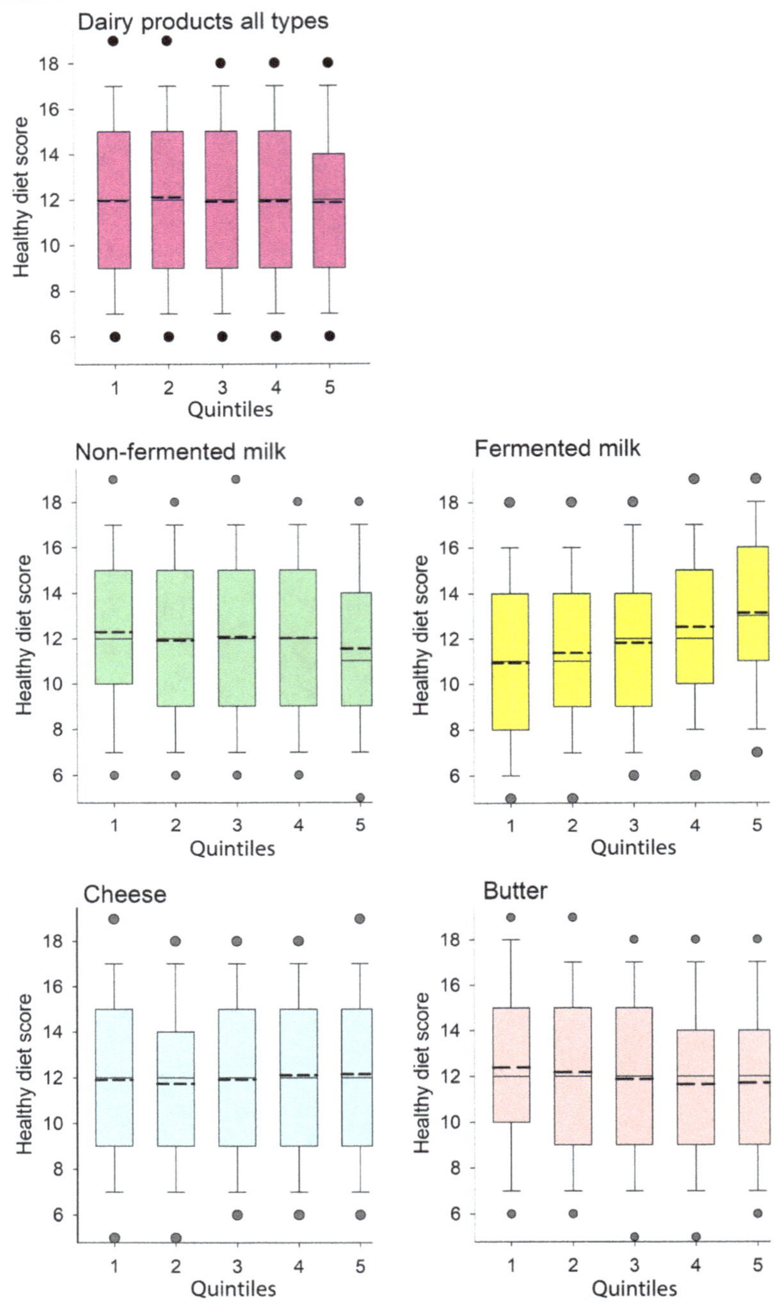


**Fig. 2** Healthy Diet Score by dairy intake. Box plots illustrating the median (straight line) and mean (dotted line) scores for quintile groups based on reported intake of total dairy products, non-fermented and fermented milk, cheese and butter. Whiskers represent the 25th and 75th percentile values, and dots represent the 5th and 95th percentile values

cross-sectional and longitudinal evaluation of associations between non-fermented milk and other dairy products and biological and lifestyle risk markers for cardiometabolic diseases [34] was performed in one of the three cohorts [14]. The study revealed an unfavourable profile of lifestyle factors in the present population, such as preference for butter, cream, sweet products, and use of tobacco products in high fat (3% fat) non-fermented milk and butter consumers. Further, some dairy products were associated with higher risk to have elevated cardio-metabolic risk factors, like BMI in high non-fermented milk consumers, and serum cholesterol in high consumers of total dairy products and butter, which, for butter, was confirmed in a prospective evaluation. These findings possibly support a contribution of

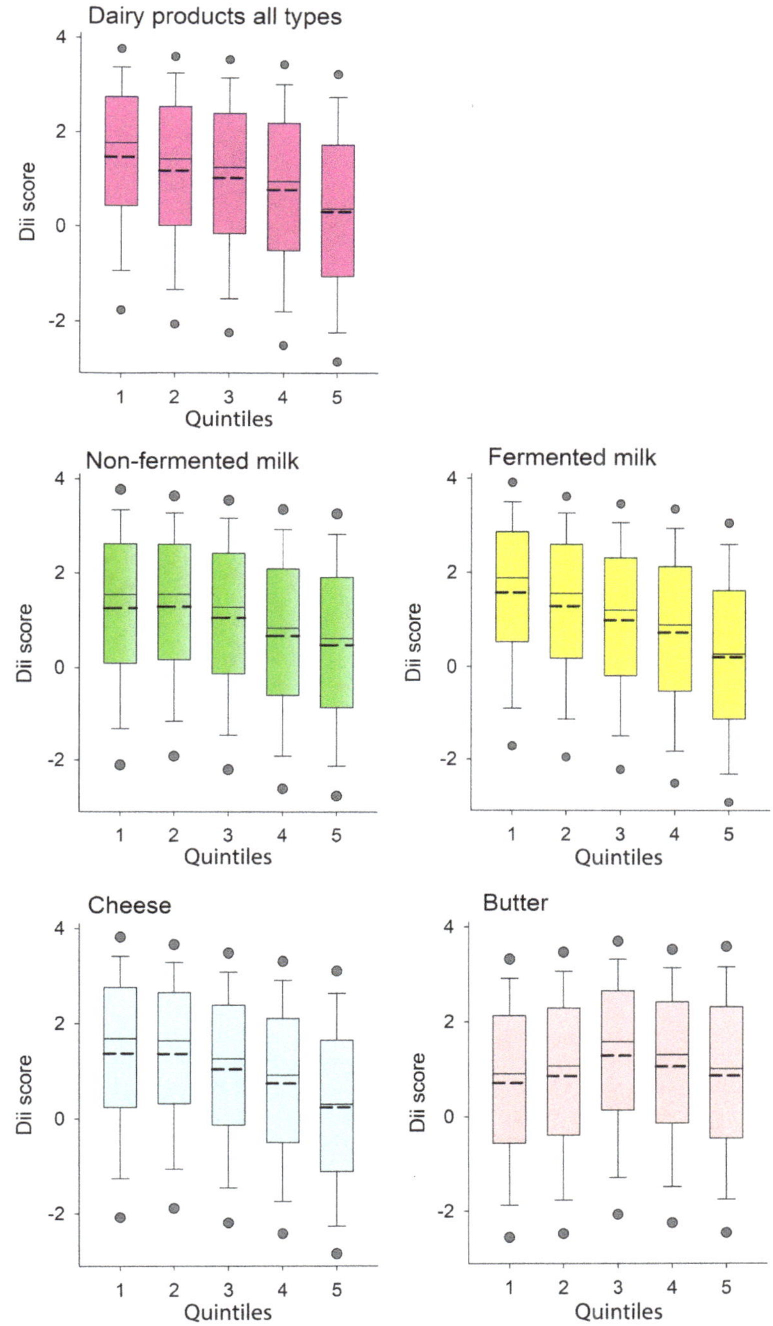


**Fig. 3** Diet Inflammation Index (DII) by dairy intake. Box plots illustrating the median (straight line) and mean (dotted line) scores for quintile groups based on reported intake of total dairy products, non-fermented and fermented milk, cheese and butter. Whiskers represent the 25th and 75th percentile values, and dots represent the 5th and 95th percentile values

confounding factors to the described association between total non-fermented milk intake and mortality in the same population [12, 14, 15].

In the present cohort, increasing reported intake of total dairy products and butter in both men and women and cheese in women was associated with decreased odds of having a BMI ≥ 25. Mean BMI was also lower in individuals who reported exclusive intake of high or middle fat non-fermented milk than in those with an intake of low fat non-fermented milk. These inverse associations have previously been reported in several cross-sectional studies [7, 36, 37]. However, Nordic and

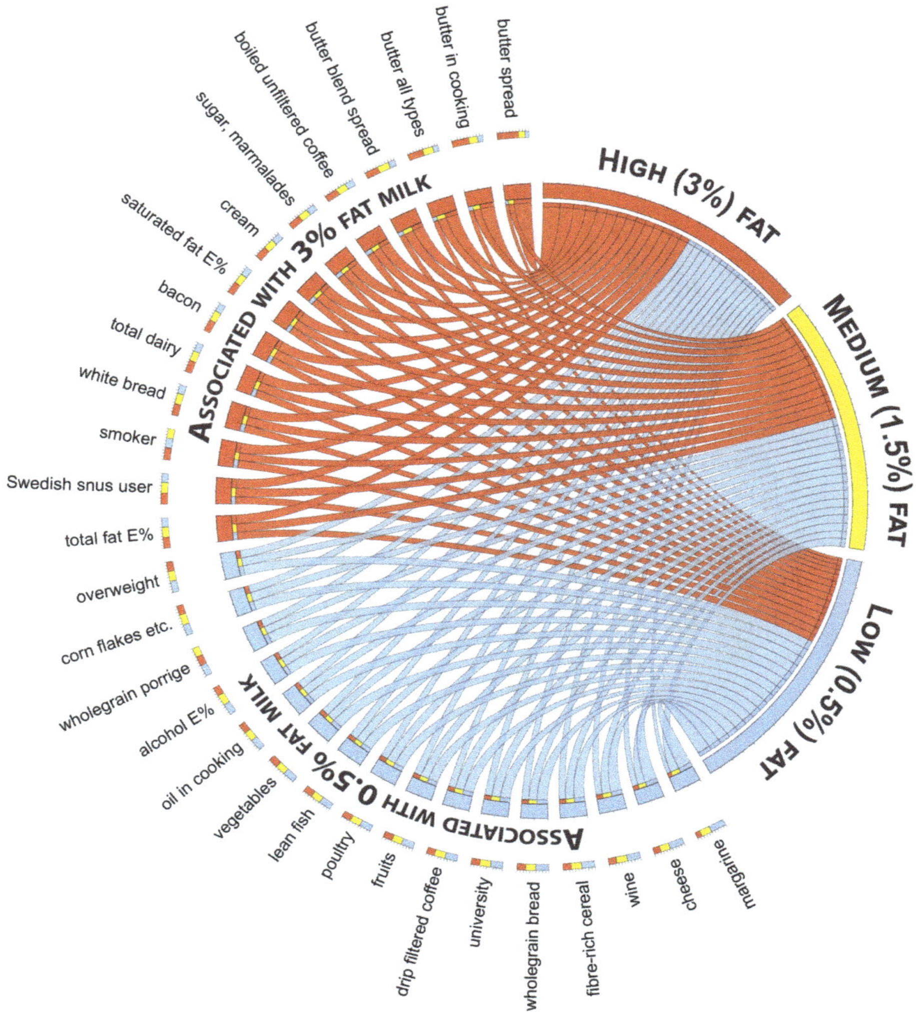


**Fig. 4** Circos plot for foods associated with non-fermented milk intake. The plot illustrates associations between cardiometabolic risk factors and sex, age, BMI, and reported energy adjusted intake of food items identified with a significant correlation with intake of non-fermented milk of different fat content. The lines illustrate the relationship between intake of high (3%) fat (red), medium (1.5%) fat (yellow), and low (0.5%) fat (blue) milk, respectively, and the outer circle reflects the proportion of the influential foods and cardiometabolic risk factors association with each of the three types of milk. Each food and cardiometabolic risk factor is color labeled as indicated above and sorted by strength of association to type of non-fermented milk consumed

international dietary guidelines recommend low fat dairy intake for weight control [16, 17] and encourage overweight subjects to favour low fat dairy foods. Thus, the identified association may reflect reversal causality, a hypothesis supported by the fact that consumption of all types of dairy food variants exhibited no association with weight increase when analysed prospectively over 8–12 years. Further, three large-scale studies using genetically determined dairy intake as an instrumental variable in Mendelian randomization found higher consumption of total dairy [38] or non-fermented milk [39, 40] to be associated with significantly increased odds for overweight/obesity, supporting a causal association between consumption of these products and higher body weight.

The trend analysis for intake of total dairy and specific dairy groups showed that the intake of butter products increased continuously from 2007 onward. This finding was paralleled by an increased intake of high fat non-fermented milk (3% fat), whereas the intake of lower fat alternatives decreased. This trend is likely a result from the fatty-diet supporting trend in Swedish media for a period [19] combined with the inherent palatability of fatty and creamy foods [41]. Notably, choosing butter and high fat non-fermented milk was also associated with a panel of other less healthy food choices and worse scores on both healthy diet and inflammatory diet indices. Based on the present results with increased odds of having undesirable cholesterol levels (total and LDL) and hazard

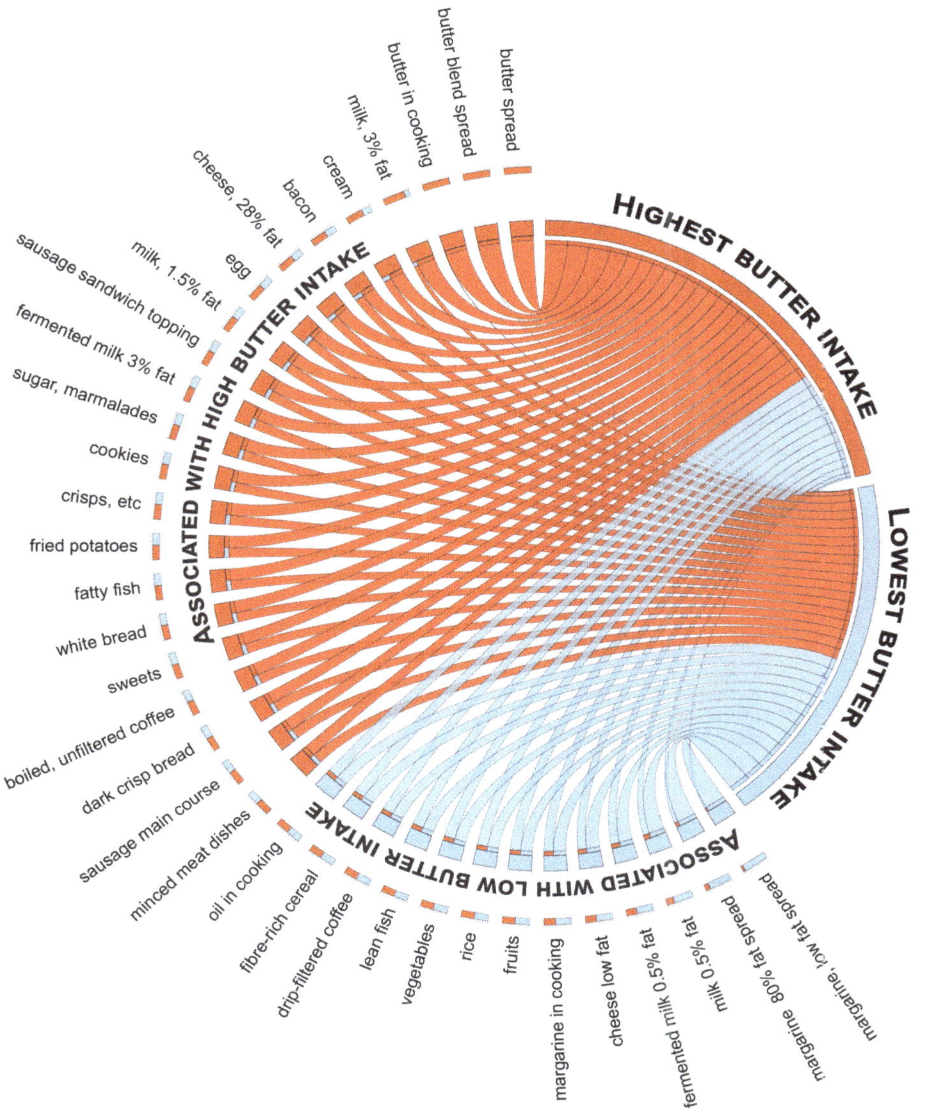


**Fig. 5** Circos plot for foods associated with highest or lowest butter intake. The plot illustrates associations between cardiometabolic risk factors and sex, age, BMI, and reported energy adjusted intake of food items identified with a significant correlation with intake of butter intake. The lines illustrate the relationship for those with the highest (red) versus lowest (blue) butter intake, respectively, and the outer circle reflects the proportion of the influential foods and cardiometabolic risk factors association with each of the butter intake levels. Each food and cardiometabolic risk factor is color labeled as indicated above and sorted by strength of association to butter consumption

of deterioration of S-cholesterol levels over a decade, this trend seems unfortunate, and the impact on disease development must be monitored.

The strengths of the present study relate to the large study cohort with cross-sectional and longitudinal data in a population that is genetically and culturally homogenous for most of the participants. This strength is manifested in that 75% of participants reported an intake of non-fermented milk at least every third day and that 99% reported an intake of any dairy product every day. However, we cannot exclude some selection bias since the respondents had to be able to visit their local health clinic during working hours. However, validation efforts have not found any evidence for systematic bias [23, 24], and the large cohort likely compensates for random errors to some degree. Further, the well-known risk for measurement errors in diet intake data also exist here. Finally, there is an evident risk of reversed causality for BMI and dairy intake in cross-sectional analysis as discussed above, and residual confounding cannot be excluded.

Though several recent studies using genes as proxies for milk or dairy intake do not support a causal association with cardiometabolic risk factors or medical emergencies [2, 3, 38–40, 42], causal contributions cannot be fully excluded [43] and should be a target for further studies. However, the present results and those from other publications, support that confounding factors likely contribute to, and possibly explain, the demonstrated association between high dairy intake and unfavourable medical outcomes in populations that are similar to the one studied, leaving counselling on a healthy lifestyle overall as valid as ever. Importantly, type of diary product should be evaluated separately in future studies as these likely have different biological impacts and are proxies for different lifestyle patterns.

## Conclusions

Confounding factors likely contribute to the demonstrated association between dairy intake and mortality, and other medical conditions reported in populations like the one studied and the results support that future analyses should be stratified by dairy type.

## Additional files

**Additional file 1:** Reported dairy product intake presented as servings/day among all 29- to 65-year-old women and men at their first visit to the health screening. The study population lived in northern Sweden and data were collected from 1991 through 2016. Data are presented as means (95% CI limits) adjusted for BMI, estimated non-alcohol energy intake and screening year. Differences between age groups were tested with ANOVA in the general linear modeling procedure, and means differed significantly for all variables, i.e. all *p*-values < 0.001.

**Additional file 2:** Odds ratio (95% CI limits) from multivariable logistic regression models for the association of being identified with an undesirable level of blood sugar (≥6.1 mmol/l) and increasing quintile groups (Q1 to Q5) for intake of dairy products. Q1, which represents the lowest intake, is the reference category. Statistically significant *p*-values are given in superscript.

**Additional file 3:** Odds ratio (95% CI limits) from multivariable logistic regression models for the association of being classified with an undesirable level of blood pressure (defined as diastolic blood pressure ≥ 130 or systolic blood pressure ≥ 80) and increasing quintile groups (Q1 to Q5) for intake of dairy products. Q1, which represents the lowest intake, was the reference category. Statistically significant *p*-values are given in superscript.

**Additional file 4:** Odds ratio (95% CI limits) from multivariable logistic regression models for the association of being classified with an undesirable level of HDL (defined as < 1 mmol/l) and increasing quintile groups (Q1 to Q5) for intake of dairy products. Data were collected from 2010 through 2016. Q1, which in the basic models represents the lowest intake and is the reference category. Statistically significant *p*-values are given in superscript.

**Additional file 5:** Odds ratio (95% CI limits) from multivariable logistic regression models for the association of being classified with an undesirable level of LDL (defined as > 3 mmol/l) and increasing quintile groups (Q1 to Q5) for intake of dairy products. Data were collected from 2010 through 2016. Q1, which represents the lowest intake, was the reference category. Statistically significant *p*-values are given in superscript.

#### Abbreviations

BMI: Body Mass Index; DII: Dietary Inflammatory Index; FIL: Food Intake Level; HR: Hazard ratio; kCal: kilo calories; NSDD: the Northern Sweden Diet Database; NSHDS: The Northern Sweden Health and Disease Study; OR: Odds ratio; S-Cholesterol: Serum cholesterol; S-HDL: Serum high density lipoprotein; S-LDL: Serum low density lipoprotein; S-Triglycerides: Serum triglycerides; VIP: Västerbotten Intervention Program

#### Acknowledgements

The authors want to acknowledge professor Göran Hallmans for initiating and creating NSHDS, teams at Västerbotten County Council for collecting data and the organizing VIP, and the personnel at the Department of Biobank Research, Umeå University for data maintenance and administrative support.

#### Funding

The Northern Sweden Diet Database was supported by the Swedish Research Council for Health, Working Life and Welfare (FORTE) and Vetenskapsrådet (the Swedish Research Council). The present study was supported by the Swedish Research Council for Health, Working Life and Welfare (FORTE).

#### Authors' contributions

IJ and AW designed the project; IJ analysed the data; IJ and AW drafted the manuscript; JHJ contributed special medical interpretation of the results and LMN, AE, AW and IJ contributed interpretation of other aspects; All authors participated in manuscript revision and all approved the final manuscript.

#### Competing interests

The authors declare that they have no competing interests.

#### Author details

[1]Department of Nutritional Research, Umeå University, Umeå, Sweden. [2]Department of Odontology, Umeå University, Umeå, Sweden. [3]Department of Public Health and Clinical Medicine, Research Unit Skellefteå, Umeå University, Umeå, Sweden. [4]Department of Internal Medicine and Clinical Nutrition, Sahlgrenska Academy, University of Gothenburg, Gothenburg, Sweden.

#### References

1. Larsson SC, Crippa A, Orsini N, Wolk A, Michaelsson K. Milk consumption and mortality from all causes, cardiovascular disease, and Cancer: a systematic review and meta-analysis. Nutrients. 2015;7:7749–63. https://doi.org/10.3390/nu7095363.
2. Bergholdt HK, Nordestgaard BG, Varbo A, Ellervik C. Milk intake is not associated with ischaemic heart disease in observational or Mendelian randomization analyses in 98,529 Danish adults. Int J Epidemiol. 2015;44:587–603. https://doi.org/10.1093/ije/dyv109.
3. Bergholdt HKM, Nordestgaard BG, Varbo A, Ellervik C. Lactase persistence, milk intake, and mortality in the Danish general population: a Mendelian randomization study. Eur J Epidemiol. 2017. https://doi.org/10.1007/s10654-017-0328-x.
4. Olds LC, Sibley E. Lactase persistence DNA variant enhances lactase promoter activity in vitro: functional role as a cis regulatory element. Hum Mol Genet. 2003;12:2333–40. https://doi.org/10.1093/hmg/ddg244.
5. Kuokkanen M, Enattah NS, Oksanen A, Savilahti E, Orpana A, Jarvela I. Transcriptional regulation of the lactase-phlorizin hydrolase gene by polymorphisms associated with adult-type hypolactasia. Gut. 2003;52:647–52.

6. Food balance sheets [http://www.fao.org/faostat/en/#data/FBS]. Accessed 6 Feb 2018.
7. Larsson SC, Virtamo J, Wolk A. Dairy consumption and risk of stroke in Swedish women and men. Stroke. 2012;43:1775–80. https://doi.org/10.1161/strokeaha.111.641944.
8. Patterson E, Larsson SC, Wolk A, Akesson A. Association between dairy food consumption and risk of myocardial infarction in women differs by type of dairy food. J Nutr. 2013;143:74–9. https://doi.org/10.3945/jn.112.166330.
9. Warensjö E, Smedman A, Stegmayr B, Hallmans G, Weinehall L, Vessby B, Johansson I. Stroke and plasma markers of milk fat intake--a prospective nested case-control study. Nutr J. 2009;8:21. https://doi.org/10.1186/1475-2891-8-21.
10. Warensjö E, Jansson JH, Cederholm T, Boman K, Eliasson M, Hallmans G, Johansson I, Sjogren P. Biomarkers of milk fat and the risk of myocardial infarction in men and women: a prospective, matched case-control study. Am J Clin Nutr. 2010;92:194–202. https://doi.org/10.3945/ajcn.2009.29054.
11. Sonestedt E, Wirfalt E, Wallstrom P, Gullberg B, Orho-Melander M, Hedblad B. Dairy products and its association with incidence of cardiovascular disease: the Malmo diet and cancer cohort. Eur J Epidemiol. 2011;26:609–18. https://doi.org/10.1007/s10654-011-9589-y.
12. Michaëlsson K, Wolk A, Langenskiold S, Basu S, Warensjo Lemming E, Melhus H, Byberg L. Milk intake and risk of mortality and fractures in women and men: cohort studies. BMJ. 2014;349:g6015. https://doi.org/10.1136/bmj.g6015.
13. Michaëlsson K, Wolk A, Melhus H, Milk BL. Fruit and vegetable, and Total antioxidant intakes in relation to mortality rates: cohort studies in women and men. Am J Epidemiol. 2017;185:345–61. https://doi.org/10.1093/aje/kww124.
14. Tognon G, Nilsson LM, Shungin D, Lissner L, Jansson JH, Renstrom F, Wennberg M, Winkvist A, Johansson I. Nonfermented milk and other dairy products: associations with all-cause mortality. Am J Clin Nutr. 2017;105:1502–11. https://doi.org/10.3945/ajcn.116.140798.
15. Tognon G, Rothenberg E, Petrolo M, Sundh V, Lissner L. Dairy product intake and mortality in a cohort of 70-year-old swedes: a contribution to the Nordic diet discussion. Eur J Nutr. 2017. https://doi.org/10.1007/s00394-017-1556-2.
16. Nordic Council of Ministers. Nordic nutrition recommendations 2012 : integrating nutrition and physical activity: Nordic Council of Ministers; 2014. p. 627.
17. Sacks FM, Lichtenstein AH, Wu JHY, Appel LJ, Creager MA, Kris-Etherton PM, Miller M, Rimm EB, Rudel LL, Robinson JG, et al. Dietary fats and cardiovascular disease: a presidential advisory from the American Heart Association. Circulation. 2017;136:e1–e23. https://doi.org/10.1161/cir.0000000000000510.
18. Johansson I, Nilsson LM, Stegmayr B, Boman K, Hallmans G, Winkvist A. Associations among 25-year trends in diet, cholesterol and BMI from 140,000 observations in men and women in northern Sweden. Nutr J. 2012;11:40. https://doi.org/10.1186/1475-2891-11-40.
19. Mann J, Nye ER. Fad diets in Sweden, of all places. Lancet. 2009;374:767–9. https://doi.org/10.1016/s0140-6736(09)61575-0.
20. Hao L, Huang H, Gao J, Marshall C, Chen Y, Xiao M. The influence of gender, age and treatment time on brain oxidative stress and memory impairment induced by D-galactose in mice. Neurosci Lett. 2014;571:45–9. https://doi.org/10.1016/j.neulet.2014.04.038.
21. Chakrabarti S, Jahandideh F, Wu J. Food-derived bioactive peptides on inflammation and oxidative stress. Biomed Res Int. 2014;2014:608979. https://doi.org/10.1155/2014/608979.
22. de Goede J, Soedamah-Muthu SS, Pan A, Gijsbers L, Geleijnse JM. Dairy consumption and risk of stroke: a systematic review and updated dose-response meta-analysis of prospective cohort studies. J Am Heart Assoc. 2016;5. https://doi.org/10.1161/jaha.115.002787.
23. Weinehall L, Hallgren CG, Westman G, Janlert U, Wall S. Reduction of selection bias in primary prevention of cardiovascular disease through involvement of primary health care. Scand J Prim Health Care. 1998;16:171–6.
24. Pukkala E, Andersen A, Berglund G, Gislefoss R, Gudnason V, Hallmans G, Jellum E, Jousilahti P, Knekt P, Koskela P, et al. Nordic biological specimen banks as basis for studies of cancer causes and control--more than 2 million sample donors, 25 million person years and 100,000 prospective cancers. Acta Oncol. 2007;46:286–307. https://doi.org/10.1080/02841860701203545.
25. Johansson I, Hallmans G, Wikman A, Biessy C, Riboli E, Kaaks R. Validation and calibration of food-frequency questionnaire measurements in the northern Sweden health and disease cohort. Public Health Nutr. 2002;5:487–96. https://doi.org/10.1079/PHNPHN2001315S136898000200068X [pii].
26. Johansson I, Van Guelpen B, Hultdin J, Johansson M, Hallmans G, Stattin P. Validity of food frequency questionnaire estimated intakes of folate and other B vitamins in a region without folic acid fortification. Eur J Clin Nutr. 2010;64:905–13. https://doi.org/10.1038/ejcn.2010.80.
27. Wennberg M, Vessby B, Johansson I. Evaluation of relative intake of fatty acids according to the northern Sweden FFQ with fatty acid levels in erythrocyte membranes as biomarkers. Public Health Nutr. 2009;12:1477–84. https://doi.org/10.1017/S1368980008004503.
28. Klingberg S, Winkvist A, Hallmans G, Johansson I. Evaluation of plant sterol intake estimated with the northern Sweden FFQ. Public Health Nutr. 2013;16:460–7. https://doi.org/10.1017/s1368980012003151.
29. Nettleton JA, Hivert MF, Lemaitre RN, McKeown NM, Mozaffarian D, Tanaka T, Wojczynski MK, Hruby A, Djousse L, Ngwa JS, et al. Meta-analysis investigating associations between healthy diet and fasting glucose and insulin levels and modification by loci associated with glucose homeostasis in data from 15 cohorts. Am J Epidemiol. 2013;177:103–15. https://doi.org/10.1093/aje/kws297.
30. Shivappa N, Steck SE, Hurley TG, Hussey JR, Hebert JR. Designing and developing a literature-derived, population-based dietary inflammatory index. Public Health Nutr. 2014;17:1689–96. https://doi.org/10.1017/s1368980013002115.
31. Bodén S, Wennberg M, Van Guelpen B, Johansson I, Lindahl B, Andersson J, Shivappa N, Hebert JR, Nilsson LM. Dietary inflammatory index and risk of first myocardial infarction : a prospective population-based study. Nutr J. 2017;16. https://doi.org/10.1186/s12937-017-0243-8.
32. Winkvist A, Klingberg S, Nilsson LM, Wennberg M, Renstrom F, Hallmans G, Boman K, Johansson I. Longitudinal 10-year changes in dietary intake and associations with cardio-metabolic risk factors in the northern Sweden health and disease study. Nutr J. 2017;16:20. https://doi.org/10.1186/s12937-017-0241-x.
33. WHO. Definition and diagnosis of diabetes mellitus and intermediate hyperglycaemia : report of a WHO/IDF consultation / World Health Organization, international diabetes federation. Geneva: World Health Organization; 2006. p. 46.
34. Graham I, Atar D, Borch-Johnsen K, Boysen G, Burell G, Cifkova R, Dallongeville J, De Backer G, Ebrahim S, Gjelsvik B, et al. European guidelines on cardiovascular disease prevention in clinical practice: executive summary. Atherosclerosis. 2007;194:1–45. https://doi.org/10.1016/j.atherosclerosis.2007.08.024.
35. Schoenfeld D. Chi-squared goodness-of-fit tests for the proportional hazards regression model. Biometrika. 1980;67:145–53. https://doi.org/10.2307/2335327.
36. Romaguera D, Angquist L, Du H, Jakobsen MU, Forouhi NG, Halkjaer J, Feskens EJ, van der AD, Masala G, Steffen A, et al. Food composition of the diet in relation to changes in waist circumference adjusted for body mass index. PLoS One. 2011;6:e23384. https://doi.org/10.1371/journal.pone.0023384.
37. Beydoun MA, Gary TL, Caballero BH, Lawrence RS, Cheskin LJ, Wang Y. Ethnic differences in dairy and related nutrient consumption among US adults and their association with obesity, central obesity, and the metabolic syndrome. Am J Clin Nutr. 2008;87:1914–25.
38. Mendelian Randomization of Dairy Consumption Working Group. Dairy consumption and body mass index among adults: Mendelian randomization analysis of 184802 individuals from 25 studies. Clin Chem. 2018;64:183–91. https://doi.org/10.1373/clinchem.2017.280701.
39. Hartwig FP, Horta BL, Smith GD, de Mola CL, Victora CG. Association of lactase persistence genotype with milk consumption, obesity and blood pressure: a Mendelian randomization study in the 1982 Pelotas (Brazil) birth cohort, with a systematic review and meta-analysis. Int J Epidemiol. 2016;45:1573–87. https://doi.org/10.1093/ije/dyw074.
40. Bergholdt HK, Nordestgaard BG, Ellervik C. Milk intake is not associated with low risk of diabetes or overweight-obesity: a Mendelian randomization study in 97,811 Danish individuals. Am J Clin Nutr. 2015;102:487–96. https://doi.org/10.3945/ajcn.114.105049.
41. Manabe Y, Matsumura S, Fushiki T. Frontiers in neuroscience preference for high-fat food in animals. In: Montmayeur JP, le Coutre J, editors. Fat

detection: taste, texture, and post ingestive effects. Boca Raton: CRC Press/ Taylor & Francis Taylor & Francis Group, LLC; 2010.

42. Ding M, Huang T, Bergholdt HK, Nordestgaard BG, Ellervik C, Qi L. Dairy consumption, systolic blood pressure, and risk of hypertension: Mendelian randomization study. BMJ. 2017;356:j1000. https://doi.org/10.1136/bmj.j1000.
43. Timpson NJ. Commentary: one size fits all: are there standard rules for the use of genetic instruments in Mendelian randomization? Int J Epidemiol. 2016;45:1617–8. https://doi.org/10.1093/ije/dyw197.

# 15

# Co-morbidity, treatment outcomes and factors affecting the recovery rate of under-five children with severe acute malnutrition admitted in selected hospitals from Ethiopia

Behailu Derseh*, Kalayu Mruts, Takele Demie and Tesfay Gebremariam

**Abstract**

**Background:** In spite of the availability of guidelines for the management of severe acute malnutrition (SAM) in Ethiopia, high comorbidity and poor treatment outcomes are still observed in therapeutic feeding centers among under -five children with SAM. The aim of this study was to assess comorbidity, treatment outcomes and factors affecting the recovery rate of children aged 1–59 months with SAM admitted into Therapeutic Feeding Centers (TFCs).

**Methods:** A total of 413 records of children with SAM admitted in three selected hospitals from July 2013 to July 2015 G.C were retrospectively reviewed. Descriptive analysis was used to compare performance indicator values with SPHERE project reference standards (the minimum standard to be attained during nutritional therapy). Cox-proportional hazard regression analysis was performed to estimate the predictors of recovery rate at $p$-value < 0.05.

**Result:** The mean age of children was 16 months (95% CI, 15.0, 17.0). Out of 413 children with SAM, 231 (55.9%) recovered, 24 (5.8%) died and 16.3% were defaulted from TFCs. The mean weight gain (in gram per weight of kilogram per day) for recovered children was 15.61 g/kg/day (95% CI, 14.15, 17.07). The overall median recovery time for these children was 12 days (95% CI, 11.22, 12.78). Moreover, most (77.5%) of children admitted with SAM were marasmic followed by Kwash (16%). Pneumonia (54.8%), diarrhea (41.8%) and rickets (21.4%) were co-morbidities which affected SAM children. A child being admitted at Mehal Meda Hospital (Adjusted Hazard Ratio (AHR) = 2.01; 95% CI: 1.34, 2.91), edematous form of malnutrition (AHR = 0.59; 95% CI: 0.39, 0.90) and being a child infected with pneumonia (AHR = 0.71; 95% CI: 0.51, 0.98) were predictors of nutritional recovery rate.

**Conclusion:** Under five pneumonia, diarrhea and rickets were co-morbidities that should be prevented. Recovery rate was poor when compared to SPHERE project reference value (which is > 75%). Predictors, namely presence of pneumonia and edematous form of malnutrition reduced nutritional recovery rate. Whereas, being admitted at Mehal Meda Hospital improved recovery rate. Therefore, hospitals should work in collaboration with health extension workers to prevent co-morbidities and strengthen screening and referral of malnutrition cases at community level. Moreover, Zonal Health Department and District Health Offices should facilitate experience sharing among health facilities.

**Keywords:** Co-morbidity, Kwashiorkor, Severe acute malnutrition, Treatment outcomes

* Correspondence: minastariku@gmail.com
Department of Public Health, College of Health Sciences, Debre Berhan University, P.O. Box 445, Debre Berhan, Ethiopia

## Introduction

Malnutrition is an abnormal physiological condition caused by deficiencies or imbalances in energy, protein and/or other nutrients. It is also explained as "a state in which the physiology of an individual is impaired to the point where he/she can no longer maintain adequate bodily performance, like growth and recovering from disease" [1–3]. According to World Health Organization, Severe Acute Malnutrition (SAM) is defined as a Weight-for-Height value < − 3 Z scores or Middle Upper Arm Circumference (MUAC) < 115 mm or children having bilateral pitting edema. This form of malnutrition is caused by poor-quality diets, weak care for mothers and children, insufficient access to health services, and unsanitary or unhealthy environments [3]. Severe acute malnutrition is the common cause of morbidity and mortality among under-five children all over the world and with the highest concentration in Sub Saharan Africa and South-East Asia [1–3]. According to 2017 global nutrition report, 52 million children are wasted (SAM) and it is the main challenge to achieve the sustainable development goals [4]. Moreover, it is a risk factor for more than 50% of 11 million deaths annually and the number-one driver of the global burden of disease [5, 6].

Severely malnourished children typically are brought to medical attention when a health crisis, such as an infection, precipitates the transition between marasmus (a state of nutritional adaptation) and kwashiorkor, in which adaptation is no longer adequate [5–7]. However, the clinical assessment of the child with malnutrition includes distinguishing between marasmus and kwashiorkor, assessing the severity of malnutrition, and identifying acute life-threatening complications, including sepsis, acute dehydration, and other complications. These children are also at risk for micronutrient deficiencies. An intensive and comprehensive approach is required to reduce the mortality rate associated with this condition and improvement in recovery rate is compulsory [7].

Considering the high burden of the problem, the seriousness and complicated condition, and the management and outcome, children with severe acute malnutrition should be properly and promptly treated in a suitable health facility at therapeutic feeding centers. It was seen that over the last several decades of the twentieth century, the median case fatality rate in developing countries remained unacceptable and relatively higher rates for edematous cases [8]. Despite the efforts made so far, Ethiopia has a high burden of under-five malnutrition (stunting 38%, underweight 24% and wasting 10%) which is an indication of the high magnitude of severe acute malnutrition in the country. Beyond its long-term preventive measures, the country has established different therapeutic feeding centers that can reduce under-five morbidity and mortality attributed to SAM [9].

Several studies have been reported on the magnitude of co-morbidity with SAM which ranges from 1.9% (hypothermia) to 72.9% (diarrhea) and recovery rate which ranges from 60.4 to 87% [10–16]. Co-morbidity, health facility, forms of malnutrition and age were factors associated with recovery rate among under-five children with SAM in Some TFCs of selected hospitals in Ethiopian and elsewhere. These findings in general showed inconsistent evidence across different geographic areas and time of events [10–16]. Besides, studies done so far in Ethiopia are limited to show all components of treatment outcomes and inadequate to compare treatment outcomes from adjacent health facilities.

Furthermore, since the establishment of therapeutic feeding centers in Debre Berhan referral Hospital, Enat general and Mehal Meda primary hospitals, data from therapeutic feeding centers was not analyzed or interpreted. But it is evident that comprehensive data analysis helps to evaluate the effectiveness of TFCs and identify determinant factors that affect treatment outcomes of TFCs. Therefore, the purpose of this study was to assess comorbidity status, treatment outcomes and to identify factors affecting the recovery rate of under-five children with SAM in TFCs. The result of this study also will be used as an input for improving the management of severe acute malnutrition in the selected TFCs and other similar settings in Ethiopia.

## Methodology

### Study design and settings

Retrospective follow up study was conducted at Debre Berhan referral hospital, Enat general and Mehal Meda primary hospitals. Debre Berhan hospital was the only referral hospital in North Shoa Zone and provides services for 2.4 million people in the catchment area. In these hospitals, Severely Malnourished children are admitted in Therapeutic Feeding Centers (TFCs) and further diagnosed and treated by pediatricians, general practitioners, health officers and nurses [17].

### Study participants and data sources

Study participants were severely malnourished children admitted in TFCs based on the Protocol for the Management of SAM in Ethiopia [18, 19]. These participants were under five children with SAM admitted from July 1, 2013 to July 31, 2015. The admission criteria for participants (whose age > 6 months to 59 months) were Weight/Height value < 70% or Middle Upper Arm Circumference (MUAC) < 110 mm or children having bilateral pitting edema. Similarly, participants less than 6 months could be admitted if they are too weak to suckle breast milk or weight/length < 70% or presence of bilateral edema. Data was collected using data extraction form designed for this specific study from inpatient therapeutic feeding registration book, multi-charts and medical records. A total of 413 children documents were considered in this study after diagnosing the completeness of the records.

The outcome variable called recovery rate from SAM was obtained by computing the number of patients discharged for recovery divided by the total number of discharges. Similarly, time-to-cure from SAM was calculated by subtracting the start of treatment date from the date of cure or censored (in days). Since our statistical analysis technique was survival analysis, we recoded treatment outcomes into two categories: Event (Recovery Rate = 1) and all the remaining outcomes considered as censored (Censored = 0). Cured children according to SAM treatment protocol are defined as children who have a weight- for- height > 85% and no bilateral edema. Children were considered to be cured and discharged, which is our event of interest if they fulfilled the discharging criteria for SAM [15]. However, the time-to-cure were censored for those children transferred to other wards, dropped treatment, died, did not cure at the end of the study. The following variables were considered for their influence on the recovery rate from SAM; age, sex, health facility, edema, Naso-gastric tube insertion, and co-morbidity. For age, we used three categories; Less than 12 months, 12–24 months and greater than 24 months. Health facilities had three categories; Debre Berhan Referral, Enat and Mehal Meda Hospitals. Bilateral edema was categorized based on whether the child had an edematous form of malnutrition or not. Co-infection was categorized based on whether the child has coinfection such as anemia, pneumonia, measles and giardiasis or not. The phrase, performance indicator used to mean the character which monitors the performance of TFC and indicates the quality of care provided in terms of attributes (Cure rate, death rate, defaulter rate and etc.) [20].

### Data collection and quality assurance

A structured data extraction form was designed to collect data from the registration book, inpatient multi -chart, and patient medical records. Patient's medical record number was obtained from therapeutic feeding registration book, so that their records were easily retrieved from medical record units to predict the survival status and the outcome of interest between July 2013–2015.

Data was collected by BSc nurses who had been working in the same health facilities after training on the techniques of data collection. Prior to actual data collection, a pre-test was carried out to check the functionality of data extraction form. The completeness of data was checked by three trained supervisors so as to provide feedback in the data collection process and to provide appropriate measures when necessary. Furthermore, every day after data collection, data collectors, supervisors and principal investigators discussed on quality of data and exchanged information to increase the validity and consistency of the data.

### Data processing and analysis

Data were entered, cleaned and checked for the completeness using EpiData software version 3.1. Errors related to inconsistency were verified using data exploration techniques. Then, data were exported to Statistical Product for Service Solution (SPSS) version 16 software (Release 16.0.0, September 13, 2007, Copyright (c) SPSS, Inc., 1989_2007). Subsequently, data were recoded and checked to facilitate analysis. The Shapiro-Wilk's test ($p > 0.05$) and a visual inspection of histogram, normal Q-Q plot, normal P-P plot and Box and Whisker plot were used to check the normality of distributions for continuous variables. Descriptive statistical analysis was done using percentages for categorical data and mean/ median for continuous variables. Recovery rate, defaulter rate, non-responder rate and case fatality rate of children with SAM were computed. Average weight gain and median length of stay were calculated. Treatment outcomes and other performance indicator values were compared with the SPHERE project reference standards as described in the 2007 SAM management protocol of Ethiopia [19]. The SPHERE standards for performance indicator were the minimum standards for food security, nutrition and food aid that follow the principles and rights of humanitarian charter [20]. Additionally, survival probability was estimated using the Kaplan-Meier method and survival curves were verified by Log-Rank test. Cox-proportional regression analysis was used to measure the association of each independent characteristic with recovery rate. Factors that were associated with time to recovery at 25% [21] significance level in the "Univariate" analysis were included in the final multiple analysis. Statistical significance was declared at *p*-value less than 0.05.

## Results

### Socio -demographic characteristics of SAM children

Out of 413 children with SAM, 229 (56%) were males and the majority (70.8%) of these children was in the age group of 6 to 24 months with the mean age of 16 months (95% CI, 15–17.1). The majority (71.7%) of participants was from Debre Berhan Referral Hospital and 93.7% were Amhara in Ethnicity.

### Medical condition and complications

Of the admitted children with SAM, most (77.5%) had Marasmus and 66(16%) had Kwashiorkor. Concerning co-morbidity, almost all (94%) of admitted children had at least one medical conditions or complications with pneumonia 54.8% followed by diarrhea (41.8%) and Rickets 21.4% "Table 1".

#### Management of medical complications

The study presented that different clinical management was made to improve the health status of children. Among these, a parenteral antibiotic was given to 88.8% of the children, nasogastric tube and intravenous infusions were given for 55.5 and 15.3% of children with SAM, respectively. Nearly 10% of children also received blood transfusion.

**Table 1** Co-morbidity and medical conditions among study participants in TFCs of Debre Berhan Referral, Enat General and Mehal Meda Primary Hospitals, 2013–2015

| Medical conditions | N (%) |
|---|---|
| Type of Malnutrition | |
| *Marasmus* | 320 (77.5) |
| *Kwashiorkor* | 66 (16.0) |
| *Marasmic Kwashiorkor* | 27 6.5) |
| Admission type | |
| *New* | 383 (92.7) |
| *Readmission* | 30 (7.3) |
| Edema at admission | |
| *Present* | 89 (21.8) |
| *Absent* | 320 (78.2) |
| Grade of edema at admission | |
| *Plus one (+)* | 28 (32.2) |
| *Plus two (++)* | 29 (33.3) |
| *Plus three (+++)* | 30 (34.5) |
| Breast fed during stay | |
| *Yes* | 246 (71.5) |
| *No* | 105 (28.5) |
| Immunization status | |
| *Fully vaccinated* | 184 (63.4) |
| *On immunization* | 63 (21.7) |
| *Partially immunized* | 23 (7.9) |
| *Not immunized* | 20 (6.9) |
| Co-morbidity | |
| *Present* | 378 (94.0) |
| *Absent* | 24 (6.0) |
| Major co-morbidities | |
| Tuberculosis | 20 (5.3) |
| Pneumonia | 207 (54.8) |
| HIV/AIDS | 10 (2.6) |
| Anemia | 62 (16.4) |
| Diarrhea | 158 (41.8) |
| Rickets | 81 (21.4) |
| Hypothermia (Temp < 35 °C) | 13 (3.3) |
| Fever (Temp > 38.5 °C) | 24 (6.2) |

#### Treatment outcomes

Concerning the treatment outcomes of children with SAM at discharge, 231 (55.9%) recovered, 24 (5.8%) died, 16.3% defaulted from TFCs. Moreover, the mean weight gain for recovered children was estimated to be 15.6 g/kg/day. The overall performance indicators for respective hospitals were displayed below with its SPHERE project reference values "Table 2".

#### Descriptive survival analysis

In the first week of admission, only 11 (3%) of children were recovered while 132 (43%) within 2 weeks. The percentage of recovery within 3 weeks of admission was estimated to be 53%. The median recovery time was 15 days (95% CI: 14.09, 15.908) "Table 3".

#### Kaplan Meier analysis of nutritional recovery time

The overall median recovery time was 12 days (95% CI: 11.22, 12.78), whereas the median recovery time for edematous and wasted children were 16 days (95% CI: 14.27, 17.73) and 11 days (95% CI: 10.21, 11.79), respectively.

#### Predictors of recovery rate among under- five children with SAM

After controlling for confounding factors, being treated at Mehal Meda hospital, an edematous form of malnutrition and presence of pneumonia remained the predictors of recovery rate. Children treated in Mehal Meda Hospital were 2 times more likely to recover as compared to those children treated in Debre Berhan Referral hospital (AHR = 2.01; 95% CI: 1.34, 2.91), edematous children were 41% less likely to recover as compared to children without edema (AHR = 0.59; 95% CI: 0.39, 0.90). Additionally, children who had pneumonia were 29% less likely to recover as compared to children who had no pneumonia (AHR = 0.71; 95% CI: 0.51, 0.98) "Table 4".

## Discussion

This study was intended to assess the co-morbidity status, treatment outcomes and factors affecting nutritional recovery rate of children with SAM treated in TFCs of three hospitals from Ethiopia. The main findings indicated that in spite of using updated guideline recommended for inpatient management of severely malnourished under -five children [19, 22], co-morbidities were impairing nutritional recovery, treatment outcomes were poor and predictors, like pneumonia, edematous form of malnutrition reduced recovery rate. Whereas, a child being admitted at Mehal Meda hospital improved recovery rate by two- fold.

**Table 2** Performance indicators of TFCs of Debre Berhan Referral, Enat General and Mehal-Meda Primary Hospitals as compared to SPHERE project reference values, 2013–2015

| Performance indicators | Performance by Health facilities | | | Overall performance | The SPHERE project reference values | |
|---|---|---|---|---|---|---|
| | Debre Berhan RH | Enat General hospital | Mehal Meda General hospital | | Acceptable | Alarming |
| Recovery rate | 51.7% | 58% | 79.2% | 55.9% | > 75% | < 50% |
| Death rate | 6.4% | 4.3% | 4.2% | 5.8% | < 10% | > 15% |
| Defaulter rate | 19.6% | 10.1% | 4.2% | 16.3% | < 15% | > 25% |
| Mean weight gain | 14.5 | 22.2 | 16.3 | 15.6 | ≥8 g/kg/day | < 8 g/kg/day |
| Mean length of stay | 13.8 | 13.3 | 10.6 | 13.2 | < 28 days | > 42 days |

Thus, in this study, Marasmus was the most common (77.5%) form of severe acute malnutrition followed by Kwashiorkor (16%) and Marasmic Kwashiorkor (6.5%). Similar findings were reported by different scholars from different parts of Ethiopia, Tanzania and Ghana [23–30]. This implies that in some parts of our study setting the land is degraded and the soil has lower fertility, yielding low crop productivity. In contrast, studies conducted in Southern Ethiopia [16, 31], Malawi [32], Zambia [33] and Uganda [34] reported that the edematous form of malnutrition was the most common. Because of the difference in food security status, feeding practice and socio-cultural factors, it is not unique to have different forms of childhood nutritional problem among different geographic areas.

There was a statistical difference ($p$-value $< 0.05$) between the median recovery time for edematous children (16 days) and their counterparts (11 days). Furthermore, this study depicted that those children who were diagnosed as wasted were more likely to recover earlier than those children diagnosed with edematous. This could be due to edematous children being prone to developing a metabolic complication and fluid overload with chronic diseases. Moreover, children with bilateral edema are more likely to be diseased than Marasmic children; as a result, their condition is more severe and would take longer to recover [35].

Poor recovery rate (55.9%) was projected as one of the treatment outcomes as previously reported from different TFCs in Ethiopia; (such as Felege Hiwot Hospital [25]; Gondar University Tertiary Hospital [26]; Sekota Hospital [27]; Gedeo Zone [31] and other facilities like Tamale Teaching Hospital from Ghana [30], Allahabad Hospital from India [11] and Hospital from North Uganda [34]. On the other hand, retrospective studies from different part of Ethiopia (Yirgalem hospital [28], Woldia hospital [15], Wolisso hospital [36], Jimma specialized hospital [37], hospitals from Southern region of Ethiopian [10]) and a study in Malawi [32] reported that recovery rate was within an acceptable range as compared to the minimum standard of SPHERE project reference values [20]. This could be due to higher defaulter rate in our study compared to other studies, which could decrease the chance of recovery. Additionally, since one of the study areas (DBRH) being a referral hospital, due to patient overload, high burden of co-morbidities and the late arrival of cases (after the development of complication) might also be the explanation for poor recovery rate.

The study showed that severely malnourished children who were treated at Mehal Meda TFC had significantly higher nutritional recovery rate than children treated in Debre Berhan TFC. This was consistent with other findings where nutritional recovery rate might be different among TFCs as explained by Teferi et al. [10], Gebremichael [16], Grum T et al. [31], Chiwaula Maggie [32] and Ngallaba Sospatro et al. [38]. This could be due to malnourished children coming to TFC and being admitted

**Table 3** Actuarial Life table analysis of children with SAM in TFCs of Debre Berhan Referral, Enat General and Mehal Meda Primary Hospitals, from 2013 to 2015

| Interval start time (in days) | Subjects entered interval | Subjects censored | Subjects exposed to risk | Subjects recovered | Probability of recovery |
|---|---|---|---|---|---|
| 0–7 | 413 | 57 | 384.5 | 11 | 0.03 |
| 7–14 | 345 | 74 | 308 | 132 | 0.43 |
| 14–21 | 139 | 31 | 123.5 | 66 | 0.53 |
| 21–28 | 42 | 14 | 35 | 12 | 0.34 |
| 28–35 | 16 | 4 | 14 | 7 | 0.50 |
| 35–42 | 5 | 1 | 4.5 | 1 | 0.22 |
| 42–49 | 3 | 1 | 2.5 | 1 | 0.40 |
| > 49 days | 1 | 0 | 1 | 1 | 1.00 |

**Table 4** Univariate and Multiple analyses for predictors of recovery rate for children with SAM in TFCs of selected hospital, Ethiopia, 2013–2015

| Covariates | Recovered Frequency | Censored Frequency | Crude HR (95% CI) | *p*-value | Adjusted HR (95% CI) |
|---|---|---|---|---|---|
| Age group | | | | | |
| Less than 12 months | 102 | 85 | 1 | | 1 |
| 12–24 months | 92 | 68 | 0.73 (0.55, 0.97) | 0.032* | 0.78 (0.53, 1.14) |
| More than 24 months | 27 | 27 | 0.85 (0.55, 1.29) | 0.440 | 1.08 (0.62, 1.79) |
| Health Facility | | | | | |
| Debre Berhan RH | 153 | 136 | 1 | | 1 |
| Enat General H | 40 | 25 | 1.60 (1.12, 2.28) | 0.009* | 0.91 (0.47, 1.72) |
| Mehal Meda PH | 38 | 7 | 1.80 (1.29, 2.50) | 0.000* | 2.01 (1.34, 2.91)** |
| Complementary fed | | | | | |
| Yes | 143 | 136 | 1.46 (1.05, 2.01) | 0.023* | 0.89 (0.57, 1.41) |
| No | 50 | 16 | 1 | | 1 |
| Pneumonia | | | | | |
| Present | 111 | 86 | 0.79 (0.6, 1.04) | 0.098* | 0.71 (0.51, 0.98)** |
| Absent | 95 | 72 | 1 | | 1 |
| Anemia | | | | | |
| Present | 28 | 23 | 1.34 (0.89, 1.99) | 0.155* | 0.94 (0.61, 1.46) |
| Absent | 177 | 125 | 1 | | 1 |
| Rickets | | | | | |
| Present | 51 | 28 | 0.683 (0.49,0.94) | 0.020* | 1.41 (0.98, 2.04) |
| Absent | 151 | 127 | 1 | | 1 |
| NG tube inserted | | | | | |
| Yes | 103 | 97 | 1.26 (0.95, 1.66) | 0.112* | 0.84 (0.60, 1.17) |
| No | 94 | 60 | 1 | | 1 |
| Bilateral edema | | | | | |
| Present | 42 | 188 | 0.50 (0.35, 0.71) | 0.000* | 0.59 (0.39, 0.90)** |
| Absent | 47 | 132 | 1 | | 1 |

N.B: (*) indicates that significant variables in Univariate analysis at 25% level of significance
(**) indicates that significant variables in Multiple analysis at 5% level of significance

after a complication had occurred. Since DBRH_TFC is used as referral health institution, cases may have come in increased severity, which was not the case for Mehal Meda TFC. In addition, this result could be due to the increased caseload of SAM since more children were admitted at Debre Berhan referral hospital than Mehal Meda TFC. In general, we can explain the difference in terms of difference in study settings, case load and severity of cases.

This study also showed that children with SAM who developed pneumonia had a significantly lower nutritional recovery rate than children without pneumonia. This could be explained in terms of the synergistic relationship between pneumonia and malnutrition, which has been well recognized by Cervantes and San [39]. Moreover, children with pneumonia may have an increased respiratory rate and use of accessory muscles of respiration thereby needing to stay longer in therapeutic feeding centers to recover. In addition, the presence of co-morbid conditions characterized by inadequate food intake may lead to fast depletion of nutrients and delayed nutritional recovery.

Increasing evidence suggests that malnutrition is the underlying reason for the increased susceptibility to pneumonia which results in a vicious cycle [35]. This indicates that hospitalized children experiencing malnutrition need an early diagnosis of co-morbidity and prompt treatment before developing a complication, many of which make them more vulnerable and reduce the chance of nutritional recovery. Similar findings were observed in Tanzania [29]. In our study, 94% of the cases developed at least one form of co-morbidity, which may have been due to their poor immunity to prevent nosocomial infection. Additionally, it may also be due to small bowel bacterial overgrowth and parasitic infections that commonly occur in SAM cases. These children are also the leading harbors of parasites that directly consume nutrients and prevent nutrient absorption [36]. This also explains the decrease in nutritional recovery rate in the present study.

Overall, this study is able to show co-morbidities, treatment outcomes and predictors of recovery rate among under-five children with SAM in three selected TFCs of North Shewa Zone, Amhara regional State of Ethiopia. Since these three TFCs are catchment areas for millions of people in the zone, it has paramount importance in recognizing the performance of TFCs and take remedial actions for better survival.

In spite of its strength, this study has limitations. It used staffs working in the same therapeutic feeding centers as data extractors from records, inpatient multi-charts, and medical records. However, to avoid subjectivity most of the variables reviewed as associated factors for treatment outcomes of SAM were objective in type. Moreover, since the study fully relied on secondary data, it is impossible to include essential risk factors that could have further explained the association among independent factors and recovery rate.

## Conclusion and recommendations

In conclusion, nutritional recovery rate in our study is poor when compared to the SPHERE project reference value. Additionally, the defaulter rate in the Debre Berhan referral hospital TFC needs to be improved. Regarding other performance indicators, mortality rate, mean weight gain and mean length of hospitalization were in the acceptable range of international standards in all three hospitals. This study summarizes the presence of pneumonia, the presence of edema reduced nutritional recovery rate whereas a child being admitted at Mehal Meda Hospital TFC improved recovery rate. Moreover, this study presents the high rate of co-morbidity that hinders nutritional recovery rate. Therefore, to prevent complications, improve recovery rate and decrease defaulter rate, emphasis should be given to improving early detection and treatment of severely malnourished children in the catchment areas. This can be done by creating a strong community- based screening and referral of malnutrition cases with the support of health extension workers. In addition, Zonal Health Department and District Health Offices should support and coordinate experience sharing among health facilities. Finally, combating childhood illness particularly pneumonia, diarrhea, rickets and to detect malnutrition early before developing complications should be done.

#### Abbreviations

AHR: Adjusted hazard ratio; CI: Confidence interval; DBRH: Debre Berhan Referral Hospital; ICU: Intensive care unit; IMNCI: Integrated maternal, neonatal and childhood illness; SAM: Severe acute malnutrition; SPSS: Statistical package for social sciences TFC: Therapeutic feeding center

#### Acknowledgments

Our great appreciation go to Debre Berhan referral hospital, Enat and Mehal Meda hospital's pediatric ward staffs for their unreserved support beginning with the conceptualization of ideas through data collection. Particularly, we would like to acknowledge Sr. Wagaye (DERH) for her kind assistance during the work of this project. Finally, our great gratitude also goes to data collectors and the DBU Health Science Col ege Research and Community Service Coordination Office for their efforts.

#### Funding

The field work of the research was sponsored by Debre Berhan University.

#### Authors' contributions

BTD conceived and designed the study. BTD, KBM and TGD supervised the acquisition of the data. BTD analyzed and interpreted the data. BTD drafted the manuscript. KBM, TGD and TBG critically revised the manuscript. All authors read and approved the manuscript.

#### Competing interests

The authors declare that they have co competing interests.

#### References

1. Global Nutrition Report 2015: Actions and accountability to advance nutrition and sustainable development. This report is found the link (URL): http://ebrary.ifpri.org/utils/getfile/collection/p15738coll2/id/129444/filename/129655.pdf.
2. Collins S, Dent N, Binns P, Bahwere P, Sadler K, Hallam A. Management of severe acute malnutrition in children. [review] [117 refs]. Lancet. 2006;368: 1992–2000.
3. World Health Organization. Management of severe malnutrition: a manual for physicians and other senior health workers. Geneva: WHO; 1999. http://apps.who.int/iris/bitstream/handle/10665/41999/a57361.pdf;jsessionid=27B7925804557EB3F112594A1377E695?sequence=1.
4. GNP. Global Nutrition Report 2017: Nourishing the SDGs. 2017. https://doi.org/10.1891/1058-1243.21.1.9.
5. Black RE, Morris SS, Bryce J. Where and why are 10 million children dying every year? Lancet. 2003;361:2226–34. https://doi.org/10.1016/S0140-6736(03)13779-8.
6. Black RE, Allen LH, Bhutta ZA, Caulfield LE, de Onis M, Ezzati M, et al. Maternal and child undernutrition: global and regional exposures and health consequences. Lancet. 2008;371:243–60.
7. BL Nichols. Malnutrition in developing countries: Clinical assessment. UpToDate 19.3. 2011. http://cursoenarm.net/UPTODATE/contents/mobipreview.htm?6/5/6224?source=see_link. Accessed 1 Jan 2017.
8. Schofield C, Ashworth A. Why have mortality rates for severe malnutrition remained so high? Bull World Health Organ. 1996;74:223–9.
9. Central Statistical Agency [Ethiopia] and ICF International. Federal Democratic Republic of Ethiopia Ethiopia Demographic and Health Survey 2016 Key Indicators Report. 2016. https://www.usaid.gov/sites/default/files/documents/1860/EthiopiaDHS2016KIR-Final10-17-2016.pdf.
10. Teferi E, Lera M, Sita S, Bogale Z, Datiko DG, Yassin MA. Treatment outcome of children with severe acute malnutrition admitted to therapeutic feeding centers in southern region of Ethiopia. Ethiop J Heal Dev. 2010;24:234–8.
11. Manisha M, Singh DK, Ruchirai PCM, Srivastava A. An experience of Facility-based Management of Severe Acute Malnutrition in children aged between 6-59 months adopting the World Health Organization recommendations. Indian J Pediatr. 2014;51:481–3.
12. Ahmed AU, Ahmed TU, Uddin MS, Chowdhury MHA, Rahman MH, Hossain MI. Outcome of standardized case Management of Under-5 children with severe acute malnutrition in three hospitals of Dhaka City in Bangladesh. Bangladesh J Child Heal. 2013;37:5–13. https://doi.org/10.3329/bjch.v37i1.15345.

13. Munthali T, Jacobs C, Sitali L, Dambe R, Michelo C. Mortality and morbidity patterns in under-five children with severe acute malnutrition (SAM) in Zambia: a five-year retrospective review of hospital-based records (2009–2013). Arch Public Heal. 2015;73:23. https://doi.org/10.1186/s13690-015-0072-1.
14. Ubesie AC, Ibeziako NS, Ndiokwelu CI, Uzoka CM, Nwafor CA. Under-five Protein Energy Malnutrition Admitted at the University of in Nigeria Teaching Hospital, Enugu: A 10 year retrospective review. Nutr J. 2012;11:1. https://doi.org/10.1186/1475-2891-11-43.
15. Chane T, Oljira L, Atomesa GE, Agedew E. Treatment Outcome and Associated Factors among Under-Five Children with Severe Acute Malnutrition Admitted to Therapeutic Feeding Unit in Woldia Hospital, North Ethiopia. J Nutr Food Sci. 2014;4:329. https://doi.org/10.4172/2155-9600.1000329.
16. Gebremichael DY. Predictors of nutritional recovery time and survival status among children with severe acute malnutrition who have been managed in therapeutic feeding centers, Southern Ethiopia: retrospective cohort study. BMC Public Health. 2015;15:1267. https://doi.org/10.1186/s12889-015-2593-5.
17. Embassy of United State, Addis Abeba, Ethiopia; Press releases 2013, retrieved from https://www.ethiosports.com/2013/06/25/u-s-government-supports-renovation-of-debre-berhan-hospital-laboratory/ retrieved date; Thu Feb 11 2016 23:35:22 GMT-0800 (Pacific Standard Time).
18. Ethiopian Federal Ministry of Health. Training Course On The Management Of Severe Acute Malnutrition. Federal democratic Republic of Ethiopia: Ministry of Health; 2013.
19. Chamois S, Golden M, Grellety Y. The protocol for management of severe acute malnutrition: Ethiopian Federal Minister of Health; 2007.
20. The SPHERE Project: Humanitarian Charter and Minimum Standards in Humanitarian Response. 2011.
21. Mickey RM, Greenland S. The impact of confounder selection criteria on effect estimation. Am J Epidemiol. 1989;129:125–37. https://doi.org/10.1093/oxfordjournals.aje.a115101.
22. Ashworth A, Schofield C, Sultana K, Alan J. Guidelines for the inpatient treatment of severely malnourished children. 2003. Report No.: ISBN 92 4 1546093.
23. Ahmed M. Managment outcome of severe acute malnutrition from 6 months to 5 years of age children admitted to Yekatit 12 hospital: Addis Ababa University; 2014.
24. Mekuria G, Derese T, Hailu G. Treatment outcome and associated factors of severe acute malnutrition among 6--59 months old children in Debre Markos and Finote Selam hospitals, Northwest Ethiopia: a retrospective cohort study. BMC Nutr. 2017;3(1):42. https://doi.org/10.1186/s40795-017-0161-3.
25. Desyibelew HD, Fekadu A, Woldie H. Recovery rate and associated factors of children age 6 to 59 months admitted with severe acute malnutrition at inpatient unit of Bahir Dar Felege Hiwot Referral hospital therapeutic feeding unite, northwest Ethiopia. PLoS One. 2017;12:2. https://doi.org/10.1371/journal.pone.0171020.
26. Terefe AA. Analysis of hospital records on treatment outcome of severe acute malnutrition: the case of Gondar University tertiary hospital. Pediatr Ther. 2016;6:3–7. https://doi.org/10.4172/2161-0665.1000283.
27. Shitaye DK. Survival Status and Predictors of Mortality among Children Aged 0–59 Months with Severe Acute Malnutrition Admitted to Stabilization Center at Sekota Hospital Waghemra Zone. J Nutr Disord Ther. 2015;5:168.
28. Kabeta A, Bekele G. Factors associated with treatment outcomes of under-five children with severe acute malnutrition admitted to therapeutic feeding unit of Yirgalem hospital. Clinics Mother Child Health. 2017;14:261. https://doi.org/10.4172/2090-7214.1000261.
29. Ahmed MM, Hokororo A, Kidenya BR, Kabyemera R, Kamugisha E. Prevalence of undernutrition and risk factors of severe undernutrition among children admitted to Bugando medical Centre in Mwanza, Tanzania. BMC Nutr. 2016;2(1):49. https://doi.org/10.1186/s40795-016-0090-6.
30. Saaka M, Osman SM, Amponsem A, Ziem JB, Abdul-Mumin A, Akanbong P, et al. Treatment outcome of severe acute malnutrition cases at the tamale teaching hospital. J Nutr Metab. 2015;2015:1–8. https://doi.org/10.1155/2015/641784.
31. Girum T, Kote M, Tariku B, Bekele H. Survival status and predictors of mortality among severely acute malnourished children < 5 years of age admitted to stabilization centers in Gedeo Zone : a retrospective cohort study. Ther Clin Risk Manag. 2017;13:101–10.
32. Chiwaula MP. Critical appraisal of the management of severe acute malnutrition in Malawi : a case of two hospitals in Zomba: University of Malawi; 2011.
33. Munthali T, Jacobs C, Sitali L, Dambe R, Michelo C. Mortality and morbidity patterns in under-five children with severe acute malnutrition (SAM) in Zambia: a five-year retrospective review of hospital-based records (2009–2013). Arch Public Health. 2015;73(1):23. https://doi.org/10.1186/s13690-015-0072-1.
34. Nyeko R, Calbi V, Ssegujja BO, Ayot GF. Treatment outcome among children under-five years hospitalized with severe acute malnutrition in St. Mary's hospital Lacor, Northern Uganda. BMC Nutr. 2016;2(1):19. https://doi.org/10.1186/s40795-016-0058-6.
35. Fauci AS, Braunwald E, Kasper DL, Hauser SL, Longo DL, Jameson JL, et al. Harrison's Manual of Medicine. In: Fauci AS, Braunwald E, Kasper DL, Hauser SL, Longo DL, Larry Jameson JL J, editors. . 17th ed. New York; 2009.
36. Berti A, Bregani ER, Manenti F, Pizzi C. Outcome of severely malnourished children treated according to UNICEF 2004 guidelines: a one-year experience in a zone hospital in rural Ethiopia. Trans R Soc Trop Med Hyg. 2008;102:939–44. https://doi.org/10.1016/j.trstmh.2008.05.013.
37. Misganaw C, Megdelawit M. Retrospective study on outcome of in-patient treatment of severe acute malnutrition in Jimma University specialized hospital from September 2011-September 2012. J Diagnostics. 2014;1:18–28.
38. Ngallaba SE, Makerere DJ, Kapesa A, Mongela S, Namanya B. Outcome and Effectiveness of Inpatient Care of Malnourished under Five Children in District Hospitals of Mwanza Region, North Western Tanzania. Open J Prev Med. 2014;4:293–8.
39. Cervantes E, San A. Malnutrition and gastrointestinal and respiratory infections in children : a public health problem. Int J Environ Res Public Health. 2011;8(1):1174–205.

16

# Nutritional status of in-school children and its associated factors in Denkyembour District, eastern region, Ghana: comparing schools with feeding and non-school feeding policies

Mavis Pearl Kwabla[1*], Charlotte Gyan[2] and Francis Zotor[2]

**Abstract**

**Background:** Childhood malnutrition still remains a major public health problem impacting negatively on the academic aptitude of school-aged children (SAC) particularly in limited resource countries. The Government of Ghana in collaboration with the Dutch Government introduced the school feeding programme (SFP) to boost the nutritional status of SAC in the country. This study sought to compare the nutritional status of SAC enrolled in schools with the SFP and SAC enrolled in schools without the SFP in place for the purpose of identifying which group has the higher rate of malnutrition.

**Methods:** A multi-stage sampling was used to select 359 SAC between 5 and 12 years who are enrolled in primary one to six. Twelve public schools were selected, of which 6 schools benefit from the SFP and the other six do not. Anthropometric measurements were conducted for the subjects and SPSS version 20.0 was used for data entry and analysis. Chi square test was carried out to determine the difference between the two groups of schools.

**Results:** Of the total of 359 subjects, 55.1% were from schools that do not implement the SFP and 44.9% were from schools that implement the SFP. The prevalence of stunting among children in schools on the SFP was 16.2% compared with 17.2% among children in schools that do not implement the SFP. The prevalence of thinness was two times higher (9.3%) among children in schools on the SFP than in children in schools that do not implement the SFP (4.6%) ($p = 0.028$). The prevalence of overweight among children in schools on the SFP was 1.9% and 0.0% for children in schools that do not implement the SFP. Sub district, sex, age of pupil, area of residence and community type were significantly associated with stunting ($p = 0.002$), ($p = 0.008$), ($p = 0.008$), ($p < 0.001$) and ($p = 0.007$) respectively.

**Conclusion:** Overweight and thinness were higher among children in schools on SFP than in children in schools without SFP. An evaluation of the implementation of the school feeding programme is recommended for future studies.

**Keywords:** Malnutrition, School-age children, Stunting, Thinness, Overweight

* Correspondence: mkwabla@uhas.edu.gh
[1]Department of Epidemiology and Biostatistics, School of Public Health, University of Health and Allied Sciences, Ho, Ghana
Full list of author information is available at the end of the article

## Background

Good nutrition is the foundation to proper growth and development in every human, the absence of which individuals are subjected to multiple health complications. Malnutrition still remains a significant problem all over the world, especially among children [1] . Childhood malnutrition continues to be a public health problem of school-aged children in limited resource countries [2]. Of the total of 7.6 million deaths reported by the World Health Organization (WHO) in 2010, 64% were attributable to infectious causes [3] but their severity was greater when confounded by malnutrition especially in children who are unable to mount an effective immune response [4, 5]. In 2014, an estimated 95 million children under five years of age in less developed regions were underweight with the highest prevalence rates in Southern Asia (28%), followed by Western Africa (20%) [1]. In 2012 also, there was a recorded 6.6 million deaths among children below five years as a result of malnutrition [1]. Malnutrition leads to delay in physical growth and motor development, lower intelligent quotient, behavioural problems and poor social skills and an increase in the risk of morbidity and mortality [6].

Childhood malnutrition is triggered by multiple risk factors which when tackled can lead to a significant reduction in cases as seen in children. The common causes of malnutrition are frequent infections and lack of access to nutritious foods [1].

In response to the high incidents of diseases caused by malnutrition among children, interventions such as school-based nutrition education, deworming, food fortification, supplementation and school feeding programmes were introduced. [1]. Majority of these interventions have proven to be effective since their implementation. National-scale fortification for instance which includes the addition of micronutrients to staple foods in factories has proven to be an effective method to improve the health of populations [2]. The Ghana school feeding programme (GSFP) introduced in 2005 in some selected schools is one of such interventions to enhance nutrition and improve school attendance and education outcomes [7]. In resource limited nations, majority of school-aged children often walk long distances to school without having a morning and midday meal due to poverty [8]. The school feeding programme therefore offers these children with at least one free meal during school hours. However, because resources are generally limited in the poorest countries and providing food can be expensive, targeting communities that lack the resources to adequately provide for their school-age children is a critical element in improving the impact and penetration of school feeding programmes [9]. It was against this background that the school feeding programme in Ghana has not been scaled up to cover all schools in the country so that the programme can provide the greatest benefit to those most in need [9].

On a global scale, an estimated 60 million children attend school hungry every day with about 40% in Africa [9] whereas 65 million children suffer from chronic under nutrition globally due to inadequate food intake, frequent infection or both. Efforts by the World Food Programme (WFP) has helped in providing school meals to between 20 and 25 million children across 63 countries each year, often in the hardest-to-reach areas. Lunch programmes in schools have improved school enrolment, increased attendance, decreased dropout rates and raised nutrition levels among the children [2].

Following the implementation of the school feeding programme in Ghana, numerous challenges emerged including challenges of linking the program with local farmers, delay in the release of funds, inadequate resources for effective monitoring and inadequate training for caterers on health and nutrition related issues [10]. In addition, findings about the benefits of the SFP appear inconclusive. Whilst some studies found the SFP to impact positively on the nutritional status of SAC, others have not witness any significant difference in the nutritional status of children in schools on the feeding programme compared with those in schools that do not implement the school feeding programme [11, 12]. The GSFP has been in implementation for over 10 years now and as such, its impacts on the nutritional status of children can be well ascertained. Hence the study assessed the nutritional status of children in schools on the school feeding programme and those in schools that do not implement the feeding programme in Denkyembour District.

## Methods

### Study area

Denkyembour District is one of the 26 Administrative Districts in the Eastern Region of Ghana. It is located at the South-Western part of the Eastern Region and shares boundaries with Kwaebibirem and Akyemansa Districts to the North, West Akim Municipality to the South and Birim Central Municipality to the South-West.

The district has 78 Communities with an estimated population of 78,841 according to the Ghana 2010 population and housing census. It has a population growth rate of 2.3%. The district is a food and cash crop growing area with major cultivations being palm fruits and plantain. The district comprises of 6 sub districts and 23 public basic schools, of which 11 are on the school feeding programme and 12 do not implement the school feeding programme. The district was chosen based on the implementation of the school feeding programme in some selected public schools. This situation therefore provides the settings for evaluating the school feeding programme.

### Study population

This comprised of school children between ages 5 to 12 years who were in primary 1–6 and registered in the school for at least one academic year and whose parents or guardians provided consent for participation in the study. The children were interviewed together with their parents/teachers after which their anthropometric measurements were taken. Children with known health problems were excluded from the study.

### Study design

A cross-sectional study using multi-stage sampling was carried out from February to March 2016 to assess nutritional status of primary school-age children from 12 public schools in Denkyebour district of Ghana.

### Sample size determination

The sample size of 359 participants was determined using the formula:

$$n = \frac{z^2 * p(q)}{d^2}$$

Where, n is the desired sample size, z is the standard normal deviate, p is the estimated prevalence of stunting, q is 1.0 – p, and d is degree of accuracy desired. With the regional prevalence of stunting (17%), which is the highest among all the indicators, the calculation was based on stunting prevalence with confidence level of 95%.

Using a prevalence of stunting of 17% (DHS, 2015), z = 1.96, $p = 0.28$, q = 0.83 and d = 0.05 at a 95% confidence level,

$$n = \frac{1.96^2(0.17)\ (0.83)}{0.05^2}$$

$$n = 217$$

With the extra uncertainty about the true prevalence of stunting, design effect was considered in the sample size calculation. Therefore, the sample size was n*design effect (which is 1.5 in this case),

$$n = 217 \times 1.5$$

$$n = 326$$

For a 10% non-response rate, the sample size was upwardly adjusted and rounded to 359 participants. This sample size was to ensure that, with probability of 95%, the estimated prevalence will fall within ±5% of the true population prevalence.

### Sampling

Respondents for the study comprised of school age children aged 5–12 years from two categories of Public schools (schools that implement the school feeding programme (SFP) and those that do not). They were selected from six stratified sub-districts using a multi-stage sampling technique. A list and population of all public schools on the SFP and those that do not implement SFP was obtained from the district education office following which 3 sub districts were purposively selected. For each sub district, two schools (one with the SFP and one without the SFP) were randomly selected. Proportionate sampling was used to determine the exact number of respondents to be recruited from each school. Respondents from the various schools were then selected based on balloting. A ballot involving the selection of a YES or NO was made for pupils in the selected schools who were in primary 1–6. Respondents who picked YES were the only ones interviewed together with their parents and or teachers.

### Data collection

After a pre-testing and training of research assistants, we used face-to-face interviews to administer the questionnaires to the pupils and or parents and teachers alike. Questionnaires administered to pupils solicited information about their personal characteristics (sex, age, area of residence, religion, and ethnicity) and dietary habits (number of meals intake per day and whether or not children receive money for food on school days) whereas that to the parents solicited information mainly about their occupation. Anthropometric measurements were taken using standard procedures. Weight and height readings were taken using a battery powered digital Seca 803 weighing scale (Medical measuring systems and scales, Hammer Steindamm 3–25, 22,089 Hamburg, Germany) and Seca 216 portable stadiometer (Medical measuring systems and scales, Hammer Steindamm 3–25, 22,089 Hamburg, Germany) respectively. Weight measurement was taken in duplicates and the average weight recorded. Before taking weight measurement, respondents were not permitted to wear shoes and heavy clothing except their school uniforms. Each school child was made to stand on the scale without holding onto any support with feet closed, hands by the sides and head in a forward position. Weight was then read immediately and recorded to the nearest 0.1 kg. Height was measured to the nearest 0.1 cm with a well mounted stadiometer. Before taking the measurements, respondents were asked to take off all foot wears and head gears or hats if any. Each pupil was made to stand with back against a wall, heels together and in line with the buttocks, shoulders and head. With a horizontal line of sight to the respondent, the head piece of the stadiometer was used to ensure that the top of the head was measured at right angle to the wall.

### Data analysis

Data was entered twice and checked using SPSS version 20.0. Chi square test was used for categorical variables to establish the differences between the 2 groups (schools with the school feeding programme and those without the school feeding programme). Multiple logistic regression analysis was used to confirm associations between dependent (nutritional status) and the independent variables (age, sex, mother's occupation and community type).

## Results

A total of 359 school aged children (SAC) from 6 sub-districts were recruited for the study of which 55.2% were from schools that do not implement the school feeding programme and 44.9% were from schools on the school feeding programme. The mean age of the school aged children was 9.8 ± 1.9 years. It was found that most of the participants (69.4%) were from the rural communities with 72.1% staying with their biological parents. Majority (56.3%) of the participants were in the age category of 5–9 years with almost equal proportion of both sexes. Background and demographic data of participants is shown in Table 1 below.

### Dietary history of the participants

All participants in both schools on the school feeding programme and those in schools without the school feeding programme eat between 2 and 3 times (including snacks) in a day. Majority, 348 (96.9) frequently eat 3 times in a day whilst the rest eat 2 times in a day. None was reported to have taken less than one meal in a day. Of the 3 meals taken in a day, breakfast 269 (74.9) and lunch 78 (21.7) were normally taken at school whilst supper 232 (64.5) was taken at home. About 94% of pupils were given money to purchase food at school.

### Prevalence of stunting, thinness and overweight among the participants

Approximately, 16.7, 6.7 and 0.8% of all the respondents were stunted (HAZ), thin (WHZ) and overweight (BAZ) respectively and 0.6% found to be of tall stature or well nourished (Table 2).

### Comparison of the levels of stunting, thinness, and overweight among study participants

The Prevalence of stunting was found to be higher among children in schools without the school feeding

**Table 1** Background and demographic characteristics of participants

Mean age ± SD =9.8 ± 1.9

| Attribute | Frequency ($N = 359$) | Percent |
|---|---|---|
| Sub-district | | |
| Akwatia | 97 | 27.0 |
| Topremang | 121 | 33.7 |
| Okumaning | 141 | 39.3 |
| Sex of pupil | | |
| Male | 171 | 47.6 |
| Female | 188 | 52.4 |
| Age of pupil(years) | | |
| 5–9 | 202 | 56.3 |
| 10–12 | 157 | 43.7 |
| Area of residence | | |
| Rural | 249 | 69.4 |
| Urban | 110 | 30.6 |
| Community type | | |
| Mining | 126 | 35.1 |
| Farming | 233 | 64.9 |
| Religion | | |
| Christian | 327 | 91.1 |
| Islam | 31 | 8.6 |
| Ethnicity | | |
| Akan | 238 | 66.3 |
| Ewe | 58 | 25.3 |
| Ga | 9 | 2.5 |
| Northerners | 24 | 6.7 |
| Others | 30 | 8.4 |
| Child lives with: | | |
| Both parents | 259 | 72.1 |
| Mother alone | 43 | 12.0 |
| Father alone | 13 | 3.6 |
| Other relations | 44 | 12.3 |
| Guardian's Occupation | | |
| Father's occupation | | |
| Farming | 129 | 35.9 |
| Mining | 45 | 12.5 |
| Civil/public servant | 34 | 9.5 |
| trading | 19 | 5.3 |
| Others | 74 | 20.6 |
| Unemployed | 28 | 7.8 |
| Mother's occupation | | |
| Farming | 69 | 19.2 |
| Mining | 29 | 8.1 |

**Table 1** Background and demographic characteristics of participants *(Continued)*

| Mean age ± SD =9.8 ± 1.9 | | |
|---|---|---|
| Attribute | Frequency (*N* = 359) | Percent |
| Civil/public servant | 18 | 5.0 |
| trading | 189 | 52.7 |
| Others | 26 | 7.2 |
| Unemployed | 28 | 7.8 |
| Receive money for school | | |
| Yes | 332 | 92.5 |
| No | 26 | 7.2 |
| Frequency of meal intake per day | | |
| < 1 | 0 | 0.0 |
| > 2 | 359 | 100 |
| Amount of money(Cedis) for school | | |
| < 1.00 | 89 | 24.8 |
| 1.00–1.99 | 240 | 66.9 |
| 2.00–3.00 | 6 | 1.7 |
| no money | 24 | 6.7 |
| Feeding type | | |
| School feeding | 161 | 44.9 |
| Non-school feeding | 198 | 55.2 |

programme (17.2%) than in children in schools on the feeding programme (16.2%) but there was no significant difference ($p = 0.284$). The prevalence of thinness was about twice higher (9.3%) in children with the school feeding programme than in those without the programme (4.6%), ($p = 0.028$). Unfortunately, 1.9% of children in schools with the feeding programme were found to be overweight. Summary of the comparison can be found in Table 3 below.

**Table 2** Nutritional status of the pupils

| Attribute | All | |
|---|---|---|
| | Frequency | Percentage (%) |
| Height for age z-score (HAZ) | | |
| Normal | 297 | 82.7 |
| Tall | 2 | 0.6 |
| Stunted | 60 | 16.7 |
| Total | 359 | (100.0) |
| Body mass index for age z-score (BAZ) | | |
| Normal | 332 | 92.5 |
| Overweight | 3 | 0.8 |
| Thinness | 24 | 6.7 |
| Total | 359 | (100.0) |

### Risk factors associated with malnutrition among school age children

The study explored possible risk factors associated with malnutrition in school age children. Overweight, thinness and stunting were the outcome variables measured. In exploring the possible risk factors associated with malnutrition, the study reveals that occupation of mother affects the overweight status of the child, a chi squared test performed at a significant level of 0.05, revealed a strong significant association between the two variables ($\chi^2 = 15.37$, $p = 0.009$, $\alpha = 5\%$).

With regards to thinness, sex and age were proven to be significantly associated with thinness with a chi square and $p$-value of ($\chi^2 = 5.55$, $p = 0.018$, $\alpha = 5\%$) and ($\chi^2 = 5.48$, $p = 0.019$, $\alpha = 5\%$) respectively, however a logistic regression performed to test the strength of the association indicated that female is a strong indicator of thinness as females are 2.7 times likely to become thin as compared to males [OR = 2.7 (95% CI = 1.70–6.70), $p = 0.023$].

With respect to stunting, Sub district, sex of pupil, age of pupil, area of residence and community type were significantly associated with stunting at bivariate analysis level, with a chi square values and $p$-values of ($\chi^2 = 12.29$, $p = 0.002$, $\alpha = 5\%$), ($\chi^2 = 7.12$, $p = 0.008$, $\alpha = 5\%$), ($\chi^2 = 6.94$, $p = 0.008$, $\alpha = 5\%$), ($\chi^2 = 12.20$, $p < 0.001$, $\alpha = 5\%$) and ($\chi^2 = 7.21$, $p = 0.007$, $\alpha = 5\%$) respectively.

However logistic regression revealed that only sub district and sex of pupils were strong indicators of stunting with odds ratio of [OR = 1.7 (95% CI = 0.16–18.60), $p = 0.001$] and [OR = 2.0 (95% CI = 1.12–3.67), $p = 0.007$] respectively. Refer Table 4 below.

## Discussion

The study sought to compare nutritional status of school age children (SAC) enrolled in schools benefiting from the school feeding programme and those that do not for the purpose of identifying which group has the higher rate of malnutrition. Anthropometric measurements of respondents were taken to evaluate the health and nutritional status of the children and the indices that directly reflect the socio-economic status of the family, health and social wellbeing of the population. Overweight, thinness and stunting were the anthropometric indicators used to measure malnutrition in the children.

Our study found an over-all prevalence of 0.8% for overweight among the school children in the Denkyembour District. This prevalence is lower compared to what was found in other studies [2, 12–14]. On the contrary, as high as 67% of children in schools on school feeding programme in the La-Nkwatanang Madina District were found to be stunted, underweight and anaemic [15]. The differences observed may be attributed to geographical differences: participants in this current study were from a rural setting where majority of the populace were

**Table 3** Nutritional status (comparison of school feeding and non- school feeding)

| Attribute | All Frequency (%) | School feeding Frequency (%) | Non- school feeding Frequency (%) | *p*-value |
|---|---|---|---|---|
| Height for age z-score(HAZ) | | | | |
| Normal | 297 (82.7) | 133 (82.6) | 164 (82.8) | |
| Tall | 2 (0.6) | 2 (1.2) | 0 (0.0) | |
| Stunted | 60 (16.7) | 26 (16.2) | 34 (17.2) | |
| Total | 359 (100.0) | 16 1(100.0) | 198 (100) | 0.284 |
| Body mass index for age z-score(BAZ) | | | | |
| Normal | 332 (92.5) | 143(88.8) | 189 (95.5) | |
| Overweigh0074 | 3 (0.8) | 3 (1.9) | 0 (0.0) | |
| Thinness | 24 (6.7) | 15 (9.3) | 9 (4.6) | |
| Total | 359 (100.0) | 161 (100.0) | 198 (100.0) | 0.028 |

farmers and may tend to consume more energy dense foods whereas La-Nkwatanang is a peri-urban area. The different makes of weighing instruments used in the measurement of weight and the different methods used in the classification of weight status by the different authors may also play a role.

The nutritional status of school aged children in the two genre of schools recruited for this study revealed an overweight prevalence of 1.9% among pupils in schools on the school feeding programme compared to 0.0% for those in schools without the feeding programme. Surprisingly, prevalence of thinness was also found to be higher among children in schools with the feeding programme (9.3%) than in those in schools without the feeding programme (4.6%) which concur with result of a similar study done in the Nkwanta South District [16]. On the contrary, a study conducted in Kenya [17] reported that Children participating in the school feeding programme were less wasted than children in the control group ($P = 0.002$).

The higher prevalence of overweight among children in schools with the school feeding programme compared to those in schools without the programme found in this study could be due to parents' lack of adequate knowledge on good nutrition practices to provide their children with healthy foods. This could also be as a result of the nutritional transition characterised by consumption of a more energy and high fat diet coupled with low physical activity in such schools. Furthermore, a more worrying findings in this study was the high prevalence of thinness found among children in schools on school feeding programme as compared with children in schools without school feeding programmes since it is expected that children in feeding programme receive supplementary food intended to improve their nutrition. This result confirms the findings of a study where the food being served by the school feeding programme was found not to meet the recommended energy from macronutrient intake as set by World Food Programme [18]. This could be as a result of the high level of poverty in the communities selected for the feeding programme since one of the aims of the feeding programme was to target communities that lack adequate resources to provide for their school age children. A report by the GSFP also indicated that the feeding programme is faced with numerous operational challenges including inconsistent release of funds making feeding irregular and the food not meeting the recommended energy and micronutrient levels [9, 10, 19] and this could also be a contributing factor.

The study found an association between overweight and parent's occupation ($p = 0.009$) which is in conformity with a similar study (13), which reported a significant association between overweight/obesity and father's occupation (<0.05). Their study also found overweight and obesity to be more prevalent in children belonging to affluent and higher socioeconomic group or families. This could mean that children from affluent homes have more fat and protein components in their diet with neglect to physical activity. Excessive consumption of calories from carbohydrate intake by these children could play a role in their overweight status. Consequently, their energy intake is more than energy expenditure, hence the accumulation of fat.

## Limitation

Cross-sectional design used in the study was not appropriate to establish a causal relationship between provision of school meals and nutritional status (stunting, thinness, and underweight). We could not also estimate the effect of challenges facing the feeding programme such as missed and irregular meals. Impact assessment was not also undertaken as a result of the

**Table 4** Factors associated with malnutrition among school age children

| Attribute | N (%) | N (%) | Pearson chi-square | | AOR (95% CI) |
|---|---|---|---|---|---|
| | | | $X^2$ | *P*-value | |
| Overweight status | | | | | |
| Occupation of mother | Not Overweight | Overweight | | | |
| Mining | 27 (93.1) | 2 (6.9) | 15.37 | 0.009 | 0.637 |
| Farming | 68 (98.6) | 1 (1.4) | | | |
| Trading | 189 (100.0) | 0 (0.0) | | | |
| Civil/public servant | 18 (100.0) | 0 (0.0) | | | |
| Other | 26 (100.0) | 0 (0.0) | | | |
| Unemployed | 28 (100.0) | 0 (0.0) | | | |
| Thinness | | | | | |
| sex | Not Thin | Thin | | | |
| Males | 181 (96.3) | 7 (3.7) | 5.55 | 0.018 | 1 |
| Female | 154 (90.1) | 17 (9.9) | | | 2.7 (1.08–6.70) |
| Age (years) | | | | | |
| 5–9 | 183 (90.6) | 19 (9.4) | 5.48 | 0.019 | 1 |
| 10–12 | 152 (96.8) | 5 (3.2) | | | 0.3 (0.12–0.93) |
| Stunting | | | | | |
| Sub-district | Not stunted | Stunted | | | |
| Akwatia | 91 (93.8) | 6 (6.2) | 12.29 | 0.002 | 1 |
| Topremang | 100 (82.6) | 21 (17.4) | | | 1.7 (0.16–18.60) |
| Okumaning | 108 (76.6) | 33 (23.4) | | | |
| sex of pupil | | | | | |
| Male | 166 (88.3) | 22 (11.7) | 7.12 | 0.008 | 1 |
| Female | 133 (77.8) | 38 (22.2) | | | 2.0 (1.12–3.67) |
| Age of pupil (years) | | | | | |
| 5–9 | 159 (78.7) | 43 (21.3) | 6.94 | 0.008 | 1 |
| 10–12 | 140 (89.2) | 17 (10.8) | | | 0.5 (0.27–0.96) |
| Area of residence | | | | | |
| Rural | 196 (78.7) | 53 (21.3) | 12.20 | <0.001 | 1 |
| Urban | 103 (93.6) | 7 (6.4) | | | 0.4 (0.05–3.20) |
| Community type | | | | | |
| Mining | 185 (79.4) | 48 (20.6) | 7.21 | 0.007 | 1 |
| Farming | 114 (90.5) | 12 (9.5) | | | 0.n (0.36–2.73) |

Chi-square test, significance defined as $p < 0.05$. Stunting defined as HAZ < −2 Wasting defined as WHZ < −2 and Overweight/Obesity defined as BMI-for-Age > +1SD

unavailability of baseline information about the nutrition status of the children at the start of the feeding program.

## Conclusion

The overall prevalence of overweight was low compared to that found in other studies. However, prevalence rates of overweight and thinness were found to be higher among children in schools on the school feeding programme compared to children in schools without the feeding programme. An evaluation of the implementation of the school feeding programme is recommended for future studies.

### Abbreviations

GSFP: Ghana school feeding programme; SAC: School age children; SFP: School feeding programme; WFP: World food programme

### Acknowledgements

We wish to thank Mr. Wisdom Takramah, Mr. Appiah Kubi Prince, Mr. Norbert Amuna and Mr. Nyinaku Elorm Kwame, all of School of Public Health of the University of Health and Allied Sciences as well as the Denkyembour District Directors of Education and Health.

**Funding**
The research work was self-sponsored by the authors.

**Authors' contributions**
This work was carried out in collaboration with all authors. CG drafted the protocol and carried out the study in partial fulfilment of the requirement for the award of Bachelor of Public Health Degree by the School of Public Health of the University of Health and Allied Sciences. MPK and FBZ participated in the study design. All authors CG, MPK and FBZ did the statistical analysis and literature searches. Author MPK drafted the manuscript which was reviewed by authors CG and FBZ.

**Competing interests**
All authors declare that they have no competing interests.

**Author details**
[1]Department of Epidemiology and Biostatistics, School of Public Health, University of Health and Allied Sciences, Ho, Ghana. [2]Department of Family and Community Health, School of Public Health, University of Health and Allied Sciences, Ho, Ghana.

**References**
1. M Do, Monteiro C, Akré J, Clugston G. Global Database on Child Growth and Malnutrition The worldwide magnitude of protein energy malnutrition : an overview from the WHO Global Database on Child Growth. Bull World Health Organ. 2015; 2015.
2. Lardner D, Giordano J, Jung MK, Passafaro MD, Small A, Haar M, et al. Evaluation of nutritional status among school-aged children in rural Kwahu-Eastern region, Ghana; anthropometric measures and environmental influences. AJFANDce. 2015;15(3):9996–10012. Available from :http://ovidsp.ovid.com/ovidweb.cgi
3. Liu L, Johnson HL, Cousens S, Perin J, Scott S, Lawn JE, et al. Global, regional, and national causes of child mortality: an updated systematic analysis for 2010 with time trends since 2000. Lancet. 2012;379(9832): 2151–61. Available from: http://www.ncbi.nlm.nih.gov/pubmed/22579125
4. Rice AL, Sacco L, Hyder A, Black RE. Malnutrition as an underlying cause of childhood deaths associated with infectious diseases in developing countries. Bull World Health Organ. 2000;78(10):1207–21.
5. Rayhan MI, Khan MSH. Factors causing malnutrition among under five children in Bangladesh. Pak J Nutr. 2006;5(6):558–62.
6. UNICEF. Improving child nutrition: The achievable imperative for global progress. In: Division of Communication UNICEF; 2013. p. 1–132.
7. Gelli A, Masset E, Folson G, Kusi A, Arhinful DK, Asante F, et al. Evaluation of alternative school feeding models on nutrition, education, agriculture and other social outcomes in Ghana: rationale, randomised design and baseline data. Trials. 2016;17(1):37. Available from: http://trialsjournal.biomedcentral.com/articles/10.1186/s13063-015-1116-0
8. Intiful FD, Lartey A. Breakfast habits among school children in selected communities in the eastern region of Ghana. Ghana Med J. 2014;48(2):71–7.
9. Buhl A. Meeting Nutritional Needs Through School Feeding: A Snapshot of Four African Nations. Report. 2010; (c).
10. WHO. The world health report 2006: working together for health. World Health. 2006;19:237. Available from: http://www.who.int/whr/2006/whr06_en.pdf
11. Quaye W, Essegbey G, Frempong G, Ruivenkamp G. Understanding the concept of food sovereignty using the Ghana school feeding Programme (GSFP). Int Rev Sociol. 2010;20(3):427–44.
12. Danquah AO, Amoah AN, Steiner-Asiedu M, Opare-Obisaw C. Nutritional Status of Participating and Non-participating Pupils in the Ghana School Feeding Programme. J Food Res. 2012;1(3):263. Available from: http://www.ccsenet.org/journal/index.php/jfr/article/view/19250
13. Vohra R, Bhardwaj P, Srivastava JP, Srivastava S, Vohra A. Overweight and obesity among school-going children of Lucknow city. J Fam Community Med. 2011;18(2):59–62.
14. Ghana Statistical Service. Ghana Demographic and Health Survey 2014: Ghana statistical service, Ghana Health Service. In: Ghana Statistical Service (GSS) Ghana Demographic and Health Survey; 2014.
15. Owusu JS, Colecraft EK, Aryeetey R, Vaccaro JA, Huffman FG. Nutrition Intakes and Nutritional Status of School Age Children in Ghana. J Food Res. 2017;6(2) Available from: https://doi.org/10.5539/jfr.v6n2p11
16. Prince A, Laar A. Nutritional Status of School-Age Children in the Nkwanta South District -Volta Region of Ghana. Eur Scientif J. 2014, 1010:1857–7881. Available from: http://www.eujournal.org/index.php/esj/article/view/4462/4272.
17. Neervoort F, von Rosenstiel I, Bongers K, Demetriades M, Shacola M, Wolffers I. Effect of a school feeding programme on nutritional status and anaemia in an urban slum: a preliminary evaluation in Kenya. J Trop Pediatr. 2013;59(3):165–74.

# 17

# Effect of soy lecithin on fatigue and menopausal symptoms in middle-aged women: a randomized, double-blind, placebo-controlled study

Asuka Hirose[1,2], Masakazu Terauchi[2*], Yurika Osaka[1], Mihoko Akiyoshi[1], Kiyoko Kato[2] and Naoyuki Miyasaka[1]

**Abstract**

**Background:** Lecithin is a complex mixture of phospholipids which compose lipid bilayer cell membranes. Lipid replacement therapy, or administration of phospholipids for the purpose of repairing the dmaged cell membranes, had been shown to alleviate fatigue. The present study aimed to investigate the effect of soy lecithin on fatigue in middle-aged women, as well as other menopausal symptoms and various health parameters.

**Methods:** This randomized, double-blind, placebo-controlled study included 96 women aged 40 to 60 years who complained of fatigue. The participants were randomized to receive active tablets containing high-dose (1200 mg/day; $n = 32$) or low-dose (600 mg/day; $n = 32$) soy lecithin, or placebo ($n = 32$), for 8 weeks. The following parameters were evaluated: age, menopausal status, lifestyle factors, physical and psychological symptoms of menopause, subjective symptoms of insomnia and fatigue, body composition, cardiovascular parameters, and physical activities and objective sleep states obtained from actigraphy before and 4 and 8 weeks after treatment. Fatigue was evaluated using the Profile of Mood States (POMS)-brief, Menopausal Health-Related Quality of Life questionnaire, Chalder Fatigue Scale, and Brief Fatigue Inventory.

**Results:** Eighty-nine women completed the study. There were no significant differences in the changes in Chalder Fatigue Scale score (placebo vs low-dose vs high-dose groups: $-2.9 \pm 1.1$, $-3.2 \pm 1.1$, and $-3.5 \pm 1.0$; $P = 0.79$). On the other hand, the improvements were greater in the high-dose group compared with the placebo group concerning vigor scores in the POMS-brief ($1.9 \pm 0.7$ vs $0.2 \pm 0.6$; $P = 0.02$), diastolic blood pressure ($-4.1 \pm 1.8$ vs $1.2 \pm 1.9$; $P = 0.05$), and cardio-ankle vascular index ($-0.4 \pm 0.2$ vs $0.07 \pm 0.1$; $P = 0.03$) after 8 weeks of treatment.

**Conclusions:** High-dose (1200 mg/day) soy lecithin not only increases vigor, but also lowers the diastolic blood pressure and cardio-ankle vascular index in middle-aged women who present with fatigue.

**Keywords:** Atherosclerosis, Cardiovascular risks, Fatigue, Lipid replacement therapy, Menopausal symptoms, Psychological symptoms, Soy

* Correspondence: teragyne@tmd.ac.jp
[2]Department of Women's Health, Tokyo Medical and Dental University, Yushima 1-5-45, Bunkyo, Tokyo 113-8510, Japan
Full list of author information is available at the end of the article

## Background

Middle-aged women are bothered by various symptoms such as hot flashes, night sweats, anxiety, depression, insomnia, and fatigue. A previous study revealed that 86% of Japanese middle-aged women who visited our menopausal clinic felt tiredness more than once a week, and 49% felt it almost every day [1]. Another study revealed that 85% of Japanese and 82% of Australian middle-aged women felt fatigue, at least to some extent [2]. Compared to the patients attending a primary care clinic of whom 14% complained of fatigue [3], apparently more middle-aged women are bothered by the symptom.

Lecithin is a complex mixture of phospholipids found mainly in egg yolks, soy, and coleseeds. Phospholipids such as phosphatidyl choline, phosphatidyl ethanolamine, phosphatidyl inositol, phosphatidyl serine, and phosphatidyl glycerol compose the lipid bilayer of the cellular membrane structure. Membrane lipids are used for energy storage necessary for membrane biogenesis [4–6]. The matrix of cellular membranes is formed by polar lipids, which consist of a hydrophobic and hydrophilic portion and segregate the internal and external environment [6]. Furthermore, membrane lipids act as first and second messengers in signal transduction and molecular recognition pathways [4, 6], implying the variability of their biological roles. The administration of fresh phospholipids to replace damaged cell membranes and restore the structure and function of the cellular membrane is called lipid replacement therapy (LRT). LRT has been shown to improve fatigue, and is expected to be effective for the treatment of degenerative diseases, metabolic syndrome, diabetes, and cardiovascular diseases [4, 7]. However, previous studies have demonstrated the effects of LRT using a supplement containing not only phospholipids but also other active ingredients. To the best of our knowledge, this study is the first to examine the effects of soy lecithin on fatigue.

The present study aimed to investigate the effect of soy lecithin on menopausal symptoms including fatigue and other various health parameters in Japanese middle-aged women.

## Methods

### Study population

We performed a randomized, double-blind, placebo-controlled study from February to July 2015 at the Menopause Clinic of Tokyo Medical and Dental University. The study protocol was reviewed and approved by the Tokyo Medical and Dental University Review Board, and written informed consent was obtained from all the participants. The present study was conducted in accordance with the Declaration of Helsinki.

Ninety-six Japanese women aged 40 to 59 years who complained of fatigue participated in this study. Fatigue was evaluated using the item about fatigue in the Menopausal Health-Related Quality of Life (MHR-QOL) questionnaire. The participants were recruited through advertisements posted in our hospital and in the patients' social network. Those who were receiving menopausal hormone therapy, herbal medicine, or psychotropic drugs were excluded. Collected data included age, menopausal status, lifestyle factors, physical and psychological symptoms of menopause, subjective symptoms of insomnia and fatigue, body composition, cardiovascular parameters, and physical activities and objective sleep states obtained from actigraphy. The data were evaluated before and 4 and 8 weeks after treatment. Regarding menopausal status, participants were classified as follows: premenopausal (regular menstrual cycles in the past 3 months), perimenopausal (a menstrual period within the past 12 months but a missed period or irregular cycles in the past 3 months), postmenopausal (no menstrual period in the past 12 months), or surgically induced menopause (hysterectomy).

### Randomization and intervention

The participants were randomized into 1 of 3 groups to receive active tablets containing high-dose (1200 mg/day; $n = 32$) or low-dose (600 mg/day; $n = 32$) soy lecithin, or placebo (n = 32) for 8 weeks. The high-dose and low-dose soy lecithin and placebo tablets, indistinguishable in shape, weight, and color, were manufactured and packaged by Kikkoman Corporation (Noda, Japan). The tablet contained phospholipids in the form of phosphatidylcholine, 24%; phosphatidylethanolamine, 20%; and phosphatidylinositol, 12%. The women were instructed to take six tablets per day after breakfast. Medication adherence was evaluated by collecting the packages of the supplements from participants. The participants were sequentially numbered, and received supplement packages with the corresponding number. The content of each package, namely high-dose or low-dose soy lecithin, or placebo, was known only by the manufacturers. Thus, allocation was concealed from both the participants and the investigators. Safety was assessed by patient-reported treatment-emergent adverse events.

### Menopausal symptoms

Menopausal symptoms were evaluated using the Menopausal Health-Related Quality of Life (MHR-QOL) questionnaire, Hospital Anxiety and Depression Scale (HADS), and Athens Insomnia Scale (AIS). The MHR-QOL questionnaire, developed and validated at our clinic [8, 9], is a modification of the Women's Health Questionnaire [10, 11], and contains 38 items scored on a 4-point or binary scale covering four major domains (physical symptoms, psychological symptoms, life satisfaction, and social involvement) of a woman's health during menopause. The

HADS [12] is a reliable instrument for screening clinically significant anxiety and depression in women visiting a general medicine clinic. The translated Japanese version of the HADS [13] was used in the present study. The AIS was developed as a brief and easy-to-administer self-assessment questionnaire for determining the severity of insomnia defined according to the International Classification of Diseases 10th Revision. The internal consistency and test-retest reliability of the AIS have been confirmed previously [14]. Detailed information about the MHR-QOL questionnaire, HADS, and AIS is provided elsewhere [8].

#### Fatigue and mood states

Fatigue and mood states were evaluated by the Profile of Mood States (POMS)-brief, Chalder Fatigue Scale (CFS), and Brief Fatigue Inventory (BFI). The POMS is a psychological rating scale used to assess feelings and mood states. The original version of the POMS consists of 65 items, while the POMS-brief, a shortened version, includes 30 items covering six major domains (tension, depression, anger, vigor, fatigue, and confusion). Because the latter is easier to complete and its validity has been demonstrated [15], it is now more widely used than the original form. The POMS-brief was translated into Japanese, and its reliability and validity were confirmed previously [16]. The CFS is a self-administered questionnaire with 14 items which evaluates fatigue-related symptoms by using a 4-point Likert scale for the extent or frequency of the symptoms [17]. Although originally developed to measure fatigue symptoms in clinical settings, the scale is now more widely used [18]. The BFI, a self-rating assessment composed of 9 items using a numerical scale of 0 to 10, was developed for the rapid assessment of fatigue severity in cancer patients [19]. It was translated into Japanese, and its reliability and validity were confirmed previously [20].

#### Body composition and cardiovascular parameters

Height, weight, body mass index, and body composition including fat mass, and fat free mass, was assessed using a body composition analyzer (MC190-EM; Tanita, Tokyo, Japan). Cardiovascular parameters, including systolic and diastolic blood pressure, heart rate, and the cardio-ankle vascular index (CAVI), were measured using a vascular screening system (VS-1000; Fukuda Denshi Co., Tokyo, Japan).

#### Physical activities and objective sleep states

We investigated physical activities and objective sleep states using the actigraphy system that is loaded with a miniature triaxial acceleration sensor (Wrist-worn Accelerometers; Hitachi Ltd., Tokyo, Japan). It measured motion with accelerometers and sleep–wake identification was automatically performed by using the Cole–Kripke algorithm. The outcome measures included zero-crossing (ZC) and metabolic equivalents (METs) during the awake and sleep phase, total sleep time, day-to-day variation of sleep time, episodes of nocturnal awakening, sleep latency, and sleep efficiency. ZC is the rate of signal changes from the triaxial acceleration sensor, representing the frequency of wrist motion. METs are calculated as the ratio of metabolic rate relative to that in resting, representing the intensity of exercise. We define sleep latency as the time from time in bed to the start of identification of sleep. Sleep efficiency is calculated as pure sleep time (time in bed minus awake time) divided by time in bed. Participants were requested to wear a wrist actigraph device for 72 h on their non-dominant arms except during bathing time. The analysis of the actigraphy data was performed at 'blinded for peer review'.

#### Statistical analyses

The baseline characteristics of the participants who completed the 8-week treatment were compared using one-way analysis of variance, $\chi 2$ test, and Kruskal-Wallis test. Then, the changes from baseline to 8 weeks of treatment in all of the collected data were evaluated using Mann-Whitney test and unpaired t-test. All statistical analyses were performed with GraphPad Prism version 5.02 (GraphPad Software Incorporated, CA, USA). A $P$-value <0.05 was considered statistically significant.

### Results

A total of 96 middle-aged women were enrolled in the study and were randomized to the high-dose ($n = 32$), low-dose (n = 32), or placebo groups ($n = 32$); of these, 89 (94%) completed the 8-week treatment period (Fig. 1). During the study period, seven women dropped out of the study. Five of them did not continue to take the supplements, and two did not have an examination at our clinic. The baseline characteristics of the participants who completed the 8-week treatment are shown in Table 1. The group mean age ranged from 49 to 51 years. The proportion of women who were premenopausal, perimenopausal, postmenopausal, and had surgically induced menopause ranged from 22 to 52%, 7 to 22%, 41 to 53%, and 0 to 7%, respectively. The weight, body mass index, and body fat mass were significantly higher in the high-dose group than the other groups ($P = 0.018$, 0.012, and 0.008, respectively).

The mean ± SEM CFS scores significantly decreased after 8 weeks of treatment in all the groups, and there were no significant differences among the groups (placebo vs low-dose vs high-dose groups: −2.9 ± 1.1, −3.2 ± 1.1, and −3.5 ± 1.0, respectively; $P = 0.79$, Kruskal-Wallis test, Fig. 2a). After 8 weeks of treatment, the mean ± SEM POMS-vigor score was significantly higher in the high-

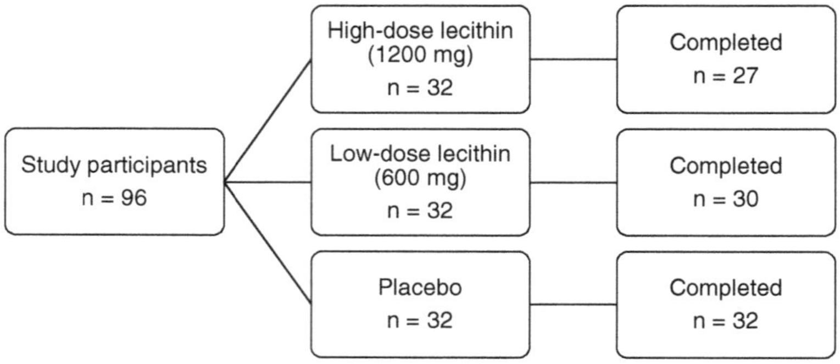


**Fig. 1** Participant disposition

dose group than the placebo group (1.9 ± 0.7 vs 0.2 ± 0.6, respectively; $P = 0.02$, Mann-Whitney test, Fig. 2b). The mean ± SEM diastolic blood pressure (−4.1 ± 1.8 vs 1.2 ± 1.9; $P = 0.05$, unpaired t-test, Fig. 2c) and CAVI (−0.4 ± 0.2 vs 0.07 ± 0.1; $P = 0.03$, unpaired t-test, Fig. 2d) significantly decreased after 8 weeks of treatment in the high-dose group compared with the placebo group. Neither the body composition parameters nor the actigraphic parameters changed significantly in any of the groups (data not shown).

During the whole study period, no treatment-emergent adverse event was reported by the participants, even though laboratory tests were not routinely performed.

## Discussion

In this randomized, double-blind, placebo-controlled study, the effect of soy lecithin on menopausal symptoms including fatigue and other various health parameters in Japanese middle-aged women was investigated. The results showed that high-dose (1200 mg/day) soy lecithin not only increases vigor, but also lowers the diastolic blood pressure and CAVI in Japanese middle-aged women who complained of fatigue.

LRT is a concept proposed by Nicolson et al. [4]. The mitochondrion is the site where adenosine triphosphate (ATP) is synthesized aerobically, and the inner and outer membrane of the organelle are composed by phospholipids. Reactive oxygen species (ROS) are generated in the process of uncoupling the electron transport chain from ATP generation, with the inner mitochondrial membrane being the most important source of ROS [4, 21]. When mitochondrial membranes are damaged by ROS, energy production by the organelle is decreased, which could lead to fatigue, as well as aging and various diseases. In previous animal [22] and clinical studies [23], LRT was demonstrated to improve mitochondrial function assessed by transport and reduction of the dye Rhodamine-123, mitochondrial membrane potentials assessed by flow cytometry, and mitochondrial DNA deletions [24].

Lecithin is particularly abundant in egg yolks, soybeans, organ and lean meats, and fish. The total phospholipids contained in 100 g of egg yolk and soybeans are 31.8 g and 20.8 g, respectively [25], and the normal dietary intake of phospholipids is estimated as 2–8 g per day [26]. Most previous studies [4, 7, 26] have used the dosage of 1 to 3 g per day of oral supplementation of lecithin, exhibiting its effects for inflammatory diseases, hyperlipidemia, cardiovascular diseases, cognitive impairment, and fatiguing illnesses. Oral administration of phospholipids has been shown to be generally safe [4]. For example, in phase I and II clinical trials in patients with cardiovascular diseases, over 5 g of soy phospholipids were administered with no apparent toxicity [27]. Referring to older studies, a daily dosage of as much as 54 g has been administered without any apparent adverse effects [28]. Regarding the duration of the treatment, most of the previous studies investigating the effects of dietary LRT supplement on fatigue examined for 8 weeks, meanwhile some examined for 1 or 12 weeks [4].

In this study, the effect of soy lecithin on fatigue and other factors was investigated, and our findings showed that lecithin promotes vigor assessed by the POMS-brief questionnaire. Previous studies have demonstrated the effect of phospholipids on cancer-associated fatigue and adverse chemotherapy effects, such as nausea, diarrhea, constipation, and fatigue [29, 30], using NT Factor® (Nutritional Therapeutics, Inc., Hauppauge, NY.), an oral supplement containing phospholipids, glycolipids, and other membrane lipids [23]. Feelings of fatigue and loss of vigor are similar and the difference is ambiguous, and our result can be understood in the same context. In this study, significant differences in the fatigue scores among the groups could not be shown. The reason for this may be the placebo effect because the fatigue scores were improved in all groups, and it was explained to the participants that lecithin might improve fatigue. Other reasons why the improvement of fatigue was not different among the groups might be

**Table 1** Background characteristics of the participants

| | Placebo (*n* = 32) | Low-dose lecithin (*n* = 30) | High-dose lecithin (*n* = 27) | *P* value |
|---|---|---|---|---|
| Age, y | 51.2 ± 5.2 | 50.3 ± 5.8 | 49.3 ± 4.8 | 0.423[a] |
| Menopausal status, n (%) | | | | |
| Premenopausal | 7 (21.9) | 10 (33.3) | 14 (51.9) | 0.222[b] |
| Perimenopausal | 7 (21.9) | 5 (16.7) | 2 (7.4) | |
| Postmenopausal | 17 (53.1) | 13 (43.3) | 11 (40.7) | |
| Surgically induced menopause | 1 (3.1) | 2 (6.7) | 0 (0) | |
| Questionnaire | | | | |
| MHR-QOL physical symptom score | 21.2 ± 3.5 | 21.9 ± 2.9 | 20.6 ± 3.2 | 0.406[c] |
| MHR-QOL psychological symptom score | 27.1 ± 8.0 | 29.7 ± 6.7 | 30.0 ± 5.5 | 0.328[c] |
| HADS-anxiety subscale score | 5.8 ± 2.9 | 5.3 ± 3.3 | 4.9 ± 2.7 | 0.549[c] |
| HADS-depression subscale score | 5.5 ± 3.7 | 4.8 ± 3.7 | 4.7 ± 3.1 | 0.679[c] |
| AIS score | 5.0 ± 3.0 | 4.0 ± 2.9 | 4.1 ± 2.6 | 0.443[c] |
| Chalder Fatigue Scale | 18.7 ± 8.3 | 17.1 ± 5.3 | 17.6 ± 5.6 | 0.628[c] |
| Brief Fatigue Inventory | 2.7 ± 1.9 | 3.0 ± 1.7 | 3.0 ± 2.0 | 0.575[c] |
| POMS-tension | 6.1 ± 4.9 | 5.5 ± 4.3 | 4.3 ± 3.1 | 0.461[c] |
| POMS-depression | 3.9 ± 3.9 | 2.5 ± 3.1 | 2.5 ± 2.6 | 0.217[c] |
| POMS-anger | 5.1 ± 4.2 | 3.7 ± 3.1 | 2.8 ± 2.5 | 0.104[c] |
| POMS-vigor | 7.7 ± 4.1 | 7.2 ± 3.6 | 6.1 ± 3.5 | 0.179[c] |
| POMS-fatigue | 6.8 ± 4.4 | 7.8 ± 4.3 | 6.4 ± 3.6 | 0.727[c] |
| POMS-confusion | 5.0 ± 2.8 | 4.8 ± 2.4 | 3.8 ± 2.2 | 0.323[c] |
| Body composition | | | | |
| Height, cm | 157.6 ± 4.6 | 158.4 ± 5.1 | 158.0 ± 3.8 | 0.817[a] |
| Weight, kg | 52.8 ± 7.5 | 52.6 ± 6.0 | 58.3 ± 11.1 | 0.018[a] |
| Body mass index, kg/cm$^2$ | 21.2 ± 2.8 | 21.0 ± 2.5 | 23.3 ± 4.0 | 0.012[a] |
| Body fat mass, kg | 14.0 ± 5.1 | 13.7 ± 4.4 | 18.5 ± 8.5 | 0.008[a] |
| Fat free mass, kg | 36.5 ± 2.8 | 36.6 ± 2.2 | 37.6 ± 2.8 | 0.222[a] |
| Waist:hip ratio, % | 80.6 ± 6.1 | 81.7 ± 4.8 | 83.4 ± 6.2 | 0.191[a] |
| Body temperature, °C | 36.3 ± 0.33 | 36.4 ± 0.42 | 36.3 ± 0.41 | 0.701[a] |
| Cardiovascular parameters | | | | |
| Systolic blood pressure, mmHg | 122.7 ± 15.7 | 119.3 ± 16.1 | 119.9 ± 13.6 | 0.668[a] |
| Diastolic blood pressure, mmHg | 69.2 ± 12.1 | 67.8 ± 13.6 | 68.7 ± 13.6 | 0.919[a] |
| Heart rate, beats/min | 77.2 ± 8.0 | 76.9 ± 12.7 | 80.1 ± 12.4 | 0.504[a] |
| Cardio-ankle vascular index | 7.19 ± 0.79 | 7.24 ± 0.79 | 7.14 ± 0.78 | 0.967[a] |
| Actigraphy | | | | |
| Active ZC (/min) | 156.6 ± 26.2 | 148.0 ± 31.8 | 149.0 ± 34.0 | 0.506[a] |
| Sleep ZC (/min) | 4.3 ± 1.1 | 4.3 ± 1.8 | 4.7 ± 1.7 | 0.606[a] |
| Active METs | 1.6 ± 0.15 | 1.5 ± 0.14 | 1.6 ± 0.21 | 0.674[a] |
| Sleep METs | 1.1 ± 0.015 | 1.1 ± 0.015 | 1.1 ± 0.019 | 0.580[a] |
| Sleep time (min/day) | 372.1 ± 70.6 | 371.4 ± 60,6 | 367.8 ± 54.8 | 0.687[a] |
| Sleep efficiency (%) | 97.2 ± 1.4 | 97.4 ± 1.7 | 97.5 ± 1.8 | 0.719[a] |
| Episodes of nocturnal awakening (>1 min) (/day) | 1.7 ± 1.2 | 1.8 ± 1.4 | 1.8 ± 1.5 | 0.676[a] |
| Lifestyle factors, % | | | | |
| Exercising regularly | 50.0 | 46.7 | 51.9 | 0.923[b] |
| Smoking | 6.25 | 10.0 | 7.4 | 0.856[b] |
| Drinking alcohol (daily / by chance / not at all) | 15.6 / 68.8 / 15.6 | 20.0 / 63.3 / 16.7 | 29.6 / 59.3 / 11.1 | 0.749[b] |

Values are presented as mean ± SD unless otherwise indicated
*AIS* Athens Insomnia Scale, *CAVI* cardio-ankle vascular index, *HADS* Hospital Anxiety and Depression Scale, *METs* metabolic equivalents, *MHR-QOL* Menopausal Health-Related Quality of Life, *POMS* Profile of Mood States, *ZC*, zero-crossing
[a]One-way analysis of variance
[b]Chi-square test
[c]Kruskal-Wallis test

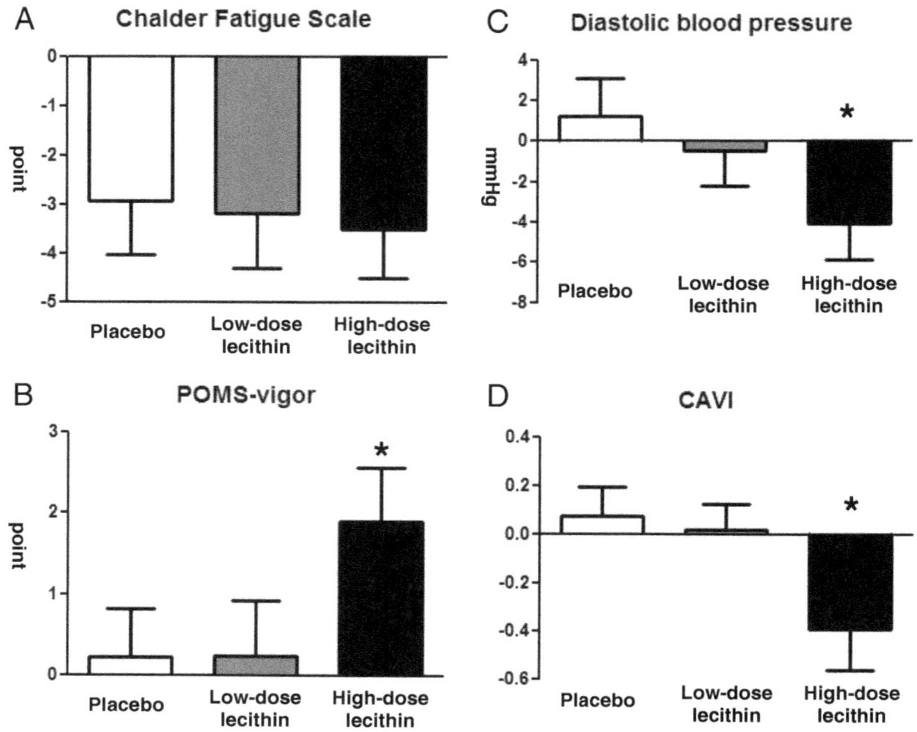


**Fig. 2** The changes from baseline after 8 weeks of intervention in: (**a**) the Chalder Fatigue Scale scores; (**b**) the Profile of Mood States (POMS)-vigor scores; (**c**) diastolic blood pressure; and (**d**) cardio-ankle vascular index (CAVI). Data are presented as means and standard errors. **P* < 0.05 vs placebo, Mann-Whitney test or unpaired t-test

that the participants were relatively healthy and the baseline fatigue scores were not high enough, or that some portion of the fatigue experienced by the participants was derived from pathological conditions, such as infection, inflammation, and sleep disorders.

The present study also revealed that lecithin decreases the diastolic blood pressure and CAVI. The risk of cardiovascular diseases (CVDs), including central obesity, hypertension, dyslipidemia, and diabetes, increases after menopause [31–34], partly as a result of diminished estrogen production [35]. CVD is rare in young women, but it is the second leading cause of death among the 45–64 year age group in the United States after cancer, and it has become the leading cause after the age of 65 years [36]. Especially in women, the treatment of arterial hypertension and diabetes is considered important for the prevention of CVD [37]. Several studies demonstrated that lecithin lowered total cholesterol in patients with primary hyperlipidemia [38, 39], and a mini-pig study showed that LRT reduced atherosclerotic plaques in the aortas and heart valves [40]. There is a possibility that lecithin lowers cardiovascular risks, although the mechanisms are yet to be elucidated. This is the first study showing the effects of lecithin on the diastolic blood pressure and CAVI. Further study is warranted to corroborate the findings and also to examine the effect on systolic blood pressure. In the present study, there was statistically significant differences in the baseline characteristics among the study groups, that is weight, body mass index, and body fat mass were significantly higher in the high-dose group. On the other hand, there was no significant difference in the POMS-vigor score, diastolic blood pressure, and CAVI that changed significantly after the 8-week treatment, therefore we consider that the differences in the baseline characteristics would have a small influence on the results of the present study.

The present study has some limitations. First, the sample size was relatively small and the study period was as short as 8 weeks, and all the participants were relatively healthy women. Second, mitochondrial function was not evaluated, and the results could not be directly explained by the functional improvement of the mitochondria. Finally, we set the full dose as 1200 mg in this study, which might not be sufficient. Further studies with longer duration enrolling more patients with severe fatigue, hypertension, or established atherosclerosis are warranted in order to corroborate our findings concerning the effects of soy lecithin on vigor and cardiovascular risks. Higher doses of lecithin and simultaneous assessment of the mitochondrial function may be needed to evaluate the effects of the compound.

## Conclusions

High-dose (1200 mg/day) soy lecithin not only increases vigor, but also lowers the diastolic blood pressure and CAVI in middle-aged women who present with fatigue. Further studies with longer duration enrolling more patients with severe fatigue are warranted in order to corroborate our findings.

### Abbreviations

AIS: Athens insomnia scale; ATP: Adenosine triphosphate; BFI: Brief fatigue inventory; CAVI: Cardio-ankle vascular index; CFS: Chalder fatigue scale; CVD: Cardiovascular disease; HADS: Hospital anxiety and depression scale; LRT: Lipid replacement therapy; MET: Metabolic equivalent; MHR-QOL: Menopausal health-related quality of life; POMS: Profile of mood states; ROS: Reactive oxygen species; ZC: Zero-crossing

### Acknowledgements

Not applicable.

### Funding

MT received an unrestricted research grant from Kikkoman Corporation.

### Authors' contributions

AH and MT were responsible for project development, data collection, and data analysis. YO, MA, and KK were responsible for data collection. NM participated in the project development and supervision. All authors contributed to reviewing, editing, and approving the final manuscript.

### Competing interests

The authors declare that they have no competing interests.

### Author details

[1]Department of Obstetrics and Gynecology, Tokyo Medical and Dental University, Yushima 1-5-45, Bunkyo, Tokyo 113-8510, Japan. [2]Department of Women's Health, Tokyo Medical and Dental University, Yushima 1-5-45, Bunkyo, Tokyo 113-8510, Japan.

### References

1. Terauchi M, Hiramitsu S, Akiyoshi M, Owa Y, Kato K, Obayashi S, et al. Effects of the kampo formula tokishakuyakusan on headaches and concomitant depression in middle-aged women. Evid Based Complement Alternat Med. 2014;2014:593560.
2. Anderson D, Yoshizawa T, Gollschewski S, Atogami F, Courtney M. Menopause in Australia and Japan: effects of country of residence on menopausal status and menopausal symptoms. Climacteric. 2004;7:165–74.
3. Cathébras PJ, Robbins JM, Kirmayer LJ, Hayton BC. Fatigue in primary care: prevalence, psychiatric comorbidity, illness behavior, and outcome. J Gen Intern Med. 1992;7:276–86.
4. Nicolson GL, Ash ME. Lipid replacement therapy: a natural medicine approach to replacing damaged lipids in cellular membranes and organelles and restoring function. Biochim Biophys Acta. 1838;2014:1657–79.
5. Shevchenko A, Simons K. Lipidomics: coming to grips with lipid diversity. Nat Rev Mol Cell Biol. 2010;11:593–8.
6. van Meer G, Voelker DR, Feigenson GW. Membrane lipids: where they are and how they behave. Nat Rev Mol Cell Biol. 2008;9:112–24.
7. Küllenberg D, Taylor LA, Schneider M, Massing U. Health effects of dietary phospholipids. Lipids Health Dis. 2012;11:3.
8. Terauchi M, Horiguchi N, Kajiyama A, Akiyoshi M, Owa Y, Kato K, et al. Effects of grape seed proanthocyanidin extract on menopausal symptoms, body composition, and cardiovascular parameters in middle-aged women: a randomized, double-blind, placebo-controlled pilot study. Menopause. 2014;21:990–6.
9. Terauchi M, Obayashi S, Akiyoshi M, Kato K, Matsushima E, Kubota T. Insomnia in Japanese peri- and postmenopausal women. Climacteric. 2010; 13:479–86.
10. Hunter M, Battersby R, Whitehead M. Relationships between psychological symptoms, somatic complaints and menopausal status. Maturitas. 1986;8: 217–28.
11. Hunter M. The south-east England longitudinal study of the climacteric and postmenopause. Maturitas. 1992;14:117–26.
12. Zigmond AS, Snaith RP. The hospital anxiety and depression scale. Acta Psychiatr Scand. 1983;67:361–70.
13. Zigmond AS, Snaith RP, Kitamura T. The hospital anxiety and depression scale (in Japanese). Seisinka-Sindangaku 1993;4:371–2.
14. Soldatos CR, Dikeos DG, Paparrigopoulos TJ. Athens insomnia scale: validation of an instrument based on ICD-10 criteria. J Psychosom Res. 2000; 48:555–60.
15. Yeun EJ, Shin-Park KK. Verification of the profile of mood states-brief: cross-cultural analysis. J Clin Psychol. 2006;62:1173–80.
16. Yokoyama K, Araki S, Kawakami N, Tkakeshita T. Production of the Japanese edition of profile of mood states (POMS): assessment of reliability and validity. Nihon Koshu Eisei Zasshi. 1990;37:913–8.
17. Chalder T, Berelowitz G, Pawlikowska T, Watts L, Wessely S, Wright D, et al. Development of a fatigue scale. J Psychosom Res. 1993;37:147–53.
18. Jackson C. The Chalder fatigue scale (CFQ 11). Occup Med (Lond). 2015;65:86.
19. Mendoza TR, Wang XS, Cleeland CS, Morrissey M, Johnson BA, Wendt JK, et al. The rapid assessment of fatigue severity in cancer patients: use of the brief fatigue inventory. Cancer. 1999;85:1186–96.
20. Okuyama T, Wang XS, Akechi T, Mendoza TR, Hosaka T, Cleeland CS, et al. Validation study of the Japanese version of the brief fatigue inventory. J Pain Symptom Manag. 2003;25:106–17.
21. Kalogeris T, Bao Y, Korthuis RJ. Mitochondrial reactive oxygen species: a double edged sword in ischemia/reperfusion vs preconditioning. Redox Biol. 2014;2:702–14.
22. Seidman MD, Khan MJ, Tang WX, Quirk WS. Influence of lecithin on mitochondrial DNA and age-related hearing loss. Otolaryngol Head Neck Surg. 2002;127:138–44.
23. Agadjanyan M, Vasilevko V, Ghochikyan A, Berns P, Kesslak P, Settineri RA, et al. Nutritional supplement (NT factor™) restores mitochondrial function and reduces moderately severe fatigue in aged subjects. J Chronic Fatigue Syndr. 2003;11:23–36.
24. Kim M, Cooper DD, Hayes SF, Spangrude GJ. Rhodamine-123 staining in hematopoietic stem cells of young mice indicates mitochondrial activation rather than dye efflux. Blood. 1998;91:4106–17.
25. Cohn JS, Kamili A, Wat E, Chung RW, Tandy S. Dietary phospholipids and intestinal cholesterol absorption. Nutrients. 2010;2:116–27.
26. Cohn JS, Wat E, Kamili A, Tandy S. Dietary phospholipids, hepatic lipid metabolism and cardiovascular disease Curr Opin Lipidol. 2008;19:257–62.
27. Pandey NR, Sparks DL. Phospholipids as cardiovascular therapeutics. Curr Opin Investig Drugs. 2008;9:281–5.
28. Knuiman JT, Beynen AC, Katan MB. Lecithin intake and serum cholesterol. Am J Clin Nutr. 1989;49:266–8.
29. Nicolson GL, Ellithorpe R. Lipid replacement and antioxidant nutritional therapy for restoring mitochondrial function and reducing fatigue in chronic fatigue syndrome and other fatiguing illnesses. Chronic Fatigue Syndr. 2006;13:57–68.
30. Nicolson GL, Conklin KA. Reversing mitochondrial dysfunction, fatigue and the adverse effects of chemotherapy of metastatic disease by molecular replacement therapy. Clin Exp Metastasis. 2008;25:161–9.
31. Carr MC. The emergence of the metabolic syndrome with menopause. J Clin Endocrinol Metab. 2003;88:2404–11.
32. Rosano GM, Vitale C, Tulli A. Managing cardiovascular risk in menopausal women. Climacteric. 2006;9(Suppl 1):19–27.
33. Lizcano F, Guzmán G. Estrogen deficiency and the origin of obesity during menopause. Biomed Res Int. 2014;2014:757461.
34. Collins P, Rosano G, Casey C, Daly C, Gambacciani M, Hadji P, et al. Management of cardiovascular risk in the peri-menopausal woman: a

consensus statement of European cardiologists and gynaecologists. Eur Heart J. 2007;28:2028–40.
35. Rosano GM, Vitale C, Marazzi G, Volterrani M. Menopause and cardiovascular disease: the evidence. Climacteric. 2007;10(Suppl 1):19–24.
36. Leading Causes of Death in Females. Centers for Disease Control and Prevention. https://www.cdc.gov/dhdsp/data_statistics/fact_sheets/fs_women_heart.htm Accessed 1 Aug 2017.
37. Vitale C, Miceli M, Rosano GM. Gender-specific characteristics of atherosclerosis in menopausal women: risk factors, clinical course and strategies for prevention. Climacteric. 2007;10(Suppl 2):16–20.
38. Simons LA, Hickie JB, Ruys J. Treatment of hypercholesterolaemia with oral lecithin. Aust NZ J Med. 1977;7:262–6.
39. Wojcicki J, Pawlik A, Samochowiec L, Kaldonska M, Mysliwiec Z. Clinical evaluation of lecithin as a lipid-lowering agent. Phytother Res. 1995;9:597–9.
40. Samochowiec L, Kadlubowska D, Rozewicka L, Kuzna W, Szyszka K. Investigations in experimental atherosclerosis .2. Effect of phosphatidylcholine (EPL) on experimental atherosclerotic changes in miniature pigs. Atherosclerosis. 1976;23:319–31.

# 18

# Vitamin D status and dental caries in healthy Swedish children

Johanna Gyll[1], Karin Ridell[2], Inger Öhlund[3], Pia Karlsland Åkeson[4], Ingegerd Johansson[5] and Pernilla Lif Holgerson[1*]

**Abstract**

**Background:** Vitamin D is crucial for mineralized tissue formation and immunological functions. The purpose of this study was to evaluate the association between vitamin D status and dental status in healthy children with vitamin D supplementation in infancy and at 6 years of age.

**Method:** Eight-year-old children who had participated in a vitamin D intervention project when they were 6 years old were invited to participate in a dental follow-up study. They had fair or darker skin complexion and represented two geographically distant parts of Sweden. 25-hydroxy vitamin D in serum had been measured at 6 years of age and after a 3-month intervention with 25, 10 or 2 (placebo) µg of vitamin $D_3$ per day. Two years later, caries and enamel defects were scored, self-reported information on e.g., oral behavior, dietary habits and intake of vitamin D supplements was collected, and innate immunity peptide LL37 levels in saliva and cariogenic mutant streptococci in tooth biofilm were analyzed. The outcome variables were caries and tooth enamel defects.

**Results:** Dental status was evaluated in 85 of the 206 children in the basic intervention study. Low vitamin D levels were found in 28% at baseline compared to 11% after the intervention, and 34% reported continued intake of vitamin D supplements. Logistic regression supported a weak inverse association between vitamin D status at 6 years of age and caries 2 years later (odds ratio 0.96; $p = 0.024$) with minor attenuation after an adjustment for potential confounders. Multivariate projection regression confirmed that insufficient vitamin D levels correlated with caries and higher vitamin D levels correlated with being caries-free. Vitamin D status at 6 years of age was unrelated to enamel defects but was positively associated with saliva LL37 levels.

**Conclusion:** An association between vitamin D status and caries was supported, but it was not completely consistent. Vitamin D status at 6 years of age was unrelated to enamel defects but was positively associated with LL37 expression.

**Keywords:** Vitamin D – Children – caries – enamel defects – LL37

## Background

Vitamin D is associated with a broad spectrum of biological functions owing to its endocrine, autocrine and paracrine activities [1]. Its reported functions include the regulation of calcium and phosphate metabolism and their deposition in mineralized tissues [2, 3], effects on innate immunity effectors [4], involvement in cognitive functions, roles in blood pressure maintenance and effects related to health outcomes (cardiometabolic conditions, total mortality and aging) [5, 6]. Children and adolescents are particularly vulnerable to the clinical manifestations of insufficient vitamin D because of its central role in bone and tooth formation [3].

Generally, serum 25-hydroxy vitamin D [S-(25(OH)D] levels below <30 nmol/L are considered deficient, 50 nmol/L are insufficient, and >75 nmol/L are suggested as optimal for health [7–9]. According to epidemiological studies, insufficient levels of vitamin D are common in children and adolescents [10] with a higher prevalence reported in areas with less sunshine and in populations with

* Correspondence: pernilla.lif@umu.se
[1]Department of Odontology, Section of Paediatric Dentistry, Faculty of Medicine, Umeå University, 90185 Umeå, Sweden
Full list of author information is available at the end of the article

protection against sun exposure or with dark skin complexions [11, 12]. 25-hydroxyvitamin D status is determined by measuring its circulating forms in serum, including the $D_2$ and $D_3$ variants [2, 7]. Most foods contain relatively small amounts of vitamin *D. major* natural sources include oily fish and eggs, which contain $D_3$, and many countries, including Sweden, fortify table spreads and milk with vitamin $D_3$.

The function of vitamin D in tooth development implies that impaired tooth composition is more prevalent in subjects with vitamin D deficiency [13], but the association may be overlooked since clinical manifestations appear after a significant delay [10, 14]. Based on the effects of vitamin D on tooth quality and the innate immune system, including the defensins and cathelicidins (LL37) [4], studies have evaluated the association between vitamin D levels and dental caries; however, the results are conflicting. Thus, according to some studies, low vitamin D levels/intakes are associated with higher caries prevalence [14–16], but other studies have not observed an association [17]. A recent systematic review of clinical trials assessing the effect of vitamin D on the prevention of dental caries yielded a weak positive effect of vitamin D supplementation with no clear difference in the positive effect between supplementation route, i.e., vitamin $D_2$, vitamin $D_3$, or ultraviolet radiation [18]. Other studies have assessed associations between vitamin D receptor (VDR) polymorphisms or a combined genetic risk score and dental caries, but these studies have also produced conflicting results [15, 19, 20]. Therefore, further clarification is needed to determine the reasons for the conflicting results, such as studies targeting defined populations and careful monitoring of confounding factors and sufficient variations in vitamin D status.

The primary aim of the present study was to evaluate the association between the vitamin D status of 6-year-old children and their caries status 2 years later. A secondary goal was to evaluate associations of vitamin D status with tooth enamel disturbances and levels of the innate immunity peptide LL37.

## Methods

### Ethical approval

The basic intervention study (DViSUM) was registered at ClinicalTrials.gov (NCT01741324) and approved by the Regional Ethical Review board at Umeå University (Reference: 2012–158-31 M). An addendum was approved (Reference: 2014–103-32 M) for the present dental follow-up study. Data were collected and analyzed according to the guidelines of the Declaration of Helsinki (including written consent from caretakers and children for participation), the Swedish Law on personal data act (PuL) and Law on biobanking, and the guidelines of the Swedish Data Inspection Board.

### Subjects

The present study recruited 8-year-old children who had participated in an intervention study on milk-based vitamin D supplementation at 6 years of age (DViSUM) [21, 22]. DViSUM included 206 children who were proportionally distributed across different living regions [northern Sweden (Umeå, 63°N; $n$ = 85) and southern Sweden (Malmö, 55°N; $n$ = 121)] and were selected to represent both fair ($n$ = 108) and darker skin ($n$ = 98) complexions. To be included, the children had to be regular milk consumers. Baseline examinations in DViSUM occurred in November and December of 2012 and included anthropometric measures, blood sampling and questionnaires on information about diet intake and socioeconomic conditions. At the first visit in DViSUM, children were randomly assigned to receive 25, 10 or 2 (placebo group), µg of vitamin $D_3$ per day in a milk-based supplement for 3 months. Follow-up blood samples were collected when the 3-month intervention period was completed.

Of the 206 children who participated in DViSUM, 85 (41%) consented to participate in an examination of their dental status. Of the 85 children, 37 (42%) in the 25 µg per day group, 38 (45%) in the 10 µg per day group, and 10 (12%) were in the placebo group, and compared to 42%, 39% and 19%, respectively, in the basic study [22]. Dental follow-up occurred in the latter half of 2014. The major reason for non-participation was that the children's caretakers had moved out of the specified geographic areas. A flow diagram is shown in Fig. 1.

The general characteristics of the study population were low to moderate caries activity and organized dental care from 2 to 3 years of age, including compulsory caries prevention programs. Furthermore, supplementation with vitamin D3 drops (10 µg/day) was strongly encouraged from birth to 2 years of age and up to 5 years in children with dark skin complexions [23].

### Dental examination and data collection

All children were examined by an experienced dentist (JG or KR) for dental caries and enamel defects. At this visit, a questionnaire on tooth brushing and other dental health-related behaviors, including diet with focus on sugar and vitamin D containing foods/food aggregates, use of fluoride and supplements, and health status, medication, and socio-economic information, was administered. All examinations were performed in well-equipped dental offices with good lighting conditions. Caries status was determined by the surface-related decayed-missing-filled index [24], but the missing component was not included since teeth were not lost because of caries. Initial caries and fissure sealants were not included in the decayed and filling components, respectively. Therefore, the permanent dentition $D_{3\text{-}4}FS$ and the primary dentition $d_{3\text{-}4}$ fs were

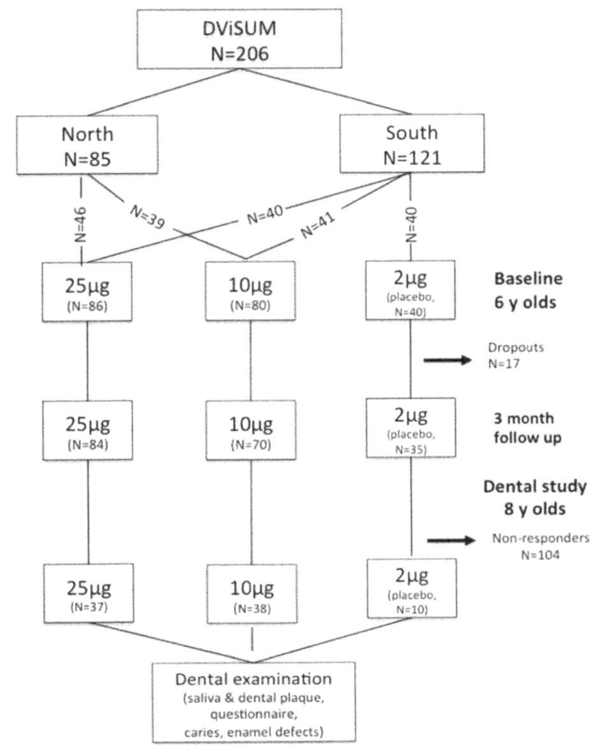


**Fig. 1** Flow diagram of the numbers of children in the basic intervention DViSUM and placebo groups at baseline, 3 month follow up and at the dental follow up at 8 years of age

scored (scores 3–4 represent caries lesions into the dentine). The combined measures of $D_{3-4}$FS and $d_{3-4}$ fs are hereafter referred to as dfs/DFS. Bitewing radiographs were captured for special indications, such as when approximal tooth surfaces were unavailable for visual inspection.

Enamel defects were documented and evaluated from photos captured during the clinical examination using criteria defined by the Commission on Oral Health, Research & Epidemiology [25]. Enamel defects, i.e., opacities and signs of enamel hypoplasia, were scored on a 6-level scale, where a score of 0 represents sound enamel and scores of 1–6 represent increasing severity of opacities and hypoplasia. The number of permanent first molars and central upper and lower incisors with a score of 0 or ≥1 were registered.

The scoring of enamel defects was trained and calibrated among two evaluating dentists (JG and KR) and a senior consultant in pediatric dentistry (PLH). Training was conducted with intra-oral photos from anonymous, non-study patients with various manifestations of enamel defects. Diverging scores were discussed to reach a consensus. Reproducibility rates were calculated for the occurrence of enamel defects. The intra-examiner weighted kappa-values (κ) ranged between 0.96 and 0.98. Inter-examiner agreement for the scoring of enamel defects was evaluated using photographs from 10 randomly selected participating children with a κ-value of 0.81.

### Tooth biofilm and saliva sampling and analyses

Tooth biofilm was collected for PCR detection of the caries associated *Streptococcus mutans* and *Streptococcus sobrinus*. Samples were collected from all available supra-gingival tooth surfaces using sterilized toothpicks, pooled for each participant and stored in TE buffer (10 mM Tris and 1 mM EDTA, pH 7.6) at −80 °C. Genomic DNA was extracted and quality controlled as previously described [26]. The presence of *S. mutans* and *S. sobrinus* was detected using SmF5 and SmR4 primers for *S. mutans* and SsF3 and SsR1 primers for *S. sobrinus* [27].

Paraffin chewing-stimulated whole saliva (3 mL) was collected into ice-chilled test tubes for the analysis of LL37 levels. Samples were aliquoted and stored at −80 ° C until further analysis.

### Anthropometric measures

Height and body weight were measured at the baseline DViSUM visit [21, 22], and body mass index, BMI (kg/m$^2$), was calculated and converted to a BMI z-score based on WHO reference data for children and adolescents aged 5 to 19 years [28].

### Serum and plasma analyses

Serum 25(OH)D and vitamin D-related components, i.e., calcium, phosphate, magnesium, parathyroid hormone (PTH), alkaline phosphatase (ALP), and osteocalcin in plasma, were analyzed before and after the intervention period as previously described [21, 22]. Briefly, venous blood samples were collected at least 2 h after a meal. The samples were light protected, centrifuged after 30 min, and stored at −20 °C for up to a week and then at -80 °C. S- 25(OH) vitamin D2 and S-25(OH) vitamin D3 levels were analyzed by mass spectrometry on an API 4000 LC/MS/MS system (AB Sciex, Framingham, MA). All other components were analyzed in plasma on Cobas 6000/8000 analyzers (Roche Diagnostics, Mannheim, Germany). Serum levels of 25(OH)D < 50 nmol/L were considered insufficient, and levels <30 nmol/L were considered deficient [29].

### LL37 analysis in saliva

LL37 levels were analyzed using the LL37 Human ELISA kit (HK321, Hycult Biotech, Uden, The Netherlands) according to the manufacturer's instructions. Briefly, thawed samples were centrifuged, and the supernatant was transferred to antibody-coated microtiter wells to capture LL37, incubated with a biotinylated secondary antibody and detected by streptavidin-peroxidase.

### Data handling and statistical analyses

Continuous, normally distributed variables are presented as the means with 95% confidence limits (CI). Differences between group means were either evaluated with Student's t-test for comparisons between two groups and ANOVA for more than two groups. Differences in dietary intake were tested with the Mann-Whitney non-parametric test. When appropriate, mean values were standardized for potential confounders, such as living region, skin type, and vitamin D supplement intake, using general linear modeling (glm). Categorical variables are presented as numbers or proportions, and the Chi$^2$ test was used to determine differences in distributions. All tests were two-sided, and $p$-values <0.05 were considered statistically significant.

Logistic regression analysis was used to evaluate the adjusted odds ratio (OR) and 95% confidence limits (CI) for caries with vitamin D status as the independent variable and potential confounders included as covariates. Vitamin D was evaluated as a continuous measure. A dichotomous caries classification (caries-free or caries-affected) was used to account for zero-inflated dfs/DFS scores. Three models were evaluated: model 1 (basic model) was adjusted for the number of teeth, tooth brushing (once or twice a day), presence or absence of *S. mutans*, father's education level (<12 years or ≥12 years of school attendance), and region of residence; model 2 also included BMI (z-scores) and intake of a vitamin D supplement at the time of the dental examination; and model 3 also included skin type. Since all blood samples were collected in the same season, adjustment for season was not needed. Further adjustments, including the parents' country of origin and reported intake of various sweet products, were tested, but they did not affect the results. Firth's penalized likelihood approach was used to address the small group sizes using proc. logistic in SAS 9.4 (SAS Institute Inc., Cary, NC, USA) and odds ratios with and without correction are presented.

Multivariate principal component analysis (PCA) and partial least square (PLS) regression analyses were used to search for clustering of subjects and variables associated with caries (yes/no) and number of teeth with defective enamel, respectively. Following a screening step in which variables that were influential in explaining the variation in the dependent variables, i.e., Variable Importance in Projection (VIP) values >1 among all serum/plasma components, anthropometric measures, diet, oral health behavior, socio-economic, and medical variables ($n$ = 106) were identified. These variables were then entered into final PCA/PLS models for caries and enamel defects.

Analyses were performed using SPSS version 23 (IBM Corporation, Armonk, NY, USA). SIMCA P+ version 12.0 (Umetrics AB, Umeå, Sweden) was used for PCA and PLS modeling.

### Power calculation

Dental caries was the primary outcome measure, and secondary outcomes were enamel defects and LL37 levels in saliva. G*Power (http://www.gpower.hhu.de/) was used to calculate the power to find a statistically significant difference in mean vitamin D levels between children with or without caries given the number and distribution of participants. With 85 participants, $\alpha$ = 0.05, an effect size of 0.6 (difference in group means = 12 and SD = 18 based on the distribution of all serum values), and two-tailed testing, we have 77% power to detect a statistically significant difference.

## Results

### Vitamin D status and other participants' characteristics

Vitamin D status before and after the intervention in the basic DViSUM cohort ($n$ = 206) and the children in the dental subgroup ($n$ = 85) are presented in Table 1 together with information on dietary intake. Additional information for the DViSUM basic study is found in Karlsland Åkeson et al. and Öhlund et al. [21, 22]. The overall (n = 206) mean vitamin D level was 55.4 nmol/L (95% CI: 52.8, 58.0) at baseline with a mean increase of 30% in the high and 19% in the low intervention groups and no change in the placebo group (23). This result were in accordance with the levels found in the subgroup employed in the present study, i.e., 60.4 nmol/L (95% CI: 56.4, 64.3) and 76.3 nmol/L (95% CI: 72.2, 80.3) at baseline and follow-up, respectively (Table 1). However, children who participated in the dental follow-up study had 8 nmol/L higher vitamin D levels at baseline and 3-month follow-up than those who did not (both $p$ = 0.002). Skin complexion and vitamin D intake from fortified milk and spreads were identified as the major determinants for vitamin D status in the DViSUM cohort [21]. A larger proportion of children who participated in the dental follow-up study had fair skin compared to those who did not (68 and 41%, respectively; $p$ = 0.001), but their reported milk and fish intakes were similar (Table 1). Intake of sweet products was not monitored at 6 years of age, but at 8 years of age, intake of several sweet products was common. Mean intake of products with added sucrose was 1.7 times per day (Table 1).

Similar to in the basic DViSUM cohort [21, 22], serum 25 (OH)D levels varied by skin type and region of residence in the dental subgroup. Thus, children with darker skin ($n$ = 27) had significantly lower 25 (OH)D levels than children with fair skin ($n$ = 58) (mean (95% CI): 49.4 (42.0, 56.8) and 65.4 (61.3, 69.6) nmol/L, respectively, $p$ < 0.001). In the former group, 59.3% had insufficient levels compared with 13.8% in the latter group (p < 0.001). Further, children in southern Sweden had significantly lower S-25

**Table 1** Vitamin D status and diet intake in 6 year olds in the DViSUM study group ($n$ = 206) and in the nested dental study sub-group ($n$ = 85). Data are presented as mean with 95% CI. ND = not determined

| | DViSUM | Dental study sub-group | |
|---|---|---|---|
| | 6 years of age n = 206 | 6 years of age n = 85 | 8 years of age n = 85 |
| Vitamin D status, nmol/L | | | |
| at baseline | 55.4 (52.8, 58.0) | 60.4 (56.4, 64.3) | ND |
| after intervention | 71.5 (68.6, 74.3) | 76.3 (72.2, 80.3) | ND |
| Intake of vitamin D foods | | | |
| Milk[a], mL/day | 535 (484, 587) | 562 (478, 646) | 574 (521, 629) |
| Cheese[b], g/day | 20.0 (13.5, 26.5) | 14.7 (9.9, 19.2) | 17 (12, 22) |
| Eggs, g/day | 13.4 (8.2, 18.5) | 14.4 (12.5, 17.6) | ND |
| Fatty fish, g/day | 14 (11.7, 17.5) | 14.2 (12.6, 17.2) | 13 (9, 16) |
| Table spreads, g/day | 19.7 (17.9, 21.5) | 20.9 (17.9, 23.9) | ND |
| Vitamin D supplement, % with reported intake | 14 | 10 | 34 |
| Intake of sweet products | | | |
| Sum of sucrose product, frequency/day | ND | ND | 1.7 (1.1, 2.3) |
| Sodas with sucrose, frequency/day | ND | ND | 0.4 (0.3, 0.5) |
| Cookies and sweet buns, frequency/day | ND | ND | 0.53 (0.28, 0.79) |
| Non-sweet snacks, frequency/day[c] | ND | ND | 0.15 (0.12, 0.18) |
| Fruits, frequency/day | ND | ND | 1.5 (1.3, 1.7) |

[a]including non-fermented milk, sour milk, and yoghurt (natural and sweetened)
[b]including cheese, and cottage cheese
[c]including crisps, cheese doodles, popcorn

(OH)D levels than children in northern Sweden (mean (95% CI): 54.7 (48.9, 60.4) and 64.9 (59.7, 70.1), respectively; $p$ = 0.009). Insufficient S-25 (OH)D levels were seen in 42.1% in the former compared to 17.0% in the latter group ($p$ = 0.011).

### Vitamin D and caries status

Caries-affected children had a mean of 4.5 decayed or filled tooth surfaces (dfs/DFS) (95% CI: 3.3, 5.8) at 8 years of age (Table 2). In univariate analyses, vitamin D levels did not differ between children with or without caries, although the proportion with <50 nmol/L of S-25[OH]D tended to be higher among children with caries (Table 2). dfs/DFS scores did not differ significantly between the three vitamin D intervention groups [2.5 (0, 6.3), 2.1 (1.0, 3.1) and 1.7 (0.7, 2.7) for 2, 10 and 25 µg, respectively; $p$ = 0.758]. Children with <50 nmol/l of S-25[OH]D after the intervention had a mean dfs/DFS of 5.8 compared to 1.4 for those with >50 nmol/L ($p$ = 0.001). The trend was similar for the baseline S-25[OH]D strata (2.9 versus 1.6: $p$ = 0.086). A darker skin complexion was significantly more common among those with caries than without ($p$ = 0.014, Table 2). No association was seen between caries status and reported intake frequency of any sweet or other food item assessed in the questionnaire (data not shown). The proportions reporting vitamin D supplement intake did not differ between caries groups (Table 2) or vitamin D intervention groups (data not shown), but it was more common among children who had an insufficient vitamin D status or not at baseline (58% and 25%, $p$ = 0.004) and after the intervention (78% and 30%, $p$ = 0.005). Notably, after the second blood analyses, parents were informed about the child's vitamin D status and supplements were recommended for those with low levels. This recommendation was reflected in that at 8 years of age, 34% reported intake of a vitamin D supplement compared to 14% before the intervention started (Table 1).

As a next step, we evaluated the risk of developing caries according to vitamin D levels (continuous measure) at baseline and after the 3-month intervention using a logistic regression model that included potential confounders. In the basic model (model 1), higher baseline vitamin D levels were significantly associated with less caries [OR (95% CI) 0.961 (0.929, 0.995; $p$ = 0.024)] which remained after Firth's correction (Table 3). Additional adjustments for BMI and reported intake of vitamin D supplement at caries examination attenuated the results slightly (0.967 (0.931, 1.005; $p$ = 0.085); Table 3) and they were no longer statistically significant after Firth's correction. The results were similar when vitamin D levels at follow-up were used as the independent variable (Table 3). Backward elimination indicated that S-

**Table 2** Characteristics of dental study group participants by caries status. Data are presented as mean with 95% CI for continuous measures and proportion (%) for categorical measures. Differences between groups were tested with Students t-test and Chi-square test, respectively

| | Caries-free $n = 48$ | Caries $n = 37$ | p-value |
|---|---|---|---|
| Baseline | | | |
| Age years, mean (95% CI) | 6.4 (6.2, 6.6) | 6.3 (6.0, 6.5) | 0.259 |
| Boys, % | 52.1 | 32.4 | 0.070 |
| Region, south; north, % | 52.1; 47.9 | 35.1; 64.9 | 0.119 |
| Fair; darker skin, % | 79.2; 20.8 | 54.1; 45.9 | 0.014 |
| Mother education, % ≥12 years | 56.3 | 51.4 | 0.653 |
| Father education, % ≥12 years | 68.1 | 51.4 | 0.126 |
| BMI, z-score | 0.23 (−0.06, 0.52) | 0.29 (−0.03, 0.62) | 0.764 |
| Vitamin D supplement, % with reported intake | 31.3 | 38.9 | 0.466 |
| Insufficient vitamin D status, % | 20.8 | 37.8 | 0.084 |
| S-25(OH) D, nmol/L | 62.6 (57.3, 67.8) | 57.4 (51.3, 63.5) | 0.195 |
| S-Calcium, mmol/L | 2.43 (2.41, 2.45) | 2.45 (2.43, 2.47) | 0.339 |
| S-Phosphate, mmol/L | 1.57 (1.53, 1.61) | 1.51 (1.46, 1.55) | 0.033 |
| S-Magnesium, mmol/L | 0.88 (0.86, 0.89) | 0.85 (0.84, 0.87) | 0.015 |
| Parathyroid hormone (PTH), pmol/L | 3.86 (3.47, 4.30) | 3.68 (3.32, 4.04) | 0.512 |
| Osteocalcin, µg/L | 86.2 (79.1, 93.4) | 81.3 (73.1, 89.6) | 0.364 |
| Alkaline phosphatase, µkat/L | 3.94 (3.71, 4.16) | 3.99 (3.62, 4.35) | 0.812 |
| Dental examinations | | | |
| Age, years | 8.3 (8.1, 8.5) | 8.1 (7.8, 8.3) | 0.258 |
| Number of teeth | | | |
| total number | 23.5 (23.2, 23.7) | 22.9 (22.4, 23.5) | 0.059 |
| deciduous teeth | 11.5 (10.7, 12.3) | 11.5 (10.6, 12.5) | 0.968 |
| permanent teeth | 12.0 (11.2, 12.7) | 11.4 (10.5, 12.4) | 0.368 |
| Caries status score (dfs/DFS) | 0 | 4.5 (3.3, 5.8) | <0.001 |
| Enamel defects | | | |
| single tooth, % | 62.5 | 63.9 | 0.896 |
| multiple teeth, % | 45.8 | 44.4 | 0.899 |
| Tooth brushing twice a day, % | 88.9 | 94.3 | 0.397 |
| Saliva analyses | | | |
| LL37, ng/mL | 1.01 (0.74, 1.29) | 1.56 (1.24, 1.88) | 0.012 |
| *S. mutans*, % positive by PCR | 27.1 | 33.3 | 0.535 |
| *S. sobrinus* % positive by PCR | 0 | 0 | — |

25[OH]D levels at baseline, tooth brushing, number of teeth, and living region were independently associated with having caries ($p = 0.01$, Table 3).

Finally, PLS modeling was applied with caries status (yes/no) as dependent variables and variables with a screening VIP value > 1 in the independent block. PLS identified one significant component with an explanatory ($R^2$) and predictive ($Q^2$) capacity of 29.8% and 12.1%, respectively. Having caries was significantly associated with number of siblings, skin color and type, and having less than 50 nmol/l of 25(OH)D levels in serum (Fig. 2). Being caries-free was significantly associated with higher levels of magnesium, phosphate and 25(OH)D in serum (Fig. 2).

### Vitamin D status and enamel defects

The prevalence of enamel defects on the permanent first molars and central upper and lower incisors did not differ between children with insufficient and sufficient vitamin D levels at 6 years of age. Six children had serum vitamin D levels corresponding to a vitamin D deficiency, i.e., <30 nmol/L, and 4 of

**Table 3** Odds ratios to have dental caries or not by increasing vitamin D status. Serum vitamin D levels are at 6 years of age and caries status at 8 years of age

| | Logistic regression | | | | | |
|---|---|---|---|---|---|---|
| | Baseline | | | 3 months after intervention | | |
| | Odds ratio | 95% CI | p-value | Odds ratio | 95% CI | p-value |
| Method: Variables entered | | | | | | |
| Model 1[a] | 0.961 | 0.929, 0.995 | 0.024 | 0.966 | 0.936, 0.997 | 0.030 |
| Model 2[b] | 0.962 | 0.928, 0.998 | 0.037 | 0.971 | 0.939, 1.003 | 0.075 |
| Model 3[c] | 0.967 | 0.931, 1.005 | 0.085 | 0.975 | 0.943, 1.009 | 0.148 |
| With Firth's correction | | | | | | |
| Model 1[a] | 0.966 | 0.935, 0.998 | 0.040 | 0.969 | 0.940, 0.999 | 0.044 |
| Model 2[b] | 0.970 | 0.935, 1.008 | 0.117 | 0.975 | 0.943, 1.008 | 0.134 |
| Model 3[c] | 0.973 | 0.936, 1.010 | 0.153 | 0.979 | 0.947, 1.013 | 0.232 |
| Method: Backward elimination (variables retained in final model) | | | | | | |
| D vitamin status | 0.958 | 0.926, 0.990 | 0.01 | 0.971 | 0.940, 1.003 | 0.08 |
| Number of teeth | 0.666 | 0.412, 1.061 | 0.087 | 0.598, | 0.366, 0.975 | 0.039 |
| Living region[d] | 3.13 | 1.05, 9.33 | 0.040 | 2.62 | 0.842, 8.16 | 0.096 |
| Tooth brushing[d] | 0.099 | 0.008, 1.16 | 0.065 | Not retained | | |
| Skin type[d] | Not retained | | | 3.08 | 1.02, 9.35 | 0.047 |

[a]Model 1 with caries (yes/no) as dependent variables and serum levels of vitamin D, number of teeth, tooth brushing, *S. mutans*, parental education, and living region as covariates
[b]model 1+ BMI, and reported intake of vitamin D supplement at the caries examination
[c]model 2 + skin type
[d]The reference categories were southern Sweden (living region), brushing <twice a day (tooth brushing), and fair skin (skin type)

these children had multiple enamel defects on the assessed teeth, but 2 did not. Thus, in this population, baseline levels of S-25 (OH)D or any of the other serum components did not differ between the children with or without enamel defects on the permanent first molars and central upper and lower incisors (data not shown).

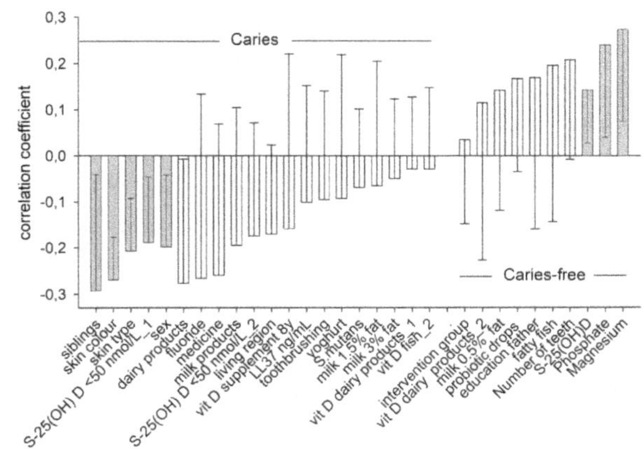


**Fig. 2** PLS correlation coefficients from multivariate modelling with caries status (yes/no) as dependent variables. Correlation coefficients with 95% CI for the variables in the final mode are presented. Bars for which the 95% whisker do not pass zero are statistically significant

PLS modeling only identified intake of a vitamin D supplement at 8 years of age as associated with having defects, which likely reflects reversed causality.

### Vitamin D status and LL37 levels in saliva

LL37 is an innate immunity peptide for which expression has been linked to vitamin D status [4]. In the dental study group, region-adjusted mean LL37 levels were lower in children with insufficient serum vitamin D status than in children with serum 25(OH)D levels ≥50 nmol/L after the 3-month intervention [1.09 (0.87, 1.30)] and [2.38 (1.77, 2.99), respectively; $p < 0.001$]. No difference was observed in LL37 levels between children who reported vitamin D supplement intake at 8 years of age or not. The mean LL37 levels in saliva (adjusted for region of residence) were higher among children who had caries at 8 years of age.

## Discussion

The primary goal of the present study was to evaluate the association between vitamin D status and prospective caries status in children selected from a population with overall low caries prevalence, high milk consumption and vitamin D supplementation in infancy [21, 30]. The results support an inverse association between vitamin D status and caries, i.e., higher vitamin D and less caries, although the results were not fully consistent. No association was found with enamel defects.

Most studies evaluating the association between vitamin D status and dental caries use a cross-sectional design [14, 31]. Caries development is normally a slow process with several years of delay before a cavity is observed. Therefore, the serum 25(OH)D level at the time of caries scoring may or may not be representative of the period when caries symptoms developed [14]. Therefore, we examined the participants' caries status 2 years after vitamin D levels were assessed. Although the participants' vitamin D status was not followed during the two years between the initial vitamin D measurement and dental examination, information on vitamin D supplement intake at the time of the dental examination was available. The children in the present study were nested in a study in which vitamin D status was analyzed before and after a 3-month treatment with milk-based supplements with different vitamin D concentrations at 6 years of age. When the follow-up blood samples were analyzed, parents of children with serum levels <50 nmol/L were advised to administer a vitamin D supplement to their children. We have no information on individual compliance with this advice, but at the time of dental examination, 78% of children with <50 nmol/L (insufficient vitamin D status) in their second blood sample reported that the child was given a vitamin D supplement. Therefore, one might hypothesize that the serum 25(OH)D levels measured after the intervention would better reflect the levels over the 2-year interval for most study subjects. On the other hand, the results from the models employing the baseline values may better reflect habitual levels and the situation during the period between 2 and 6 years of age when teeth mineralized and caries development likely began. However, to be able to assess the associations properly, the question should be addressed in a longitudinal study with repeated measures of both serum 25(OH)D levels and caries status from early childhood to the age of caries scoring and should include children with more selective diets. In the present study, consuming milk was an inclusion criterion.

The saliva LL37 concentration was lower in children who had an insufficient D vitamin levels than in children who had sufficient serum levels at follow-up. This result was stable in sensitivity analyses stratified by supplement intake at 8 years of age. LL37, a 37-amino acid peptide generated from proteolytic cleavage of the extracellular domain of the 18-kDa hCAP18 protein from epithelial cells and neutrophils [32, 33], is the only cathelicidin-derived antibacterial peptide in humans. Vitamin D has been shown to have a specific role in the expression of the cathelicidins, and several studies have confirmed the association between vitamin D and LL37 levels [4]. LL37 has been linked to several biological innate immune functions, including those in periodontal disease and psoriasis [34, 35]. LL37 has also been implicated in the oral microbiota, but the results from studies on its association with dental caries are inconsistent [36, 37]. In the present study, children with caries had higher LL37 levels, which may indicate oral microbiota-induced expression. Although these findings are consistent with some previous publications [38, 39], the results should be interpreted with caution and evaluated in a larger study in which vitamin D status is measured closer to the time of LL37 analysis.

According to previous studies, enamel defects in the form of opacities and hypomineralization are more prevalent in patients with vitamin D deficiency [40]. In the present population, the prevalence of enamel defects on permanent first molars or central incisors did not differ between children with serum levels <50 nmol/L at 6 years of age and children with sufficient vitamin D at this age. This finding was expected since the evaluated teeth were mineralized during the first years of life, and all parents in Sweden are encouraged to provide vitamin $D_3$ supplements of 10 μg/day in drop form to their children from birth to 2 years of age. The drops are available free of charge. Children with dark skin, or those with little outdoor activity, and children who do not receive fortified products or eat fish are advised to continue taking the vitamin D drops up to 5 years of age [29, 41]. Therefore, during these early years, intake from supplements rather than UV light exposure is likely to be the major determinant of vitamin D status. This hypothesis was also supported by the finding that the prevalence of enamel defects on the specified teeth did not differ between children with fair or dark skin in the present study, even though their vitamin D status differed at 6 years of age.

The strengths of the present study include that vitamin D status was measured and not based on self-reported intake only, that caries were evaluated prospectively and were scored by experienced pediatric dentists who took X-rays when approximal surfaces were not accessible and that the study group was very well characterized. However, there are limitations that should be acknowledged when the results are interpreted. The study group is small with limitations in stratification, vitamin D status was not reanalyzed later than the intervention follow-up, and there is a potential risk of response bias in the questionnaire replies. It should also be acknowledged that the study group represents populations characterized by vitamin D supplementation in the first living years and regular dental care.

## Conclusions

Based on the present results, we conclude that the results from Schroth et al. [14] of an inverse association between vitamin D status and caries were supported. However, the comparably small study group and weak association with attenuation from confounder adjustment suggest the need for replication. Vitamin D status was unrelated to enamel defects on permanent incisors and molars in the present circumstances, whereas an association between vitamin D status and LL37 levels was supported.

### Abbreviations

ALP: Alkaline Phosphatase; BMI: Body Mass Index; CI: Confidence Interval limit; DFS: Decayed Filled Surface; GLM: General Linear Modelling; OR: Odds ratio; PCA: Principal Component Analysis; PCR: Polymerase Chain Reaction; PLS: Partial Least Square Regression analysis; PTH: ParaThyroid Hormone; PuL: Swedish law on personal data act

### Acknowledgements

The basic DViSUM study was funded by grants from Dr. Per Håkansson Foundation, the Fanny Ekdahl foundation, the Samariten Foundation, the Oskar Foundation, the Jerring Foundation, and through Västerbotten County Council in the field of Medicine, Odontology, and Health (ALF) and the present dental follow-up study by Umeå University and TUA, the Västerbotten County Council, Sweden. Funders had no role in study design, data collection and analysis, decision to publish, or preparation of the manuscript. Carina Öhman and Agneta Rönnlund are acknowledged for skilful laboratory work.

### Funding

The present study was funded by Umeå University, and TUA, the County Council of Västerbotten, Sweden.

### Authors' contributions

PLH designed the study, JG and KR performed the clinical examination and JG, KR and PLH analysed the photos, IÖ and PKÅ were responsible for the basic study from which participants were recruited and serum and some questionnaire data were obtained, IJ performed the data analyses and wrote the manuscript, and all authors read and approved of the final article.

### Competing interest

The authors declare that they have no competing interests.

### Author details

[1]Department of Odontology, Section of Paediatric Dentistry, Faculty of Medicine, Umeå University, 90185 Umeå, Sweden. [2]Department of Paediatric Dentistry, Faculty of Odontology, Malmö University, Malmö, Sweden. [3]Department of Clinical Sciences/Section of Paediatric Medicine, Faculty of Medicine, Umeå University, Umeå, Sweden. [4]Department of Clinical Sciences, Pediatrics, Lund University, Lund, Malmö, Sweden. [5]Department of Odontology/Section of Cariology, Faculty of Medicine, Umeå University, Umeå, Sweden.

### References

1. Reichrath J, Saternus R, Vogt T. Challenge and perspective: the relevance of ultraviolet (UV) radiation and the vitamin D endocrine system (VDES) for psoriasis and other inflammatory skin diseases. Photochem Photobiol Sci. 2017;16:433–44.
2. Svensson D, Nebel D, Nilsson B-O. Vitamin D3 modulates the innate immune response through regulation of the hCAP-18/LL-37 gene expression and cytokine production. Inflamm Res. 2016;65:25–32.
3. Davideau JL, Lezot F, Kato S, Bailleul-Forestier I, Berdal A. Dental alveolar bone defects related to vitamin D and calcium status. J Steroid Biochem Mol Biol. 2004;89:615–8.
4. Raftery T, Martineau AR, Greiller CL, et al. Effects of vitamin D supplementation on intestinal permeability, cathelicidin and disease markers in Crohn's disease: results from a randomised double-blind placebo-controlled study. United European Gastroenterol J. 2015;3:294–302.
5. Abhimanyu, Coussens A. The role of UV radiation and vitamin D in the seasonality and outcomes of infectious disease. *Photochem Photobiol Sci* 2017;16:314–38.
6. Skaaby T, Nystrup Husemoen LL, Pisinger C, et al. Vitamin D status and incident cardiovascular disease and all-mortality: a general population study. Endocrine. 2013;43:618–25.
7. Institute of Medicine. Dietary reference intakes for calcium and vitamin D. Washington (DC): The National Academic Press. 2011.
8. Greer FR. 25-Hydroxyvitamin D: functional outcomes in infants and young children. Am J Clin Nutr. 2008;88:529S–33S.
9. Vieth R. Why the minimum desirable serum 25-hydroxyvitamin D level should be 75 nmol/L(30 ng/ml). Best Pract Res Clin Endocrinol Metab. 2011; 25:681–91.
10. Prentice A, Goldberg GR, Schoenmakers I. Vitamin D across the lifecycle: physiology and biomarkers. Am J Clin Nutr. 2008;88:500S–6S.
11. Clemens TL, Adams JS, Henderson SL, Holick MF. Increased skin pigment reduces the capacity of skin to synthesise vitamin D3. Lancet. 1982;1:74–6.
12. Öhlund I, Silfverdal SA, Hernell O, Lind T. Serum 25-hydroxyvitamin D levels in preschool children in northern Sweden are inadequate after summer and diminish further during winter. J Pediatr Gastroenterol Nutr. 2013;56:551–5.
13. Schroth RJ, Lavelle C, Tate R, Bruce S, Billings RJ, Moffatt MEK, Prenatal Vitamin D. Dental caries in infants. Pediatrics. 2014;133:277.
14. Schroth RJ, Rabbani R, Loewen G, Moffatt ME. Vitamin D and Dental caries in children. J Dent Res. 2016;95:173–9.
15. Dudding T, Thomas SJ, Duncan K, Lawlor DA, Timpson NJ. Re-examining the association between vitamin D and childhood caries. PLoS One 2015;21: 10:e0143769.
16. Herzog K, Scott JM, Hujoel P, Seminario AL. Association of vitamin D and dental caries in children: findings from the National Health and nutrition examination survey, 2005-2006. J Am Dent Assoc. 2016;147: 413–20.
17. Theodoratou E, Tzoulaki I, Zgaga L, Ioannidis JP, Vitamin D. Multiple health outcomes: umbrella review of systematic reviews and meta-analyses of observational studies and randomised trials. BMJ. 2014;348:2035.
18. Hujoel PP, Vitamin D. Dental caries in controlled clinical trials: systematic review and meta-analysis. Nutr Rev. 2013;71:88–97.
19. Karpiński M, Galicka A, Milewski R, Popko J, Badmaev V, Stohs SJ. Association between vitamin D receptor polymorphism and serum vitamin D levels in children with low-energy fractures. J Am Coll Nutr. 2017;9:1–8.
20. Mäkinen M, Mykkänen J. Koskinen *et al.* serum 25-hydroxyvitamin D concentration in children progressing to autoimmunity and clinical type 1 diabetes. J Clin Endocrinol Metab. 2016;101:723–9.
21. Åkeson PK, Lind T, Hernell O, Silfverdal SA, Öhlund I, Serum Vitamin D. Depends less on latitude than on skin color and dietary intake during early winter in northern Europe. J Pediatr Gastroenterol Nutr. 2016;62:643–9.
22. Öhlund I, Lind T, Hernell O, Silfverdal SA, Karlsland Åkeson P. Increased vitamin D intake differentiated according to skin color is needed to meet requirements in young Swedish children during winter: a double-blinded randomized clinical trial. *Am J Clin Nutr.* 2017;jun 14. ajcn147108.
23. www.livsmedelsverket.se/globalassets/english/food-habits-health-environment/dietary-guidelines/good-food-for-children-1-2-years (2017–06-09).
24. World Health Organization. Oral health surveys: basic methods 4th edition 1997. World Health Organization, Geneva.
25. A review of the developmental defects of enamel index (DDE-Index). Commission on Oral Health, Research & Epidemiology. Report of an FDI Working Group. *Int Dent J.* 1992; 42:411–26.
26. Lif Holgerson P, Harnevik L, Hernell O, Tanner AC, Johansson I. Mode of

birth delivery affects oral microbiota in infants. J Dent Res. 2011;90:1183–8.
27. Yano A, Kaneko N, Ida H, Yamaguchi T, Hanada N, Real-time PCR. For quantification of Streptococcus Mutans. FEMS Microbiol Lett. 2002;19: 23–30.
28. de Onis M, Onyango AW, Borghi E, Siyam A, Nishida C, Siekmann J. Development of a WHO growth reference for school-aged children and adolescents. Bull World Health Organ. 2007;85:660–7.
29. Ross AC, Manson JE, Abrams SA, et al. The 2011 report on dietary reference intakes for calcium and vitamin D from the Institute of Medicine: what clinicians need to know. J Clin Endocrinol Metab. 2011;96:53–8.
30. Nordic Council of Ministers. Nordic Nutrition Recommendations 2012. *Nordic Nutrition Recommendations 2012* 2012;5(11):1.
31. Guizar JM, Muñoz N, Amador N, Garcia G. Association of Alimentary Factors and Nutritional Status with caries in children of Leon, Mexico. Oral Health Prev Dent. 2016;14:563–9.
32. Larrick JW, Hirata M, Balint RF, Lee J, Zhong J, Wright SC. Human CAP18: a novel antimicrobial lipopolysaccharide-binding protein. Infect Immun. 1995; 63:1291–7.
33. Yamasaki K, Schauber J, Coda A, et al. Kallikrein-mediated proteolysis regulates the antimicrobial effects of cathelicidins in skin. FASEB J. 2006;20: 2068–80.
34. Gomes Pde S, Fernandes MH. Defensins in the oral cavity: distribution and biological role. J Oral Pathol Med. 2010;39:1–9.
35. Lande R, Botti E, Jandus C, et al. The antimicrobial peptide LL37 is a T-cell autoantigen in psoriasis. Nat Commun. 2014;5:5621.
36. Tao R, Jurevic RJ, Coulton KK. Salivary antimicrobial peptide expression and dental caries experience in children. Antimicrob Agents Chemother. 2005; 49:3883–8.
37. Phattarataratip E, Olson B, Brofitt B, et al. Streptococcus Mutans strains recovered from caries-active or caries-free individuals differ in sensitivity to host antimicrobial peptides. Mol Oral Microbiol. 2011;26:187–99.
38. Colombo NH, Ribas LF, Pereira JA, et al. Antimicrobial peptides in saliva of children with severe early childhood caries. Arch Oral Biol. 2016;69:40–6.
39. Malcolm J, Sherriff A, Lappin DF, et al. Salivary antimicrobial proteins associate with age-related changes in streptococcal composition in dental plaque. Mol Oral Microbiol. 2014;29:284–93.
40. Künisch J, Thiering E, Kratzsch J, Heinrich- Weltzien R, Hickel R, Heinrich J. Elevated serum 25(OH)-vitamin D levels are negatively correlated with molar-incisor hypomineralisation. J Dent Res. 2015;94:381–7.
41. https://www.livsmedelsverket.se/livsmedel-och innehall/naringsamne/vitaminer-och-antioxidanter/vitamin-d/ (2017–01–27).

# 19

# Association between time perspective and organic food consumption in a large sample of adults

Marc Bénard[1*], Julia Baudry[1], Caroline Méjean[1,2], Denis Lairon[3], Kelly Virecoulon Giudici[1], Fabrice Etilé[4], Gérard Reach[5], Serge Hercberg[1,6,7], Emmanuelle Kesse-Guyot[1] and Sandrine Péneau[1]

**Abstract**

**Background:** Organic food intake has risen in many countries during the past decades. Even though motivations associated with such choice have been studied, psychological traits preceding these motivations have rarely been explored. Consideration of future consequences (CFC) represents the extent to which individuals consider future versus immediate consequences of their current behaviors. Consequently, a future oriented personality may be an important characteristic of organic food consumers. The objective was to analyze the association between CFC and organic food consumption in a large sample of the adult general population.

**Methods:** In 2014, a sample of 27,634 participants from the NutriNet-Santé cohort study completed the CFC questionnaire and an Organic-Food Frequency questionnaire. For each food group (17 groups), non-organic food consumers were compared to organic food consumers across quartiles of the CFC using multiple logistic regressions. Moreover, adjusted means of proportions of organic food intakes out of total food intakes were compared between quartiles of the CFC. Analyses were adjusted for socio-demographic, lifestyle and dietary characteristics.

**Results:** Participants with higher CFC were more likely to consume organic food (OR quartile 4 (Q4) vs. Q1 = 1.88, 95% CI: 1.62, 2.20). Overall, future oriented participants were more likely to consume 14 food groups. The strongest associations were observed for starchy refined foods (OR = 1.78, 95% CI: 1.63, 1.94), and fruits and vegetables (OR = 1.74, 95% CI: 1.58, 1.92). The contribution of organic food intake out of total food intake was 33% higher in the Q4 compared to Q1. More precisely, the contribution of organic food consumed was higher in the Q4 for 16 food groups. The highest relative differences between Q4 and Q1 were observed for starchy refined foods (22%) and non-alcoholic beverages (21%). Seafood was the only food group without a significant difference.

**Conclusions:** This study provides information on the personality of organic food consumers in a large sample of adult participants. Consideration of future consequences could represent a significant psychological determinant of organic food consumption.

**Keywords:** Organic food consumption, Nutrition, Consideration of future consequences, Psychology

* Correspondence: m.benard@eren.smbh.univ-paris13.fr

[1]Equipe de Recherche en Epidémiologie Nutritionnelle, Centre de Recherche en Epidémiologie et Statistique Sorbonne Paris Cité, INSERM U1153, INRA U1125, Cnam, Université Paris 13, 74, rue Marcel Cachin, 93017 Bobigny, France

Full list of author information is available at the end of the article

## Background

The demand of organic foods has been notably increasing over the past years. In France, sales of organic products represented 5.5 billion euros in 2014 corresponding to a 10% increase from the previous year as it was the case in most European countries [1]. The major reasons regarding the purchase of organic foods include altruistic motives such as environmental and ethics aspects [2–7], and self-centered motives such as health, food safety, and sensory aspects [2, 4, 6, 8, 9]. Despite individual differences concerning these motivations, specific psychological traits which could lead to these motivations, and thus to an organic food consumption oriented behavior, have rarely been explored.

Consideration of Future Consequences (CFC) is a construct which measures "the extent to which individuals consider the potential distant outcomes of their current behaviors and the extent by which they are influenced by these potential outcomes [10]." Individuals with a low CFC are expected to act on their immediate needs and concerns whereas individuals with a high CFC are expected to consider the future implication of their behavior and to use their distant goals as guides for their current actions. Higher CFC have been shown to be associated with healthy and environmentally friendly behaviors [10]. In particular, several studies found that future oriented individuals were more likely to have a health oriented behavior, such as exercising more [11, 12], presenting healthy eating attitudes and intentions [13], being more sensitive to health communications to get tested for colorectal cancer [14], and participating in diabetes screening [15]. A meta-analysis measuring time perspective with different constructs found that future time perspective influenced individual attitudes and behaviors towards the environment [16], such as environmental preservation [17], recycling and waste reduction [18], and water conservation [19]. Finally, a study reported future oriented consumers to be more careful about organic labels, suggesting a higher interest in health related and sustainability issues [20]. However, to our knowledge no data are available on the relationship between time orientation and organic food intakes.

The aim of this study was therefore to analyze the association between consideration of futures consequences and the consumption of 17 organic food groups in a sample of the general population participating in the NutriNet-Santé cohort study by taking into account sociodemographic, lifestyle and dietary characteristics. Firstly, we wanted to assess whether organic food consumers were more likely to be future oriented compared to nonorganic food consumers. Then, we quantitatively analyzed intakes of organic food according to the individual level of consideration of future consequences.

## Methods

### Population

This study was conducted as part of the NutriNet-Santé study, which is a large ongoing web-based prospective cohort started in France in May 2009.The rationale, design and methods of the study have been described elsewhere [21]. Its overall aim is to explore the relationships between nutrition and health and the determinants of eating behavior and nutritional status. Participants are adult volunteers (age ≥ 18 years) of the general French population with a scheduled follow-up of at least 10 years. At inclusion, participants have to complete several self-reported web-based questionnaires to assess their diet, their physical activity, anthropometric measures, lifestyle characteristics, socioeconomic conditions and health status. Participants complete this set of questionnaires every year after inclusion. Finally, another set of optional questionnaires related to determinants of eating behaviors, nutritional status, and specific aspects related to health are sent to every participant each month. A flowchart of the participants included in this study is available as Additional file 1.

This study was conducted in accordance with the guidelines of the Declaration of Helsinki, and all procedures were approved by the International Research Board of the French Institute for Health and Medical Research (IRB Inserm n° 0000388FWA00005831) and the Commission Nationale Informatique et Libertés (CNIL n° 908450 and n° 909216). Electronic informed consent was obtained from all participants.

### Data collection

#### *Consideration of future consequences*

Consideration of Future Consequences was assessed with the French version of the CFC-12 questionnaire [22] over a 6-month period from June to November 2014. The CFC-12 is a 12-item self-report questionnaire [10] developed to measure the extent to which individuals consider distant versus immediate consequences of their behavior. Each item is measured on a 5-point Likert scale ranging from "extremely uncharacteristic" to "extremely characteristic". An example of the items of the CFC-12 is as followed: *I consider how things might be in the future, and try to influence those things with my day to day behavior*. The total score is obtained by summing each item ratings leading to a possible range from 12 to 60 (higher scores indicating greater consideration of future consequences). Participants were divided into 4 categories determined by quartiles of the total score (Q1, Q2, Q3, and Q4). A good internal consistency was obtained in our sample with a Cronbach's $\alpha$ of 0.79.

### *Dietary intake*

To assess their organic food consumption, participants completed a semi-quantitative organic food frequency questionnaire (Org-FFQ) by providing the frequency and portion sizes of consumed foods and beverages. The Org-FFQ was administered over a 5-month period from June to October 2014. This questionnaire was based on a validated food frequency questionnaire [23] supplemented by a section pertaining to the frequency of organic food consumption. More precisely, participants were asked to report their frequency of consumption and the quantity consumed over the past year for 264 items allowing to assess total food intakes (g/d). In addition, the frequency of organic food consumption for each item was assessed with a 5-point Likert scale ranging from never to always. Organic food intake (g/d) was obtained for each item by applying a weight of 0, 0.25, 0.5, 0.75 and 1 to the five respective categories of frequency (never, rarely, half the time, often and always). A full description of the Org-FFQ as well as sensitivity analyses pertaining to weighting can be found elsewhere [24].

Beverage and food items were aggregated into 17 food groups: fruits and vegetables (including juices and soups); seafood; meat, poultry and processed meat; eggs; dairy products; starchy refined foods; whole-grain products; legumes; fats (oil, butter, and margarine); fatty sweets (including cake, chocolate, ice cream, and pancakes); non-fatty sweets (including honey, jelly, sugar, and candy); alcoholic beverages; non-alcoholic beverages; fast food; snacks (including chips and salted biscuits); dressings and sauces; and dairy products and meat substitutes (including soya-based products). For each food group, contribution of organic food consumed was estimated by computing the organic food intake of the food group (g/d) out of the total food intake of the food group (g/d) multiplied by 100. Total energy intake (kcal/day) was also calculated using a validated composition table [25]. Participants with unlikely estimates of energy intake were identified as under- and over-reporting participants against estimated energy requirement. Basal metabolic rate (BMR) was calculated according to age, gender, weight and height using Schofield's equations [26]. The ratio between energy intake and estimated energy requirement (physical activity level x BMR, with physical activity level set by default at 1.55) was calculated and individuals with ratios below the 1st percentile (0.35) or above the 99th percentile (1.93) were excluded. These cutoffs were calculated on the validated FFQ for usual dietary intake used in the NutriNet-Santé cohort [23].

### *Socio-demographic, economic, anthropometric and lifestyle characteristics*

Potential confounders of the relationship between CFC and organic food consumption were collected based on information provided yearly by the participants after their inclusion: age (years), gender, education level (primary, secondary, undergraduate, and postgraduate), occupational status (unemployed, student, self-employed and farmer, employee and manual worker, managerial staff and intellectual profession, intermediate profession, and retired), monthly income per household unit, place of residence (rural community, urban unit with a population < 20,000 inhabitants, urban unit with a population between 20,000 and 200,000 inhabitants, and urban unit with a population > 200,000 inhabitants), and BMI (kg/m$^2$). More precisely, monthly income per household unit was calculated with information about income and composition. The number of people of the household was converted into a number of consumption units (CU) according to a weighting system: one CU is attributed for the first adult in the household, 0.5 for other persons aged 14 or older and 0.3 for children under 14 [27]. Categories of income were defined as followed: < 1200; 1200–1799; 1800–2299; 2300–2699; 2700–3699; and > 3700 euros per household unit as well as "unwilling to answer".

The Programme National Nutrition Santé Guidelines Score (PNNS-GS), which is an a priori nutritional diet quality score reflecting the adherence to the French nutritional recommendations of the participants [28], was considered as a confounder in the analyses. The original score includes 13 components: eight refer to food serving recommendations, four refer to moderation of nutrients or food, and one refers to physical activity. Points are deducted for overconsumption of salt and sweets. Points are also deducted from the total when energy intake exceeds the energy needs by more than 5%. A modified version of the PNNS-GS (mPNNS-GS) that did not include the physical activity component was used in this study. The score has a range of 0 to 13.5 points, with a higher score indicating a better overall nutritional quality of the diet.

### Statistical analysis

The characteristics of the sample across quartiles of the CFC-12 were compared with linear contrast tests for continuous variables, and with Mantel-Haenszel chi-square tests for categorical variables. Logistic regression models were performed between organic food consumption as a dependent variable (organic food consumer versus non-organic food consumer (reference)) for each of the 17 food groups) and the four categories (quartile, Q) of the CFC-12 as the main independent variable (Q1 as reference). The strength of the association was estimated by calculating odds ratios (ORs) and 95% confidence intervals (95% CI). Furthermore, adjusted means of proportions of the contribution of organic food to the total food intake by food group were compared across categories of the CFC-12 for the 17 food groups among organic food consumers only. A percentage of the relative difference between adjusted means of Q4 and Q1 was calculated to estimate the effect size of the differences. For every analysis on each food group, participants who did not report to consume at least one food item of the group (organic or non-organic food intakes) were excluded from the analysis of this food group. Since socio-economic positions are associated with CFC [29] and dietary intakes, all adjusted models included the following confounders: age, gender, education level, occupational status, monthly income per household unit, and place of residence. In addition, it has been suggested that time perspective can predict or be predicted by health behaviors [12]. Moreover, BMI, energy intake, mPNNS-GS (diet quality), and total food intake of the food group all predict the level of organic food consumption and were thus taken into account. No significant interaction terms were found between the CFC-12 and confounders. Missing data on confounding variables were handled with multiple imputation by chained eqs. (20 imputed datasets) [30].

All tests of statistical significance were 2-sided and significance was set at 5%. A Hochberg procedure was applied to correct for multiple testing. Statistical analyses were performed using SAS software (SAS Institute Inc., version 9.4).

## Results

### Description of the sample

A total of 33,384 participants of the NutriNet-Santé cohort study completed the Org-FFQ. Among these participants 2097 underreporters and overreporters were excluded, as well as 2320 individuals with missing covariates (which are required to assess inappropriate energy intake), and 722 participants residing in overseas territories. From those 28,245 individuals, 27,843 completed the CFC-12. Then, 209 participants who presented an acquiescence bias (agreeing to all questions without consideration of reversed items) in answers of the CFC-12 were excluded, leaving 27,634 participants in the final analysis. A total of 51,394 participants from the NutriNet-Santé study completed the CFC-12 questionnaires. Compared to excluded participants, the 27,634 participants in the final analysis were older (53.2 ± 14.1 years old for included participants vs 47.1 ± 14.5 years old for excluded participants, $p < .0001$), more often men (25.6% vs. 20.5%, $p < .0001$), had less often a university education (34.6% vs. 40.5%, $p < .0001$). In average, included participants had a lower CFC score (40.5 ± 7.1 vs. 40.9 ± 6.9, $p < .0001$). This marginal difference was likely to be significant due to the large sample size.

Table 1 shows characteristics of the sample according to the 4 categories determined by quartiles of the CFC-12. Overall, apart from energy intake, there was a significant linear trend between every variable analyzed and the categories of the CFC-12 (all $P < .0001$). Compared to Q1, participants in higher categories of CFC consumed more organic food (overall), were younger, were less often women, had more often a high level of education, were less often unemployed, employee, manual worker or retired and were more often student, self-employed, farmer, from managerial staff or intellectual professions, had more often a high monthly income per household, lived more often in large urban units, had a lower BMI, and had a higher mPNNS-GS.

Table 2 shows the percentages of organic food consumers in the 17 food groups according to CFC-12 categories. A significant linear trend was observed for every food group (all $P < .0001$).

### Association between consideration of future consequences and organic food consumption

Table 3 presents the results of logistic regression models between categories of the CFC-12 and organic food consumption and shows significant linear trends for most food groups. Overall, future oriented participants were more likely to consume organic foods. In particular, compared to Q1, participants in higher categories of the CFC-12 were more likely to consume organic: fruits and vegetables, eggs, dairy products, starchy refined foods, whole-grain products, legumes, fats, fatty sweets, non-fatty sweets, alcoholic beverages, non-alcoholic beverages, fast food, snacks, and dressing and sauces. Three food groups did not present a significant linear trend: seafood, meat, poultry and processed meat, and dairy products and meat substitutes. Comparing Q4 vs. Q1, the strongest associations were found for starchy refined foods (OR = 1.78, 95% CI: 1.63, 1.94), fruits and vegetables (OR = 1.74, 95% CI: 1.58, 1.92), and non-alcoholic beverages (OR = 1.72, 95% CI: 1.59, 1.85).

Table 4 focuses on organic consumers and shows the proportions of organic food consumed out of the total intake across categories of the CFC-12. The ratio of total organic food intakes out of total intakes significantly increased from 20.39% (Q1) to 27.12% (Q4) with a relative difference of 33%. There was a significant increase of the proportion of organic food consumed (on total intakes) for almost every group: fruits and vegetables, seafood, meat, poultry and processed meat, eggs, dairy products, starchy refined foods, whole-grain products, legumes, fats, fatty sweets, non-fatty sweets, alcoholic beverages, non-alcoholic beverages, fast food, snacks, dressings and sauces, and dairy products and meat substitutes. Seafood was the only food group without a statistical significant $p$-value for linear trend. The highest relative differences between Q4 and Q1 were observed for starchy refined foods (22%), and non-alcoholic beverages (21%); whereas

**Table 1** Individuals characteristics of the participants of the according to categories of the CFC

| | All | Quartiles of Consideration of Future Consequences | | | | $P^a$ |
|---|---|---|---|---|---|---|
| | | Q1 | Q2 | Q3 | Q4 | |
| | | < 36 | 36–40 | 41–46 | > 46 | |
| n | 27,634 | 6670 | 7107 | 6964 | 6893 | |
| % | 100 | 24.1 | 25.7 | 25.2 | 24.9 | |
| CFC-12 (12–60) | 40.5 ± 7.1 | 31.3 ± 3.7 | 38.0 ± 1.4 | 43.0 ± 1.4 | 49.4 ± 3.0 | |
| Total organic food intake (g/d) | 760.3 ± 799.7 | 625.8 ± 738.5 | 717.3 ± 779.5 | 775.0 ± 789.4 | 920.1 ± 857.4 | < .0001 |
| Age (years)[b] | 53.2 ± 14.1 | 55.9 ± 13.2 | 54.6 ± 13.8 | 51.6 ± 14.2 | 50.5 ± 14.5 | < .0001 |
| Gender (%) | | | | | | < .0001 |
| Women | 74.4 | 76.0 | 74.9 | 74.0 | 72.7 | |
| Men | 25.6 | 24.0 | 25.1 | 26.0 | 27.3 | |
| Education level (%) | | | | | | < .0001 |
| Primary | 2.8 | 5.5 | 3.2 | 1.7 | 1.0 | |
| Secondary | 32.9 | 46.6 | 38.2 | 27.2 | 20.1 | |
| Undergraduate | 29.6 | 27.1 | 30.7 | 31.5 | 29.1 | |
| Postgraduate | 34.6 | 20.8 | 27.8 | 39.7 | 49.8 | |
| Occupational status (%) | | | | | | < .0001 |
| Unemployed | 8.8 | 9.9 | 8.6 | 8.1 | 8.6 | |
| Student | 1.2 | 0.6 | 0.9 | 1.3 | 2.0 | |
| Self-employed, farmer | 1.7 | 1.5 | 1.6 | 1.7 | 2.2 | |
| Employee, manual worker | 14.2 | 17.2 | 14.8 | 13.8 | 11.2 | |
| Intermediate professions | 13.8 | 11.2 | 13.7 | 15.9 | 14.1 | |
| Managerial staff, intellectual profession | 21.0 | 12.5 | 16.9 | 24.8 | 29.4 | |
| Retired | 39.3 | 47.0 | 43.5 | 34.5 | 32.4 | |
| Monthly income (%)[c] | | | | | | < .0001 |
| < 1200€ | 10.1 | 12.2 | 10.1 | 8.8 | 9.3 | |
| 1200–1799€ | 20.9 | 23.0 | 21.3 | 20.6 | 18.7 | |
| 1800–2299€ | 15.3 | 16.2 | 16.3 | 14.8 | 13.9 | |
| 2300–2699€ | 10.3 | 10.1 | 10.3 | 10.6 | 10.2 | |
| 2700–3699€ | 17.7 | 14.3 | 17.1 | 18.6 | 20.9 | |
| > 3700€ | 13.2 | 9.1 | 11.4 | 14.8 | 17.2 | |
| Unwilling to answer | 12.3 | 14.9 | 13.4 | 11.5 | 9.5 | |
| Missing data | 0.2 | 0.2 | 0.2 | 0.3 | 0.3 | |
| Place of residence (%) | | | | | | < .0001 |
| Rural community | 22.0 | 22.7 | 22.5 | 21.3 | 21.5 | |
| Urban unit with a population < 20,000 inhabitants | 15.5 | 16.8 | 16.0 | 14.6 | 14.4 | |
| Urban unit with a population between 20,000 and 200,000 inhabitants | 18.0 | 18.7 | 18.4 | 18.0 | 17.0 | |
| Urban unit with a population > 200,000 inhabitants | 44.5 | 41.8 | 43.1 | 46.0 | 47.1 | |
| BMI (kg/m$^2$)[b] | 24.2 ± 4.5 | 25.0 ± 5.0 | 24.4 ± 4.6 | 24.0 ± 4.4 | 23.3 ± 4.0 | < .0001 |
| Energy intake (kcal/d)[b] | 1994 ± 629 | 2017 ± 646 | 1982 ± 632 | 1975 ± 615 | 2002 ± 620 | .32 |
| mPNNS-GS[b] | 8.5 ± 1.8 | 8.4 ± 1.8 | 8.5 ± 1.8 | 8.5 ± 1.7 | 8.6 ± 1.7 | < .0001 |

mPNNS-GS, modified Programme National Nutrition Santé Guideline Score

[a] *p*-value based on linear trend for continuous variables or Mantel-Haenszel chi-square test for categorical variables (corrected for multiple testing with a Hochberg procedure)

[b] Mean ± SD

[c] Monthly income represents the household income per month calculated by consumption unit (CU). The number of people of the household was converted into a number of CU according to a weighting system: one CU is attributed for the first adult in the household, 0.5 for other persons aged 14 or older and 0.3 for children under 14 [27]

**Table 2** Percentages of organic food consumers by food group according to quartiles of the CFC

| | All | | Quartiles of consideration of future consequences | | | | $P^a$ |
|---|---|---|---|---|---|---|---|
| Food groups (%) | n | % | Q1 | Q2 | Q3 | Q4 | |
| All | 27,634 | 93.5 | 90.4 | 92.8 | 94.6 | 96.0 | < .0001 |
| Fruits and vegetables (including juices and soups) | 27,618 | 83.0 | 77.3 | 81.7 | 84.9 | 87.8 | < .0001 |
| Seafood | 26,579 | 50.8 | 45.3 | 50.7 | 52.7 | 54.2 | < .0001 |
| Meat, poultry, and processed meat | 26,550 | 73.3 | 68.2 | 72.3 | 75.6 | 77.1 | < .0001 |
| Eggs | 26,494 | 76.6 | 71.2 | 75.4 | 78.5 | 81.5 | < .0001 |
| Dairy products | 27,177 | 69.7 | 62.6 | 68.1 | 72.1 | 75.8 | < .0001 |
| Starchy refined foods | 27,603 | 77.5 | 70.4 | 75.6 | 80.1 | 83.6 | < .0001 |
| Whole-grain products | 22,527 | 71.4 | 63.9 | 69.6 | 73.8 | 77.2 | < .0001 |
| Legumes | 24,811 | 55.0 | 47.2 | 52.5 | 57.0 | 62.5 | < .0001 |
| Fats (oil, butter, and margarine) | 27,537 | 71.3 | 64.4 | 69.9 | 73.1 | 77.6 | < .0001 |
| Fatty sweets (including cake, chocolate, ice cream, and pancakes) | 27,501 | 69.1 | 61.1 | 67.2 | 72.1 | 75.7 | < .0001 |
| Non-fatty sweets (including honey, jelly, sugar, and candy) | 26,296 | 69.7 | 63.1 | 68.2 | 71.9 | 75.3 | < .0001 |
| Fast food | 26,838 | 53.0 | 45.1 | 51.4 | 56.0 | 59.2 | < .0001 |
| Snacks (including chips and salted biscuits) | 25,902 | 47.0 | 39.1 | 45.5 | 49.1 | 54.0 | < .0001 |
| Dressings and sauces | 27,126 | 55.7 | 48.7 | 54.5 | 57.7 | 61.5 | < .0001 |
| Dairy products and meat substitutes (including soya-based products) | 11,382 | 85.7 | 82.0 | 84.8 | 86.5 | 88.3 | < .0001 |
| Non-alcoholic beverages | 27,552 | 67.1 | 58.9 | 64.7 | 69.8 | 74.7 | < .0001 |
| Alcoholic beverages | 25,417 | 58.7 | 50.5 | 56.6 | 61.5 | 65.7 | < .0001 |

[a] *p*-value is based on $\chi^2$ test and adjusted for multiple testing with a Hochberg procedure

the lowest relative differences were observed for dairy products and meat substitutes (6%), and eggs (7%).

## Discussion

Overall, analyses performed in this study showed higher organic food consumption among future oriented individuals compared to less future oriented participants independently of socioeconomic, lifestyle and dietary characteristics. First, individuals with a high consideration of future consequences were found more likely to eat organic foods. Then, among organic food consumers, future oriented individuals were also found in average to have a higher contribution of organic foods in their diet.

### Characteristics of future oriented individuals

Our results supported previous data of the literature indicating that future oriented individuals were younger [29], had more often a high education level [31], and had a lower BMI [12, 29], compared with less future oriented individuals.

### Association between consideration of future consequences and organic food consumption

Overall, results of the association between consideration of future consequences and organic food consumption showed that future oriented individuals were more likely to consume organic food. Moreover, when considering consumers of organic food groups specifically, the more participants were future oriented, the higher was the average contribution of organic foods in their diet (for almost every food group considered). Therefore, these analyses, focusing either on the whole sample or on organic food consumers specifically, both show a link between CFC and organic food intake. No significant interaction was found between gender and CFC in our study, suggesting no moderation effect of gender on the relationship between CFC and organic food intakes. To our knowledge, our study is the first to take into account the CFC-12 or any other measure of time perspective to assess the likelihood of organic food consumption. One study showed evidence that preferences for food products with an organic logo varied according to the level of future orientation [20].

**Table 3** Logistic regression models between CFC and the likelihood to consume organic foods

| | | Quartiles of consideration of future consequences[a] | | | | |
|---|---|---|---|---|---|---|
| | | Q1 | Q2 | Q3 | Q4 | $P^b$ |
| Food groups | n | Ref. | OR (95% CI) | OR (95% CI) | OR (95% CI) | |
| All | 27,634 | 1 | 1.24 (1.09, 1.40) | 1.51 (1.32, 1.74) | 1.88 (1.62, 2.20) | .0043 |
| Fruits and vegetables (including juices and soups) | 27,618 | 1 | 1.22 (1.12, 1.33) | 1.46 (1.33, 1.60) | 1.74 (1.58, 1.92) | < .0001 |
| Seafood | 26,579 | 1 | 1.20 (1.12, 1.29) | 1.26 (1.18, 1.36) | 1.30 (1.21, 1.39) | .32 |
| Meat, poultry, and processed meat | 26,550 | 1 | 1.15 (1.07, 1.24) | 1.31 (1.21, 1.42) | 1.34 (1.23, 1.46) | .08 |
| Eggs | 26,494 | 1 | 1.18 (1.09, 1.27) | 1.34 (1.23, 1.46) | 1.53 (1.40, 1.67) | .0008 |
| Dairy products | 27,177 | 1 | 1.20 (1.11, 1.29) | 1.36 (1.26, 1.47) | 1.55 (1.43, 1.68) | .0003 |
| Starchy refined foods | 27,603 | 1 | 1.22 (1.13, 1.32) | 1.49 (1.38, 1.62) | 1.78 (1.63, 1.94) | < .0001 |
| Whole-grain products | 22,527 | 1 | 1.25 (1.15, 1.36) | 1.49 (1.37, 1.62) | 1.66 (1.52, 1.82) | .0002 |
| Legumes | 24,811 | 1 | 1.18 (1.09, 1.27) | 1.35 (1.25, 1.46) | 1.55 (1.44, 1.68) | < .0001 |
| Fats (oil, butter, and margarine) | 27,537 | 1 | 1.22 (1.13, 1.31) | 1.38 (1.28, 1.49) | 1.67 (1.54, 1.81) | < .0001 |
| Fatty sweets (including cake, chocolate, ice cream, and pancakes) | 27,501 | 1 | 1.23 (1.15, 1.33) | 1.48 (1.37, 1.60) | 1.67 (1.55, 1.81) | < .0001 |
| Non-fatty sweets (including honey, jelly, sugar, and candy) | 26,296 | 1 | 1.22 (1.13, 1.31) | 1.42 (1.32, 1.54) | 1.62 (1.49, 1.75) | < .0001 |
| Fast food | 26,838 | 1 | 1.24 (1.16, 1.33) | 1.44 (1.34, 1.55) | 1.57 (1.46, 1.69) | .0002 |
| Snacks (including chips and salted biscuits) | 25,902 | 1 | 1.26 (1.17, 1.36) | 1.42 (1.32, 1.53) | 1.63 (1.51, 1.76) | < .0001 |
| Dressings and sauces | 27,126 | 1 | 1.23 (1.15, 1.32) | 1.40 (1.30, 1.50) | 1.58 (1.47, 1.70) | < .0001 |
| Dairy products and meat substitutes (including soya-based products) | 11,382 | 1 | 1.19 (1.02, 1.38) | 1.36 (1.17, 1.59) | 1.51 (1.28, 1.77) | .30 |
| Non-alcoholic beverages | 27,552 | 1 | 1.20 (1.12, 1.29) | 1.44 (1.33, 1.55) | 1.72 (1.59, 1.85) | < .0001 |
| Alcoholic beverages | 25,417 | 1 | 1.21 (1.13, 1.30) | 1.40 (1.30, 1.51) | 1.59 (1.48, 1.72) | < .0001 |

[a]Model 2: model adjusted on age, gender, education level, occupational status, monthly income per household unit, place of residence, BMI, energy intake, mPNNS-GS (modified Programme National Nutrition Santé Guideline Score), and total food intake of the food group considered in the model
[b]adjusted *p*-value for trend (correction for multiple testing with a Hochberg procedure)

Although very little data is available on association between psychological traits and organic consumption, many studies have investigated how psychological traits influence motives behind organic food choices. A large list of motives has been found to predict organic food intake, such as environmental and ethics aspects [2–7, 32, 33], or health, food safety and sensory aspects [2, 4, 6, 8, 9, 32, 33]. Broadly, these motives could be divided into two categories: environmental concerns (considered as altruistic motives), and individual concerns such as health (self-centered motives) [34]. Future time perspective has been shown to lead to a pro-environmental behavior [16] and to more health oriented behaviors [11, 12, 14, 15]. Consideration of future consequences could therefore be a psychological construct predicting organic food consumption through altruistic or self-centered motives (or both), which could explain the higher proportion of organic food consumers among future oriented participants. Significant linear trends showing increases of proportions of organic food intakes among organic food consumers across categories of the CFC strengthened this hypothesis.

#### Food group differences

Future oriented individuals were more likely to consume organic foods, but strengths of the association varied depending on the food group. The strongest associations were found for starchy refined foods, fruits and vegetables, and non-alcoholic beverages. No associations were found for seafood, meat, poultry and processed meat, and dairy products and meat substitutes. Specific factors could play an important role and weaken the relationship between time perspective and the consumption of these organic food groups. For example, constraints like price or origin of the product represent important factors in food choices and purchases [35]. Organic products with the highest differences in price between the organic and the conventional version such as meat, poultry and processed meat [36] could be consumed less because the price constraint would be too important [37]. Moreover, differences in the availability across products could also explain these different associations [38]. For example, less available products could be less purchased and less likely to be consumed. Some studies showed that fruits and vegetables intake in the diet was the most popular organic foods in proportion, whereas meat products and fishes were the least popular products [5, 39]. Our results also suggest that the strongest associations were found in the food groups which show or which are thought to have the greatest benefits for the environment or health (or both) when consumed in

**Table 4** Adjusted proportions of organic food intake out of total food intake, by food group, among consumers of organic foods

| Food groups | n | Q1 mean[b] | Q1 SE | Q2 mean[b] | Q2 SE | Q3 mean[b] | Q3 SE | Q4 mean[b] | Q4 SE | Relative difference between Q4-Q1 (%) | $P^a$ |
|---|---|---|---|---|---|---|---|---|---|---|---|
| All | 25,828 | 20.39 | 0.26 | 22.40 | 0.25 | 23.89 | 0.25 | 27.12 | 0.25 | 33 | < .0001 |
| Fruits and vegetables (including juices and soups) | 22,921 | 37.57 | 0.40 | 39.56 | 0.37 | 41.09 | 0.37 | 44.64 | 0.37 | 19 | < .0001 |
| Seafood | 13,491 | 31.92 | 0.46 | 31.94 | 0.41 | 31.79 | 0.41 | 33.41 | 0.42 | 5 | 0.13 |
| Meat, poultry, and processed meat | 19,464 | 29.34 | 0.38 | 30.52 | 0.35 | 30.48 | 0.35 | 33.16 | 0.36 | 13 | < .0001 |
| Eggs | 20,307 | 69.32 | 0.44 | 69.83 | 0.41 | 71.06 | 0.40 | 74.22 | 0.41 | 7 | < .0001 |
| Dairy products | 18,936 | 36.50 | 0.47 | 38.16 | 0.43 | 40.24 | 0.43 | 43.59 | 0.43 | 19 | < .0001 |
| Starchy refined foods | 21,385 | 34.05 | 0.42 | 35.86 | 0.39 | 37.47 | 0.38 | 41.41 | 0.38 | 22 | < .0001 |
| Whole-grain products | 16,089 | 53.28 | 0.54 | 53.67 | 0.48 | 55.56 | 0.46 | 59.96 | 0.46 | 13 | < .0001 |
| Legumes | 13,646 | 56.23 | 0.57 | 57.04 | 0.51 | 58.38 | 0.49 | 62.47 | 0.47 | 11 | < .0001 |
| Fats (oil, butter, and margarine) | 19,635 | 47.52 | 0.49 | 48.40 | 0.45 | 51.31 | 0.44 | 55.35 | 0.44 | 16 | < .0001 |
| Fatty sweets (including cake, chocolate, ice cream, and pancakes) | 19,000 | 29.06 | 0.41 | 30.56 | 0.37 | 31.88 | 0.36 | 34.72 | 0.36 | 19 | < .0001 |
| Non-fatty sweets (including honey, jelly, sugar, and candy) | 18,336 | 52.19 | 0.49 | 53.12 | 0.45 | 55.05 | 0.44 | 58.63 | 0.44 | 12 | < .0001 |
| Fast food | 14,224 | 32.28 | 0.49 | 33.67 | 0.44 | 34.09 | 0.42 | 37.94 | 0.42 | 18 | < .0001 |
| Snacks (including chips and salted biscuits) | 12,183 | 41.84 | 0.57 | 41.64 | 0.50 | 43.74 | 0.49 | 47.81 | 0.47 | 14 | < .0001 |
| Dressings and sauces | 15,099 | 38.79 | 0.54 | 40.06 | 0.49 | 41.64 | 0.48 | 46.18 | 0.47 | 19 | < .0001 |
| Dairy products and meat substitutes (including soya-based products) | 9758 | 77.45 | 0.66 | 77.87 | 0.60 | 79.00 | 0.56 | 82.39 | 0.53 | 6 | < .0001 |
| Non-alcoholic beverages | 18,487 | 17.74 | 0.29 | 19.21 | 0.26 | 19.53 | 0.26 | 21.40 | 0.25 | 21 | < .0001 |
| Alcoholic beverages | 14,908 | 28.41 | 0.42 | 28.54 | 0.38 | 28.80 | 0.37 | 31.20 | 0.37 | 10 | < .0001 |

Q1–Q4: Categories of consideration of future consequences

*SE* standard error
[a]adjusted *p*-value for trend (correction for multiple testing with a Hochberg procedure)
[b]adjusted for age, gender, education level, occupational status, monthly income per household unit, place of residence, BMI, energy intake, mPNNS-GS (modified Programme National Nutrition Santé Guideline Score), and total food intake of the food group considered in the model

their organic version compared to their conventional versions, and inversely for some of the weakest associations. Maximum residue level exceedances are higher in conventionally produced products compared to organic products [40].

In addition, among consumers of organic food products, the highest relative differences in proportions of organic intakes between Q4 and Q1 were found for starchy refined foods, non-alcoholic beverages, while the weakest variation were found for dairy products and meat substitutes, and eggs. The strength of the associations found for this analysis was similar to previous results. Similarly, observed differences between food groups could be explained by constraints regarding price, access, and environment, even among organic food consumers [38].

### Strengths and limitations

The main strength of this study is its large sample size with subjects of various socio-demographic characteristics which allows controlling for confounding factors while keeping a reasonable statistical power. Yet, other potential confounders were not taken into account, such as environmental factors and the availability of organic food. The second strength of this study was the use of a semi-quantitative food frequency questionnaire of 264 items which allowed a reliable estimation of usual diet over the previous year for conventional and organic intakes, despite a possibility of overestimation of intakes. The two complementary analyses, on the whole sample, and on organic food consumers specifically, bring more confidence on the relationship between consideration of future consequences and organic food intake. Questions concerning frequency of organic food consumption were not validated and could have led to misestimate the percentages of organic food consumer or proportions of organic food consumption in the diet. However, the estimation of organic food consumers was not substantially modified in a sensitivity analysis assessing the robustness of the scale [24]. In addition, considering that the completion of the Org-FFQ was optional and the long set of items of the questionnaire, participants with more sustainable food concerns could be more likely to complete it compared to other participants of the cohort. Finally, a high proportion of women and of individuals with a high level of education was included in our analysis, whom have been shown to have greater sustainable consumption [41, 42].

A selection bias could be present because of the method used to recruit participants, which is based on volunteering. The NutriNet-Santé being a cohort focusing on nutrition, its participants are more likely to be interested in nutrition-related issues. Consequently, our subjects may have high health awareness, and a high interest toward organic food and sustainability issues compared to the general population; meaning that percentages of organic food consumers were probably not representative of the general population. Another limitation of this study is its design, which is a cross-sectional analysis within a cohort, and thus does not allow us to assess causality. Moreover, all collected data were self-reported which could have led to measurement errors. The CFC questionnaire has been widely used with health and environmental outcomes. Recent studies reported a two-factor structure of the CFC, distinguishing immediate and future subscales [43]. Even though there is no consensus on the use of the CFC [44], a two-dimension analysis could have added another perspective in our interpretation of the results.

## Conclusions

This study showed that consideration of future consequences could be considered as a construct associated with consumption of organic food. For the majority of the assessed food groups, participants with the highest future orientation were more often consumers of organic foods, and when consuming these foods consumed a higher quantity of them. More generally, time perspective could be a personality trait predicting environmental and health concerns, and could be a key psychological factor influencing dietary behaviors and in particular organic food intake. These findings could explain the cognitive process underlying organic food choices and show the importance to take individual's psychological factors into account regarding overall food choices. Promoting the importance of future outcomes and long-term benefits could represent an approach of public health programs aiming at encouraging intake of organic food or more generally health promotion and chronic disease prevention.

### Abbreviations

CFC: Consideration of future consequences; CNIL: Commission Nationale Informatique et Libertés; CU: Consumption unit; IRB: International Research Board of the French Institute for Health and Medical Research; mPNNS-GS: Modified Programme National Nutrition Santé Guidelines Score; Org-FFQ: Organic food frequency questionnaire

### Acknowledgements

We thank Younes Esseddik, Thi Duong Van, Frédéric Coffinieres, Mac Rakotondrazafy, Régis Gatibelza and Paul Flanzy (computer scientists); and Nathalie Arnault, Véronique Gourlet, Dr. Fabien Szabo, Julien Allegre, Anouar Nechba and Laurent Bourhis (data-manager/biostatisticians) for their technical contribution to the NutriNet-Santé study. We thank all the volunteers of the NutriNet-Santé cohort.

### Sources of support

This study was supported by the BioNutriNet project. The BioNutriNet-Santé project is a research supported by the French National Research Agency (ANR) in the context of the 2013 Programme de Recherche Systèmes Alimentaires Durables (ANR-13-ALID-0001). The NutriNet-Santé Study is supported by the French Ministry of Health (DGS), the Santé Publique France agency, the French National Institute for Health and Medical Research (INSERM), the French National Institute for Agricultural Research (INRA), the National Conservatory for Arts and Crafts (CNAM), the Medical Research Foundation (FRM), and the University of Paris 13.

This research was part of the FOODPOL project, which was supported by the French National Institute for Agricultural Research (Institut National de la Recherche Agronomique) in the context of the 2013–2017 Metaprogramme "Diet impacts and determinants: Interactions and Transitions".

### Authors' contributions

MB conducted the literature review and drafted the manuscript. MB performed analyses. MB, JB, CM, DL, KVG, FE, GR, SH, EK-G, and SP were involved in interpreting results and critically reviewed the manuscript. CM, SH, EK-G, and SP were responsible for developing the design and protocol of the study. MB, JB, CM, DL, KVG, FE, GR, SH. All authors read and approved the final manuscript.

### Competing interests

The authors declare that they have no competing interests.

### Author details

[1]Equipe de Recherche en Epidémiologie Nutritionnelle, Centre de Recherche en Epidémiologie et Statistique Sorbonne Paris Cité, INSERM U1153, INRA U1125, Cnam, Université Paris 13, 74, rue Marcel Cachin, 93017 Bobigny, France. [2]INRA, UMR1110 MOISA, F-34000 Montpellier, France. [3]Aix Marseille Université, Nutrition Obésité et Risque Thrombotique (NORT), INSERM UMR S 1062, INRA 1260, Marseille, France. [4]Paris School of Economics and INRA, UMR1393 PjSE, 48 Boulevard Jourdan, 75014 Paris, France. [5]Service d'Endocrinologie, Diabétologie, Maladies Métaboliques, Hôpital Avicenne, Bobigny, France. [6]Unité de Surveillance en Epidémiologie Nutritionnelle, Institut de Veille Sanitaire, Université Paris 13, Bobigny, France. [7]Département de Santé Publique, Hôpital Avicenne, Bobigny, France.

### References

1. Willer H, Schaack D, Lernoud J. Organic Farming and Market Development in Europe and the European Union. World Org Agric-Stat Emerg Trends 2017 [Internet]. FiBL and IFOAM-Organics International; 2017. p. 206–243. Available from: http://orgprints.org/31187/. Accessed 8 Mar 2017.
2. Brown E, Dury S, Holdsworth M. Motivations of consumers that use local, organic fruit and vegetable box schemes in Central England and southern France. Appetite. 2009;53:183–8.
3. Honkanen P, Verplanken B, Olsen SO. Ethical values and motives driving organic food choice. J Consum Behav. 2006;5:420–30.

4. Lea E, Worsley T. Australians' organic food beliefs, demographics and values. Br Food J. 2005;107:855–69.
5. Oates L, Cohen M, Braun L. Characteristics and consumption patterns of Australian organic consumers. J Sci Food Agric. 2012;92:2782–7.
6. Pino G, Peluso AM, Guido G. Determinants of regular and occasional consumers' intentions to buy organic food. J Consum Aff. 2012;46:157–69.
7. Torjusen H, Lieblein G, Wandel M, Francis CA. Food system orientation and quality perception among consumers and producers of organic food in Hedmark County, Norway. Food Qual Prefer. 2001;12:207–16.
8. de Magistris T, Gracia A. The decision to buy organic food products in southern Italy. Br Food J. 2008;110:929–47.
9. Schifferstein HN, Ophuis PAO. Health-related determinants of organic food consumption in the Netherlands. Food Qual Prefer. 1998;9:119–33.
10. Strathman A, Gleicher F, Boninger DS, Edwards CS. The consideration of future consequences: weighing immediate and distant outcomes of behavior. J Pers Soc Psychol. 1994;66:742–52.
11. Ouellette JA, Hessling R, Gibbons FX, Reis-Bergan M, Gerrard M. Using images to increase exercise behavior: prototypes versus possible selves. Personal Soc Psychol Bull. 2005;31:610–20.
12. Adams J, Nettle D. Time perspective, personality and smoking, body mass, and physical activity: an empirical study. Br J Health Psychol. 2009;14:83–105.
13. Joireman J, Shaffer MJ, Balliet D, Strathman A. Promotion orientation explains why future-oriented people exercise and eat healthy evidence from the two-factor consideration of future consequences-14 scale. Personal Soc Psychol Bull. 2012;38:1272–87.
14. Orbell S, Perugini M, Rakow T. Individual differences in sensitivity to health communications: consideration of future consequences. Health Psychol. 2004;23:388.
15. Crockett RA, Weinman J, Hankins M, Marteau T. Time orientation and health-related behaviour: measurement in general population samples. Psychol Health. 2009;24:333–50.
16. Milfont TL, Wilson J, Diniz P. Time perspective and environmental engagement: a meta-analysis. Int J Psychol. 2012;47:325–34.
17. Milfont TL, Gouveia W. Time perspective and values: an exploratory study of their relations to environmental attitudes. J Environ Psychol. 2006;26:72–82.
18. Ebreo A, Vining J. How similar are recycling and waste reduction? Future orientation and reasons for reducing waste as predictors of self-reported behavior. Environ Behav. 2001;33:424–48.
19. Corral-Verdugo V, Fraijo-Sing B, Pinheiro JQ. Sustainable behavior and time perspective: present, past, and future orientations and their relationship with water conservation behavior. Int J Psychol. 2006;40:139–47.
20. De Marchi E, Caputo V, Nayga RM, Banterle A. Time preferences and food choices: evidence from a choice experiment. Food Policy. 2016;62:99–109.
21. Hercberg S, Castetbon K, Czernichow S, Malon A, Mejean C, Kesse E, et al. The Nutrinet-Santé study: a web-based prospective study on the relationship between nutrition and health and determinants of dietary patterns and nutritional status. BMC Public Health. 2010;10:242.
22. Demarque C, Apostolidis T, Chagnard A, Dany L. Adaptation et validation française de l'échelle de perspective temporelle «Consideration of future consequences»(CFC). Bull Psychol. 2010;5:351–60.
23. Kesse-Guyot E, Castetbon K, Touvier M, Hercberg S, Galan P. Relative validity and reproducibility of a food frequency questionnaire designed for French adults. Ann Nutr Metab. 2010;57:153–62.
24. Baudry J, Méjean C, Allès B, Péneau S, Touvier M, Hercberg S, et al. Contribution of organic food to the diet in a large sample of French adults (the NutriNet-Santé cohort study). Nutrients. 2015;7:8615–32.
25. Nutrinet-Santé E. Table de composition des aliments de l'étude Nutrinet-Santé (Nutrinet-Santé Study Food Composition Database). Economica. 2013. https://www.economica.fr/livre-table-de-composition-des-aliments-etude-nutrinet-sante,fr,4,9782717865370.cfm.
26. Schofield WN. Predicting basal metabolic rate, new standards and review of previous work. Hum Nutr Clin Nutr. 1984;39:5–41.
27. INSEE (Institut national de la statistique et des études économiques) [National Institute of Statistics and Economic Studies]. Unités de consommation [consumption units] [Internet]. Available from: http://www.insee.fr/en/methodes/default.asp?page=definitions/unite-consommation.htm. Accessed 8 Mar 2017.
28. Estaquio C, Kesse-Guyot E, Deschamps V, Bertrais S, Dauchet L, Galan P, et al. Adherence to the French Programme National Nutrition Sante Guideline Score is associated with better nutrient intake and nutritional status. J Am Diet Assoc. 2009;109:1031–41.
29. Adams J, White M. Time perspective in socioeconomic inequalities in smoking and body mass index. Health Psychol. 2009;28:83–90.
30. Van Buuren S. Multiple imputation of discrete and continuous data by fully conditional specification. Stat Methods Med Res. 2007;16:219–42.
31. Peters BR, Joireman J, Ridgway RL. Individual differences in the consideration of future consequences scale correlate with sleep habits, sleep quality, and GPA in university students. Psychol Rep. 2005;96:817–24.
32. Baudry J, Péneau S, Allès B, Touvier M, Hercberg S, Galan P, et al. Food choice motives when purchasing in organic and conventional consumer clusters: focus on sustainable concerns (the NutriNet-Santé cohort study). Nutrients. 2017;9:88.
33. Michaelidou N, Hassan LM. The role of health consciousness, food safety concern and ethical identity on attitudes and intentions towards organic food. Int J Consum Stud. 2008;32:163–70.
34. McEachern M, Seaman C, Padel S, Foster C. Exploring the gap between attitudes and behaviour: understanding why consumers buy or do not buy organic food. Br Food J. 2005;107:606–25.
35. Hughner RS, McDonagh P, Prothero A, Shultz CJ, Stanton J. Who are organic food consumers? A compilation and review of why people purchase organic food. J Consum Behav. 2007;6:94–110.
36. Hamm U, Gronefeld F, others. The European market for organic food: revised and updated analysis. Eur Mark Org Food Revis Updat Anal [Internet]. 2004; Available from: https://www.cabdirect.org/cabdirect/abstract/20043156600. Accessed 27 Mar 2017.
37. Marian L, Chrysochou P, Krystallis A, Thøgersen J. The role of price as a product attribute in the organic food context: an exploration based on actual purchase data. Food Qual Prefer. 2014;37:52–60.
38. Buder F, Feldmann C, Hamm U. Why regular buyers of organic food still buy many conventional products: product-specific purchase barriers for organic food consumers. Br Food J. 2014;116:390–404.
39. Baudry J, Touvier M, Allès B, Péneau S, Méjean C, Galan P, et al. Typology of eaters based on conventional and organic food consumption: results from the NutriNet-Santé cohort study. Br J Nutr. 2016;116:700–9.
40. European Food Safety Authority. The 2014 European Union report on pesticide residues in food. EFSA J. 2016;14:n/a-n/a.
41. Panzone L, Hilton D, Sale L, Cohen D. Socio-demographics, implicit attitudes, explicit attitudes, and sustainable consumption in supermarket shopping. J Econ Psychol. 2016;55:77–95.
42. Gilg A, Barr S, Ford N. Green consumption or sustainable lifestyles? Identifying the sustainable consumer. Futures. 2005;37:481–504.
43. Joireman J, Balliet D, Sprott D, Spangenberg E, Schultz J. Consideration of future consequences, ego-depletion, and self-control: support for distinguishing between CFC-immediate and CFC-future sub-scales. Personal Individ Differ. 2008;45:15–21.
44. Joireman J, King S. Individual differences in the consideration of future and (more) immediate consequences: a review and directions for future research. Soc Personal Psychol Compass. 2016;10:313–26.

# 20

# Resistant starch lowers postprandial glucose and leptin in overweight adults consuming a moderate-to-high-fat diet

Mindy Patterson Maziarz[1], Sara Preisendanz[2], Shanil Juma[2], Victorine Imrhan[2], Chandan Prasad[2,3] and Parakat Vijayagopal[2*]

**Abstract**

**Background:** High-amylose maize resistant starch type 2 (HAM-RS2) stimulates gut-derived satiety peptides and reduces adiposity in animals. Human studies have not supported these findings despite improvements in glucose homeostasis and insulin sensitivity after HAM-RS2 intake which can lower adiposity-related disease risk. The primary objective of this study was to evaluate the impact of HAM-RS2 consumption on blood glucose homeostasis in overweight, healthy adults. We also examined changes in biomarkers of satiety (glucagon-like peptide-1 [GLP-1], peptide YY [PYY], and leptin) and body composition determined by anthropometrics and dual-energy x-ray absorptiometry, dietary intake, and subjective satiety measured by a visual analogue scale following HAM-RS2 consumption.

**Methods:** Using a randomized-controlled, parallel-arm, double-blind design, 18 overweight, healthy adults consumed either muffins enriched with 30 g HAM-RS2 ($n$ = 11) or 0 g HAM-RS2 (control; $n$ = 7) daily for 6 weeks. The HAM-RS2 and control muffins were similar in total calories and available carbohydrate.

**Results:** At baseline, total PYY concentrations were significantly higher 120 min following the consumption of study muffins in the HAM-RS2 group than control group ($P = 0.043$). Within the HAM-RS2 group, the area under the curve (AUC) glucose ($P = 0.028$), AUC leptin ($P = 0.022$), and postprandial 120-min leptin ($P = 0.028$) decreased independent of changes in body composition or overall energy intake at the end of 6 weeks. Fasting total PYY increased ($P = 0.033$) in the HAM-RS2 group, but changes in insulin or total GLP-1 were not observed. Mean overall change in subjective satiety score did not correlate with mean AUC biomarker changes suggesting the satiety peptides did not elicit a satiation response or change in overall total caloric intake. The metabolic response from HAM-RS2 occurred despite the habitual intake of a moderate-to-high-fat diet (mean range 34.5% to 39.4% of total calories).

**Conclusion:** Consuming 30 g HAM-RS2 daily for 6 weeks can improve glucose homeostasis, lower leptin concentrations, and increase fasting PYY in healthy overweight adults without impacting body composition and may aid in the prevention of chronic disease. However, between-group differences in biomarkers were not observed and future research is warranted before specific recommendations can be made.

**Trial registration:** None.

**Keywords:** Resistant starch, Satiety, Overweight, Gut peptides, Fiber, Leptin, PYY

* Correspondence: pvijayagopal@twu.edu
[2]Department of Nutrition and Food Sciences, Texas Woman's University, P.O Box 425888, Denton, TX 76204, USA
Full list of author information is available at the end of the article

## Introduction

Epidemiological observations show that consuming a diet high in fiber can lower the risk for obesity, obesity-related comorbidities, and reduce all-cause mortality [1, 2]. One systematic review that examined the effects of dietary fiber on body weight reported that a 0.4% reduction in body weight can be achieved by consuming most dietary fibers for 4 weeks [3]. However, the amount of weight lost was dependent on the physiochemical properties (solubility, fermentability, and viscosity) of each type of fiber [3].

The purported mechanisms by which fiber contributes to weight loss such as altering gut motility, attenuating nutrient absorption, and lowering overall caloric intake are also associated with the physiochemical properties [2, 4]. Fermentable fibers are receiving attention because the metabolites produced from bacterial fermentation in the gastrointestinal (GI) tract can influence body weight. These fibers produce short chain fatty acids (SCFA; acetate, propionate, butyrate) in the distal intestine that stimulate the release of glucagon-like peptide-1 (GLP-1) and peptide YY (PYY) that act synergistically with leptin, an adipokine primarily released from adipose tissue, to induce satiety and regulate energy expenditure through central nervous system actions [5–7].

Despite increased SCFA production from fiber fermentation, the relationship between GLP-1 and PYY on satiety and food intake in humans is inconsistent. After consuming a standardized breakfast on the morning immediately following 3 days of consecutive intake of a barley kernel-based bread with resistant starch, fasting plasma GLP-1 and postprandial PYY concentrations increased in healthy middle-aged adults [8]. However, changes in appetite sensations (satiety, hunger, and desire to eat) did not occur [8]. Similarly, overweight women did not elicit a postprandial subjective satiety response despite improvements of GLP-1 and PYY after consuming an enzyme-hydrolyzed arabinoxylan from wheat or intact arabinoxylan from flax at breakfast [9]. In contrast, in healthy adults, the upregulation of GLP-1 and PYY corresponded with enhanced subjective satiety immediately after resistant maltodextrin intake [10]. However, subsequent energy intake was not suppressed despite these improvements. One recent trial found improvements in the area under the curve (AUC) PYY that corresponded with satiety and a 14% reduction in food intake in healthy adults consuming 15 g unripe banana flour rich in resistant starch for 6 weeks [11]. The different satiety peptides and satiation responses may be related to fermentability patterns, the type, amount, and duration of fiber intake, and the gut microbiota composition of individuals. Also, blood gut peptides may be too low in concentration to cross the blood brain barrier or the individuals may have hypothalamic resistance, which can occur from a high-fat diet even in lieu of obesity [12].

High-amylose maize resistant starch type 2 (HAM-RS2) is an insoluble, nonviscous fermentable fiber that has been shown to improve glucose homeostasis and/or peripheral insulin sensitivity among individuals who were healthy with normal glucose homeostasis [13] or those with metabolic syndrome [14–16]. However, many of these trials of longer duration did not report or show improvements in blood concentrations of gut peptides, satiety responses, or changes in food intake. HAM-RS2 may exert its benefits on glucose metabolism by increasing SCFA in the blood to alter free fatty acid and glycerol release from adipocytes and increased fat oxidation [17], modulate bile acid metabolism [18], or alter the gut microbiota profile [19].

Most previous trials reported the impact of HAM-RS2 on glucose homeostasis in either healthy individuals or those with metabolic syndrome [12–15]. Therefore, our primary aim was to determine the impact of the daily consumption of 30 g HAM-RS2 incorporated into muffins for 6 weeks on glucose homeostasis in normoglycemic, healthy overweight adults at risk for developing glycemic abnormalities. We also measured fasting and postprandial biomarker concentrations known to influence satiety (GLP-1, PYY, and leptin), subjective satiety, dietary intake, and body composition in these individuals.

## Materials and Methods

### Participants

Healthy overweight adults with a body mass index (BMI) $\geq 28$ kg/m$^2$ between 18 and 50 years of age of any race or ethnicity were recruited from Denton, Texas and the surrounding area. Participants were sedentary (<20 min of activity no more than 2 days per week) for at least 6 months prior to enrollment in the study. Exclusion criteria included those diagnosed with or taking medication(s) for chronic conditions, such as diabetes, hypertension, cancer, diseases of the liver, kidney, or heart, or other metabolic disorders. Participants were also excluded if they gained or lost a significant amount of weight or followed a special diet $\leq 3$ months prior to enrollment, consumed vitamins, minerals, or antioxidants in excess of amounts found in a daily multivitamin tablet, or dietary supplements known to alter metabolism, had an intolerance to the study foods, or smoked. Women who were pregnant, lactating, or interested in becoming pregnant were not eligible. The study was approved by the Institutional Review Board at Texas Woman's University. All participants provided written consent prior to study enrollment.

### Protocol

The study was a randomized-controlled, parallel-arm, double-blind design lasting 6 weeks. Individuals who met the screening criteria and agreed to participate in the study were randomized to either the HAM-RS2 group or control group using a random numbers generator from SPSS version 19 (IBM Corporation, Armonk, NY, USA).

Prior to participant randomization, the study muffins were formulated at the University food preparation laboratory. The treatment muffins were developed to provide 50 g Hi-Maize® 260 resistant starch (~30 g HAM-RS2, ~20 g equal mixture slowly and rapidly digestible starch; Ingredion Incorporated, Westchester, IL, USA) daily. The control muffins (0 g HAM-RS2) were developed to contain similar amounts of available carbohydrate and minimal differences in total calories than the treatment muffins (Table 1). Each 60 g treatment muffin contained 16.7 g Hi-Maize® 260 resistant starch to provide 10 g HAM-RS2, therefore three muffins (180 g cooked) were required to obtain 30 g HAM-RS2 daily as indicated in the protocol. No difference in overall muffin likeability was found based on sensory evaluations of HAM-RS2 and control muffins using a 9-point hedonic scale prior to the implementation of this study [20]. All study muffins were prepared, packaged, and labeled by culinary and nutrition students twice per week to ensure freshness and quality. Two flavors of the treatment and control muffins were developed, pumpkin spice and cranberry spice. The different flavors of muffins were administered on alternating weeks to alleviate monotony and improve compliance. The two flavors of muffins were closely matched for total calories and macronutrients. The cranberry spice muffins included 4.3 g dried cranberries, but no pumpkin puree. The pumpkin spice muffins included 6.8 g pumpkin puree without dried cranberries. Different amounts of dried cranberries and pumpkin puree were added so the caloric value of each muffin type was similar.

The participants arrived for baseline data collection following an overnight fast. Anthropometric measurements were obtained in triplicate followed by the baseline blood collection (time 0). Participants consumed all three of their respective study muffins within 15 min along with 6 oz of orange juice. Immediately following muffin intake the participants completed a visual analogue scale (VAS). Four additional postprandial blood samples were collected at 15, 30, 60, and 120 min. Nutrition education and body composition analysis occurred between blood collections. Participants were instructed by a Registered Dietitian Nutritionist (RDN) to follow a balanced diet according to the Dietary Guidelines for Americans 2010 [21] adjusted for the caloric value of the study muffins and to remain sedentary during the study. Body composition was determined by whole body dual-energy x-ray absorptiometry (DXA) using the Lunar DPX NT model (GE Healthcare, Fairfield, CT, USA). Body composition analysis and blood collections were repeated using the same protocol as baseline at the end of the intervention (week 6).

**Table 1** Comparison of nutrients between muffins[a]

| Nutrient | HAM-RS2 | Control |
|---|---|---|
| Energy (kcal)[b] | 349.6 | 389.1 |
| Available carbohydrate (g)[c] | 70.5 | 71.6 |
| Protein (g) | 5.4 | 10.6 |
| Fat (g) | 5.1 | 6.6 |
| Fiber (g) | 30.9 | 11.4 |

[a]Nutrient analysis based on the amount consumed daily by each participant; 180 g cooked (baked) weight. Analysis conducted by Pope Labs, Irving, Texas using the following Official AOAC Methods: moisture 925.10; oil 923.03; ash 923.03; nitrogen 988.05A; total dietary fiber 991.43
[b]Energy does not include contribution from short chain fatty acids associated with fermentation
[c]Available carbohydrate excludes fiber

### Dietary intake and bowel habits

Three days prior to baseline measurements, at midpoint (week 3), and the end of the study (week 6) all participants completed bowel habit logs and dietary intake journals for 3 days as instructed by a RDN. Dietary intake was analyzed using the United States Department of Agriculture National Nutrient Database for Standard Reference [22]. The bowel habit logs evaluated tolerance and potential adverse events from study muffin consumption by asking a series of questions adapted from Lewis et al. [23], such as "describe the consistency of your stools," and provided a space for comments. Participants were instructed to contact investigators immediately if abnormal changes in bowel habits, or the presence of blood or mucus, were observed. Muffin intake compliance was assessed through food intake journals.

### Subjective satiety measurements

Each VAS was 100 mm in length with questions at each end to indicate feelings of subjective satiety ranging from "not at all" to "very much or a lot". The 7 questions were adapted from Flint et al. [24] and included "how hungry are you?", "how satisfied do you feel?", "how full do you feel?", "how much do you think you can eat?", "how pleasant would you find eating another mouthful of this food?" "would you like to eat something sweet?", and "would you like to eat something fatty?".

### Biomarkers

A phlebotomist drew approximately 12 mL of blood at each time point into EDTA vacutainers (BD Diagnostics, Franklin Lakes, NF, USA). The tubes were centrifuged at 3,200 rpm for 12 min at 4 °C. Plasma was immediately aliquoted into 1.5 mL Eppendorf microcentrifuge tubes and stored at −80 °C until analyzed for glucose, insulin, GLP-1, PYY, and leptin. Glucose was determined using a hexokinase colorimetric method (Stanbio Laboratory, Boerne, TX, USA) with an intra-assay coefficient of variation (CV) <6%. Total insulin (CV < 8%; Alpco, Salem, NH, USA), leptin (CV < 6%; Raybiotech, Norcross, GA, USA), and total PYY ($PYY_{(1-36)}$ and PYY $_{(3-36)}$; CV < 6%; EMD Millipore, Billerica, MA, USA) were measured using an enzyme-linked immunosorbent (ELISA) technique. Total GLP-1 (GLP-$1_{(7-36)}$ and GLP-1 $_{(9-36)}$; CV < 7%; Raybiotech, Norcross, GA, USA) concentrations were determined by an enzyme immunoassay protocol.

### Statistical analysis

To assess differences between and within the HAM-RS2 and control groups, change from mean baseline and final scores were calculated for anthropometric, body composition, satiety (after three questions were reverse coded), and biomarker concentrations from each individual blood collection time points (fasting, 15, 30, 60, and 120 min). Due to limited sample size and potential deviations from normality, primary analyses were conducted using nonparametric tests. The Wilcoxon Signed Ranked test compared differences within groups, while the Mann–Whitney *U* test examined between group differences. The total area under the curve (AUC) was calculated for all plasma biomarkers using the trapazoidal rule and was compared using the nonparametric tests described above. Pearson's correlation coefficient examined associations between dependent outcomes. Data are presented as mean ± standard error of the mean (SEM), unless otherwise noted. SPSS version 19 (IBM Corporation, Armonk, NY, USA) and statistical significance was achieved with a $P$-value ≤ 0.05.

## Results

### Participants

Twenty-five participants were enrolled in the study; however, only 18 (83% female) completed the protocol and were included in the data analysis (Fig. 1). Baseline characteristics of the participants who completed the study and were included in the data analysis did not differ between groups (Table 2).

### Dietary intake and compliance

Energy and macronutrient (carbohydrate, protein, lipid) intake were similar between groups throughout the study (Table 3). Mean daily fiber intake significantly increased by 113% at midpoint in the HAM-RS2 group. At week 6, the mean fiber intake in the HAM-RS2 group increased 100% from baseline indicating fiber intake was sustained throughout the study. In contrast, the control group had a significant reduction in both fiber and carbohydrate intake from midpoint to the end of the study. Dietary fiber intake was considerably higher in the HAM-RS2 group at midpoint and the end of the study than the control. An unexplained reduction in dietary carbohydrate and fiber intake occurred from week 3 to week 6 in the control group. At baseline the HAM-RS2 group consumed a high fat diet averaging 95.8 ± 29.5 g/d (39.3% of total calories), which was non-significantly reduced to 82.1 ± 25.1 g/d (34.8% of total calories) at week 6. Based on data from the food intake journals, the HAM-RS2 and control groups consumed 94 and 98% of the study muffins, respectively, at midpoint suggesting high compliance. Compliance decreased to 85% in the HAM-RS2 group and 73% in the control group at the end of the study.

### Tolerance to study muffins

In both groups, stool consistency was relatively stable throughout the study. No differences in reaching the bathroom in time, usage of toilet paper, or marks on undergarments occurred across groups at any time point. One participant in the HAM-RS2 group recorded the presence of blood or mucus in stool on two separate occasions; one prior to receiving the

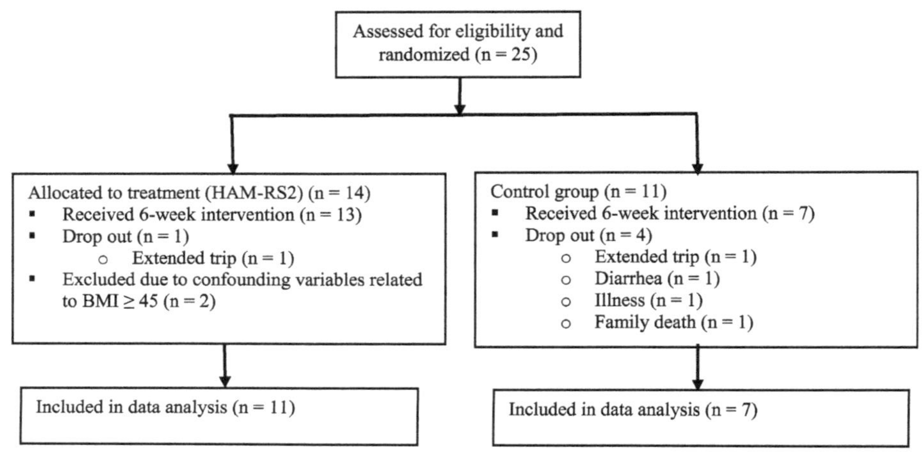


**Fig. 1** Consort Diagram

**Table 2** Baseline participant characteristics

| Characteristic | HAM-RS2 (*n* = 11) | Control (*n* = 7) | *P* value[a] |
|---|---|---|---|
| Female, n (%) | 9 (81.8) | 6 (85.7) | |
| Age, years | 31.0 ± 3.0 | 31.2 ± 4.2 | 0.973 |
| Body mass index (kg/m$^2$) | 34.8 ± 1.5 | 30.6 ± 1.5 | 0.085 |
| Waist circumference (cm) | 99.1 ± 3.7 | 91.6 ± 3.3 | 0.151 |
| Total body fat mass (kg)[b] | 42.8 ± 3.1 | 34.6 ± 3.0 | 0.085 |
| Total body lean mass (kg)[b] | 47.3 ± 1.8 | 43.7 ± 2.3 | 0.179 |
| Trunk total mass (kg)[b] | 47.1 ± 3.6 | 43.9 ± 6.0 | 0.285 |
| Trunk fat mass (kg)[b] | 22.2 ± 2.1 | 19.8 ± 3.0 | 0.285 |
| Trunk lean mass (kg)[b] | 23.8 ± 1.8 | 23.1 ± 2.9 | 0.479 |
| Android fat (kg)[b] | 50.8 ± 2.1 | 50.1 ± 0.8 | 0.791 |
| Gynoid fat (kg)[b] | 52.2 ± 2.6 | 49.6 ± 1.0 | 0.285 |
| Visceral adipose tissue (in$^3$)[b] | 76.8 ± 13.9 | 63.0 ± 18.1 | 0.417 |

Data presented as mean ± SEM except for qualitative values. All body composition measurements were obtained in triplicate after fasting for ≥8 h
[a]Between group differences determined by Mann–Whitney *U* test
[b]Measured by dual-energy x-ray absorptiometry (Lunar DPX NT model, GE Healthcare, Fairfield, CT, USA)

intervention and the other at midpoint. This participant was 89% compliant with muffin consumption at midpoint based on food records suggesting intake remained adequate. Overall, the HAM-RS2 and control muffins were well tolerated and few changes in bowel habit indicators were documented throughout the study.

### Subjective satiety

Mean overall satiety score did not differ within or between groups ($P = 0.230$). The mean score for the question "how full do you feel?" in the HAM-RS2 group increased from baseline to the end of the study and approached significance ($P = 0.058$) (data not shown).

### Body composition

Consuming muffins with HAM-RS2 did not significantly change body composition. A decrease ($P = 0.043$) in total trunk mass and a near significant decrease in lean trunk mass ($P = 0.063$) occurred in the control group (data not shown). At baseline the HAM-RS2 group had higher total leg mass ($P = 0.011$) than the control group, and the difference was sustained at the end of the intervention ($P = 0.02$) (data not shown).

### Biomarkers

Changes from baseline to week 6 in the AUC for the plasma biomarkers are shown in Table 4. At the end of the 6-week treatment, the AUC change from baseline was not significantly different between HAM-RS2 and control groups for any biomarker measures. However, a significant within-group decrease in both AUC glucose ($P = 0.028$) and AUC leptin ($P = 0.022$) was observed from baseline to week 6 in the HAM-RS2 group. There were no changes from baseline to the end of the intervention in the AUC for any biomarker in the control group. Within-group comparisons for biomarkers collected at each time point at the end of the intervention are shown in Fig. 2. Only one biomarker differed between groups

**Table 3** Changes in mean macronutrient intake between HAM-RS2 and control groups[1,2]

| Nutrient | HAM-RS2 | | | Control | | | *P* value** |
|---|---|---|---|---|---|---|---|
| | Baseline | Week 3 | Week 6 | Baseline | Week 3 | Week 6 | |
| Calories | 2190 ± 564 | 2193 ± 397 | 2123 ± 424 | 2091.1 ± 455.3 | 2046. ± 1337 | 1910.5 ± 648.7 | 0.256 |
| Carbohydrate (g) | 257.5 ± 84.8 | 283.0 ± 73.2 | 268.7 ± 62.6 | 294.3 ± 90.4 | 289.4 ± 173.7[a] | 261.7 ± 84.0[a] | 1.000 |
| Protein (g) | 82.7 ± 15.3 | 78.0 ± 13.2 | 78.4 ± 24.7 | 88.0 ± 11.1 | 74.8 ± 48.3 | 67.4 ± 32.7 | 0.462 |
| Lipid (g) | 95.8 ± 29.5 | 82.5 ± 20.7 | 82.1 ± 25.1 | 75.5 ± 23.9 | 70.1 ± 52.4 | 70.8 ± 27.0 | 0.462 |
| Fiber (g) | 21.5 ± 13.9[a,b] | 45.7 ± 8.2[1*] | 43.1 ± 6.7[b] | 29.5 ± 14.5 | 30.2 ± 18.0[a*] | 23.8 ± 6.8[a] | 0.001 |

[1]Dietary analysis software used is United States Department of Agriculture (USDA) National Nutrient Database for Standard Reference (http://ndb.nal.usda.gov)
[2]Within group values with the same letter superscript ([a,b]) in the same row are statistically different ($P < 0.05$)
*Between group values are statistically different ($P < 0.05$) by Mann–Whitney *U* test
**Between group comparisons at week 6 analyzed by Mann–Whitney *U* test

**Table 4** Mean AUC biomarker comparisons within and between groups

| Biomarkers | HAM-RS2 | | Control | | *P* value[1] |
|---|---|---|---|---|---|
| | Change from baseline to week 6 | *P* value[2] | Change from baseline to week 6 | *P* value[2] | |
| Glucose | −1588 ± 545 | 0.028 | −790 ± 706 | 0.310 | 0.285 |
| Insulin | −908 ± 941 | 0.333 | 518 ± 1197 | 1.000 | 0.425 |
| GLP-1 | 120 ± 94 | 0.139 | 208 ± 127 | 0.176 | 0.791 |
| PYY | 438 ± 719 | 0.285 | 954 ± 1465 | 0.866 | 0.085 |
| Leptin | −664 ± 235 | 0.022 | −191 ± 230 | 0.398 | 0.425 |

Data presented as mean ± SEM
[1]Between group comparisons at week 6 by Mann–Whitney *U* test
[2]Within group comparisons from baseline to week 6 by Wilcoxon Signed-Ranked test

when examining single blood collection time points. The 120 min postprandial concentration of PYY ($P = 0.043$) was higher in the HAM-RS2 group than the control group at baseline. Within-group differences in leptin and PYY were found from baseline to week 6 in the HAM-RS2 group. A decrease in postprandial leptin ($P = 0.028$) occurred at 120 min in the HAM-RS2 group. A within-group change in PYY was also observed in the HAM-RS2 group where fasting concentrations increased ($P = 0.033$) from baseline to the end of the intervention. Within the control group, no differences in the individual time points or AUC for any biomarker occurred.

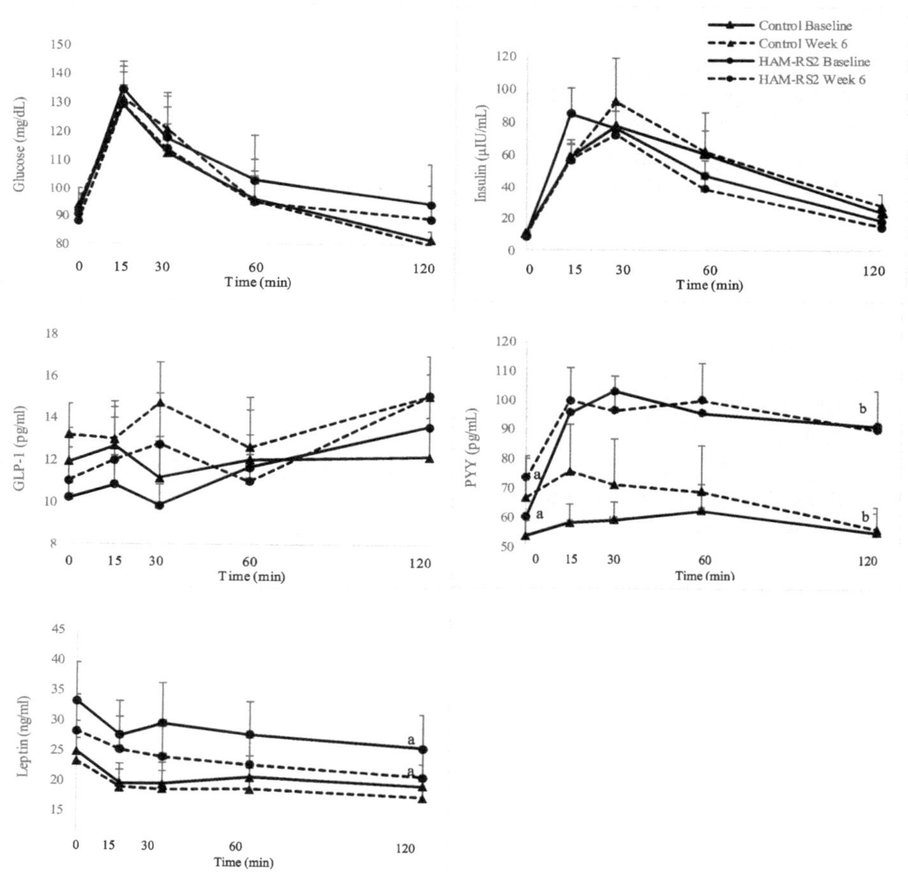


**Fig. 2** Change in biomarker concentrations from baseline to week 6 in the HAM-RS2 and control groups. This figure shows within-group comparisons from Wilcoxon Signed Ranked tests and between-group comparisons from Mann–Whitney *U* tests. [a]Indicates significant within-group changes in biomarkers from baseline to week 6. Fasting PYY increased ($P = 0.033$) while leptin decreased ($P = 0.028$) 120 min after study foods were consumed in the HAM-RS2 group. A near-significant decrease ($P = 0.062$) in leptin also occurred 60 min after study foods were consumed in the HAM-RS2 group. [b]Indicates significant difference at baseline between groups in 120 min postprandial PYY concentrations ($P = 0.043$)

**Relationship between subjective satiety and biomarkers of satiety**

Correlations between the mean AUC for each biomarker and the mean score for each VAS question were not found in either the control or HAM-RS2 group at the end of the intervention; however, correlations between body composition measurements and the AUC for several biomarkers were found. In the HAM-RS2 group, BMI (r = 0.655; $P = 0.029$), percent total fat (r = .889; $P <$ 0.001), total trunk mass (r = 0.851; $P = 0.001$); trunk fat (r = 0.700; $P = 0.017$); trunk lean (r = 0.795; $P = 0.003$) were associated with the AUC glucose. The percent total body fat correlated (r = 0.652; $P = 0.030$) with AUC leptin. In the control group AUC glucose was associated with BMI (r = 0.814; $P = 0.026$), total fat (r = 0.801; $P = 0.030$), percent fat (r = 0.879; $P = 0.009$), and percent trunk fat (r = 0.772; $P = 0.042$). Total trunk lean mass correlated with the AUC insulin (r = 0.792; $P = 0.034$) in the control group. The AUC glucose was associated with the AUC insulin in both the HAM-RS2 (r = 0.710; $P = 0.014$) and control (r = 0.785; $P = 0.036$) groups.

## Discussion

Our primary aim was to examine changes in glucose homeostasis after consuming 30 g HAM-RS2 for 6 weeks in overweight adults. We also measured the plasma biomarkers (GLP-1, PYY, and leptin) and subjective satiety which could alter dietary intake and body composition. We found significant reductions in AUC glucose and AUC leptin in the HAM-RS2 group although differences between groups did not occur. In addition, a significant increase in fasting PYY occurred within the HAM-RS2 group after consuming the treatment muffins for 6 weeks. Interestingly, the favorable changes in biomarkers in the HAM-RS2 group did not elicit changes in overall mean subjective satiety score or body composition at the end of the intervention. Only one biomarker differed between groups throughout the duration of the study. Baseline PYY 120-min post-muffin intake was significantly higher in the HAM-RS2 group which may be attributed to initial HAM-RS2 fermentation. Increasing the duration of the. intervention or sample size may have produced additional between-group changes in biomarkers.

The decrease in AUC glucose in the HAM-RS2 group occurred under normoglycemic conditions and no change in overall mean carbohydrate intake suggesting other contributing mechanisms. One mechanism could be due to the SCFA produced from the fermentation of HAM-RS2 by bacteria in the lower GI tract. Butyrate and propionate are substrates for intestinal gluconeogenesis [25]. The newly synthesized glucose from the intestine reduces overall hepatic gluconeogenesis through portal vein sensors that contribute to overall blood glucose control [25].

Interestingly, HAM-RS2 lowered glucose AUC in the presence of a high-fat diet. At baseline habitual dietary fat intake in the HAM-RS2 group was 39.4% of total calories (~95 g per day). It is well established that diets high in fat consisting of large amounts of saturated and omega-6 polyunsaturated fatty acids and lower omega-3 polyunsaturated fatty acids contribute to chronic inflammation [26] and the development of chronic disease. Interestingly when dietary composition contains only 30.4% of calories from fat, HAM-RS2 can suppress inflammation and normalize glucose by mediating gluconeogenesis potential and altering hepatic fuel usage from lipids to carbohydrate [27]. Despite observing an improvement in AUC glucose in the HAM-RS2 group, we did not see changes in plasma insulin or insulin sensitivity (determined by Homeostasis Model Assessment estimates) that have been reported in human trials [13–15]. We did, however, observe a positive correlation between AUC glucose and AUC insulin in both groups.

A novel finding from our study is that AUC leptin significantly decreased from baseline to the end of the intervention in the HAM-RS2 group independent of changes in body composition. We also found a significant postprandial reduction at 120 min and near significant postprandial reductions at 30 ($P = 0.074$) and 60 min ($P = 0.062$) in leptin. Leptin is primarily produced by adipocytes and blood concentrations correlate with adipocyte size and percent body fat. One plausible mechanism could be enhanced fat oxidation which has been observed in healthy adults where postprandial fat oxidation increased 23% after 5.4% of dietary carbohydrate, but not 10.7%, was consumed acutely as HAM-RS2 [17]. Approximately 11% of mean daily carbohydrate intake was in the form of HAM-RS2 in our study; however, our population and study duration differed from Higgins et al. [17]. Another study found increased fat oxidation when resistant starch type 4 (RS4) plus whey protein was administered to healthy overweight and lean women [28]. Increased fat oxidation and resting energy expenditure also occurred in healthy lean males following consumption of 38 g RS4 in a mixed meal [29]. In addition, a fermentable cereal fiber reduced leptin by enhancing the gene expression of several enzymes involved in fat oxidation [30]. Similar to our findings, So et al. [31] reported lower leptin in addition to smaller adipocyte size in mice consuming HAM-RS2 compared to mice on a low resistant starch diet even though body composition did not differ between the groups. In contrast, no change in adipose leptin mRNA expression or plasma leptin concentrations occurred after a meal tolerance test in healthy males who consumed 30 g HAM-RS2 over 4 weeks [13]. The study by Robertson et al. examined healthy individuals with an average BMI of 23.7 kg/m$^2$ which is much lower than our mean baseline BMI of 34.8 kg/m$^2$, and our intervention was longer in duration. This suggests that duration of HAM-RS2 consumption and degree of adiposity may also be important in modulating leptin. Differences in adiposity (mean total body fat mass) between HAM-RS2 and control groups ($P = 0.085$) may explain why leptin did not differ between groups in our study, or that changes in leptin are more sensitive in individuals with higher fat mass.

The reduction in leptin after HAM-RS2 intake may benefit individuals with leptin resistance. Leptin resistance can develop from consuming high fat diets [12, 32] and sustained elevated leptin concentrations [33]. In our study, the HAM-RS2 group had a mean fasting leptin concentration of 33 ± 6 ng/mL. Fasting leptin concentrations of ≥15 ng/mL have been described as the cutoff value to predict insulin resistance [34]. Although we did not observe insulin resistance in the HAM-RS2 group, it is plausible that the study participants in our study were resistant to leptin due to high blood leptin concentrations and consumption of a high-fat diet at baseline. We observed significant reductions in leptin, but also a non-significant mean reduction (5.5%) in total calories from fat, but not overall total calories, in the HAM-RS2 group. This decrease in dietary fat is not likely responsible for the decrease in AUC leptin concentrations [35]. Similar to our results, leptin decreased with the addition of a fermentable soluble fiber in obese rats ingesting a high-fat diet [36]. Interestingly, the decrease in leptin in this study did not induce an orexigenic effect since overall caloric intake did not change and was similar to the control.

Our study also found an increase in total fasting PYY but not postprandial or AUC PYY in the HAM-RS2 group at the end of the study. The increase may be related to the carry-over fermentation effects of prior-day HAM-RS2 intake. Increased PYY has been observed with fermentable fiber consumption in animal studies [37]. PYY binds to the Y2 receptors of the arcuate nucleus to elicit a satiation response alongside increased energy expenditure [38]. Two isoforms of PYY exist: $PYY_{1-36}$ and $PYY_{3-36}$. $PYY_{1-36}$ predominates under fasting conditions and has a lower affinity to the Y2 receptor. This may explain why we did not see a relationship between total PYY and satiety. At baseline, PYY was significantly higher ($P = 0.043$) in the HAM-RS2 group than control 120 min after the consumption of the study muffins and may be due to the initial fermentation of HAM-RS2 following intake. A similar increase in PYY occurred in healthy adults consuming resistant starch and whey protein 180 min after intake [28]. We did not observe improvements in GLP-1, which is consistent with several human studies examining HAM-RS2 intake in overweight adults for ≥4 weeks [39, 40].

This study has several limitations. First, only inactive concentrations of GLP-1 and total PYY ($PYY_{(1-36)}$ + $PYY_{(3-36)}$) were measured. We were not able to determine the exact PYY isoform which may have explained why subjective satiety did not change. Another limitation includes the lack of adding di-peptidyl peptidase-4 inhibitors (DPP-IV) following blood collection. DPP-IV rapidly degrades GLP-1, thus we were not able to measure the physiologically active form of GLP-1 [41]. Also, the participants consumed the study muffins at any time during the day. Consuming the muffins at one meal or equally distributed throughout the day could impact metabolic response. In addition, the participants consumed the study muffins prior to postprandial blood collection instead of an isocaloric mixed meal equal in macronutrient composition. Thus, the plasma biomarker response is reflective of study muffin consumption. However, a between group 120-min improvement in PYY was observed in the HAM-RS2 group indicating fermentation can upregulate this satiety peptide. Lastly, a significant reduction in daily fiber intake from midpoint to week 6 occurred in the control group indicating the control muffins replaced other high-fiber foods in the diet.

## Conclusion

In conclusion, daily consumption of 30 g of HAM-RS2 in muffins over 6 weeks can decrease leptin concentrations, assist with blood glucose homeostasis, and improve fasting PYY in healthy overweight adults. These findings occurred without changes in total caloric intake or body composition. Adding HAM-RS2 to the diet can improve fiber intake to enhance overall diet quality. However, strong conclusions cannot be made due to small sample size and between group differences in biomarkers were not observed at the end of the intervention. The mechanisms associated with biomarker changes in the HAM-RS2 group are likely related to the fermentation of HAM-RS2 by gut microbiota, but additional research is needed to determine the type, amount, and duration of resistant starch that would provide the most advantageous physiological results.

### Abbreviations

AUC: Area under the curve; BMI: Body mass index; DXA: Dual-energy X-ray absorptiometry; GI: Gastrointestinal; GLP-1: Glucagon-like peptide-1; HAM-RS2: High-amylose maize resistant starch type 2; PYY: Peptide YY; RDN: Registered Dietitian Nutritionist; SCFA: Short chain fatty acids; SEM: Standard error of the mean; VAS: Visual analogue scale

### Acknowledgements

None

### Funding

This research was funded by the Office of Research and Sponsored Programs at Texas Woman's University through the Research Enhancement Program and Ingredion Incorporated. Ingredion Incorporated supplied the Hi-Maize® 260 resistant starch.

**Authors' contributions**
PV, SJ, VI, and CP conceived and designed the experiments; MPM and SP collected data and performed the experiments; MPM and SP analyzed the data; MPM wrote the manuscript; PV, SJ, VI, and CP commented on and approved the manuscript. All authors read and approved the final manuscript.

**Competing interests**
The authors declare that they have no competing interests.

**Author details**
[1]Department of Nutrition and Food Sciences, Institute of Health Sciences, Texas Woman's University, 6700 Fannin Street, Houston, TX 77030, USA. [2]Department of Nutrition and Food Sciences, Texas Woman's University, P.O Box 425888, Denton, TX 76204, USA. [3]Department of Medicine (Endocrinology), Louisiana State University Health Science Center, New Orleans, LA 70112, USA.

**References**

1. Yang Y, Zhou LG, Wu QJ, Ma X, Xiang YB. Association between dietary fiber and lower risk of all-cause mortality: a meta-analysis of cohort studies. Am J Epidemiol. 2015;181(2):83–91. doi:10.1093/aje/kwu257.
2. Slavin JL. Dietary fiber and body weight. Nutrition. 2005;21(3):411–8.
3. Wanders AJ, van den Borne JJ, de Graaf C, Hulshof T, Jonathan MC, Kristensen M, Mars M, Schols HA, Feskens EJM. Effects of dietary fibre on subjective appetite, energy intake and body weight: a systematic review of randomized controlled trials. Obes Rev. 2011;12(9):724–39.
4. Lattimer JM, Haub MD. Effects of dietary fiber and its components on metabolic health. Nutrients. 2010;2(12):1266–89. doi:10.3390/nu2121266.
5. Guyenet SJ, Schwartz MW. Regulation of food intake, energy balance, and body fat mass: implications for the pathogenesis and treatment of obesity. J Clin Endocrin Metab. 2012;97(3):745–55.
6. Malijaars P, Peters H, Mela D, Masclee A. Ileal break: a sensible food target for appetite control. A review. Physiol Behav. 2008;95(3):271–81.
7. Murphy KG, Bloom SR. Gut hormones and the regulation of energy homeostasis. Nature. 2006;444(7121):854–9.
8. Nilsson AC, Johansson-Boll EV, Bjorck IME. Increased gut hormones and insulin sensitivity index following a 3-d intervention with a barley kernel-based product: a randomized cross-over study in health middle-aged subjects. Br J Nutr. 2015;114(6):899–907. doi:10.1017/S0007114515002524.
9. Lanfond DW, Greaves KA, Maki KC, Leidy HJ, Romsos DR. Effects of two dietary fibers as part of ready-to-eat cereal (RTEC) breakfasts on perceived appetite and gut hormones in overweight women. Nutrients. 2015;7(2): 1245–66. doi:10.3390/nu7021245.
10. Ye Z, Arumugam V, Haugabrooks E, Williamson P, Hendrich S. Soluble dietary fiber (Fibersol-2) decreased hunger and increased satiety hormones in humans when ingested with a meal. Nutr Res. 2015;35(5):393–400. doi:10.1016/j.nutres.2015.03.004.
11. Sarda FAH, Giuntini EB, Gomez ML, Lui MCY, Negrini JAE, Tadini CC, Lajolo FM, Menezes EW. Impact of resistant starch from unripe banana flour on hunger, satiety, and glucose homeostasis in healthy volunteers. J Func Foods. 2016;24:63–74.
12. Vasselli JR, Scarpace PJ, Harris RBS, Banks WA. Dietary components in the development of leptin resistance. Adv Nutr. 2013;4:164–75.
13. Robertson MD, Bickerton AS, Dennis AL, Vidal H, Frayn KN. Insulin-sensitizing effects of dietary resistant starch and effects on skeletal muscle and adipose tissue metabolism. Am J Clin Nutr. 2005;82(3):559–67.
14. Maki KC, Pelkman CL, Finocchiaro ET, Kelley KM, Lawless AL, Schild AL, Rains TM. Resistant starch from high-amylose maize increases insulin sensitivity in overweight and obese men. J Nutr. 2012;142(4):717–23.
15. Robertson MD, Wright JW, Loizon E, Debard C, Vidal H, Shojaee-Moradie F, Russell-Jones D, Umpleby AM. Insulin-sensitizing effects on muscle and adipose tissue after dietary fiber intake in men and women with metabolic syndrome. J Clin Endocrin Metabol. 2012;97(9):3326–32.
16. Johnston K, Thomas E, Bell J, Frost G, Robertson M. Resistant starch improves insulin sensitivity in metabolic syndrome. Diab Med. 2010;27(4):391–7.
17. Higgins JA, Higbee DR, Donahoo WT, Brown IL, Bell ML, Bessesen DH. Resistant starch consumption promotes lipid oxidation. Nutr Metab. 2004; 1(1):8. doi:10.1186/1743-7075-1-8.
18. Ebihara K, Shiraishi R, Okuma K. Hydroxypropyl-modified potato starch increases fecal bile acid excretion in rats. J Nutr. 1998;128:848–54.
19. Venkataraman A, Sieber JR, Schmidt AW, Waldron C, Theis KR, et al. Variable responses of human microbiomes to dietary supplementation with resistant starch. Microbiome. 2016;4:33. doi:10.1186/s40168-016-0178-x.
20. Maziarz M, Sherrard M, Juma S, Prasad C, Imrhan V, Vijayagopal P. Sensory characteristics of high-amylose maize resistant starch in three food products. Food Sci Nutr. 2012;1(2):117–24.
21. US Department of Agriculture, US Department of Health and Human Services. Dietary Guidelines for Americans. 7th ed. Washington DC: US Government Printing Office; 2010.
22. United States Department of Agriculture National Nutrient Database for Standard Reference. http://ndb.nal.usda.gov. Accessed 15 Jan 2014.
23. Lewis S, Heaton K. Stool form scale as a useful guide to intestinal transit time. Scandinav J Gastroenterol. 1997;32(9):920–4.
24. Flint A, Raben A, Blundell J, Astrup A. Reproducibility, power and validity of visual analogue scales in assessment of appetite sensations in single test meal studies. Int J Obes Rel Metab Disord. 2000;24(1):38–48.
25. De Vadder F, Kovatcheva-Datchary P, Goncalves D, Vinera J, Zitoun C, et al. Microbiota-generated metabolites promote metabolic benefits via gut-brain neural circuits. Cell. 2014;156:84–96.
26. Teng KT, Change CY, Chang LF, Nesaretnam K. Modulation of obesity-induced inflammation by dietary fats: mechanisms and clinical evidence. Nutr J. 2014;13:12. doi:10.1186/1475-2891.
27. Polakof S, Diaz-Rubio ME, Dardevet D, Martin JF, Pujos-Guillot E, Scalbert A, Sebedio JL, Mazur A, Comte B. Resistant starch intake partly restores metabolic and inflammatory alterations in the liver of high-fat-diet-fed rats. J Nutr Biochem. 2013;24:1920–30.
28. Gentile CL, Ward E, Holst JJ, Astrup A, Ormsbee MJ, Connelly S, Arciero PJ. Resistant starch and protein intake enhances fat oxidation and feelings of fullness in lean and overweight/obese women. Nutr J. 2015;14:113. doi:10.1186/s12937-015-0104-2.
29. Shimotoyodome A, Suzuki J, Kameo Y, Hase T. Dietary supplementation with hydroxypropyl-distarch phosphate from waxy maize starch increases energy expenditure by lowering the postprandial glucose-dependent insulinotropic polypeptide response in humans. Br J Nutr. 2011;106:96–104.
30. Han S, Jia J, Zhang W, Xu J, Wan Z, et al. Dietary fiber prevents obesity-related lipid toxicity by modulating sterol-regulator element binding protein pathway in C57BL/6 J mice fed a high-fat/cholesterol diet. Sci Rep. 2015;5: 15256. 10.1038/srep15256.
31. So PW, Yu WS, Kuo TU, Wasserfall C, Goldstone AP, Bell JD, Frost G. Impact of resistant starch on body fat patterning and central appetite regulation. PLosOne. 2007;2(12):e1309. 10.1371\journal.pone.0001309.
32. Enrori PJ, Evans AE, Sinnayah P, Jobst EE Tonelli-Lemos L, Billes SK, et al. Diet-induced obesity causes severe but reversible leptin resistance in arcuate melanocortin neurons. Cell Metabol. 2007;5(3):181–94.
33. Knight AZ, Hannan KS, Greenberg ML, Friedman JM. Hyperleptinemia is required for the development of leptin resistance. PLosOne. 2010;5(6): e11376. doi:10.1371/journal.pone.0011376.
34. Askari H, Tykodi G, Liu J, Dagogo-Jack S. Fasting plasma leptin level is a surrogate measure of insulin sensitivity. J Clin Endocrinol Metab. 2010;95(8): 3836–43. doi:10.1210/jc.2010-0296.
35. Weigle DS, Duell PB, Connor WE, Steiner RA, Soules MR, Kuijper JL. Effect of fasting, refeeding, and dietary fat restriction on plasma leptin levels. J Clin Endocrin Metab. 1997;82(2):561–5.
36. Adams CL, Thomson LM, Williams PA, Ross AW. Soluble fermentable dietary fiber (pectin) decreases caloric intake, adiposity and lipidaemia in high-fat diet-induced obese rats. PLosOne. 2015 10(10):e0140392. doi:10.1371/journal.pone.0140392.

37. Zhou J, Martin RJ, Raggio AM, Shen L, McCutcheon K, Keenan MJ. The importance of GLP-1 and PYY in resistant starch's effect on body fat in mice. Mol Nutr Food Res. 2015;59:1000–3. doi:10.1002/mnfr.201400904.
38. Batterham RL, Cowley MA, Small CJ, Herzog H, Cohen MA, Dakin CL, et al. Gut hormone PYY3-36 physiologically inhibits food intake. Nature. 2002; 418(6898):650–4.
39. Bindels LB, Walter J, Ramer-Tait AE. Resistant starches for the management of metabolic disease. Curr Opin Clin Nutr Metab Care. 2015;18:559–65.
40. Keenan MJ, Zhou J, Hegsted M, Pelkman C, Durham HA, Coulon DB, Martin RJ. Role of resistant starch in improving gut health, adiposity, and insulin resistance. Adv Nutr. 2015;6:198–205. doi:10.3945/an.114.007419.
41. Holst JJ. The physiology of glucagon-like peptide-1. Physiol Rev. 2007;87:1409–39.

# 21

# Possible benefits of tomato juice consumption: a pilot study on irradiated human lymphocytes from healthy donors

Ayumi Nakamura[1], Chieko Itaki[2], Ayako Saito[3], Toko Yonezawa[3], Koichi Aizawa[4], Ayumi Hirai[4], Hiroyuki Suganuma[4], Tomisato Miura[5], Yasushi Mariya[1*] and Siamak Haghdoost[6]

**Abstract**

**Background:** Reactive oxygen species (ROS) mediate much of the DNA damage caused by ionizing radiation. Among carotenoids, lycopene and β-carotene, present in tomato juice, are known to be strong radical scavengers. The aim of the study was to investigate the effect of tomato juice intake on the levels of DNA damage and oxidative stress in human whole blood induced by in vitro exposure to X-rays.

**Methods:** Ten healthy adults were asked to drink 190 g of tomato juice, containing 17 mg lycopene and 0.25 mg β-carotene, per day for 3 weeks and then refrain from drinking it for 3 weeks. Peripheral whole blood samples were collected before and after the intake period of tomato juice and after the washout period. The blood samples were exposed in vitro to X-ray doses of 0, 0.1, 0.5, and 2 Gy. Cytogenetic damage was measured using the cytokinesis-block micronucleus (CBMN) assay and the dicentrics (DIC) assay. The level of oxidative stress was determined using serum 8-oxo-7, 8-dihydro-2-deoxyguanosine (8-oxo-dG) and plasma reactive oxygen metabolite-derived compounds (d-ROMs). The concentration of carotenoids in plasma was measured at the three time points.

**Results:** The levels of 8-oxo-dG tended to decrease during the intake period and increase during the washout period. A non-significant inverse correlation was noted between the plasma concentration of lycopene plus β-carotene and the level of 8-oxo-dG ($P = 0.064$). The radiation-induced MN and DIC frequencies increased in a dose-dependent manner, and when compared at the same dose, the MN and DIC frequencies decreased during the intake period compared with those at baseline and then increased during the washout period. The results suggest that continuous tomato juice consumption non-significantly decreases extracellular 8-oxo-dG, d-ROMs, and MN. Tomato juice intake had minimal or no effect on radiation-induced 8-oxo-dG and d-ROMs. For most radiation doses, continuously tomato juice intake lowered the levels of MN and DIC.

**Conclusion:** Tomato juice consumption may suppress human lymphocyte DNA damage caused by radiation, but further examination is required.

**Trial registration:** 2014-001 and 2014-R06.

**Keywords:** Reactive oxygen species, Tomato juice, Lycopene, β-carotene, Radioprotective effect, Human lymphocytes

* Correspondence: mariya@hirosaki-u.ac.jp
[1]Department of Radiological Life Sciences, Division of Medical Life Sciences, Hirosaki University Graduate School of Health Sciences, Aomori 036-8564, Japan
Full list of author information is available at the end of the article

## Background

Oxidative stress is generated by reactive compounds such as reactive oxygen species (ROS) and reactive nitrogen species. ROS react with biomolecules in vivo, resulting in lipid peroxidation, DNA damage, and protein modification. ROS are produced by a variety of processes such as exposure to radiation, alcohol consumption, smoking and excessive exercise. ROS are also produced during cellular metabolism and give rise to DNA damage and protein/lipid modifications. An excessive level of ROS may contribute to the development of various diseases and promotion of the aging process [1–3].

In the present study, we used X-rays to induce DNA damages. X-rays cause DNA damage directly by inducing ionization and excitation of DNA molecules and indirectly through the formation of ROS by radiolysis of cellular water molecules. The indirect action is responsible for approximately 70% of the DNA damage caused by low linear energy transfer ionizing radiation, such as X-rays. In addition to the level of ROS formed by the radiolysis of cellular water, ionizing radiation also increases the endogenous production of free radicals from e.g., mitochondria [4, 5]. Although different DNA repair systems act on the damaged DNA to restore the original DNA sequences, the repair processes are not error free and may result in mutations including deletions, point mutations, and chromosomal aberrations. The aberrations can be measured in the form of dicentrics (DIC) formed as result of mis-repaired double strand breaks [6].

In addition to the DNA molecule, ROS can also react with free DNA precursors in the cytoplasm (nucleotide pool, dNTPs) and modify their structures. Modified dNTPs can be incorporated into the DNA during replication, causing point mutations [7]. One of the most studied modifications of dNTP is 8-hydroxy-2′-deoxyguanosine-triphosphate (8-oxo-dGTP), which is formed when ROS react with deoxyguanosine triphosphate (dGTP). A protein called MTH1 dephosphorylates 8-oxo-dGTP to 8-hydroxy-2′-deoxyguanosine-monophosphate (8-oxo-dGMP). 8-oxo-dGMP will be further dephosphorylated and released from the cells as 8-oxo-7, 8-dihydro-2′-deoxyguanosine (8-oxo-dG) [4]. When endogenous antioxidant defenses are insufficient to reduce the elevated level of ROS, appropriate antioxidant interventions can inhibit, at least partly, the reaction of ROS with biomolecules, particularly DNA, thereby offering protection [8, 9].

Carotenoids, especially lycopene and β-carotene, are found primarily in red and yellow/orange fruits and vegetables such as tomato and carrots. Recent epidemiological studies indicate that the intake of carotenoid-rich foods is associated with reduced risks of chronic diseases, cancer and heart diseases. Tomato-based food products such as tomato juice are important and convenient sources of carotenoids. Tomato juice, in particular, is rich in lycopene and β-carotene. These carotenoids have strong abilities to quench singlet oxygen [10, 11]. Previously, we reported that tomato juice intake decreases oxidative stress in individuals performing extensive physical activity [12]. It was also reported that daily tomato juice consumption for 4 weeks significantly increased the levels of serum lycopene and β-carotene [13]. Therefore, we assumed that the active ingredients in tomato juice suppress excess ROS and eventually provide an antigenotoxic effect. In the present study, we investigated the effect of 3 weeks of tomato juice intake, corresponding to a daily intake of 17 mg of lycopene and 0.25 mg of β-carotene, on the levels of carotenoids and biomarkers of oxidative stress and chromosomal damage in samples of whole blood and after in vitro exposure of the samples to X-rays.

## Methods

### Subjects and blood sampling

Ten healthy donors (5 males and 5 females) aged 22–26 years (mean 23 years) were recruited and asked to drink 190 g of commercially available tomato juice ['Kagome Tomato Juice (salt added)', KAGOME CO., LTD., Nagoya, Japan] per day for 3 weeks and then to refrain from drinking it for 3 weeks. The tomato juice was prepared as per industrial standard processes and commercialized in cans. The donors were non-vegetarians, non-smokers and not pregnant. To avoid confounders that could affect the results, the donors were asked to avoid excessive physical training, alcohol consumption, intake of any vitamin supplements and exposure to radiation for diagnostic or treatment purposes during the experimental period.

The nutrition and carotenoid content of the tomato juice used in the study is presented in Table 1. Peripheral blood samples were collected before and after the intake period of tomato juice and following the washout period. Forty mL whole blood was collected at each occasion and divided in 8 tubes; 4 CPT tubes with heparin (BD Biosciences, San Jose, CA, USA) and 4 tubes without anticoagulant (BD Biosciences, Franklin Lakes, NJ, USA). This study was performed in accordance with the ethical standards and was approved by the Ethics Committee of the Hirosaki University Graduate School of Health Sciences (approval number: 2014–001) and the Ethics Committee of KAGOME CO., LTD. (receipt number: 2014-R06).

### In vitro X-ray irradiation

Four heparin tubes and four tubes without anticoagulant with 5 mL whole blood in each were cooled and irradiated on ice. The irradiation (150 kVp, 20 mA, 0.5 mm aluminum, and 0.3 mm copper filters) was performed

**Table 1** The nutrition facts and carotenoid content in the tomato juice

| (A) | | (B) | |
|---|---|---|---|
| Nutrition facts[a] | | Carotenoid content[b] | |
| Energy (kcal) | 38.0 | Lutein (mg) | 0.127 ± 0.0006 |
| Protein (g) | 1.6 | β-Cryptoxanthin (mg) | 0.042 ± 0.0035 |
| Fat (g) | 0.0 | α-Carotene (mg) | 0.074 ± 0.0003 |
| Carbohydrate (g) | 7.2 | β-carotene (mg) | 0.255 ± 0.0009 |
| Dietary fiber (g) | 1.3 | Lycopene (mg) | 16.9 ± 0.2 |
| Sodium (mg) | 210.0 | | |
| Sodium chloride equivalent (g) | 0.5 | | |
| Calcium (mg) | 13.0 | | |
| Potassium (mg) | 530.0 | | |
| Sucrose (g) | 0.0 | | |

(A) The nutrition facts (B) Carotenoid content in the tomato juice used in this experiment (190 g)
[a]Nutrition facts are according to the product label
[b]Carotenoid content is measured using HPLC (see Method section). Values are given as mean ± SE of three samples

using an X-ray generator (MBR-1520R; Hitachi Medical Co. Ltd., Tokyo, Japan) allowing a 45 cm distance between the beam focus and the samples. The doses were 0, 0.1, 0.5 and 2 Gy, delivered at a dose rate of 1 Gy/min and monitored with a thimble ionization chamber placed next to a sample.

### Isolation of plasma, lymphocytes, and serum from whole blood

Following exposure the irradiated blood samples and control samples were incubated at 37 °C in a water bath for 1 h. Plasma was collected for measuring the concentration of carotenoids, and reactive oxygen metabolites-derived compounds (d-ROMs) and serum was collected for determination of 8-oxo-dG. Mononuclear cells for the cytokinesis-block micronucleus (CBMN) assay and DIC assay were isolated with heparin using CPT tubes according to the provider's protocol.

### Quantification of carotenoids

Plasma samples of 200 μL were mixed with 10 μL 8-apocarotenal in ethanol [0.0001% (w/v), (Sigma-Aldrich, St. Luis, MO, USA)] as internal standard, 1 mL ethanol containing 0.01% (w/v) butylhydroxytoluene, and 4 mL hexane:dichloromethane [4:1 (v/v)]. The extraction process was repeated if the plasma samples contained precipitated material. After stirring and centrifugation, the supernatants rich in carotenoids were collected and kept in liquid nitrogen. Subsequently, the samples were evaporated to dryness and the residues were re-dissolved in 200 μL hexane:acetone:ethanol:toluene [10:7:6:7 (v/v/v/v)] solution and filtered through a 0.22-μm filter for high-performance liquid chromatography (HPLC) analysis. A C30 carotenoid column [S5 μm, 250 × 2.0 mm I.D. (YMC, Wilmington, NC, USA)] was used at 30 °C, and the SPD-M10 *vp* diode array detector (Shimadzu, Kyoto, Japan) was set at 460 nm. Carotenoids {[lutein, zeaxanthin, β-cryptoxanthin, α-carotene, β-carotene, and lycopene (cis- and trans-isomers)], Extrasynthese, Genay, France} were quantified by determining peak areas in the HPLC chromatograms, calibrated against known standards.

### Measurement of 8-oxo-dG

After complete coagulation of the blood samples, the blood serum was isolated. The 8-oxo-dG concentration of blood serum was measured using enzyme-linked immunosorbent assay (ELISA) as described previously [4, 14]. The ELISA kit was provided by Health Biomarkers Sweden AB (Stockholm, Sweden). Prior to ELISA, 800 μL of blood serum was filtered through a C18 solid phase extraction column (Varian, Lake Forest, CA, USA) according to a previously published method [14]. This step is necessary to remove products other than 8-oxo-dG which could cross-react with the monoclonal antibody used in the kit. A standard curve for 8-oxo-dG (0.01–10 ng/mL) was established for each plate covering the range of 8-oxo-dG in the samples. Validation of the modified ELISA method was performed by HPLC-EC ($r^2 = 0.87$, $P < 0.05$) [4]. Comparisons between the ELISA and the HPLC-EC methods showed a linear correlation in the concentration range found in human blood serum [4].

### Measurement of d-ROMs

The plasma concentration of d-ROMs was measured by a 7180 Series Automatic Biochemistry Analyzer (Hitachi, Ltd., Tokyo, Japan). In the d-ROMs test (kit from Diacron International, Grosseto, Italy), the release of the reactive oxygen metabolites (hydroperoxides primarily) and iron (by an acidic buffer) from plasma generates alkoxyl and peroxyl radicals, according to Fenton's reaction. Such radicals, in turn, oxidize an alkyl-substituted aromatic amine (N, N-dietylparaphenylendiamine) which is included in the kit, thus producing a pink-colored derivative which is photometrically quantified at 505 nm. The concentration of d-ROMs is directly associated with the color intensity and is expressed as Carratelli Units (1 CARR U corresponds to 0.08 mg hydrogen peroxide/dL).

### Cytokinesis-block micronucleus assay

The isolated lymphocytes were cultured in RPMI 1640 medium (Life Technologies, Carlsbad, CA, USA) containing 20% fetal bovine serum (FBS; Japan Bio Serum, Hiroshima, Japan), 1% penicillin/streptomycin (Life Technologies, Carlsbad, CA, USA), and 2% phytohaemagglutinin-HA15 (Remel, Lenexa, KS, USA) in a 15 mL Falcon tube. The cells were incubated in a humidified incubator at 37 °C with 5% $CO_2$ for exactly 44 h. Following the incubation, the cells were treated with Cytochalasin-B (Wako Pure Chemical Industries, Ltd., Osaka, Japan) at a final concentration of 6 μg/mL and then incubated for further 28 h in the cell culture incubator. Following the incubation, the cells were washed and suspended in RPMI 1640 medium containing 2% FBS. Further, 300 μL of cell suspension was spun onto a slide glass using Cytospin™ 4 Cytocentrifuge (Thermo Fisher Scientific, Inc., Waltham, MA, USA). The cells were fixed on the slides and stained with Diff-Quik (Sysmex, Kobe, Japan). The slides were scored at 400× magnification using a bright-field microscope (BX61: Olympus, Tokyo, Japan). At least 1000 binucleated cells (BNCs) were scored per slide and the results were expressed as number of MN/1000 BNCs.

#### Dicentric assay

The isolated lymphocytes were cultured in RPMI 1640 medium supplemented with 20% FBS, 1% penicillin/streptomycin, and 2% phytohaemagglutinin-HA15, and 0.05 μg/mL colcemid (Life Technologies, Carlsbad, CA, USA) in a 15 mL Falcon tube and incubated in a humidified incubator at 37 °C with 5% $CO_2$. Following 48 h incubation, cells were harvested, treated with 0.075 M KCl, and fixed with cold fixative (methanol: acetic acid 3:1 (v/v)). Following centrifugation, the cell pellets were resuspended in 1–2 mL of fixative. A temperature-humidity-controlled chamber (Hanabi metaphase spreader, ADSTEC, Japan) was used for spreading of the metaphases on pre-cleaned slide glass (Matsunami Glass Ind., Japan). The slides were then stained with Giemsa solution and mounted with a cover glass. The metaphase cells were found in the AutoCapt mode using two sets of AXIOImager Z.2 microscopes (Carl Zeiss AG, Oberkochen, Germany) equipped with CCD cameras and Metafer 4 software (MetaSystem GmbH, Altlusshein, Germany). Metaphases for scoring were selected in manual mode. Using the selected metaphase images, all DIC in 500 metaphases were scored. Data were presented as the number of DIC/500 metaphases. The cells were analyzed according to the criteria described by the International Atomic Energy Agency in 2011.

#### Statistical analysis

Statistical analyses were performed using the Excel 2013 software (Microsoft Corp., Redmond, WA, USA) equipped with the Statcel 3 add-in software package. Data were expressed as mean ± standard error (SE). Statistical analyses were conducted by paired $t$ test, Wilcoxon signed-ranks test, Bonferroni/Dunn test, and simple regression analysis. The linear regression analysis was performed to investigate the correlation between the plasma lycopene/β-carotene concentrations and studied biomarkers. $P$ values of less than 0.05 were considered to indicate statistical significance.

### Results

We compared values of each biomarker among three measurements, namely before and after the tomato juice intake and after the following washout period, and the measurements were defined as the "baseline," "intake," and "washout".

#### Changes in the concentration of carotenoids in blood

The plasma levels of six major carotenoids at the three different time points are shown in Table 2, and the sum of the concentrations of lycopene and β-carotene in tomato juice was calculated. The plasma concentration of lycopene significantly increased after 3 weeks of tomato juice intake (0.51 ± 0.03 μg/mL) compared with that at the baseline level (0.34 ± 0.03 μg/mL) and reduced to the baseline level after the washout period (0.34 ± 0.03 μg/mL). The concentration of β-carotene also increased from 0.35 ± 0.08 μg/mL to 0.44 ± 0.08 μg/mL due to continual intake of tomato juice and decreased to 0.32 ± 0.05 μg/mL during the washout period. Plasma levels of other carotenoids (lutein, zeaxanthin, β-cryptoxanthin, α-carotene) were not notably changed between the three measurements. Neither the concentration of lycopene nor its cis/trans ratio differed significantly between samples that received different doses of radiation and non-irradiated samples (Fig. 1a and b), indicating that radiation at doses up to 2 Gy do not degrade and/or isomerize lycopene. Also, the concentration of β-carotene in the blood remained largely unchanged by radiation (Fig. 1c).

#### Changes in the level of oxidative stress-related markers

We assessed the effect of radiation on two oxidative stress-related markers: extracellular 8-oxo-dG (Fig. 2a) in serum and d-ROMs (Fig. 2b) in plasma. In non-irradiated samples, the concentration of extracellular 8-oxo-dG decreased during the intake period (from 0.60 ± 0.16 at baseline to 0.39 ± 0.06 ng/mL) and increased after the washout period (to 0.62 ± 0.25 ng/mL), indicating that tomato juice

**Table 2** The concentration of carotenoids in the human plasma

| Carotenoids (μg/mL) | Baseline | Intake | Washout |
|---|---|---|---|
| | Mean ± SE | Mean ± SE | Mean ± SE |
| Lutein | 0.23 ± 0.03 | 0.23 ± 0.02 | 0.21 ± 0.02 |
| Zeaxanthin | 0.06 ± 0.01 | 0.05 ± 0.01 | 0.05 ± 0.01 |
| β-Cryptoxanthin | 0.12 ± 0.02 | 0.13 ± 0.02 | 0.12 ± 0.01 |
| α-Carotene | 0.15 ± 0.02 | 0.13 ± 0.02 | 0.12 ± 0.01 |
| β-Carotene | 0.35 ± 0.08 | 0.44 ± 0.08 [a, b] | 0.32 ± 0.05 |
| Lycopene | 0.34 ± 0.03 | 0.51 ± 0.03 [a, b] | 0.34 ± 0.03 |

Values are given as mean ± SE of 10 donors. [a]: different from baseline ($P < 0.05$), [b]: different from washout ($P < 0.05$) by paired $t$ test

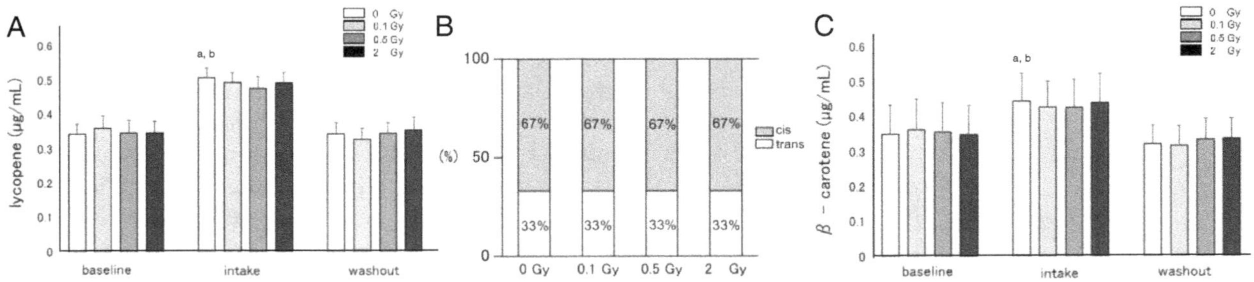

**Fig. 1** Radiation effects on the level of main carotenoids in human blood. **a** Concentration of lycopene according to radiation dose at each time point. Values are given as mean ± SE of 10 donors. **b** Structure ratio of lycopene (cis/trans) according to radiation dose. The ratio was constant between the different radiation doses. **c** Concentration of β-carotene according to radiation dose at each time point. Values are given as mean ± SE of 10 donors. a: different from baseline $P < 0.05$, b: different from washout $P < 0.05$ by Bonferroni/Dunn test. Concentrations of carotenoids after each period did not differ significantly by radiation (1**a**, 1**c**)

intake may decrease 8-oxo-dG levels in serum. However, this effect was not significant. The concentrations at baseline, intake and washout in samples exposed to 0.1 and 0.5 Gy showed a similar pattern. At 0.5 Gy the increase of 8-oxo-dG during the washout period was close to significance ($P = 0.059$). However, no protective effect was observed at 2 Gy (Fig. 2a).

Generally, it is accepted that the concentration of d-ROMs reflects oxidative stress, and we observed that the levels of d-ROMs after exposure to 0.1 and 0.5 Gy significantly decreased during the intake period compared with those at baseline (Fig. 2b). The levels of d-ROMs at 2 Gy at baseline, after intake, and after washout showed a similar pattern. However, the differences were not significant.

### Differential analysis of the lycopene plus β-carotene concentration at baseline

We analyzed correlations of the levels of circulating lycopene and β-carotene, alone or together, with all biomarkers assessed in the study. A slight inverse correlation was found only between the plasma lycopene plus β-carotene concentration and the extracellular 8-oxo-dG level (Fig. 3). This observation indicated that lycopene and β-carotene may reduce the serum levels of 8-oxo-dG ($P = 0.064$). The circulating plasma lycopene plus β-carotene concentrations at baseline in the 10 donors ranged from 0.38 to 1.24 μg/mL. Therefore, the participants were divided into two groups based on their initial plasma lycopene plus β-carotene concentrations (less than or more than 0.635 μg/mL, median value) to evaluate the differences in radiation-induced cytogenetic damage. Group A, in which the plasma lycopene plus β-carotene level exceeded 0.635 μg/mL, consisted of one male and four females, and group B (less than 0.635 μg/mL) consisted of four males and one female. Although significant differences were not observed in cytogenetic damage in Group A, there were some significant differences in Group B (Table 3). For example, the serum levels of 8-oxo-dG were significantly higher following the washout period (1.04 ± 0.21 ng/mL) than immediately after tomato juice intake (0.53 ± 0.12 ng/mL) in samples irradiated with 0.5 Gy in Group B. The number of DIC per 500 metaphases was also significantly lower following the intake (14.99 ± 1.31 ng/mL) than at baseline (18.65 ± 1.86 ng/mL) in samples irradiated with 0.5 Gy. It also increased after the washout period compared with the values immediately following the intake in samples irradiated with 0.5 Gy (from 14.99 ± 1.31 to 20.86 ± 1.96) and 2 Gy (from 85.64 ± 3.26 to 99.73 ± 5.60), but these values were not significant.

### Changes in the levels of MN and DIC

We measured the MN and DIC frequencies to assess radiation-induced cytogenetic damage in lymphocytes (Figs. 4 and 5). Tomato juice intake decreased the steady-state levels of MN per 1000 BNCs from 21.13 ± 2.00 to 16.11 ± 2.62, albeit not significantly (Fig. 4a). Decreased levels of MN following tomato juice intake were also found in the samples exposed to 0.1 Gy (non-significant effect) and 0.5 Gy (from 63.41 ± 5.54 to 52.47 ± 3.09; significant effect). No effect was found in the samples exposed to 2 Gy, indicating that the capacity of the tomato juice intake was inadequate to protect DNA against MN induction at this high dose. After the washout period, the MN frequencies per 1000 BNCs increased to the baseline levels. On comparing the levels of DIC in non-irradiated baseline samples with samples obtained after tomato juice intake and washout, no notable changes were observed (Fig. 5). The number of DIC per 500 metaphases decreased significantly during the intake period in the samples exposed to 0.5 Gy (from 19.98 ± 1.17 to 17.46 ± 1.11). Furthermore, the number of DIC per 500 metaphases increased significantly after the washout period in the samples exposed to 0.5 Gy (from 17.46 ± 1.11 to 20.99 ± 1.23) and 2 Gy (from 89.56 ± 2.86 to 102.58 ± 4.36).

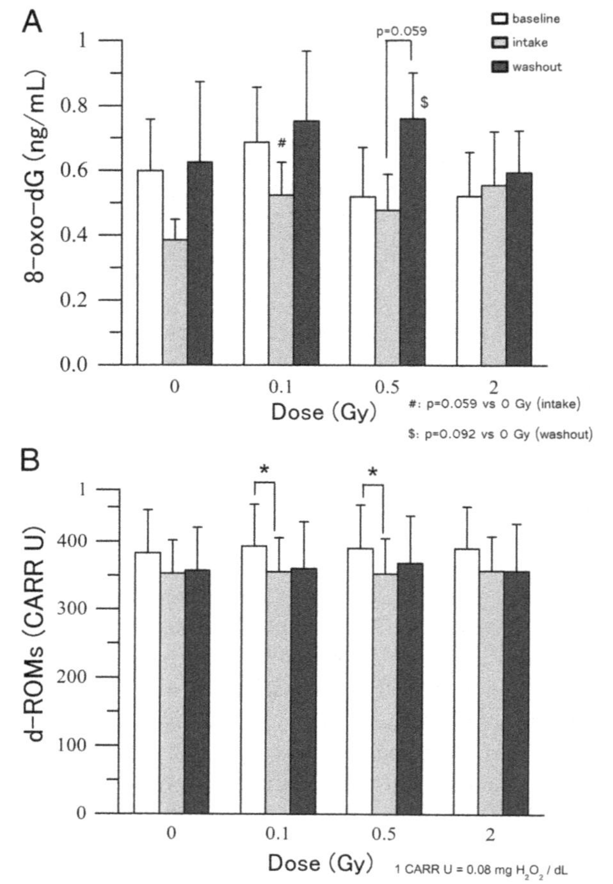


**Fig. 2** The level of oxidative stress-related markers in human blood. **a** Level of 8-oxo-dG in serum. **b** Level of d-ROMs in plasma. Values are given as mean ± SE of 10 donors. *$P < 0.05$, #: different between base line and intake period $P = 0.059$, $: different between base line and washout period $P = 0.092$ by (**a**) Wilcoxon signed-ranks test and (**b**) paired *t* test

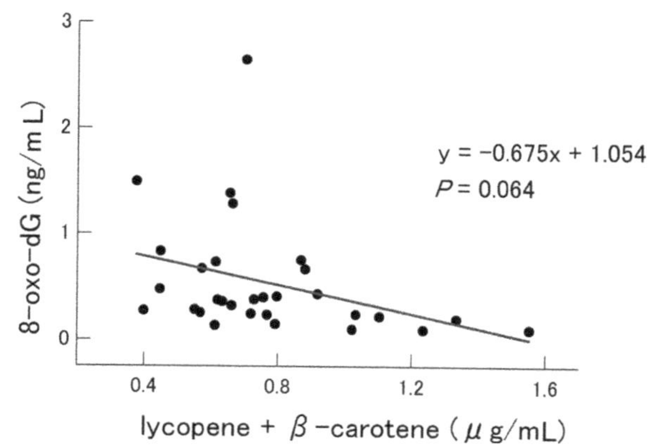


**Fig. 3** Relationship between concentration of lycopene plus β-carotene and level of 8-oxo-dG in serum in the non-irradiated samples. The *P* value was determined by linear regression analysis

## Discussion

The present study is based on a small number of healthy donors. Thus, it will be difficult to apply the findings to the general population, and our results should be considered as preliminary. Nevertheless, despite the small number of participants in the present investigation, the results indicate that drinking 190 g of tomato juice every day for 3 weeks decreases the steady state levels of 8-oxo-dG in the blood serum, as well as MN in the blood lymphocytes, although not significantly. No such effects were observed on the levels of d-ROMs. This could be due to the sensitivity of the methods, as extracellular 8-oxo-dG appears to be a more sensitive marker than d-ROMs. We did not observe any differences at the steady-state level of DIC with and without tomato juice intake. This could be due to the fact that DIC is a specific marker of radiation exposure [15]. The overall results indicate that the intake of 190 g of tomato juice per day for 3 weeks may be beneficial for healthy donors.

The baseline MN frequency in the general Japanese population has been reported to be 4–7 per 1000 BNCs [16, 17], which is lower than our observations. This could be due to differences in the protocols and slide preparation methods employed. However, in our previous publication we observed similar levels of MN as in the present investigation [18].

Next, we asked whether tomato juice intake could decrease the levels of radiation-induced oxidative stress biomarkers, namely extracellular 8-oxo-dG and d-ROMs. The reasons for choosing the stress biomarkers are: a) we know the mechanisms of radiation-induced damage in DNA and nucleotide pool [14], b) it is known that low doses of ionizing radiation induce oxidative stress [5], and c) there is worldwide concern regarding the increasing use of radiation for diagnostic purposes, especially in the low-dose region (<0.1 Gy) [19]. If tomato juice could decrease radiation-induced oxidative stress and cytogenetic damage, then it could have beneficial effects for healthy people exposed to low-dose radiation, e.g., due to medical diagnosis. For these reasons, we obtained blood samples from the donors at three time points (baseline, intake, and washout) and exposed them to 0.1, 0.5, or 2 Gy of X-rays. We observed dose-dependent increases in MN and DIC frequencies but not in extracellular 8-oxo-dG and d-ROM levels. In the case of MN and DIC, we observed that tomato juice consumption reduced radiation-induced frequencies of these biomarkers significantly at 0.5 Gy. Drinking tomato juice also resulted in decreased levels of MN and DIC upon exposure to 0.1 Gy, although the results were not statistically significant.

The levels of extracellular 8-oxo-dG in samples exposed to 0.1 and 0.5 Gy were slightly higher than those in the controls, whereas the levels of d-ROMs were

**Table 3** The level of 8-oxo-dG in human serum and cytogenetic damage in human lymphocytes in accordance with lycopene plus β-carotene concentration

| | | Dose (Gy) | Baseline Mean ± SE | Intake Mean ± SE | Washout Mean ± SE |
|---|---|---|---|---|---|
| 8-oxo-dG (ng/mL) | (A) | 0 | 0.46 ± 0.23 | 0.32 ± 0.10 | 0.28 ± 0.10 |
| | | 0.1 | 0.66 ± 0.30 | 0.52 ± 0.21 | 0.74 ± 0.35 |
| | | 0.5 | 0.58 ± 0.30 | 0.42 ± 0.20 | 0.48 ± 0.09 |
| | | 2 | 0.41 ± 0.19 | 0.34 ± 0.08 | 0.49 ± 0.17 |
| | (B) | 0 | 0.73 ± 0.22 | 0.45 ± 0.08 | 0.97 ± 0.46 |
| | | 0.1 | 0.71 ± 0.21 | 0.53 ± 0.04 | 0.76 ± 0.29 |
| | | 0.5 | 0.45 ± 0.11 | 0.53 ± 0.12 [b] | 1.04 ± 0.21 |
| | | 2 | 0.63 ± 0.20 | 0.77 ± 0.30 | 0.69 ± 0.20 |
| MN (/1000 BNC) | (A) | 0 | 22.10 ± 2.96 | 17.93 ± 4.45 | 24.07 ± 4.34 |
| | | 0.1 | 22.86 ± 1.93 | 20.54 ± 1.78 | 28.91 ± 3.59 |
| | | 0.5 | 68.98 ± 8.04 | 54.88 ± 4.87 | 57.05 ± 8.38 |
| | | 2 | 281.6 ± 15.6 | 330.7 ± 26.7 | 337.9 ± 19.9 |
| | (B) | 0 | 20.17 ± 2.97 | 14.30 ± 3.07 | 24.94 ± 5.63 |
| | | 0.1 | 22.43 ± 6.45 | 20.84 ± 4.32 | 24.27 ± 3.79 |
| | | 0.5 | 57.84 ± 7.61 | 50.06 ± 4.06 | 53.01 ± 4.19 |
| | | 2 | 286.6 ± 12.2 | 300.2 ± 26.7 | 282.6 ± 17.8 |
| DIC (/500 metaphase) | (A) | 0 | 0 | 0.18 ± 0.18 | 0 |
| | | 0.1 | 0.92 ± 0.49 | 0.38 ± 0.23 | 0.78 ± 0.20 |
| | | 0.5 | 21.31 ± 1.33 | 19.93 ± 0.87 | 21.1 ± 1.71 |
| | | 2 | 98.72 ± 6.24 | 93.47 ± 4.32 | 105.4 ± 7.1 |
| | (B) | 0 | 0.19 ± 0.19 | 0 | 0.19 ± 0.19 |
| | | 0.1 | 0.32 ± 0.32 | 0.58 ± 0.39 | 0.40 ± 0.24 |
| | | 0.5 | 18.65 ± 1.86 | 14.99 ± 1.31 [a,#] | 20.86 ± 1.96 |
| | | 2 | 89.45 ± 6.13 | 85.64 ± 3.26 [$] | 99.73 ± 5.60 |

(A) Group of individuals where the lycopene plus β-carotene concentration was higher than the median value at baseline (>0.635 μg/mL). $N = 5$ (1 male, 4 females)
(B) Group of individuals where the lycopene plus β-carotene concentration was less than the median value at baseline (<0.635 μg/mL). $N = 5$ (4 males, 1 female)
Values are given as mean ± SE of five donors. a: different from the baseline ($P < 0.05$), b: different from the washout period ($P < 0.05$), #: different from the washout ($P = 0.056$), $: different from the washout ($P = 0.056$) by Wilcoxon signed-ranks test (8-oxo-dG) and paired *t* test (MN and DIC)

unchanged following irradiation. Previously, we have shown that the major pathways that are activated in response to doses below 0.2 Gy are related to oxidative stress [4]. In contrast, most cellular response pathways following exposure to doses above 0.5 Gy are related to DNA repair, cell cycle checkpoint activation and apoptosis, due to extensive DNA damage production. Leukocytes are radiosensitive cells, so when exposed to 0.5 or 2 Gy of radiation, they will likely die through apoptosis or mitotic catastrophe rather than attempt to produce 8-oxo-dG or other stress markers. This could explain why we observed radiation-induced extracellular 8-oxo-dG production in response to 0.1 Gy of radiation. Matos et al. investigated the effect of lycopene treatment on oxidative DNA damage in the livers of male Wistar rats subjected to intraperitoneal ferric nitrilotriacetate administration. Five days of lycopene supplementation (10 mg/kg body weight/day) almost completely prevented the formation of 8-oxo-dG in the DNA of liver cells [20]. Although the applied 8-oxo-dG-forming agent and the investigated type of tissue were different from those employed in this study, these results suggest that lycopene could protect against DNA base oxidation. We also observed that tomato juice intake generally decreases the levels of d-ROMs but radiation has a minimal, if any, effect at the levels of d-ROMs. None of the oxidative stress-related markers revealed a protective effect of tomato juice in response to 2 Gy of radiation, while the analyses of cytogenetic damage disclosed an effect after this dose. In the intake period, reductions in MN frequencies were observed in the samples irradiated with 0.5 Gy, and reductions in DIC frequencies were observed in the samples irradiated with 0.5 and 2 Gy, suggesting that consumption of tomato juice protected against ionizing radiation-induced DNA damage.

It was previously reported that the addition of lycopene to cell cultures could reduce the MN frequency [21, 22]

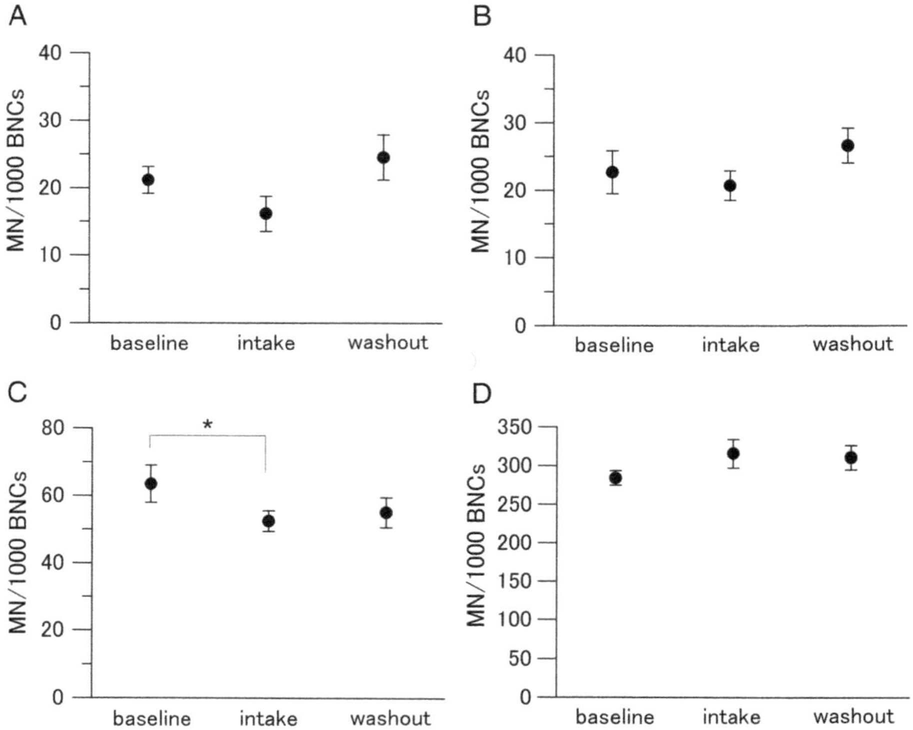


**Fig. 4** Changes in the level of MN in human lymphocytes. Values are given as mean ± SE of 10 donors. *$P < 0.05$ by paired *t* test. **a** 0 Gy. **b** 0.1 Gy. **c** 0.5 Gy. **d** 2 Gy

and DIC frequency following exposure to radiation [23]. These findings are consistent with our data suggesting that lycopene can protect against DNA damage [24–26]. Ingestion of tomato extracts has previously been reported to reduce DNA damage, and this property of tomatoes has also been attributed to components other than lycopene [25]. The present study revealed that the ingestion of tomato juice significantly increased the circulating levels of lycopene by 1.5 and β-carotene by 1.26-fold (Table 1). This result is consistent with those of previous reports [27, 28]. In addition, a non-significant inverse correlation was observed between the plasma concentrations of lycopene plus β-carotene and the levels of extracellular 8-oxo-dG (Fig. 3). A weaker and non-significant inverse correlation was observed between the plasma concentrations of lycopene plus β-carotene and the levels of MN (data not shown), whereas no correlations were found for lycopene plus β-carotene levels with d-ROMs or DIC. The results indicate that lycopene together with β-carotene may play an important role in reducing 8-oxo-dG levels. It was reported that β-carotene has radical-scavenging activity and that β-carotene supplementation decreases DNA damages in lymphocytes [29]. However, the positive health effects of β-carotene have not been fully clarified. Although several studies demonstrated that β-carotene–rich foods have positive effects on human health [29], there are indications in the literature that β-carotene supplementation can increase the risk of lung cancer among smokers and/or asbestos-exposed workers [30–32]. One possible mechanism is that β-carotene combined with cigarette smoke alters the regulation of heme oxygenase1 via its transcriptional factor Bach1, which modulates cell proliferation [33]. This aspect was considered in the present investigation, as smokers were excluded. Furthermore, tomatoes contain various antioxidants such as α-tocopherol, vitamin C, and polyphenols. Although our observations in the present study indicated that lycopene and β-carotene are active components that reduce blood oxidative stress levels, we believe that further experiments are needed to clarify the active components in tomatoes.

It has been reported that lycopene is oxidized by the addition of radicals in vitro. We assumed that lycopene thus quenched the ROS induced by radiation. However, radiation doses used in the present investigation did not degrade lycopene and the cis/trans ratio was maintained.

We compared donors with high baseline levels of lycopene and β-carotene with those with low baseline levels. Interestingly, in the former group, tomato juice consumption did not notably influence any of the parameters. However, it significantly reduced 8-oxo-dG and DIC levels in the latter group. These data indicate that it

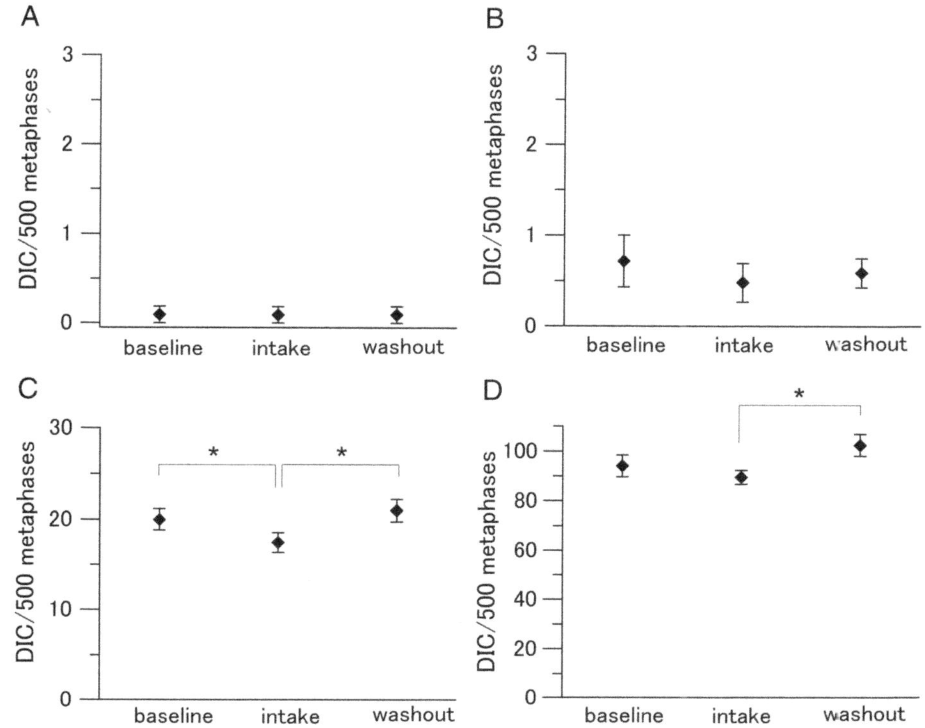


**Fig. 5** Changes in the level of DIC in human lymphocytes. Values are given as mean ± SE of 10 donors. *$P < 0.05$ by paired $t$ test. **a** 0 Gy. **b** 0.1 Gy. **c** 0.5 Gy. **d** 2 Gy

is more beneficial for people with low baseline levels of lycopene and β-carotene to drink tomato juice. Thus, when we tailor this small intervention to healthy people scheduled to undergo CT at a dose of approximately 50 mGy, they may experience the most beneficial effect by consuming tomato juice, as most of the biological effects of low-dose radiation are mediated by elevated endogenous ROS formation [5].

Additionally, healthy non-smokers with high levels of 8-oxo-dG or MN at steady state should also benefit from continuous tomato juice consumption. However, considering the small number of donors and the duration of the study, the obtained results should be considered as preliminary. It is also important to mention that ROS and other reactive species play important roles in normal physiological functions; e.g., ROS are produced by macrophages to kill bacteria and by xenobiotic systems for neutralizing toxins. A recent study demonstrated that antioxidant supplementation reduces ROS levels and DNA damage but increases tumor cell proliferation and tumor growth in mice [34]. The authors also revealed that tumor cells proliferate faster when oxidative stress is suppressed. Their explanation for these results was that a feedback mechanism in lung cancer cells downregulates the endogenous ROS defense system when ROS production is suppressed by antioxidants. However, this study used genetically modified mice that already had lung cancer as well as lung cancer cell lines in culture. The results from genetically modified mice with lung cancer and cancer cells in culture will be difficult to apply to healthy humans or considered in cancer initiation and prevention. This study provides important information regarding the negative effects of Vitamin E and NAC in people with lung cancer or an elevated risk for lung cancer, e.g., smokers. However, in the present study, we aimed to investigate the effects of tomato juice consumption in healthy individuals.

## Conclusion

In conclusion, our results suggest that continuously drinking tomato juice could decrease the steady state levels of extracellular 8-oxo-dG and MN. Generally, tomato juice intake lowered the induction of MN and DIC in exposed cells. Additionally, our results suggest that lycopene and β-carotene are active compounds in tomato juice. The juice also contains other antioxidants, the roles of which were not studied in the present investigation. It is important to mention that the obtained results are based on 10 healthy donors with great individual variation in the results, and the findings should be considered as preliminary and be verified in larger setups.

### Abbreviations

8-oxo-dG: 8-oxo-7, 8-dihydro-2′-deoxyguanosine; 8-oxo-dGMP: 8-hydroxy-2′-deoxyguanosine-monophosphate; 8-oxo-dGTP: 8-hydroxy-2′-deoxyguanosine-triphosphate; BNCs: Binucleated cells; CBMN: Cytokinesis-block micronucleus; dGTP: Deoxyguanosine triphosphate; DIC: Dicentrics; dNTP: Deoxynucleoside triphosphate; d-ROMs: Reactive oxygen metabolite-derived compounds; ELISA: Enzyme-linked immunosorbent assay; FBS: Fetal bovine serum; HPLC: High-performance liquid chromatography; MN: Micronuclei; ROS: Reactive oxygen species; SE: Standard error

### Acknowledgments

We would like to thank Ms. Yasuyo Fukushi and Mr. Yohei Fujishima for their contribution and all the volunteers who participated in this project.

### Funding

This work was funded by the Japan Society for the Promotion of Science KAKENHI Grant Number 25461900. We would also like to thank the Swedish Radiation Safety Authority (SSM) for financial support.

### Availability of data and materials

The datasets analyzed in the current study are not publicly available due to an ongoing analysis of the data, but they are available from the corresponding author upon reasonable request.

### Authors' contributions

CI, KA, HS, YM, and SH designed the research. AN, AS, TY, KA, AH, and SH conducted the research. KA, AH, HS, and SH provided essential reagents or materials. AN, KA, AH, YM, and SH analyzed the data. AN, KA, AH, and SH performed the statistical and mathematical modeling analyses. AN, KA, HS, TM, YM, and SH wrote the paper. YM had primary responsibility for the final content. All authors contributed to and approved the final version of the manuscript.

### Competing interests

The experimental food (commercially available tomato juice) used in this study was provided by KAGOME CO., LTD. There is no financial support or relationship to declare that may pose a competing interest.

### Author details

[1]Department of Radiological Life Sciences, Division of Medical Life Sciences, Hirosaki University Graduate School of Health Sciences, Aomori 036-8564, Japan. [2]Department of Disability and Health, Division of Medical Life Sciences, Hirosaki University Graduate School of Health Sciences, Aomori 036-8564, Japan. [3]Department of Clinical Laboratory Medicine, Hirosaki Central Hospital, Aomori 036-8188, Japan. [4]Nature and Wellness Research Department, Innovation Division, KAGOME CO., LTD., Tochigi 329-2762, Japan. [5]Department of Pathologic Analysis, Division of Medical Life Sciences, Hirosaki University Graduate School of Health Sciences, Aomori 036-8564, Japan. [6]Center for Radiation Protection Research, Department of Molecular Biosciences, The Wenner-Gren Institute, Stockholm University, Stockholm SE-106 91, Sweden.

### References

1. Finkel T, Holbrook NJ. Oxidants, oxidative stress and the biology of ageing. Nature. 2000;408:239–47.
2. Chakravarti B, Chakravarti DN. Oxidative modification of proteins: age-related changes. Gerontology. 2007;53:128–39.
3. Cooke MS, Evans MD, Dizdaroglu M, Lunec J. Oxidative DNA damage: mechanisms, mutation, and disease. FASEB J. 2003;17:1195–214.
4. Haghdoost S, Sjolander L, Czene S, Harms-Ringdahl M. The nucleotide pool is a significant target for oxidative stress. Free Radic Biol Med. 2006; 41:620–6.
5. Sangsuwan T, Haghdoost S. The nucleotide pool, a target for low-dose gamma-ray-induced oxidative stress. Radiat Res. 2008;170:776–83.
6. Roots R, Okada S. Protection of DNA molecules of cultured mammalian cells from radiation-induced single-strand scissions by various alcohols and SH compounds. Int J Radiat Biol Relat Stud Phys Chem Med. 1972;21:329–42.
7. Fotouhi A, Hagos WW, Ilic M, Wojcik A, Harms-Ringdahl M, de Gruijl F, Mullenders L, Jansen JG, Haghdoost S. Analysis of mutant frequencies and mutation spectra in hMTH1 knockdown TK6 cells exposed to UV radiation. Mutat Res. 2013;751–752:8–14.
8. Sies H. Oxidative stress: from basic research to clinical application. Am J Med. 1991;91:31S–8.
9. Okunieff P, Swarts S, Keng P, Sun W, Wang W, Kim J, Yang S, Zhang H, Liu C, Williams JP, et al. Antioxidants reduce consequences of radiation exposure. Adv Exp Med Biol. 2008;614:165–78.
10. Di Mascio P, Kaiser S, Sies H. Lycopene as the most efficient biological carotenoid singlet oxygen quencher. Arch Biochem Biophys. 1989;274:532–8.
11. Aizawa K, Iwasaki Y, Ouchi A, Inakuma T, Nagaoka S, Terao J, Mukai K. Development of singlet oxygen absorption capacity (SOAC) assay method. 2. Measurements of the SOAC values for carotenoids and food extracts. J Agric Food Chem. 2011;59:3717–29.
12. Harms-Ringdahl M, Jenssen D, Haghdoost S. Tomato juice intake suppressed serum concentration of 8-oxodG after extensive physical activity. Nutr J. 2012;11:29.
13. Rao AV. Processed tomato products as a source of dietary lycopene: bioavailability and antioxidant properties. Can J Diet Pract Res. 2004;65:161–5.
14. Haghdoost S, Czene S, Naslund I, Skog S, Harms-Ringdahl M. Extracellular 8-oxo-dG as a sensitive parameter for oxidative stress in vivo and in vitro. Free Radic Res. 2005;39:153–62.
15. Ray-Chaudhuri SP, Sarkar I. Frequency of dicentric bridges in Meiosis in the grasshopper Gesonia punctifrons, produced by different dosages of x-rays. Science. 1952;116:479–82.
16. Ishikawa S, Ishikawa H, Shindo T, Yoshida T, Shimoyama Y, Satomi T, Fujii S, Hamamoto Y, Iino M, Fukao A. Effects of occupational environmental controls and work management on chromosomal damage in dental technicians in Japan. Int J Hyg Environ Health. 2013;216:100–7.
17. Huang P, Huang B, Weng H, Nakayama K, Morimoto K. Effects of lifestyle on micronuclei frequency in human lymphocytes in Japanese hard-metal workers. Prev Med. 2009;48:383–8.
18. Staaf E, Brehwens K, Haghdoost S, Nievaart S, Pachnerova-Brabcova K, Czub J, Braziewicz J, Wojcik A. Micronuclei in human peripheral blood lymphocytes exposed to mixed beams of X-rays and alpha particles. Radiat Environ Biophys. 2012;51:283–93.
19. Do KH. General Principles of Radiation Protection in Fields of Diagnostic Medical Exposure. J Korean Med Sci. 2016;31 Suppl 1:S6–9.
20. Matos HR, Capelozzi VL, Gomes OF, Mascio PD, Medeiros MH. Lycopene inhibits DNA damage and liver necrosis in rats treated with ferric nitrilotriacetate. Arch Biochem Biophys. 2001;396:171–7.
21. Scolastici C, de Lima RO A, Barbisan LF, Ferreira AL, Ribeiro DA, Salvadori DM. Antigenotoxicity and antimutagenicity of lycopene in HepG2 cell line evaluated by the comet assay and micronucleus test. Toxicol In Vitro. 2008;22:510–4.
22. Scolastici C, de Lima RO A, Barbisan LF, Ferreira AL, Ribeiro DA, Salvadori DM. Lycopene activity against chemically induced DNA damage in Chinese hamster ovary cells. Toxicol In Vitro. 2007;21:840–5.
23. Srinivasan M, Devipriya N, Kalpana KB, Menon VP. Lycopene: An antioxidant and radioprotector against gamma-radiation-induced cellular damages in cultured human lymphocytes. Toxicology. 2009;262:43–9.

24. Briviba K, Kulling SE, Moseneder J, Watzl B, Rechkemmer G, Bub A. Effects of supplementing a low-carotenoid diet with a tomato extract for 2 weeks on endogenous levels of DNA single strand breaks and immune functions in healthy non-smokers and smokers. Carcinogenesis. 2004;25:2373–8.
25. Riso P, Visioli F, Erba D, Testolin G, Porrini M. Lycopene and vitamin C concentrations increase in plasma and lymphocytes after tomato intake. Effects on cellular antioxidant protection. Eur J Clin Nutr. 2004;58:1350–8.
26. Porrini M, Riso P, Brusamolino A, Berti C, Guarnieri S, Visioli F. Daily intake of a formulated tomato drink affects carotenoid plasma and lymphocyte concentrations and improves cellular antioxidant protection. Br J Nutr. 2005; 93:93–9.
27. Quilliot D, Forbes A, Dubois F, Gueant JL, Ziegler O. Carotenoid deficiency in chronic pancreatitis: the effect of an increase in tomato consumption. Eur J Clin Nutr. 2011;65:262–8.
28. Hadley CW, Clinton SK, Schwartz SJ. The consumption of processed tomato products enhances plasma lycopene concentrations in association with a reduced lipoprotein sensitivity to oxidative damage. J Nutr. 2003;133:727–32.
29. Lee HJ, Park YK, Kang MH. The effect of carrot juice, beta-carotene supplementation on lymphocyte DNA damage, erythrocyte antioxidant enzymes and plasma lipid profiles in Korean smoker. Nutr Res Pract. 2011;5: 540–7.
30. Yu N, Su X, Wang Z, Dai B, Kang J. Association of Dietary Vitamin A and beta-Carotene Intake with the Risk of Lung Cancer: A Meta-Analysis of 19 Publications. Nutrients. 2015;7:9309–24.
31. Omenn GS, Goodman GE, Thornquist MD, Balmes J, Cullen MR, Glass A, Keogh JP, Meyskens FL, Valanis B, Williams JH, et al. Effects of a combination of beta carotene and vitamin A on lung cancer and cardiovascular disease. N Engl J Med. 1996;334:1150–5.
32. The effect of vitamin E and beta carotene on the incidence of lung cancer and other cancers in male smokers. The Alpha-Tocopherol, Beta Carotene Cancer Prevention Study Group. N Engl J Med. 1994;330:1029–35.
33. Palozza P, Serini S, Curro D, Calviello G, Igarashi K, Mancuso C. beta-Carotene and cigarette smoke condensate regulate heme oxygenase-1 and its repressor factor Bach1: relationship with cell growth. Antioxid Redox Signal. 2006;8:1069–80.
34. Sayin VI, Ibrahim MX, Larsson E, Nilsson JA, Lindahl P, Bergo MO. Antioxidants accelerate lung cancer progression in mice. Sci Transl Med. 2014;6:221ra215.

22

# Plasma phospholipid fatty acid profile confirms compliance to a novel saturated fat-reduced, monounsaturated fat-enriched dairy product intervention in adults at moderate cardiovascular risk

Oonagh Markey[1,2,8], Dafni Vasilopoulou[1,2], Kirsty E. Kliem[3], Albert Koulman[4,5], Colette C. Fagan[2], Keith Summerhill[4], Laura Y. Wang[4], Alistair S. Grandison[2], David J. Humphries[3], Susan Todd[6], Kim G. Jackson[1,2], David I. Givens[7] and Julie A. Lovegrove[1,2,7*]

## Abstract

**Background:** Dairy products are a major contributor to dietary SFA. Partial replacement of milk SFA with unsaturated fatty acids (FAs) is possible through oleic-acid rich supplementation of the dairy cow diet. To assess adherence to the intervention of SFA-reduced, MUFA-enriched dairy product consumption in the RESET (**RE**placement of **S**aturat**E**d fat in dairy on **T**otal cholesterol) study using 4-d weighed dietary records, in addition to plasma phospholipid FA (PL-FA) status.

**Methods:** In a randomised, controlled, crossover design, free-living UK participants identified as moderate risk for CVD ($n = 54$) were required to replace habitually consumed dairy foods (milk, cheese and butter), with study products with a FA profile typical of retail products (control) or SFA-reduced, MUFA-enriched profile (modified), for two 12-week periods, separated by an 8-week washout period. A flexible food-exchange model was used to implement each isoenergetic high-fat, high-dairy diet (38% of total energy intake (%TE) total fat): control (dietary target: 19%TE SFA; 11%TE MUFA) and modified (16%TE SFA; 14%TE MUFA).

**Results:** Following the modified diet, there was a smaller increase in SFA (17.2%TE vs. 19.1%TE; $p < 0.001$) and greater increase in MUFA intake (15.4%TE vs. 11.8%TE; $p < 0.0001$) when compared with the control. PL-FA analysis revealed lower total SFAs ($p = 0.006$), higher total *cis*-MUFAs and *trans*-MUFAs (both $p < 0.0001$) following the modified diet.

**Conclusion:** The food-exchange model was successfully used to achieve RESET dietary targets by partial replacement of SFAs with MUFAs in dairy products, a finding reflected in the PL-FA profile and indicative of objective dietary compliance.

(Continued on next page)

* Correspondence: j.a.lovegrove@reading.ac.uk
[1]Hugh Sinclair Unit of Human Nutrition and Institute for Cardiovascular and Metabolic Research, University of Reading, Reading RG6 6AP, UK
[2]Department of Food and Nutritional Sciences, University of Reading, Reading RG6 6AP, UK
Full list of author information is available at the end of the article

(Continued from previous page)

**Trial registration:** ClinicalTrials.gov Identifier: NCT02089035, date 05-01-2014.

**Keywords:** Cardiovascular disease, Dairy products, Dietary fat composition, Food-exchange model, Fatty acids, Monounsaturated fatty acids, Nutrition assessment, Phospholipids, Saturated fatty acids

## Background

Cardiovascular diseases (CVD) are one of the leading causes of mortality in the UK [1]. As a result of the clear link between a high intake of SFAs and elevated LDL-cholesterol concentrations, dietary guidelines for CVD prevention advocate reducing SFA intake to ≤10% of total energy (%TE) [2, 3]. Despite recommendations, the UK adult population still exceeds the target for dietary SFA intake, with a mean intake of 12.1%TE [4].

Dairy products are major sources of dietary SFA and account for up to 35% of total UK SFA intake [4] and therefore reducing consumption of regular-fat dairy foods or replacing them with lower fat or fat-free alternatives is often advised [5, 6]. However, prospective studies have not presented consistent evidence for an adverse link between higher consumption of milk and dairy products and increased risk of CVD, regardless of milk fat content [7–10]. Furthermore, this rationalisation does not acknowledge the complex nature of the dairy food matrix, which may be fundamental to cardiovascular health [11]. Dairy fat contains a complex mixture of fatty acids (FA) including SFAs, MUFAs, PUFAs, *trans*-fatty acids (TFAs) and branched-chain FAs [12, 13]. Furthermore, milk is rich in micronutrients and bioactive peptides, which have been reported to exert cardio-protective effects [14, 15].

While the findings of some recent epidemiological studies have challenged the traditional link between SFA and coronary heart disease risk, and mortality [16–18], it is important to consider the macronutrient that replaces energy from dietary SFA [18, 19]. There is evidence from a randomized controlled trial (RCT) that replacement of SFA with PUFA had minimal but increased effects on CHD mortality [20]. However a more recent systematic review and meta-analysis of RCT suggests that lowering SFA intake could reduce cardiovascular events by 17%, with SFA replacement with PUFA estimated to reduce these events by 27% [21]. Despite these apparent discrepancies, current US and EU dietary guidelines recommend reduction of SFA and replacement with PUFA and/or MUFA respectively [22, 23]. In support of the latter review and dietary recommendations, a RCT illustrated that replacing SFA with *n*-6 PUFA for 16-weeks induced a reduction in serum concentration of LDL-cholesterol (a major risk factor for CVD) by 13.6%, with a comparable reduction of 11.3% on replacement of SFA with MUFA [19].

It is well documented that partial replacement of milk SFA with unsaturated FAs, predominantly in the form of MUFA, through supplementation of the dairy cow diet with plant oils or oil seeds is feasible [24–26]. At a population level, this initiative could provide a sustainable means of reducing SFA in dairy products, whilst limiting the entry of SFA into the wider food chain. While limited evidence from human studies suggest that consumption of dairy products with a modified FA profile may beneficially impact on CVD risk, there has been a heavy reliance on fasting lipid biomarkers as sole predictors of risk [27]. Further research is needed to elucidate whether FA-modified dairy product consumption has a differential effect on more novel risk markers, including endothelial function, arterial stiffness, systemic inflammation and ambulatory blood pressure, when compared with dairy products of typical milk FA composition [15, 27].

The REplacement of SaturatEd fat in dairy on Total cholesterol (RESET) study was conducted to investigate the chronic and acute effects of two iso-energetic high-fat, high-dairy diets, which varied in FA composition, on traditional and novel cardiometabolic risk markers in free-living individuals. It is important to evaluate strategies employed for the achievement of dietary targets in controlled human intervention studies [28]. The purpose of the current paper is to describe the RESET dietary exchange strategy that was developed to enable manipulation of the FA profile of the diet over two 12-week periods, through the use of SFA-reduced, MUFA-enriched (modified) dairy products and matched control dairy foods with a FA profile typical of retail products. Although it is recognised that specific plasma FA levels can be indicative of dietary FA consumption, the composition of the plasma phospholipid FA (PL-FA) fraction is believed to be a good biomarker of FA intake over recent days to weeks and an objective indicator of dietary compliance [29–31]. Thus, this paper aims to report the chronic dietary intervention food-exchange model and the compliance to the FA-modified and control dietary exchange periods using 4-d weighed dietary records, self-reported daily tick-sheets and PL-FA.

## Materials and methods

### Study participants and design

The RESET study was a double-blinded, randomised, controlled, crossover designed trial registered at Clinicaltrials.Gov as: NCT02089035. The study was given a favourable ethical opinion for conduct by the University of Reading's Research Ethics Committee (13/43) and was conducted according to the guidelines of the Declaration of Helsinki. All participants provided written informed consent prior to study entry.

Men and women aged 25–70 years were recruited from the Berkshire area of the UK in three cohorts between February 2014 and April 2016. A modified Framingham risk prediction algorithm was employed to identify individuals with moderate CVD risk [31, 32]. To meet inclusion criteria, participants were required to have ≥ 2 CVD risk points, a score that suggested a 50% greater risk of CVD development than the population mean [32]. Briefly, this score was calculated based on the existence of single or multiple CVD risk factors, including elevated fasting total cholesterol, glucose, systolic/diastolic blood pressure, low HDL-cholesterol, overweight/obesity or a family history of myocardial infarction. Potential participants were also required to meet the following inclusion criteria: BMI 19–32 kg/m$^2$; blood pressure <160/100 mmHg; total cholesterol <8 mmol/L; haemoglobin: >125 g/L for women and 135 g/L for men; normal liver and kidney function; not pregnant or lactating; no dietary supplementation; no lactose or dairy intolerances/allergies; not taking medication for hyperlipidaemia, hypertension, hypercoagulation or inflammatory conditions; no diagnosis of myocardial infarction, stroke or diabetes; participating in <20 min × 3 times/week of vigorous aerobic activity and not consuming excessive amounts of alcohol (men: <21 units/week; women: <14 units/week). If known not to interfere with study outcomes, participants continued to take their regular prescribed medication, without changes in dosage, for the duration of the study.

### Study foods

The FA composition of the dairy products (including ruminant *cis* and TFAs), along with the methods for their production, will be described in detail elsewhere (Kliem KE, Humphries DJ, Markey O, Vasilopoulou D, Fagan CC, Grandison AS, Todd S, Givens DI, Lovegrove JA: Food chain approach to lowering saturated fat in milk and dairy products: the RESET study, submitted). Based on a similar feeding strategy, it was estimated that our bovine intervention would increase *cis*-MUFA in the milk from 20 to 30 g/100 g FA, while reducing SFA from 70 to 55–60 g/100 g FA [33]. Briefly, the diet of recruited Holstein-Friesian cows was supplemented with approximately 1 kg high-oleic sunflower oil (AAK Ltd., Hull, East Yorkshire, UK) per cow per day for a ≥ 28-d period to produce milk which had a portion of SFA replaced with MUFA. Subsequently, raw milk was used to produce SFA-reduced, MUFA-enriched (modified) ultra high temperature (UHT) milk, Cheddar cheese and butter. Raw milk, provided by Arla UK Plc (Taw Valley Creamery, North Tawton, UK), was used to produce control UHT milk. Control Cheddar cheese and butter, with a FA profile typical of retail products, were also supplied by Arla UK Plc (Taw Valley Creamery, North Tawton, UK).

### Dietary intervention

The technique of minimization, controlling for gender, age, BMI and total cholesterol was used to randomly allocate participants to one of two groups in the study, with Group 1 being assigned to receive Diet A (Modified) and then Diet B (Control) during their first and second dietary intervention periods, respectively and vice-versa for Group 2 [34]. In each group, participants completed two 12-week dietary intervention periods, separated by an 8-week washout period. One dietary intervention was an iso-energetic high-fat daily dietary exchange (dietary target: 38%TE total fat) which was achieved by replacing habitual dairy foods, cooking oil and snacks with SFA-reduced, MUFA-enriched UHT milk, Cheddar cheese and butter (modified). The second dietary intervention used matched products with a FA profile typical of retail products (control). The dietary exchange periods were rich in dairy foods and were designed to give diets of equal fat content that varied in SFA and MUFA composition. The dietary target intake for total fat was 38%TE in both diets, with specific dietary FA targets for the control (19%TE SFA and 11%TE MUFA) and modified diets (16%TE SFA and 14%TE MUFA).

Measurements of circulating total cholesterol, composed of LDL and HDL-cholesterol (primary outcome), and other established and novel CVD and cardiometabolic risk markers were assessed prior to and after each dietary intervention period (chronic study). This manuscript will present the 4-d weighed dietary records, tick-sheet records, anthropometric measures, and PL-FA analysis to assess dietary compliance. The other clinical outcome measures from the RESET study will be published elsewhere.

### Food-exchange model

The RESET study food-exchange strategy for reducing SFA intake was designed based on a model adapted from both the Dietary Intervention and Vascular Function (DIVAS) study and the Reading, Imperial, Surrey, Cambridge, and Kings (RISCK) study [31, 35], which were based on the National Diet and Nutrition Survey (NDNS) for adults (aged 19–64 years) [36]. The mean habitual energy, total fat, SFA, MUFA and PUFA intakes of participants from the RISCK study were used [35], with additional TFA data obtained from the DIVAS study [31], as these dietary data represented the intake of UK adults who were at increased or moderate CVD risk. Added oils, added fats (butter and spreads), milk, cheese as well as sweet and savoury snacks were identified as 'exchangeable dietary fat' sources which could be removed from the diet and replaced with study foods. The total contribution of these 'exchangeable fat' food groups to mean daily energy, fat and FA intake were estimated, based on mean population data from the 2000/2001 NDNS 'percentage contribution of types of foods' (Table 1). The total exchangeable fat was subtracted from the RISCK/DIVAS study habitual energy, total fat and FA intake to calculate non-modifiable fat intake. This was employed to form the backbone of the food-exchange model, onto which the RESET study foods could be added to create two iso-energetic dietary exchange periods of dairy products that varied in FA composition (Table 2).

### Implementation of intervention diets

After completing baseline visits (i.e. at the beginning of each intervention period), participants were provided with 1:1 dietary advice on how to replace dietary fat sources in their habitual diets (e.g. added oils, milk, cheese, sweet and savoury snacks) with the study dairy foods. They were also given dietary guidelines and recipe suggestions to take home. Care was taken to ensure that no study visits were arranged during or immediately after the Christmas period (mid-December to mid-January). Where it was not feasible to avoid holidays and business trips during intervention periods, participants were given instructions on how to travel with the study products. This was made more convenient by providing UHT milk that did not require refrigeration. Furthermore, participants were provided with frozen butter and were advised that they could it frozen during transit, with the use of ice packs. Products were provided in plain packaging and were only identifiable by a code (A or B), to ensure that participants and researchers remained blinded to the intervention arms.

At the beginning of each intervention period, participants were given adequate study dairy foods for a 4-week period. They attended the Hugh Sinclair Unit of Human Nutrition for a food collection visit at weeks 4 and 8. During this visit, adherence to the dietary intervention was assessed by reviewing completed tick-sheet records and any issues were discussed and resolved. In addition, investigators recorded the participant's weight and any changes ≥ ± 1 kg of baseline, were addressed through advice to alter snack, meat and/or carbohydrate intake. Participants were asked to maintain their habitual physical activity levels during each intervention period. At the end of the first intervention period, participants were asked to return unopened, leftover study products and were asked not to consume any leftover study products for the duration of the washout period.

#### *Assessment of dietary intake*

Participants received verbal and written instructions by the investigators for recording 4-d weighed dietary records approximately 2 week before the first study visit (week 0). Investigators also provided participants with examples of completed diaries, including how to record recipes, and digital scales for recording food intake. Exceptions for weighing included food consumed outside of the home. On these occasions, portion-size images were used to estimate consumed portions and subsequently quantified using published food portion tables [37]. Participants completed diet diaries on four separate occasions (weeks 0, 11, 19 and 31): habitual diet intake was represented from baseline diet diaries (weeks 0 and

**Table 1** The RESET food-exchange model[a]

| | Total energy (MJ/d) | Total fat | SFA | MUFA | TFA | PUFA |
|---|---|---|---|---|---|---|
| Total habitual intake (including alcohol)[b], g/d | 8.25 | 80.1 | 29.6 | 26.6 | 1.0 | 13.1 |
| Total habitual intake, %TE | | 36.6 | 13.5 | 12.1 | 0.4 | 6.0 |
| Exchangeable fat intake | | | | | | |
| Added oils, g/d | 0.35 | 8.5 | 0.8 | 3.3 | | 4.0 |
| Added fats (butter and spreads), g/d | 0.35 | 8.6 | 3.3 | 2.9 | 0.2 | 1.7 |
| Milk, g/d | 0.45 | 4.0 | 2.4 | 1.0 | 0.0 | 0.3 |
| Cheese, g/d | 0.25 | 4.5 | 2.8 | 1.0 | 0.1 | 0.1 |
| Sweet and savoury snacks, g/d[c] | 0.87 | 10.0 | 4.4 | 3.4 | 0.1 | 0.6 |
| Total exchangeable fat intake, g/d | 2.27 | 35.5 | 13.6 | 11.6 | 0.4 | 6.6 |
| Total exchangeable fat intake adjusted for habitual intake, g/d | 2.22 | 38.5 | 14.4 | 12.5 | 0.4 | 7.3 |
| Non-exchangeable fat intake, g/d | 6.03 | 41.7 | 15.3 | 14.1 | 0.6 | 5.9 |

*TFA trans*-fatty acids, *%TE* percentage of total energy
[a]Adapted from Weech et al. [31]
[b]Mean daily dietary intakes (total energy, total fat, SFA, MUFA and PUFA) from a population with increased cardiovascular disease risk [35]. Mean daily dietary TFA intake from a population at moderate cardiovascular disease risk [31]
[c]Included buns, cakes, pastries, potato chips and chocolate confectionary

**Table 2** Replacement model for diets containing control and modified dairy products for use in the RESET study[a]

| | Quantity (g/d) | Total energy (MJ/d) | Total fat | SFA | MUFA | TFA[b] | PUFA |
|---|---|---|---|---|---|---|---|
| Non-exchangeable fat intake, g/d | | 6.03 | 41.7 | 15.3 | 14.1 | 0.5 | 5.9 |
| Control dietary exchange | | | | | | | |
| Exchangeable fat intakes[c] | | | | | | | |
| Butter, g/d | 21.5 | 0.65 | 17.4 | 11.1 | 4.5 | 0.7 | 0.6 |
| Cheese, g/d | 45.0 | 0.76 | 15.1 | 10.2 | 3.5 | 0.5 | 0.4 |
| Milk, g/d | 340.0 | 0.75 | 8.6 | 5.7 | 2.1 | 0.3 | 0.3 |
| Total intake, g/d | | 8.19 | 82.8 | 42.3 | 24.2 | 2.0 | 7.2 |
| Total intake, %TE | | | 38.1 | 19.4 | 11.1 | 0.9 | 3.3 |
| Target intake, %TE | | | 38.0 | 19.0 | 11.0 | 0.9 | |
| Modified dietary exchange | | | | | | | |
| Exchangeable fat intakes | | | | | | | |
| Butter | 25.1 | 0.76 | 20.4 | 10.2 | 8.1 | 2.1 | 0.7 |
| Cheese, g/d | 45.0 | 0.69 | 12.6 | 6.3 | 5.0 | 1.4 | 0.4 |
| Milk, g/d | 340 | 0.79 | 8.8 | 4.4 | 3.6 | 0.9 | 0.3 |
| Total intake, g/d | | 8.27 | 83.4 | 36.0 | 30.8 | 4.9 | 7.3 |
| Total intake, %TE | | | 38.0 | 16.4 | 14.0 | 2.1 | 3.3 |
| Target intake, %TE | | | 38.0 | 16.0 | 14.0 | 2.0 | |
| Mean difference between dietary exchange periods, %TE | | | −0.6 | 6.2 | −6.7 | −2.9 | −0.2 |

The FA composition of dairy products was determined using a GC-flame ionisation detection method [38], with a conversion factor of 0.933 used to estimate the proportion of FAs in the total fat content of each product [39]
%TE, percentage of total energy
[a]Total intake is the sum of exchangeable and non-exchangeable intakes based on MJ/d for energy and grams/d for FAs
[b]Total TFA intake (%TE) is calculated based on recorded energy intake at baseline (MJ/d) in Weech et al. [31]
[c]Energy and fat content of the dairy products is based on nutritional analysis conducted by SGS United Kingdom Ltd. (Ellesmere Port, Cheshire)

19), while diaries completed during weeks 11 and 31 represented participant compliance to the intervention diets. Prior to visit 1, food intake was recorded on three weekdays and one weekend day. The same days were repeated for subsequent diaries. Assessment of completion of the diaries was undertaken by the investigators during study visits. If necessary, additional information was requested to facilitate precise data entry.

Food diaries were analysed using the NDS Nutrient Database or McCance and Widdowson's (MW7) nutrient databank contained within the nutrient analysis software Dietplan 7 (Forestfield Software Ltd.). The nutritional content of the control and modified dairy products is presented in Kliem et al. (Kliem KE, Humphries DJ, Markey O, Vasilopoulou D, Fagan CC, Grandison AS, Todd S, Givens DI, Lovegrove JA: Food chain approach to lowering saturated fat in milk and dairy products: the RESET study, submitted). Energy and macronutrient content (Group 1 nutritional analysis) was performed in duplicate by SGS UK Ltd. (Ealing, London, UK; ISO 17025 accredited laboratory). Analysis of sodium, calcium, magnesium and phosphorus content was conducted in duplicate by inductively coupled plasma-optical emission spectrometry at Quaternary Scientific (QUEST, School of Archaeology, Geography and Environmental Science, University of Reading, Reading, UK). Extracted lipids from milk, cheese and butter samples were analysed in triplicate for FA composition using a GC-flame ionisation detection method [38]. A conversion factor of 0.933 was used to estimate the proportion of FAs in the total fat content of each dairy product [39]. Subsequently, the quantity of SFA, MUFA, TFA and PUFA were calculated per daily portion of each study dairy product (g/d). Nutrient composition of the study products was entered manually in Dietplan. For the purpose of analysis, the mean daily intakes of energy and macronutrients were recorded and the %TE was calculated to adjust for energy intake (EI). Dietary fibre intake was defined using the Association of Official Analytic Chemists (AOAC) method [40].

### Assessment of underestimation of energy intake

Determination of possible underestimation of dietary EI was assessed for each participant. Basal metabolic rate, based on age, gender and body weight, was estimated using the Henry equation [41]. A sedentary lifestyle was represented by a physical activity level score of 1.2 [31, 42]. The Goldberg lower 95% confidence limit was calculated as <1.132 using the CV recommended by Black

($n = 51$; 4 d) and was used to identify under-reporters of EI [42].

### Assessment of dietary compliance

As outlined in Table 2, participants were required to consume the minimum daily portions of each of the following study products: 340 g/d milk, 45 g/d cheese and 21.5 or 25.1 g/d of control or modified butter, respectively. This ensured that the intervention diets were iso-energetic and contained equal quantities of dairy fat (38%TE total fat; approx. 41 g/d). As a means of monitoring compliance with each study product type, participants were required to complete tick-sheet records on a daily basis throughout each 12-week dietary intervention period. Participants were given the option of marking the tick box if they had consumed the required portion size or could choose to record the actual weight of the product consumed. In order to calculate dietary compliance, one point was subtracted for each day that participants had not consumed a study product. These points were summed over each intervention period and were used to calculate percentage dietary compliance for each product type.

### Assessment of anthropometrics

Participants were requested to fast overnight for 12 h before each clinical visit, following consumption of a standardised low-fat evening meal (<1.46 MJ; < 7 g total fat) and low-nitrate water (Buxton Mineral Water, Nestlé Waters, Buxton, UK). At weeks 0, 12, 20 and 32, fasted measurements of BMI and waist circumference were recorded. Height was measured to the nearest 0.1 cm using a wall-mounted stadiometer (screening visit only). BMI was calculated using the Tanita BC-418 digital scale (Tanita Europe), under normal settings (standard body type and −1 kg for clothing) with participants wearing light clothing. Waist circumference was measured by a trained investigator, in triplicate, halfway between the iliac crest and the lowest rib margin to the nearest 0.5 cm [31].

### Assessment of plasma phospholipid fatty acid status

Fasting blood samples were collected into lithium heparin tubes for determination of PL-FA status prior to and after each 12-week intervention period (week 0, 12, 20, 32). Chilled samples were centrifuged at 3000 rpm (1700 g) for 15 min at 4 °C and plasma stored at −80 °C until subsequent extraction and analysis.

Sequential multipurpose sampler systems (Gerstel GmbH & Co. KG, Mülheim an der Ruhr, Germany) were employed for automated sample preparation and derivatization of FAs from the phospholipid fraction at the MRC Human Nutrition Research, Cambridge, as previously described [43]. The phospholipid fraction was isolated from plasma using solid phase extraction on $Na_2SO_4$ 50 mg/$NH_2$ 100 mg SPE cartridges (BE Gerstel; Agilent Technologies) and the FAME were produced from the phospholipid fraction according to the method published by Burge et al. [44]. The FAMEs were separated using a 30 m capillary column (HP-88; Agilent Technologies, Cheshire, UK) and detected using flame ionization. Results were expressed as molar percentage of total PL-FAs (mol%).

### Power calculation and statistical analyses

A total number of 54 participants were required for the chronic study to have sufficient power to detect a significant change in the primary and key secondary outcome measures. The primary outcome (serum total cholesterol, composed of LDL and HDL-cholesterol) was predicted to result in a ~0.3 mmol/L reduction with a population mean of 4.54 ± 0.5 mmol/L, with a power of 80% at $P < 0.05$, allowing for a 15% dropout rate. The chronic study was also powered to detect a 1.5% intergroup difference in the key secondary outcome measure, endothelial-dependent flow-mediated dilatation, with a power of 80% at $p < 0.05$ [45]. However, this paper is reporting on the food-exchange model and compliance to our high-fat, high-dairy interventions, which varied in FA composition.

Weighed dietary records, anthropometrics and PL-FA were analyzed using mixed models. Change-from-baseline for each variable of interest were modelled. Fixed effects included in the model were baseline values of the assessed variable, period, treatment, age, gender and BMI. All data were checked for normality and log transformed, if necessary. Participants were included as a fixed effect. There were no effects of the period in the model for any outcome measure.

Paired $t$-tests were used to assess differences in mean dietary compliance scores, as assessed by tick-sheet records, and underestimation of EI between the control and modified dietary interventions. For confirmation that our randomization approach was effective, differences in baseline characteristics between participants randomly assigned to the control and modified dietary intervention periods were assessed using independent $t$-tests and Chi-square tests for continuous and categorical variables, respectively. Statistical analyses were conducted using the SAS university edition statistical software (version 9.4; SAS Institute Inc., Cary, NC, USA). Results are presented as means and standard error of the mean (SEM). Differences were considered significant at $p \leq 0.01$ to account for multiplicity.

Orthogonal partial least squares discriminant analysis (PLS-DA) was applied to identify patterns between variables in our PL-FA dataset and summarised it by reducing the number of dimensions or components [46]. Measured PL-FA concentrations of 36 individual FAs

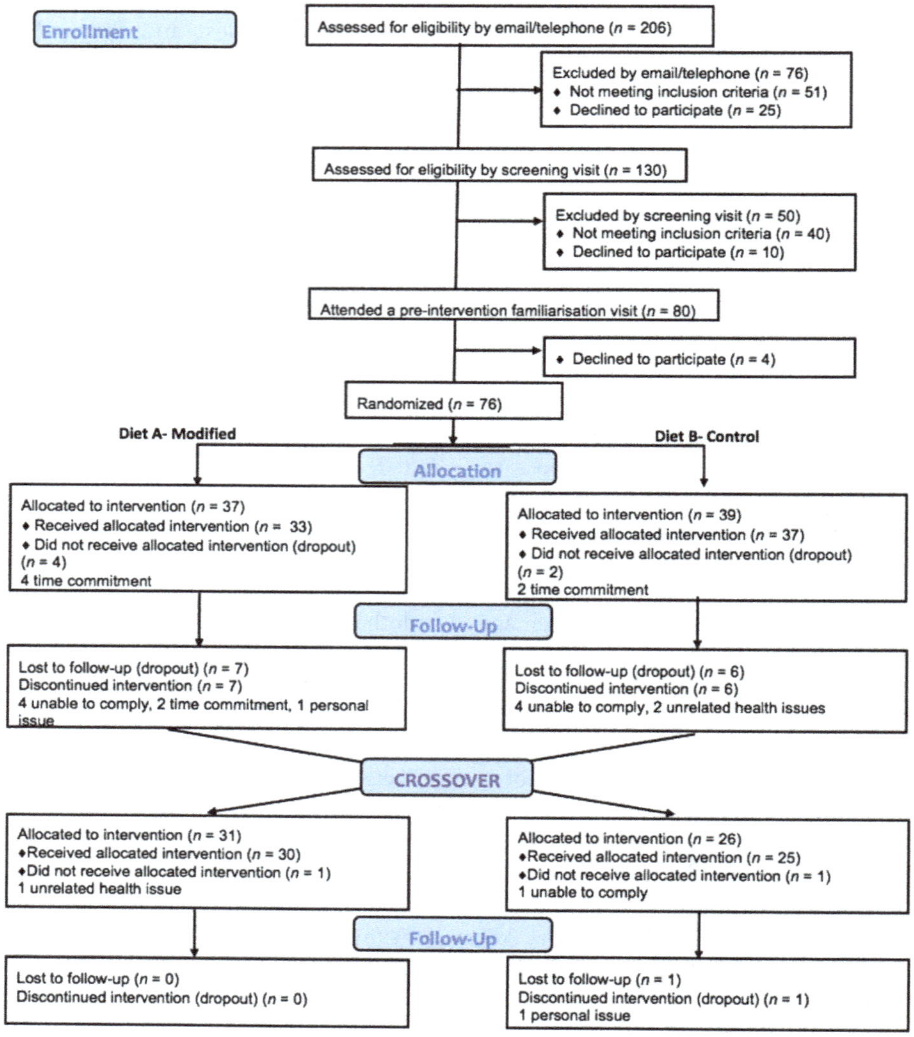


**Fig. 1** Flow of participants through the different stages of the RESET study

were subjected to orthogonal PLS-DA at: 1) baseline and 2) post-intervention using Metabolanalyst 3.0 [46]. The $R^2Y$ and $Q^2$ values represented the goodness of fit and predictability of the models, respectively. Significance of the models were tested using 1000 permutations.

## Results

Participant flow through the study is illustrated in Fig. 1. Of the 74 participants who were randomly assigned and commenced the study, 54 (31 males and 23 females) completed the study. Participants continued to take their regular prescribed medication for the duration of the study ($n = 2$ levothyroxine for hypothyroidism; $n = 1$ proton pump inhibitor for heartburn; $n = 1$ hormone replacement therapy for menopausal symptom relief; $n = 1$ tricyclic antidepressant for depression; $n = 2$ fluticasone and salmeterol for mild asthma; $n = 1$ etonogestrel contraceptive implant and $n = 1$ levonorgestrel-releasing intrauterine contraceptive device). The breakdown of the ethnicity of the study group was as follows: White, 89% ($n = 48$); Asian, 4% ($n = 2$); Black, 4% ($n = 2$) and Chinese/Far Eastern, 4% ($n = 2$). There were no significant differences between participants randomly assigned to Groups 1 and 2 at baseline (Additional file 1: Table S1). Two participants were excluded from the dietary analysis due to insufficient data.

### Dietary analysis

Recorded dietary intake at baseline and following diets that incorporated the control and modified dairy products (post-intervention) are shown in Table 3. In agreement with target intakes (Table 2), significant treatment

**Table 3** Recorded dietary intake at baseline (week 0) and following diets that incorporated the control and modified dairy products (week 12) in adults at moderate cardiovascular disease risk and target fatty acid intakes[a]

| | Control | | | | Modified | | | | |
|---|---|---|---|---|---|---|---|---|---|
| | Baseline | Post | T[b] | Δ | Baseline | Post | T | Δ | p[c] |
| Energy, MJ/d | 8.5 ± 0.4 | 9.0 ± 0.3 | | 0.5 ± 0.3 | 8.2 ± 0.3 | 9.2 ± 0.4 | | 1.0 ± 0.4 | 0.60 |
| Total fat, %TE | 36.5 ± 0.8 | 39.5 ± 0.7 | 38.0 | 3.0 ± 0.9 | 36.1 ± 0.8 | 41.1 ± 0.8 | 38.0 | 5.0 ± 1.1 | 0.03 |
| SFA, %TE | 13.9 ± 0.5 | 19.1 ± 0.4 | 19.0 | 5.2 ± 0.6 | 14.2 ± 0.5 | 16.9 ± 0.4 | 16.0 | 2.7 ± 0.6 | <0.001 |
| MUFA, %TE | 11.9 ± 0.4 | 11.8 ± 0.3 | 11.0 | −0.1 ± 0.3 | 11.7 ± 0.4 | 15.3 ± 0.4 | 14.0 | 3.6 ± 0.5 | <0.0001 |
| n-6 PUFA, %TE | 4.6 ± 0.2 | 3.3 ± 0.2 | | −1.3 ± 0.2 | 3.9 ± 0.2 | 3.4 ± 0.2 | | −0.5 ± 0.2 | 0.08 |
| n-3 PUFA, %TE | 0.8 ± 0.1 | 0.6 ± 0.0 | | −0.2 ± 0.1 | 0.7 ± 0.0 | 0.6 ± 0.0 | | −0.1 ± 0.1 | 0.34 |
| Total PUFA, %TE | 5.8 ± 0.4 | 4.4 ± 0.5 | | −1.4 ± 0.3 | 4.6 ± 0.2 | 4.0 ± 0.2 | | −0.4 ± 0.2 | 0.14 |
| TFA, %TE | 1.0 ± 0.1 | 1.3 ± 0.1 | | 0.3 ± 0.1 | 0.9 ± 0.1 | 2.5 ± 0.1 | | 1.6 ± 0.1 | <0.0001 |
| Protein, %TE | 16.3 ± 0.5 | 16.1 ± 0.4 | | −0.2 ± 0.5 | 16.9 ± 0.5 | 16.2 ± 0.3 | | −0.7 ± 0.6 | 0.80 |
| Carbohydrates, %TE | 46.3 ± 0.9 | 43.3 ± 0.9 | | −3.0 ± 0.9 | 46.6 ± 1.3 | 42.2 ± 1.0 | | −4.4 ± 1.5 | 0.19 |
| Alcohol, %TE | 3.1 ± 0.5 | 3.1 ± 0.5 | | 0.0 ± 0.4 | 2.9 ± 0.5 | 2.7 ± 0.4 | | −0.2 ± 0.5 | 0.35 |
| Dietary fiber (AOAC), g/d | 20.4 ± 1.1 | 22.0 ± 1.1 | | 1.6 ± 0.9 | 20.2 ± 1.1 | 19.4 ± 1.1 | | −0.8 ± 1.2 | 0.03 |
| Sodium, g/d | 2.7 ± 0.2 | 2.2 ± 0.1 | | −0.5 ± 0.1 | 2.5 ± 0.2 | 1.9 ± 0.1 | | −0.6 ± 0.1 | 0.03 |

Participant was included as a random effect. $p \leq 0.01$ deemed as significant

*AOAC* Association of Official Analytic Chemists, *%TE* percentage of total energy

[a]Values are means ± SEM. Dietary intakes estimated from 4-d weighed dietary records at baseline (week 0) and after intervention (week 12)

[b]Target FA intakes for the control and modified dietary exchange periods

[c]Overall effect of treatment based on change-from-baseline was calculated by mixed model analysis, with adjustments made for fixed effects of baseline values of the assessed variable, period, treatment, age, gender and BMI

effects were evident for dietary intakes of SFA and MUFA. Following introduction of the modified diet, there was a smaller increase in SFA and greater increase in MUFA and TFA, relative to baseline, when compared with the control.

#### Underestimation of energy intake

Based on the assumption that participants were in energy balance, it was estimated that recorded EI were underestimated for 35 and 22% of participants at baseline and post-intervention, respectively. Underestimation of EI was not considered further in the mixed model analysis.

#### Dietary compliance

On the basis of tick-sheet records, mean daily intake (± SEM) of the dairy products across each 12-week dietary exchange was as follows: milk (control: 343.5 ± 1.8; modified: 347.8 ± 2.8 g/d), cheese (control: 46.5 ± 0.6; modified: 45.9 ± 0.4 g/d) and butter (control: 22.0 ± 0.2; modified: 25.6 ± 0.3 g/d). Mean daily dietary compliance did not vary according to treatment: milk (control: 96.6 ± 0.01; modified: 96.5 ± 0.01%; $p = 0.92$), cheese (control: 96.6 ± 0.01; modified: 96.8 ± 0.01%; $P = 0.83$) and butter (control: 96.5 ± 0.01; modified: 97.0 ± 0.01%; $p = 0.70$).

#### Anthropometric measures

Relative to baseline, there was no significant treatment effect for BMI (control: 25.8 ± 0.5 vs. 26.2 ± 0.5 kg/m$^2$ for baseline vs. post-intervention; modified: 25.8 ± 0.5 vs. 25.9 ± 0.5 kg/m$^2$; $p = 0.13$) or waist circumference (control: 88.9 ± 1.4 vs. 89.8 ± 1.5 cm; modified: 89.3 ± 1.5 vs. 89.1 ± 1.5 cm; $p = 0.53$).

#### Plasma phospholipid FA status

After the 12-week intervention, there were significant differences in PL-FA composition between the modified and control groups ($p \leq 0.01$). Consumption of the modified dairy products led to a small but significant decrease in abundance of total SFAs from baseline (change: −0.60 ± 0.21 mol%) vs. control (change: 0.01 ± 0.17 mol%) (Table 4). Following the modified diet, there were significant increases in *cis*-MUFAs and *trans*-MUFAs from baseline vs. control (Table 4). There was a minor increase in the abundance of 16:0 from baseline following the control diet (change: 0.16 ± 0.13 mol%), while a decrease from baseline was evident following the modified diet (change: −0.46 ± 0.15 mol%) (Fig. 2b). Compared with baseline, 18 : 1*cis*-9 and 18 : 1*trans*-9 increased following the modified diet vs. control (Fig. 2b). Following the control diet, there was a significant increase in 20 : 3*n*-6 vs. the modified diet.

#### Orthogonal Partial Least Square Discriminant analysis of plasma phospholipid FA data

For the baseline PLS-DA, the first component representing the maximum differentiation between the two diets represented 4.7% of variation and was retained to

**Table 4** Plasma phospholipid fatty acids at baseline (week 0) and following diets that incorporated the control and modified dairy products (week 12) in adults at moderate cardiovascular disease risk[a]

| | Control | | | Modified | | | |
|---|---|---|---|---|---|---|---|
| mol% | Baseline | Post | Δ | Baseline | Post | Δ | $p$[b] |
| SFAs | | | | | | | |
| 11:0 | 0.0000 ± 0.0008 | 0.0013 ± 0.0008 | 0.0000 ± 0.0011 | 0.0000 ± 0.0011 | 0.0002 ± 0.0000 | 0.0025 ± 0.0010 | 0.35 |
| 12:0 | 0.0230 ± 0.0018 | 0.0242 ± 0.0015 | 0.0012 ± 0.0019 | 0.0245 ± 0.0000 | 0.0225 ± 0.0000 | 0.0019 ± 0.0016 | 0.22 |
| 13:0 | 0.00 ± 0.00 | 0.00 ± 0.00 | 0.00 ± 0.00 | 0.00 ± 0.00 | 0.00 ± 0.00 | 0.00 ± 0.00 | 0.16 |
| 14:0 | 0.35 ± 0.01 | 0.42 ± 0.02 | 0.07 ± 0.02 | 0.35 ± 0.02 | 0.38 ± 0.02 | 0.03 ± 0.01 | 0.04 |
| 15:0 | 0.23 ± 0.01 | 0.26 ± 0.01 | 0.04 ± 0.01 | 0.22 ± 0.01 | 0.24 ± 0.01 | 0.02 ± 0.01 | 0.02 |
| 16:0 | 30.70 ± 0.16 | 30.86 ± 0.17 | 0.16 ± 0.13 | 30.78 ± 0.13 | 30.32 ± 0.13 | −0.46 ± 0.15 | <0.001 |
| 17:0 | 0.39 ± 0.01 | 0.40 ± 0.01 | 0.01 ± 0.01 | 0.38 ± 0.01 | 0.38 ± 0.01 | 0.00 ± 0.01 | 0.03 |
| 18:0 | 13.95 ± 0.18 | 13.67 ± 0.14 | −0.29 ± 0.12 | 14.05 ± 0.12 | 13.83 ± 0.12 | −0.22 ± 0.13 | 0.33 |
| 20:0 | 0.14 ± 0.00 | 0.13 ± 0.00 | −0.01 ± 0.00 | 0.13 ± 0.00 | 0.12 ± 0.00 | −0.01 ± 0.00 | 0.76 |
| 21:0 | 0.0128 ± 0.0037 | 0.0130 ± 0.0043 | 0.0001 ± 0.0036 | 0.0093 ± 0.0000 | 0.0147 ± 0.0000 | 0.0054 ± 0.0034 | 0.62 |
| 22:0 | 0.23 ± 0.01 | 0.22 ± 0.01 | −0.01 ± 0.01 | 0.22 ± 0.01 | 0.22 ± 0.01 | 0.00 ± 0.01 | 0.69 |
| 23:0 | 0.10 ± 0.00 | 0.11 ± 0.00 | 0.01 ± 0.00 | 0.10 ± 0.00 | 0.11 ± 0.00 | 0.01 ± 0.00 | 0.34 |
| 24:0 | 0.25 ± 0.01 | 0.25 ± 0.01 | 0.00 ± 0.01 | 0.25 ± 0.01 | 0.24 ± 0.01 | −0.01 ± 0.01 | 0.85 |
| Total SFA[c] | 46.37 ± 0.17 | 46.36 ± 0.13 | 0.01 ± 0.17 | 46.52 ± 0.21 | 45.92 ± 0.15 | −0.60 ± 0.21 | 0.006 |
| MUFAs | | | | | | | |
| 18:1 *cis*-9 | 9.81 ± 0.15 | 9.98 ± 0.16 | 0.17 ± 0.15 | 9.99 ± 0.15 | 10.93 ± 0.15 | 0.93 ± 0.19 | <0.0001 |
| 18:1 *trans*-9 | 0.08 ± 0.00 | 0.08 ± 0.00 | 0.01 ± 0.00 | 0.07 ± 0.00 | 0.17 ± 0.00 | 0.10 ± 0.01 | <0.0001 |
| 22:1 *cis*-9 | 0.0202 ± 0.0037 | 0.0206 ± 0.0030 | 0.0004 ± 0.0045 | 0.0182 ± 0.0000 | 0.0201 ± 0.0000 | 0.0000 ± 0.0019 | 0.52 |
| Total *cis*-MUFA[d] | 11.02 ± 0.16 | 11.24 ± 0.17 | 0.21 ± 0.15 | 11.21 ± 0.18 | 12.20 ± 0.23 | 0.99 ± 0.20 | <0.0001 |
| Total *trans*-MUFA[e] | 0.12 ± 0.00 | 0.12 ± 0.00 | 0.01 ± 0.00 | 0.10 ± 0.00 | 0.23 ± 0.01 | 0.12 ± 0.01 | <0.0001 |
| PUFAs | | | | | | | |
| 18:2 n-6 | 22.26 ± 0.42 | 22.40 ± 0.37 | 0.14 ± 0.28 | 22.00 ± 0.28 | 22.29 ± 0.28 | 0.30 ± 0.29 | 0.87 |
| 18:3 n-6 | 0.08 ± 0.01 | 0.10 ± 0.01 | 0.02 ± 0.01 | 0.09 ± 0.01 | 0.09 ± 0.01 | 0.00 ± 0.01 | 0.51 |
| 18:3 n-3 | 0.31 ± 0.02 | 0.31 ± 0.01 | 0.00 ± 0.01 | 0.31 ± 0.01 | 0.29 ± 0.01 | −0.02 ± 0.01 | 0.58 |
| 20:3 n-6 | 3.07 ± 0.08 | 3.39 ± 0.11 | 0.32 ± 0.07 | 3.12 ± 0.07 | 3.17 ± 0.07 | 0.06 ± 0.06 | 0.007 |
| 20:4 n-6 | 9.88 ± 0.27 | 9.53 ± 0.22 | −0.35 ± 0.13 | 9.77 ± 0.13 | 9.41 ± 0.13 | −0.36 ± 0.21 | 0.74 |
| 20:5 n-3 | 1.27 ± 0.08 | 1.25 ± 0.06 | −0.02 ± 0.07 | 1.24 ± 0.07 | 1.14 ± 0.07 | −0.10 ± 0.07 | 0.14 |
| 22:5 n-6 | 0.20 ± 0.01 | 0.20 ± 0.01 | 0.00 ± 0.01 | 0.20 ± 0.01 | 0.20 ± 0.01 | 0.00 ± 0.01 | 0.17 |
| 22:5 n-3 | 0.99 ± 0.03 | 1.02 ± 0.02 | 0.03 ± 0.02 | 1.00 ± 0.02 | 0.95 ± 0.02 | −0.05 ± 0.03 | 0.55 |
| 22:6 n-3 | 3.77 ± 0.16 | 3.39 ± 0.13 | −0.37 ± 0.09 | 3.79 ± 0.09 | 3.44 ± 0.09 | −0.35 ± 0.10 | 0.74 |
| Total n-3 PUFA[f] | 5.35 ± 0.23 | 4.96 ± 0.17 | −0.39 ± 0.14 | 5.34 ± 0.21 | 4.87 ± 0.17 | −0.47 ± 0.14 | 0.58 |
| Total n-6 PUFA[g] | 36.15 ± 0.34 | 36.30 ± 0.27 | 0.15 ± 0.26 | 35.83 ± 0.32 | 35.86 ± 0.33 | 0.03 ± 0.33 | 0.32 |

Where no bond position is listed it is unknown [40]. 20 : 4*n*-6 + 20 : 3*n*-3 co-eluted, but as 20 : 3*n*-3 concentration in human samples is negligible, this peak was identified as 20 : 4*n*-6 [43]

[a]Values are given as means ± SEM

[b]Overall effect of treatment based on change-from-baseline was calculated by mixed model analysis, with adjustments made for fixed effects of baseline values of the assessed variable, period, treatment, age, gender and BMI. Participant was included as a random effect

[c]Total SFAs include: 11 : 0, 12 : 0, 13 : 0, 14 : 0, 15 : 0, 16 : 0, 17 : 0, 18 : 0, 20 : 0, 21 : 0, 22 : 0, 23 : 0 and 24 : 0

[d]Total *cis*-MUFAs include: 14 : 1*cis*, 15 : 1*cis*, 16 : 1*cis*, 17 : 1*cis*, 18 : 1*cis*-9, 20 : 1*cis*, 22 : 1*cis*-9 and 24 : 1*cis*. Where no bond position is listed it is unknown, as previously outlined in Wang et al. [43]

[e]Total *trans*-MUFAs include: 16 : 1*trans* (bond position unknown) and 18 : 1*trans*-9 [43]

[f]Total *n*-3 PUFAs include: 18 : 3*n*-3, 20 : 5*n*-3, 22 : 5*n*-3 and 22 : 6*n*-3

[g]Total *n*-6 PUFAs include: 18 : 2*n*-6, 18 : 2*trans*, 18 : 3*n*-6, 20 : 2, 20 : 3*n*-6, 20 : 4*n*-6 + 20:3*n*-3, 22 : 4 and 22 : 5*n*-6

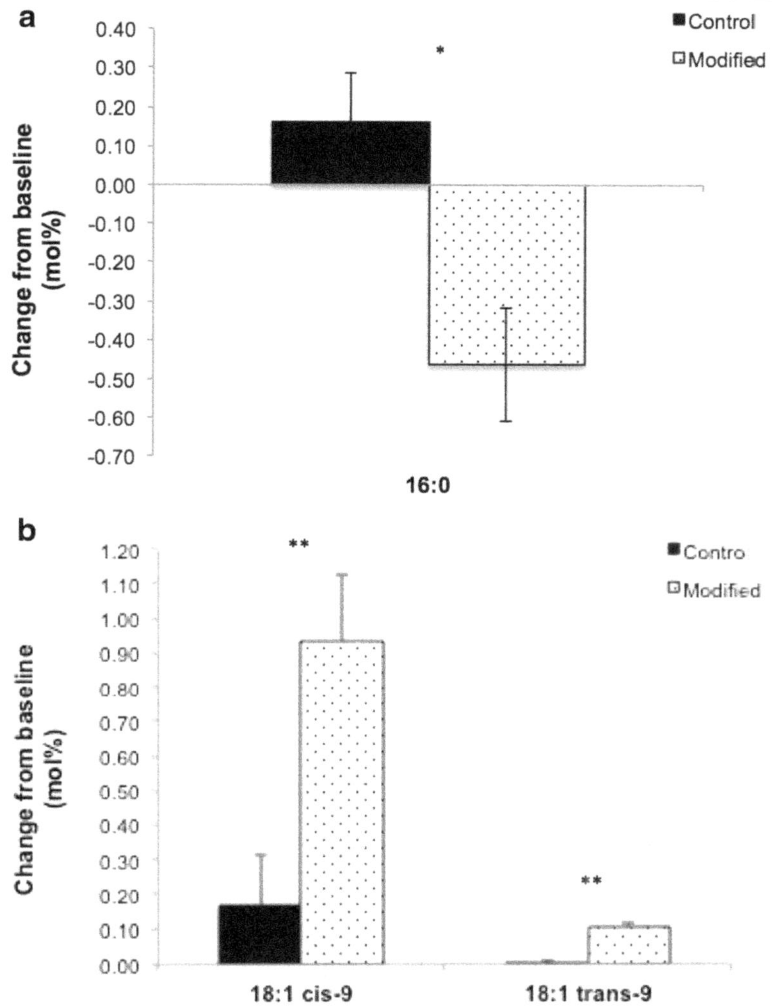


**Fig. 2** Change-from-baseline in the plasma phospholipid profile of SFA: 16 : 0 (**a**) and MUFAs: 18 : 1*cis*-9 and 18 : 1*trans*-9 (**b**) following 12-week diets that incorporated control and modified dairy products. Values are means ± SEM, $n = 54$. Significance shown as * $p < 0.001$, ** $p < 0.0001$

interpret the FA profiles of the clusters on the score plots. PLS-DA of the PL-FA data revealed a lack of distinction between the control and modified intervention groups at baseline ($R^2Y = 0.142$ and $Q^2 = -0.35$, empirical *P*-values $R^2Y$: $p = 0.99$ (986/1000) and $Q^2$: $P = 0.76$ (763/1000), suggesting that the population was indistinguishable with regard to PL-FA profiles prior to commencement of the dietary exchange periods (Fig. 3a). Additional file 2: Table S2 illustrates the loadings.

Following the intervention, the first component representing the maximum differentiation between the two diets represented 5.4% of the variability in the data. The loadings are illustrated in Additional file 2: Table S2. In contrast to baseline, the post-intervention score plot identified a clear separation ($R^2Y = 0.612$ and $Q^2 = 0.451$, empirical *p*-values $R^2Y$: $p < 0.001$ (0/1000) and $Q^2$: $p < 0.001$ (0/1000) in PL-FA profiles of participants when they were assigned to the modified and control intervention diets (Fig. 3b). The FAs that mainly contributed to this dietary status separation were: 18 : 1*trans-9*, 16 : 1*trans*, 18 : 1*cis*-9, that were higher following the modified diet, while 16 : 0, 14 : 1 *cis*, 14 : 0, 15 : 0 and 20 : 3*n*-6 were higher following the control diet.

## Discussion

The food-exchange model was used for the implementation of two iso-energetic high-fat, high-dairy diets varying in FA composition in the RESET study, through the use of SFA-reduced, MUFA-enriched dairy products and control alternatives with a FA profile typical of retail dairy products. Specific dietary targets following treatments were largely achieved in a free-living population at moderate risk of CVD. Analysis of weighed dietary records confirmed that it was possible to lower the mean SFA intake by 2.5%TE and increase MUFA intake by 3.7%TE following the diet containing modified dairy

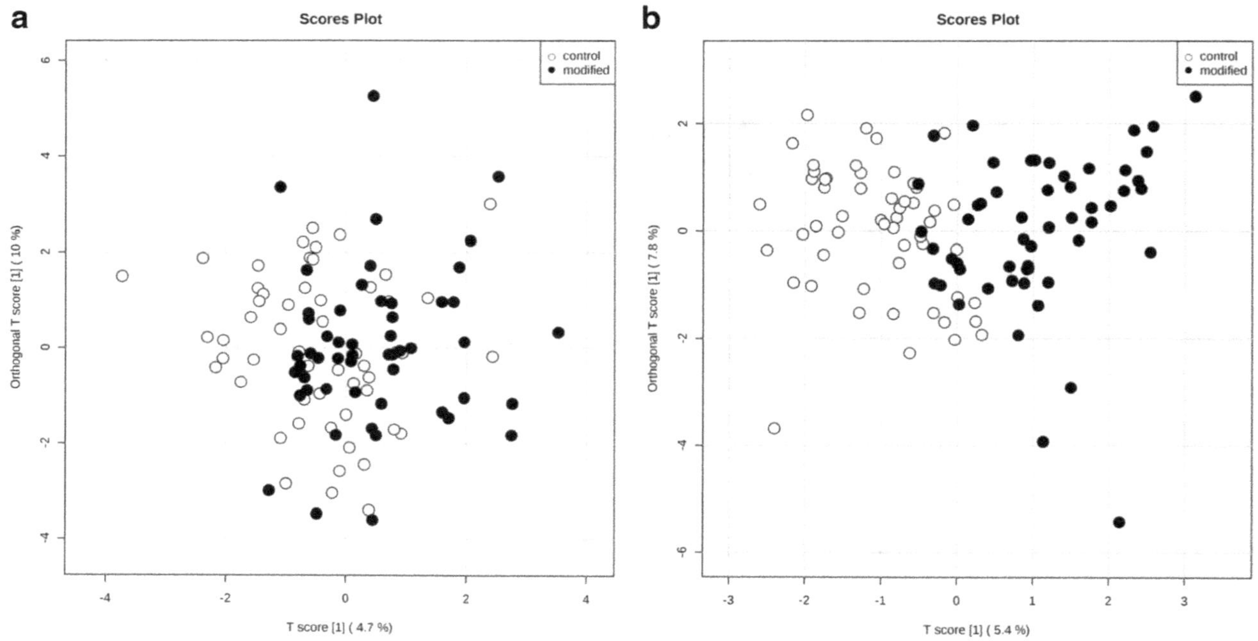


**Fig. 3** Orthogonal PLS-DA, score plots at baseline (**a**) and post-intervention (**b**) calculated using plasma phospholipid FA concentrations in adults at moderate risk of cardiovascular disease ($n = 54$). FA, fatty acid; PLS-DA, partial least squares discriminant analysis

products compared with the control products. Previously, Noakes et al. reported differences of 2.2%TE SFA and 2.8%TE MUFA (described as oleic acid intake only) following consumption of dairy products that were produced following a protein-encapsulated lipid (rapeseed and soybean oil) bovine supplementation period, when compared to control dairy foods [47]. There was a significant difference in recorded SFA intake between interventions in our study, however the reduction in SFA intake following the modified diet was slightly less than predicted by our food-exchange model. Compliance was further confirmed by assessment of dietary tick-sheet records.

To our knowledge, this is the first human study to assess the impact of modified milk, cheese and butter consumption on PL-FA concentrations, in comparison to control dairy products with a FA profile typical of retail products. In line with previous findings [31, 48–50], objective dietary compliance was confirmed by assessment of PL-FA profiles, with consumption of the control and modified dairy products leading to differential effects on total plasma phospholipid SFAs and MUFAs and their sub-classes. The consumption of the SFA-reduced, MUFA-enriched dairy products led to a small decrease in the abundance of total SFAs, and increases in total *cis*-MUFAs, including 18 : 1*cis*-9 in the PL-FA profile, when compared to the control products. These changes are comparable to the proportion of PL-FA total SFAs and MUFAs observed in the DIVAS study following a 16-week MUFA-rich diet (9%TE SFA; 19%TE MUFA; 4%TE *n*-6 PUFA) [31]. Previous literature has suggested that SFAs and MUFAs with even numbered carbon chain length can be endogenously synthesised by humans and may be less affected by dietary intake [51]. Hodson et al. suggested that this may be because it is difficult to alter the proportion of FAs that are already relatively abundant in the diet and that increases in SFA intake are not reflected in increases in the plasma FA profiles [30]. However, changes in PL-FA concentrations observed in the RESET study mirrored the FA composition of our intervention dairy foods [52]. PLS-DA provided a means for visualizing adherence to a dietary intervention. Despite using a relatively homogenous population and a modest dietary exchange, our PLS-DA plot highlighted some distinction between the PL-FA profile of the participants following the modified and control dietary exchange periods, suggesting a small but significant response to our intervention. This analysis only explained approximately 5% of the overall variability in our dataset but the affected FAs, including 18 : 1*trans*-9 and 18 : 1*cis*-9 and 16 : 0, were relevant to our interevntions. Furthermore, it provided further evidence that PL-FA were illustrative of short to medium-term FA intake [29–31].

Supplementation of the dairy cow diet with unsaturated FA leads to increased levels of ruminant *trans*-fatty acids (rTFA) in the milk and dairy products, through ruminal biohydrogenation of unsaturated FA [15, 25, 27]. There was a calculated dietary increase of 1.3%TE in total TFA intake following the modified, when compared with the control diet. It was not possible to quantify our participants' voluntary intake of specific TFA isomers (i.e. ruminant or industrial TFA intake) from weighed dietary records using our nutrient analysis software. However, based on the differences in TFA composition between our control and modified dairy products [52], it is apparent that the majority of the increased TFA intake recorded following the modified diet was derived from ruminant sources. In contrast to the recognised detrimental impact of industrially-produced TFA on cardiovascular health, consumption of rTFA may not be adversely linked to CVD risk [53], except possibly at high intakes [54, 55]. It should be noted that the calculated dietary TFA intake following our modified intervention ($2.5 \pm 0.1$%TE) exceeded the recommended population maximum of 2% food energy [3] which does not discriminate between ruminant and industrial sources, and is higher than the current mean TFA intake in UK adults (0.5%TE and 0.5% food energy) [4]. This may be in part explained by the high dairy fat content of our intervention diets. In support of this we also observed that consumption of the SFA-reduced, MUFA-enriched dairy products lead to significant increases in total *trans*-MUFA and 18:1 *trans-9* concentrations in the PL-FA. Whilst our PL-FA analysis approach was unable to identify specific *trans* isomers other than 18:1 *trans-9* [43], the detailed FA analysis of the dairy foods used in the RESET study (Kliem KE, Humphries DJ, Markey O, Vasilopoulou D, Fagan CC, Grandison AS, Todd S, Givens DI, Lovegrove JA: Food chain approach to lowering saturated fat in milk and dairy products: the RESET study, submitted) suggest there was likely to be a complex mixture of TFA in the phospholipid pool. It may be that feeding strategies that limit increases of TFA in milk fat following bovine supplementation with plant oils, such as the use of encapsulation protection technology may be advantageous [27, 56]. However, further work is justified to determine whether rTFA are detrimental to cardiovascular health [27].

Our intervention presented some challenges. Our bovine supplementation strategy was successful in altering the FA profile of the milk [52]. Alongside this, we observed a depression in milk fat content following supplementation of the bovine diet with high-oleic sunflower oil which has been reported previously [57]. As a result of this, it was necessary to standardise the fat content of the raw control milk prior to UHT so that it was equivalent to that of the modified milk. Furthermore, our modified cheese had a lower fat content compared with conventional cheese and it was necessary for our participants to consume an additional 3.6 g/d of butter during the modified dietary exchange period to standardize the fat intake of the two intervention periods.

A challenge faced by some participants was incorporating sufficient quantities of products, especially cheese, into their habitual diets on a daily basis. In line with recent NDNS data [4], some of our participants were not accustomed to consuming the quantities of dairy products that were prescribed in our food-exchange model (unpublished data obtained by food frequency questionnaire). Although it was not logistically feasible for us to include a wider range of dairy products in the RESET study, it is possible that a greater variety of items may have reduced the likelihood of 'product boredom' and minimized the potential for compliance issues [58]. Compliance with the dietary exchange was cited as the main reason for dropout by nine of our participants, predominantly in the early stages of the intervention. It should be noted that a similar number of participants withdrew from the modified and control dietary exchange periods, suggesting that the two regimens were equal in terms of acceptability. For those who completed the study, our tick-sheet records suggested that compliance to the dietary regimens was excellent and our PL-FA data provided further objective evidence of dietary adherence. It is acknowledged that there may have been discrepancies in tick-sheet recordings as a result of 'desirability bias', i.e. participants may have recorded the portions that they were required to eat as opposed to what they had actually consumed [58], and this may have led to more modest differences in PL-FA profiles between the two dietary exchange periods.

We observed a moderately high amount of under-reporting assessed by EI at baseline, however, this was similar to that observed in previous free-living populations [31, 59]. A high proportion of participants (61%; $n = 33$) in the RESET study were classified as overweight (BMI of $\geq 25.0$ kg/m$^2$). It is recognized that overweight or obese individuals may be more prone to selective bias and omission of foods with a negative health image, leading to potential under-reporting of dietary intake [60]. We observed a lower degree of under-reporting following the intervention, when our replacement model predicted that the dairy products would contribute to over 25% of daily EI. It could be speculated that participants had a greater appreciation of the importance of giving an accurate account of their dietary intake whilst on the intervention. The present study has illustrated that through the incorporation of dairy products with an altered FA profile into the habitual diet, it was possible for free-living participants to successfully improve their dietary fat quality. This was in agreement with previous successful food-exchange models [31, 35, 58]. Our dietary interventions were designed to contain a high quantity of dairy fat (~41 g/d). Both intervention periods increased relative intake of total fat and SFA over baseline. However, it is feasible that a similar, but more moderate, approach could be used for assisting in the reduction of dairy SFA intake at a population level, without reducing dairy consumption. Furthermore, we have previously reported that consumers generally accepted the SFA-reduced, MUFA-enriched dairy products, when tasted in a blinded manner (Markey O, Souroullas K, Fagan CC, Kliem KE, Vasilopoulou D, Jackson KG, Humphries DJ, Grandison AS, Givens DI, Lovegrove JA, Methven L: Consumer acceptance of dairy products with a saturated fatty acid-reduced, monounsaturated fatty acid-enriched content, In Review).

## Conclusions

We sucessfully implemented a high-fat, high-dairy food-exchange model that was suitable for replacing dairy products with a FA profile typical of retail products with SFA-reduced, MUFA-enriched alternatives over a 12-week period in a free-living population at moderate risk of CVD. Changes in the dietary intake of SFA and MUFA between our interventions was confirmed by changes in the concentrations of these FAs in the plasma phospholipid fraction, indicative of adherence to our dietary intervention.

### Abbreviations

AOAC: Association of Official Analytic Chemists; %TE: Percentage of total energy; Ca: Calcium; CVD: Cardiovascular disease; DIVAS: Dietary Intervention and Vascular Function; FA: Fatty acid; Mg: Magnesium; Na: Sodium; NDNS: National Diet and Nutrition Survey; P: Phosphorus; PC: Principal component; PL-FA: Plasma phospholipid FA; PLS-DA: Partial least squares discriminant analysis; RCT: Randomized controlled trial; RISCK: Reading, Imperial, Surrey, Cambridge, and Kings; rTFA: Ruminant *trans*-fatty acids; TFA: *Trans*-fatty acid; UHT: Ultra high temperature

### Acknowledgements

The authors gratefully acknowledge all volunteers who took part in the study. We thank S. Hargreaves, K. Jenkins, R. Mihaylova and the research students/assistants (C. Brilley, L. Bula, Y. Chatzidiakou, V. Clifton, H. Dong, A. Garcimartin, C. Holland, J. Guo, A. Kanneganti, T. Loughman, E. Mertens, J. Ryan, L. Sellem, T. Staff and H. Zhang) for their assistance.

### Funding

This work was supported by funding from the Medical Research Council (United Kingdom; Ref: MR/K020218/1). Arla Foods UK and AAK UK supplied in kind the commercially available dairy products and oils according to our specification. Arla Foods UK and AAK UK had no role in the design, analysis or writing of this article.

### Authors' contributions

The authors' contributions are as follows: JAL, DIG and KGJ: designed the human study; OM, JAL and KGJ: designed the food-exchange model; CCF, ASG, DJH and DIG: designed and produced the modified dairy products; OM and DV: conducted the research (hands-on conduct of the experiment and data collection); OM, DV, KEK and AK: analyzed data and performed statistical analysis; KEK, KS and LW: performed fatty acid analysis; ST: provided statistical advice; OM and DV: wrote the manuscript, which was modified by all co-authors; and JAL had primary responsibility for final content. All authors have read and approved the final manuscript.

### Competing interests

JAL is an expert on the UK Scientific Advisory Committee for Nutrition (SACN) Saturated Fats Working Group. There are no other competing interests.

### Consent for publication

Not applicable.

### Author details

[1]Hugh Sinclair Unit of Human Nutrition and Institute for Cardiovascular and Metabolic Research, University of Reading, Reading RG6 6AP, UK. [2]Department of Food and Nutritional Sciences, University of Reading, Reading RG6 6AP, UK. [3]Animal, Dairy and Food Chain Sciences, University of Reading, Reading RG6 6AP, UK. [4]MRC Elsie Widdowson Laboratory, 120 Fulbourn Road, Cambridge CB1 9NL, UK. [5]NIHR BRC Nutritional Biomarker Laboratory, University of Cambridge, Cambridge CB2 0QQ, UK. [6]Department of Mathematics and Statistics, School of Mathematical, Physical and Computational Sciences, University of Reading, Reading RG6 6AX, UK. [7]Institute for Food, Nutrition and Health, University of Reading, Reading RG6 6AR, UK. [8]Present address: School of Sport, Exercise and Health Sciences, Loughborough University, Loughborough LE11 3TU, UK.

### References

1. Townsend N, Bhatnagar P, Wilkins E, Wickramasinghe K. M R: Cardiovascular disease statistics. London: British Heart Foundation; 2015.
2. Mensink RP, Zock PL, Kester AD, Katan MB. Effects of dietary fatty acids and carbohydrates on the ratio of serum total to HDL cholesterol and on serum lipids and apolipoproteins: a meta-analysis of 60 controlled trials. Am J Clin Nutr. 2003;77:1146–55.
3. COMA: Department of Health—Committee on Medical Aspects of Food Policy. Dietary reference values for food energy and nutrients in the United Kingdom: report on the Panel of Dietary Reference Values of the Committee on Medical Aspects of Food Policy (Report of Health and Social Subjects, No. 41). London: The Stationary Office; 1991.
4. Bates B, Cox L, Nicholson S, Page P, Prentice A, Steer T, G S. National Diet and Nutrition Survey. Results from Years 5–6 (combined) of the Rolling Programme (2012/13 – 2013/14). [cited 21 Sept 2016]. Available from: https://www.gov.uk/government/statistics/ndns-results-from-years-5-and-6-combined. 2016.
5. USDA. Scientific Report of the 2015 Dietary Guidelines Advisory Committee. Washington: USDA and US Department of Health and Human Services; 2015.
6. Buttriss JL. The Eatwell guide refreshed. Nutr Bull. 2016;41:135–41.
7. Elwood PC, Pickering JE, Givens DI, Gallacher JE. The consumption of milk and dairy foods and the incidence of vascular disease and diabetes: an overview of the evidence. Lipids. 2010;45:925–39.
8. Soedamah-Muthu SS, Ding EL, Al-Delaimy WK, Hu FB, Engberink MF, Willett WC, Geleijnse JM. Milk and dairy consumption and incidence of cardiovascular diseases and all-cause mortality: dose–response meta-analysis of prospective cohort studies. Am J Clin Nutr. 2011;93:158–71.
9. Lamarche B, Givens DI, Soedamah-Muthu S, Krauss RM, Jakobsen MU, Bischoff-Ferrari HA, Pan A, Després J-P. Does milk consumption contribute to cardiometabolic health and overall diet quality? Can J Cardiol. 2016;32: 1026–32.
10. de Goede J, Soedamah-Muthu SS, Pan A, Gijsbers L, Geleijnse JM. Dairy consumption and risk of stroke: a systematic review and updated dose–response meta-analysis of prospective cohort studies. J Am Heart Assoc. 2016;5:e002787.
11. Huth PJ, Park KM. Influence of dairy product and milk fat consumption on cardiovascular disease risk: a review of the evidence. Adv Nutr. 2012;3:266–85.
12. Astrup A, Rice Bradley B, Brenna J, Delplanque B, Ferry M, Torres-Gonzalez M. Regular-fat dairy and human health: a synopsis of symposia presented in Europe and North America (2014–2015). Nutrients. 2016;8:463.
13. O'Donnell A, Spatny K, Vicini J, Bauman D. Survey of the fatty acid composition of retail milk differing in label claims based on production management practices. J Dairy Sci. 2010;93:1918–25.
14. Fekete ÁA, Givens DI, Lovegrove JA. The impact of milk proteins and peptides on blood pressure and vascular function: a review of evidence from human intervention studies. Nutr Res Rev. 2013;26:177–90.
15. Markey O, Vasilopoulou D, Givens DI, Lovegrove JA. Dairy and cardiovascular health: friend or foe? Nutr Bull. 2014;39:161–71.
16. Chowdhury R, Warnakula S, Kunutsor S, Crowe F, Ward HA, Johnson L, Franco OH, Butterworth AS, Forouhi NG, Thompson SG, et al. Association of dietary, circulating, and supplement fatty acids with coronary risk. A systematic review and meta-analysis. Ann Intern Med. 2014;160:398–406.

17. Siri-Tarino PW, Sun Q, Hu FB, Krauss RM. Meta-analysis of prospective cohort studies evaluating the association of saturated fat with cardiovascular disease. Am J Clin Nutr. 2010;91:535–46.
18. de Souza RJ, Mente A, Maroleanu A, Cozma AI, Ha V, Kishibe T, Uleryk E, Budylowski P, Schünemann H, Beyene J, Anand SS. Intake of saturated and trans unsaturated fatty acids and risk of all cause mortality, cardiovascular disease, and type 2 diabetes: systematic review and meta-analysis of observational studies. BMJ. 2015;351:h3978.
19. Vafeiadou K, Weech M, Altowaijri H, Todd S, Yaqoob P, Jackson KG, Lovegrove JA. Replacement of saturated with unsaturated fats had no impact on vascular function but beneficial effects on lipid biomarkers, E-selectin, and blood pressure: results from the randomized, controlled Dietary Intervention and VAScular function (DIVAS) study. Am J Clin Nutr. 2015;102:40–8.
20. Ramsden CE, Zamora D, Leelarthaepin B, Majchrzak-Hong SF, Faurot KR, Suchindran CM, Ringel A, Davis JM, Hibbeln JR. Use of dietary linoleic acid for secondary prevention of coronary heart disease and death: evaluation of recovered data from the Sydney Diet Heart Study and updated meta-analysis. BMJ. 2013;346:e8707.
21. Hooper L, Martin N, Abdelhamid A, Davey Smith G. Reduction in saturated fat intake for cardiovascular disease. Cochrane Database Syst Rev. 2015;6:Cd011737.
22. DeSalvo KB, Olson R, Casavale KO. Dietary guidelines for americans. JAMA. 2016;315:457–8.
23. WHO. Food based dietary guidelines in the WHO European Region. Copenhagen: WHO; 2003.
24. Givens DI. Session 4: challenges facing the food industry in innovating for health. Impact on CVD risk of modifying milk fat to decrease intake of SFA and increase intake of cis-MUFA. Proc Nutr Soc. 2008;67:419–27.
25. Kliem KE, Shingfield KJ. Manipulation of milk fatty acid composition in lactating cows: Opportunities and challenges. Eur J Lipid S Tech; 101002/ejlt201400543. 2016;118(11):1661–683.
26. Lock AL, Givens DI, Bauman DE. Dairy fat: perceptions and realities. In Milk and dairy products as functional foods. Chichester: Wiley. 2014: 174–197.
27. Livingstone KM, Lovegrove JA, Givens DI. The impact of substituting SFA in dairy products with MUFA or PUFA on CVD risk: evidence from human intervention studies. Nutr Res Rev. 2012;25:193–206.
28. Shaw DI, Tierney AC, McCarthy S, Upritchard J, Vermunt S, Gulseth HL, Drevon CA, Blaak EE, Saris WH, Karlstrom B, et al. LIPGENE food-exchange model for alteration of dietary fat quantity and quality in free-living participants from eight European countries. Br J Nutr. 2009;101:750–9.
29. Skeaff CM, Hodson L, McKenzie JE. Dietary-induced changes in fatty acid composition of human plasma, platelet, and erythrocyte lipids follow a similar time course. J Nutr. 2006;136:565–9.
30. Hodson L, Skeaff CM, Fielding BA. Fatty acid composition of adipose tissue and blood in humans and its use as a biomarker of dietary intake. Prog Lipid Res. 2008;47:348–80.
31. Weech M, Vafeiadou K, Hasaj M, Todd S, Yaqoob P, Jackson KG, Lovegrove JA. Development of a food-exchange model to replace saturated fat with MUFAs and n-6 PUFAs in adults at moderate cardiovascular risk. J Nutr. 2014;144:846–55.
32. Wilson PW, D'Agostino RB, Levy D, Belanger AM, Silbershatz H, Kannel WB. Prediction of coronary heart disease using risk factor categories. Circulation. 1998;97:1837–47.
33. Givens D, Kliem K, Humphries D, Shingfield KJ, Morgan R. Effect of replacing calcium salts of palm oil distillate with rapeseed oil, milled or whole rapeseeds on milk fatty-acid composition in cows fed maize silage-based diets. Animal. 2009;3:1067–74.
34. Treasure T, MacRae KD. Minimisation: the platinum standard for trials?: Randomisation doesn't guarantee similarity of groups; minimisation does. BMJ. 1998;317:362–3.
35. Moore C, Gitau R, Goff L, Lewis FJ, Griffin MD, Chatfield MD, Jebb SA, Frost GS, Sanders TA, Griffin BA, Lovegrove JA. Successful manipulation of the quality and quantity of fat and carbohydrate consumed by free-living individuals using a food exchange model. J Nutr. 2009;139:1534–40.
36. Henderson L, Gregory J, Irving K. G. S: The National Diet and Nutrition Survey: adults aged 19 to 64 years. Vol. 2, Energy, protein, carbohydrate, fat and alcohol intake. London: The Stationery Office; 2003.
37. Nelson M, Atkinson M, Meyer J. A photographic atlas of food portion sizes. London: MAFF publications; 1997.
38. Kliem KE, Shingfield KJ, Livingstone KM, Givens DI. Seasonal variation in the fatty acid composition of milk available at retail in the United Kingdom and implications for dietary intake. Food Chem. 2013;141:274–81.
39. Glasser F, Doreau M, Ferlay A, Chilliard Y. Technical note: estimation of milk fatty acid yield from milk fat data. J Dairy Sci. 2007;90:2302–4.
40. Public Health England. Scientific Advisory Committee on Nutrition Carbohydrates and Health. 2015. [cited 18 Aug 2016]. Available from: https://www.gov.uk/government/publications/sacn-carbohydrates-and-health-report.
41. Henry CJ. Basal metabolic rate studies in humans: measurement and development of new equations. Public Health Nutr. 2005;8:1133–52.
42. Black AE. Critical evaluation of energy intake using the Goldberg cut-off for energy intake:basal metabolic rate. A practical guide to its calculation, use and limitations. Int J Obes Relat Metab Disord. 2000;24:1119–30.
43. Wang LY, Summerhill K, Rodriguez-Canas C, Mather I, Patel P, Eiden M, Young S, Forouhi NG, Koulman A. Development and validation of a robust automated analysis of plasma phospholipid fatty acids for metabolic phenotyping of large epidemiological studies. Genome Med. 2013;5:39.
44. Burdge GC, Wright P, Jones AE, Wootton SA. A method for separation of phosphatidylcholine, triacylglycerol, non-esterified fatty acids and cholesterol esters from plasma by solid-phase extraction. Br J Nutr. 2000;84:781–7.
45. De Roos NM, Bots ML, Schouten EG, Katan MB. Within-subject variability of flow-mediated vasodilation of the brachial artery in healthy men and women: implications for experimental studies. Ultrasound Med Biol. 2003;29:401–6.
46. Xia J, Sinelnikov IV, Han B, Wishart DS. MetaboAnalyst 3.0-making metabolomics more meaningful. Nucleic Acids Res. 2015;43:W251–7.
47. Noakes M, Nestel PJ, Clifton PM. Modifying the fatty acid profile of dairy products through feedlot technology lowers plasma cholesterol of humans consuming the products. Am J Clin Nutr. 1996;63:42–6.
48. Katan MB, Deslypere JP, van Birgelen AF, Penders M, Zegwaard M. Kinetics of the incorporation of dietary fatty acids into serum cholesteryl esters, erythrocyte membranes, and adipose tissue: an 18-month controlled study. J Lipid Res. 1997;38:2012–22.
49. Tholstrup T, Raff M, Basu S, Nonboe P, Sejrsen K, Straarup EM. Effects of butter high in ruminant trans and monounsaturated fatty acids on lipoproteins, incorporation of fatty acids into lipid classes, plasma C-reactive protein, oxidative stress, hemostatic variables, and insulin in healthy young men. Am J Clin Nutr. 2006;83:237–43.
50. Raatz SK, Bibus D, Thomas W, Kris-Etherton P. Total Fat intake modifies plasma fatty acid composition in humans. J Nutr. 2001;131:231–4.
51. Chavarro JE, Kenfield SA, Stampfer MJ, Loda M, Campos H, Sesso HD, Ma J. Blood levels of saturated and monounsaturated fatty acids as markers of de novo lipogenesis and risk of prostate cancer. Am J Epidemiol. 2013;178:1246–55.
52. Markey O, Kliem KE, Humphries DJ, Morgan R, Vasilopoulou D, Grandison A, Fagan CC, Todd S, Jackson KG, Lovegrove LA, Givens DI. Effect of feeding high-oleic sunflower oil to dairy cows on the milk fatty acid profile – RESET study. Proc Nutr Soc. 2015;74(OCE1):E52
53. Jakobsen MU, Overvad K, Dyerberg J, Heitmann BL. Intake of ruminant trans fatty acids and risk of coronary heart disease. Int J Epidemiol. 2008;37:173–82.
54. Gebauer SK, Destaillats F, Dionisi F, Krauss RM, Baer DJ. Vaccenic acid and trans fatty acid isomers from partially hydrogenated oil both adversely affect LDL cholesterol: a double-blind, randomized controlled trial. Am J Clin Nutr. 2015;102:1339–46.
55. Motard-Belanger A, Charest A, Grenier G, Paquin P, Chouinard Y, Lemieux S, Couture P, Lamarche B. Study of the effect of trans fatty acids from ruminants on blood lipids and other risk factors for cardiovascular disease. Am J Clin Nutr. 2008;87:593–9.
56. Kliem KE, Reynolds CK, Humphries DJ, Kirkland RM, Barratt CES, Livingstone KM, Givens DI. Incremental effect of a calcium salt of cis-monounsaturated fatty acids supplement on milk fatty acid composition in cows fed maize silage-based diets. J Dairy Sci. 2013;96:3211–21.
57. Bauman DE, Griinari JM. Regulation and nutritional manipulation of milk fat. Low-fat milk syndrome. Adv Exp Med Biol. 2000;480:209–16.
58. Lockyer S, Tzanetou M, Carvalho-Wells AL, Jackson KG, Minihane AM, Lovegrove JA. SATgene dietary model to implement diets of differing fat composition in prospectively genotyped groups (apoE) using commercially available foods. Br J Nutr. 2012;108:1705–13.
59. Rennie KL, Siervo M, Jebb SA. Can self-reported dieting and dietary restraint identify underreporters of energy intake in dietary surveys? J Am Diet Assoc. 2006;106:1667–72.
60. Macdiarmid J, Blundell J. Assessing dietary intake: Who, what and why of under-reporting. Nutr Res Rev. 1998;11:231–53.

# Permissions

All chapters in this book were first published in NUTRITION, by BioMed Central; hereby published with permission under the Creative Commons Attribution License or equivalent. Every chapter published in this book has been scrutinized by our experts. Their significance has been extensively debated. The topics covered herein carry significant findings which will fuel the growth of the discipline. They may even be implemented as practical applications or may be referred to as a beginning point for another development.

The contributors of this book come from diverse backgrounds, making this book a truly international effort. This book will bring forth new frontiers with its revolutionizing research information and detailed analysis of the nascent developments around the world.

We would like to thank all the contributing authors for lending their expertise to make the book truly unique. They have played a crucial role in the development of this book. Without their invaluable contributions this book wouldn't have been possible. They have made vital efforts to compile up to date information on the varied aspects of this subject to make this book a valuable addition to the collection of many professionals and students.

This book was conceptualized with the vision of imparting up-to-date information and advanced data in this field. To ensure the same, a matchless editorial board was set up. Every individual on the board went through rigorous rounds of assessment to prove their worth. After which they invested a large part of their time researching and compiling the most relevant data for our readers.

The editorial board has been involved in producing this book since its inception. They have spent rigorous hours researching and exploring the diverse topics which have resulted in the successful publishing of this book. They have passed on their knowledge of decades through this book. To expedite this challenging task, the publisher supported the team at every step. A small team of assistant editors was also appointed to further simplify the editing procedure and attain best results for the readers.

Apart from the editorial board, the designing team has also invested a significant amount of their time in understanding the subject and creating the most relevant covers. They scrutinized every image to scout for the most suitable representation of the subject and create an appropriate cover for the book.

The publishing team has been an ardent support to the editorial, designing and production team. Their endless efforts to recruit the best for this project, has resulted in the accomplishment of this book. They are a veteran in the field of academics and their pool of knowledge is as vast as their experience in printing. Their expertise and guidance has proved useful at every step. Their uncompromising quality standards have made this book an exceptional effort. Their encouragement from time to time has been an inspiration for everyone.

The publisher and the editorial board hope that this book will prove to be a valuable piece of knowledge for researchers, students, practitioners and scholars across the globe.

# List of Contributors

**Alessandra Coscia, Enrico Bertino, Paola Tonetto, Chiara Peila, Francesco Cresi and Elena Spada**
Neonatal Unit of Turin University, City of Health and Science of Turin, Via Ventimiglia 3, 10126 Turin, Italy

**Sertac Arslanoglu and Guido E Moro**
Italian Association of Human Milk Banks, Via Libero Temolo 4, 20126 Milan, Italy

**Silvano Milani**
Unit of Medical Statistics and Biometry, Department of Clinical Sciences and Community Health, University of Milan, Milan, Italy

**Sara Antoniazzi, Amedeo Conti and Laura Cavallarin**
Institute of Sciences of Food Production, National Research Council, Largo Braccini 2, 10095 Grugliasco (TO), Italy

**Marzia Giribaldi**
Institute of Sciences of Food Production, National Research Council, Largo Braccini 2, 10095 Grugliasco (TO), Italy
Research Centre for Engineering and Agro-Food Processing, Council for Agricultural Research and Economics (CREA), Strada delle cacce 73, 10135 Turin, Italy

**Livar Frøyland, Marian Kjellevold, Maria W. Markhus, Jannike Øyen and Lisbeth Dahl**
Institute of Marine Research (IMR), 5817 Bergen, Norway

**Katina Handeland**
Institute of Marine Research (IMR), 5817 Bergen, Norway
Department of Clinical Medicine, Faculty of Medicine and Dentistry, University of Bergen, 5020 Bergen, Norway

**Ingvild E. Graff**
Institute of Marine Research (IMR), 5817 Bergen, Norway Uni Research Health, 5020 Bergen, Norway

**Øyvind Lie**
Institute of Marine Research (IMR), 5817 Bergen, Norway
Directorate of Fisheries, 5804 Bergen, Norway

**Siv Skotheim**
Regional Centre for Child and Youth Mental Health, Uni Research Health, 5020 Bergen, Norway

**Kjell M. Stormark**
Regional Centre for Child and Youth Mental Health, Uni Research Health, 5020 Bergen, Norway
Department of Health Promotion and Development, University of Bergen, N-5020 Bergen, Norway

**Valborg Baste**
Uni Research Health, 5020 Bergen, Norway

**Wendy Si Hassen, Sandrine Péneau, Anouar Nechba, Pauline Ducrot, Aurélie Lampuré and France Bellisle**
Université Paris 13, Sorbonne Paris Cité, Centre de Recherche en Epidémiologie et Statistique, Equipe de Recherche en Epidémiologie Nutritionnelle, Inserm (U1153), Inra (U1125), Cnam, 74 rue Marcel Cachin, F-93017 Bobigny, France

**Serge Hercberg**
Université Paris 13, Sorbonne Paris Cité, Centre de Recherche en Epidémiologie et Statistique, Equipe de Recherche en Epidémiologie Nutritionnelle, Inserm (U1153), Inra (U1125), Cnam, 74 rue Marcel Cachin, F-93017 Bobigny, France
Département de santé publique, Hôpital Avicenne, 125 rue de Stalingrad, F-93000 Bobigny, France

**Caroline Méjean**
Université Paris 13, Sorbonne Paris Cité, Centre de Recherche en Epidémiologie et Statistique, Equipe de Recherche en Epidémiologie Nutritionnelle, Inserm (U1153), Inra (U1125), Cnam, 74 rue Marcel Cachin, F-93017 Bobigny, France
MOISA, Université de Montpellier, INRA, CIRAD, CIHEAM-IAMM, Montpellier SupAgro, Montpellier, France

**Katia Castetbon**
Université Libre de Bruxelles, Ecole de Santé publique, Centre de Recherche en Epidémiologie, Biostatistique et Recherche Clinique, Route de Lennik 808 - CP 598, 1070 Brussels, Belgium

**Christine Tichit**
Institut National de la Recherche Agronomique (INRA) - UR 1303 Alimentation et Sciences Sociales ALISS, 65 boulevard de Brandebourg, F-94025 Ivry sur Seine, France

**Seema Mihrshahi**
School of Public Health, Faculty of Medicine, University of Sydney, Sydney, Australia

**Bindi Borg**
School of Public Health, Faculty of Medicine, University of Sydney, Sydney, Australia
C/o Pascal Marino, European Union Delegation in Cameroon, BP 847 Yaoundé, Cameroon

**Mark Griffin**
School of Public Health, University of Queensland, Brisbane, Australia

**Daream Sok**
Department of Nutrition, Exercise and Sports, Faculty of Science, University of Copenhagen, Copenhagen, Denmark
Department of Fisheries Post-Harvest Technologies and Quality Control, Fisheries Administration, Ministry of Agriculture, Forestry and Fisheries, Phnom Penh, Cambodia

**Chamnan Chhoun**
Department of Fisheries Post-Harvest Technologies and Quality Control, Fisheries Administration, Ministry of Agriculture, Forestry and Fisheries, Phnom Penh, Cambodia

**Arnaud Laillou**
Child Survival and Development Section, UNICEF, Phnom Penh, Cambodia

**Jacques Berger and Frank T. Wieringa**
UMR Nutripass, Institut de Recherche pour le Développement, IRD/UM/ SupAgro, Montpellier, France

**Mirza Bojić**
Faculty of Pharmacy and Biochemistry, Department of Medicinal Chemistry, University of Zagreb, A. Kovačića 1, 10000 Zagreb, Croatia

**Andrea Antolić**
Faculty of Science, PDS Biology, University of Zagreb, Rooseveltov trg 6, 10000 Zagreb, Croatia

**Maja Tomičić**
Department of Platelet and Leukocyte Immunology, Croatian Institute of Transfusion Medicine, Petrova 6, 10000 Zagreb, Croatia

**Željko Debeljak**
Institute of Clinical Laboratory Diagnostics, Osijek University Hospital Center, Josipa Huttlera 4, 31000 Osijek, Croatia
Faculty of Medicine, University J. J. Strossmayer of Osijek, Josipa Huttlera 4, 31000 Osijek, Croatia

**Željan Maleš**
Faculty of Pharmacy and Biochemistry, Department of Pharmaceutical Botany, University of Zagreb, Schrottova 39, 10000 Zagreb, Croatia

**Sigrun Henjum**
OsloMet - Oslo Metropolitan University, Postboks 4, St. Olavs plass, Oslo, Norway

**Ingrid Kvestad and Mari Hysing**
Regional Center for Child and Youth Mental Health and Child Welfare, West, Uni Research Health, Bergen, Norway

**Merina Shrestha, Manjeswori Ulak and Prakash S. Shrestha**
Department of Child Health, Tribhuvan University Teaching Hospital, Kathmandu, Nepal

**Ram K. Chandyo**
Department of Community Medicine, Kathmandu Medical College, Kathmandu, Nepal

**Andrew L. Thorne-Lyman**
Center for Human Nutrition, Department of International Health, Johns Hopkins Bloomberg School of Public Health, Baltimore, MD, USA
Harvard T.H. Chan School of Public Health, Boston, MA, USA

**Marian Kjellevold**
Institute of Marine Research, 5817 Bergen, Norway

**Tor A. Strand**
Division for Medical Services, Innlandet Hospital Trust, Lillehammer, Norway
The Center for International Health, University of Bergen, Bergen, Norway

**Anuraag Chaturvedi and Deepa Soni**
Public Health Foundation of India, Gurugram, India

**Ashok K. Patwari**
Hamdard Institute of Medical Sciences and Research and H.A.H.Centenary Hospital, Hamdard University, New Delhi, India

**Shivam Pandey and Jyoti Sharma**
Indian Institute of Public Health, Gurugram, India

**Audrey Prost**
University College London, London, UK

**Raj Kumar Gope and Prasanta Tripathy**
Ekjut, Chakradharpur, Jharkhand, India

**Norliza Ahmad and Munn-Sann Lye**
Department of Community Health, Faculty of Medicine and Health Sciences, Universiti Putra Malaysia, Level 1, Block B (Academic), 43400 UPM, Serdang, Selangor, Malaysia

**Zalilah Mohd Shariff**
Department of Nutrition, Faculty of Medicine and Health Sciences, Universiti Putra Malaysia, Serdang, Selangor, Malaysia

**Firdaus Mukhtar**
Department of Psychiatry, Faculty of Medicine and Health Sciences, Universiti Putra Malaysia, Serdang, Selangor, Malaysia

**Emmanuel Grellety**
Research Center Health Policy and Systems - International Health, School of Public Health, Université Libre de Bruxelles, Bruxelles, Belgium

**Michael H. Golden**
Department of Medicine and Therapeutics, University of Aberdeen, Aberdeen, Scotland

**Elieke Demmer, Christopher J. Cifelli and Jenny A. Houchins**
National Dairy Council, 10255 West Higgins Road, Suite 900, Rosemont, IL 60018-5616, USA

**Victor L. Fulgoni III**
Nutrition Impact, LLC, Battle Creek, MI 49014, USA

**Semira Ahmed**
Gambella Regional State Health Bureau, Gambella, Ethiopia

**Kalkidan Hassen and Tolassa Wakayo**
Jimma University, Faculty of Public Health, Jimma, Ethiopia

**R. Colin Carter**
Institute for Human Nutrition and Departments of Emergency Medicine and Pediatrics, Columbia University Medical Center, 3959 Broadway, CHN-1-116, New York, NY 10032, USA

**Neil C. Dodge**
Department of Psychiatry and Behavioral Neurosciences, Wayne State University School of Medicine, Detroit, USA

**Sandra W. Jacobson**
Department of Psychiatry and Behavioral Neurosciences, Wayne State University School of Medicine, Detroit, USA
Department of Psychiatry and Mental Health, University of Cape Town Faculty of Health Sciences, Cape Town, South Africa
Department of Human Biology, University of Cape Town Faculty of Health Sciences, Cape Town, South Africa

**Christopher D. Molteno**
Department of Psychiatry and Mental Health, University of Cape Town Faculty of Health Sciences, Cape Town, South Africa

**Joseph L. Jacobson**
Department of Psychiatry and Mental Health, University of Cape Town Faculty of Health Sciences, Cape Town, South Africa
Department of Human Biology, University of Cape Town Faculty of Health Sciences, Cape Town, South Africa

**Sharmilah Booley, Baheya Najaar, Ernesta M. Meintjes and Marjanne Senekal**
Department of Human Biology, University of Cape Town Faculty of Health Sciences, Cape Town, South Africa

**Lori J. Bechard and Christopher P. Duggan**
Division of Gastroenterology, Hepatology, and Nutrition, Boston Children's Hospital, Boston, USA

**Lena Maria Nilsson**
Department of Nutritional Research, Umeå University, Umeå, Sweden

**Ingegerd Johansson**
Department of Nutritional Research, Umeå University, Umeå, Sweden
Department of Odontology, Umeå University, Umeå, Sweden

**Anders Esberg**
Department of Odontology, Umeå University, Umeå, Sweden

**Jan-Håkan Jansson**
Department of Public Health and Clinical Medicine, Research Unit Skellefteå, Umeå University, Umeå, Sweden

**Anna Winkvist**
Department of Internal Medicine and Clinical Nutrition, Sahlgrenska Academy, University of Gothenburg, Gothenburg, Sweden

**Behailu Derseh, Kalayu Mruts, Takele Demie and Tesfay Gebremariam**
Department of Public Health, College of Health Sciences, Debre Berhan University, Debre Berhan, Ethiopia

**Mavis Pearl Kwabla**
Department of Epidemiology and Biostatistics, School of Public Health, University of Health and Allied Sciences, Ho, Ghana

**Charlotte Gyan and Francis Zotor**
Department of Family and Community Health, School of Public Health, University of Health and Allied Sciences, Ho, Ghana

**Yurika Osaka, Mihoko Akiyoshi and Naoyuki Miyasaka**
Department of Obstetrics and Gynecology, Tokyo Medical and Dental University, Yushima 1-5-45, Bunkyo, Tokyo 113-8510, Japan

**Asuka Hirose**
Department of Obstetrics and Gynecology, Tokyo Medical and Dental University, Yushima 1-5-45, Bunkyo, Tokyo 113-8510, Japan
Department of Women's Health, Tokyo Medical and Dental University, Yushima 1-5-45, Bunkyo, Tokyo 113-8510, Japan

**Masakazu Terauchi and Kiyoko Kato**
Department of Women's Health, Tokyo Medical and Dental University, Yushima 1-5-45, Bunkyo, Tokyo 113-8510, Japan

**Johanna Gyll and Pernilla Lif Holgerson**
Department of Odontology, Section of Paediatric Dentistry, Faculty of Medicine, Umeå University, 90185 Umeå, Sweden

**Karin Ridell**
Department of Paediatric Dentistry, Faculty of Odontology, Malmö University, Malmö, Sweden
Inger Öhlund
Department of Clinical Sciences/Section of Paediatric Medicine, Faculty of Medicine, Umeå University, Umeå, Sweden Pia Karlsland Åkeson
Department of Clinical Sciences, Pediatrics, Lund University, Lund, Malmö, Sweden

**Ingegerd Johansson**
Department of Odontology/Section of Cariology, Faculty of Medicine, Umeå University Umeå, Sweden

**Marc Bénard, Julia Baudry, Kelly Virecoulon Giudici, Emmanuelle Kesse-Guyot and Sandrine Péneau**
Equipe de Recherche en Epidémiologie Nutritionnelle, Centre de Recherche en Epidémiologie et Statistique Sorbonne Paris Cité, INSERM U1153, INRA U1125, Cnam, Université Paris 13, 74, rue Marcel Cachin, 93017 Bobigny, France

**Caroline Méjean**
Equipe de Recherche en Epidémiologie Nutritionnelle, Centre de Recherche en Epidémiologie et Statistique Sorbonne Paris Cité, INSERM U1153, INRA U1125, Cnam, Université Paris 13, 74, rue Marcel Cachin, 93017 Bobigny, France
INRA, UMR1110 MOISA, F-34000 Montpellier, France

**Serge Hercberg**
Equipe de Recherche en Epidémiologie Nutritionnelle, Centre de Recherche en Epidémiologie et Statistique Sorbonne Paris Cité, INSERM U1153, INRA U1125, Cnam, Université Paris 13, 74, rue Marcel Cachin, 93017 Bobigny, France
Unité de Surveillance en Epidémiologie Nutritionnelle, Institut de Veille Sanitaire, Université Paris 13, Bobigny, France
Département de Santé Publique, Hôpital Avicenne, Bobigny, France

**Denis Lairon**
Aix Marseille Université, Nutrition Obésité et Risque Thrombotique (NORT), INSERM UMR S 1062, INRA 1260, Marseille, France

**Fabrice Etilé**
Paris School of Economics and INRA, UMR1393 PjSE, 48 Boulevard Jourdan, 75014 Paris, France

**Gérard Reach**
Service d'Endocrinologie, Diabétologie, Maladies Métaboliques, Hôpital Avicenne, Bobigny, France

**Mindy Patterson Maziarz**
Department of Nutrition and Food Sciences, Institute of Health Sciences, Texas Woman's University, 6700 Fannin Street, Houston, TX 77030, USA

**Sara Preisendanz, Shanil Juma, Victorine Imrhan and Parakat Vijayagopal**
Department of Nutrition and Food Sciences, Texas Woman's University, Denton, TX 76204, USA

**Chandan Prasad**
Department of Nutrition and Food Sciences, Texas Woman's University, Denton, TX 76204, USA
Department of Medicine (Endocrinology), Louisiana State University Health Science Center, New Orleans, LA 70112, USA

**Ayumi Nakamura and Yasushi Mariya**
Department of Radiological Life Sciences, Division of Medical Life Sciences, Hirosaki University Graduate School of Health Sciences, Aomori 036-8564, Japan

**Chieko Itaki**
Department of Disability and Health, Division of Medical Life Sciences, Hirosaki University Graduate School of Health Sciences, Aomori 036-8564, Japan

**David J. Humphries and Kirsty E. Kliem**
Animal, Dairy and Food Chain Sciences, University of Reading, Reading RG6 6AP, UK

**Susan Todd**
School of Sport, Exercise and Health Sciences, Loughborough University, Loughborough LE11 3TU, UK

**Masoumeh Moradi**
Department of Cellular and Molecular Nutrition, School of Nutritional Sciences and Dietetics, International Campus, Tehran University of Medical Sciences, Hojatdoost Ave., Naderi St., Keshavarz Blvd., Tehran, Iran

**Fariba Koohdani**
Department of Cellular and Molecular Nutrition, School of Nutritional Sciences and Dietetics, International Campus, Tehran University of Medical Sciences, Hojatdoost Ave., Naderi St., Keshavarz Blvd., Tehran, Iran
Diabetes Research Center, Endocrinology and Metabolism Clinical Sciences Institute, Tehran University of Medical Sciences, Tehran, Iran

**Sunita Taneja and Nita Bhandari**
Centre for Health Research and Development, Society for Applied Studies, New Delhi, India

**Ranadip Chowdhury**
Department of Global Public Health and Primary Care, University of Bergen, Bergen, Norway

# Index


**A**

Adenosine Diphosphate, 40-42, 46
Alcohol Spectrum Disorders, 127-128, 137-139
Alpha-2 Acid Glycoprotein, 32, 37
Anthropometric Criteria, 90, 93
Arachidonic Acid, 10, 14-15, 17, 48, 55-56
Athens Insomnia Scale, 174, 177, 179

**B**

Bmi Z-score, 67-71, 73-74, 78, 183
Body Fat Percentage, 66-68, 70, 73-75, 78
Body Mass Index, 25, 27, 66-67, 74, 76, 140, 144, 147-148, 155, 169-170, 175, 177-178, 183, 189, 200, 202, 205, 208
Bovine Milk Proteins, 1

**C**

Cardio-ankle Vascular Index, 173, 175, 177-179
Cariogenic Mutant Streptococci, 181
Case Fatality Rates, 79, 81-82, 84-86, 89, 92
Central Nervous System, 49, 55, 202
Chalder Fatigue Scale, 173, 175, 177-179
Childhood Malnutrition, 30, 37-39, 106, 165-166
Chronic Renal Failure, 91
Cognitive Functions, 17, 53, 181
Combined Oedematous, 89
Corn-soy Blend Plus Plus, 29-30, 37
Cystic Fibrosis, 91

**D**

Diarrhea, 157-158, 160, 163, 176
Diastolic Blood Pressures, 143
Dietary Choline, 127-128, 130-132, 137-138
Dietary Diversity, 32, 35, 56, 117, 119, 121-122, 124-126
Dietary Inflammatory Index, 142, 154-155
Dietary Intervention, 8-9, 13, 17, 223-225, 232, 234-235
Docosahexaenoic Acid, 9-10, 14-15, 17-18, 48, 55-56

**E**

Epilepsy, 129
Estimated Average Requirement, 112-113, 115

**F**

Feeding Intolerance, 1, 3-6
Fetal Alcohol Syndrome, 128, 137-138
Folate Supplementation, 51, 117, 120-123, 125
Folic Acid, 33, 119, 124, 126, 131-132, 155
Food Frequency Questionnaire, 10, 16-18, 127-128, 133, 137-138, 142, 155, 191, 193, 198-200, 233

**G**

Genetic Polymorphisms, 49, 54

**H**

Hazard Ratios, 149
Hypertension, 118, 120, 122, 129, 156, 178, 202, 224
Hypothermia, 158, 160

**I**

Insulin Resistance, 74, 208, 210, 242
Intravascular Disseminated Coagulopathy, 3

**L**

Lactase-phlorizin Hydrolase, 155
Lecithin, 173-174, 176-180
Likert Scale, 175, 192-193
Lipid Replacement Therapy, 173-174, 179
Lipid-based Nutrient Supplement, 29-30, 38
Long-chain Polyunsaturated Fatty Acids, 8-9, 17, 55-56
Low Birth Weight, 1, 6, 49, 52, 54-56, 117-119, 121-122, 125-126
Low Density Lipoprotein, 143-144, 147-148, 154
Lowest Energy Intake, 20

**M**

Malnutrition Treatment Centres, 57-58, 65
Maternal Anemia, 117-120, 122, 124-126
Mean Energy Density, 23-24
Mid-upper-arm Circumference, 79-80, 87, 89-90, 105

**N**

Necrotizing Enterocolitis, 1, 3-4, 7
Non-blinded Controlled Trial, 29, 32
Non-communicable Chronic Diseases, 117-118
Nutrient-rich Beverages, 108, 114-115
Nutritional Recovery Rate, 157, 160-163

**O**

Oedema, 58, 79-81, 89-90, 92-93, 97, 101-102, 104, 106
Omega-3, 8-19, 56, 207

**P**

Paediatric Obesity, 67

Patent Ductus Arteriosus, 3

Placebo, 13, 18, 138, 173-179, 181-184

Plasma Phospholipids, 19, 48

Platelet Aggregation, 40-43, 45-47

Pneumonia, 107, 157, 159-160, 162-163, 247

Prenatal Alcohol Exposure, 127-128, 132, 137-139

**R**

Randomized Controlled Trials, 9, 18, 56, 125, 209

**S**

Sepsis, 1, 4, 7, 158

Serum Lipids, 140, 144

Severe Acute Malnutrition, 30, 32, 35, 57-58, 64-65, 79-80, 86-87, 89-90, 104-106, 157-158, 161, 163-164

Simpson's Paradox, 87, 89, 99-100, 103, 105-106

Sugar-sweetened Beverages, 67-70, 116, 142

Supercereal Plus, 30, 37

Systolic Blood Pressure, 143, 154, 156, 177-178

**T**

Thrombus Formation, 40

Total Polyphenols, 40-41, 43

Triglycerides, 140, 142-144, 147-149, 154

**U**

Urinary Iodine Concentration, 8-9, 14-17

**W**

Waist Circumference, 28, 66-75, 77, 155, 205, 227, 229

www.ingramcontent.com/pod-product-compliance
Lightning Source LLC
LaVergne TN
LVHW080919210926
848485LV00004B/684
* 9 7 8 1 6 3 9 8 9 1 8 6 3 *